Casebook of Traumatic Injury Prevention

Richard Volpe

Editor

Casebook of Traumatic Injury Prevention

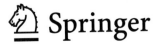 Springer

Editor
Richard Volpe
Life Span Adaptation Projects
Laidlaw Research Centre
University of Toronto
Toronto, ON, Canada

ISBN 978-3-030-27421-4   ISBN 978-3-030-27419-1   (eBook)
https://doi.org/10.1007/978-3-030-27419-1

This Springer imprint is published by the registered company Springer Nature Switzerland AG
The registered company address is: Gewerbestrasse 11, 6330 Cham, Switzerland

Acknowledgments

I want to thank the Ontario Neurotrauma Foundation for providing the funding for this research. Appreciation is also extended to members of the international community of injury prevention practitioners, especially to those who acted as representatives of the research team's external advisory group— a community who provided valuable information and resources and who helped to identify many of the programs that were brought forward for review.

The case writers were an amazing interdisciplinary and interprofessional group that wrestled complex programs into coherent and useful narratives that captured their active ingredients as exemplars.

Special thanks go out to the many key informants who shared their knowledge, time, insight, and vision about prevention programming.

The casebook finalization group of Rachel Monahan, Chelsi Major, Sabrina Amicone, and Raganya Pomanadiyil did a fantastic amount of updating and checking in a relatively short time.

Finally, the incredible sustained support of Christine Davidson and Rachel Monahan, Dr. R.G.N. Laidlaw Research Centre, University of Toronto, is gratefully acknowledged.

Contents

About the Editor

Richard Volpe, Ph.D. Dr. Richard Volpe received his Ph.D. from the University of Alberta. As a University of Alberta Pre-Doctoral Fellow at Glenrose Provincial Hospital, he did his dissertation research on the comparative social development of physically disabled and non-disabled children. Following this, he was a Laidlaw Foundation Postdoctoral Fellow, University of Toronto, Hospital for Sick Children, and the Clarke Institute of Psychiatry. Currently, he is Professor and Projects Director, Life Span Adaptation Projects, the Laidlaw Research Centre, Department of Human Development and Applied Psychology (OISE), University of Toronto.

Previously, he was Director, Dr. R.G.N. Laidlaw Research Centre, University of Toronto; Director of the Laidlaw Foundation's Evaluation and Conceptual Elaboration Unit of their Child at Risk Program; Chair of the Institute for the Prevention of Child Abuse; Co-Chair, Justice for Children and Youth; and an Organisation for Economic Co-operation and Development (OECD) Evaluation Expert. He has also been a Member of the Graduate Department of Community Health and the Institute for Life Course and Aging, University of Toronto. More recently, he was Chair of the Best Practices Committee of the Provincial Advisory Committee of the Ontario Injury Prevention Resource Centre (OIPRC) and Member of the Prevention Committee of the Ontario Neurotrauma Foundation and of the Injury Prevention Advisory Committee of the SMARTRISK Foundation. His ongoing research examines the prevention of intentional and unintentional injury and the relationship between early experience and later life.

Life Span Adaptation Projects, Laidlaw Research Centre
University of Toronto, Toronto, ON, Canada

The Challenge of Traumatic Injury Prevention

Richard Volpe

1.1 Introduction

Injury prevention occupies an increasingly important role in public policy. The general public is beginning to recognize the extent, cost, and personal burdens associated with injury, while governments and other institutions acknowledge that injuries are preventable not inevitable chance occurrences. Traumatic injury refers to physical injuries of sudden onset and severity that result from a range of both blunt and penetrating forces that cause bodily damage. Traumatic injuries can occur at work, on the street, playing field, or at home. Their magnitude, nature, and gravity are such that they are life-altering forms of injury. The case studies of exemplary traumatic injury prevention programs presented in this book are the result of more than a decade of surveying, investigating, and evaluating efforts to prevent severe sports injuries, dangerous falls, major motor vehicle crashes, violence, and other physical injuries. Although advances in the prevention and treatment of trauma have resulted in substantial decreases in mortality and severity of an injury, prevention is the only known cure.

This casebook constitutes a unique compilation of programmatic efforts to prevent traumatic injury. It provides access to comprehensive and systematic original case studies of contemporary, sustained, and historical traumatic injury prevention initiatives that can guide program planning and implementation. Despite considerable interest in injury prevention, no other collection of evidence-informed traumatic injury prevention cases is readily accessible. The investigation, analysis, and casing of these initiatives provide exemplars for further injury prevention program and policy development. They facilitate understanding of evidence of effectiveness, provide templates for replication, and afford ways to reimagine and adapt prevention efforts. Through analogical reasoning, the reader can construct what the case stories mean to the program challenges they face and transfer their understanding to their particular practice situation. These cases are written in a story format that covers a program's background, resources, implementation, and outcome. This classic outline with a beginning, middle, and end is a heuristic tool that offers the reader an opportunity to explore and imagine how they might apply to real-world problems, processes, and people. Their value is in full program description, explanatory scope, and conceptual strength, rather than as a rendering that is independent from context and generalizable. As such, they offer a way of investigating and

R. Volpe (✉)
Life Span Adaptation Projects, Laidlaw Research Centre, University of Toronto, Toronto, ON, Canada
e-mail: richard.volpe@utoronto.ca

© Springer Nature Switzerland AG 2020
R. Volpe (ed.), *Casebook of Traumatic Injury Prevention*,
https://doi.org/10.1007/978-3-030-27419-1_1

reporting both experimental and developmental program evaluations. Furthermore, they are particularly useful for studying innovation in the design and evaluation of prevention initiatives because they are rooted in actual situations and provide in-depth holistic accounts of programs.

Although prevention does work, we do not always know why. Prevention programs usually contain a multifaceted collection of strategies that involve diverse scientific disciples and practice fields. On the whole, passive engineered solutions work well in low relief and behind the scene. Sometimes, invisible technological innovation and legislative interventions are more effective than so-called active interventions based on visible attempts to change behavior. Passive solutions, however, do not work that well on their own: for example, building a safer car may contribute to driving at faster speeds. Consequently, both active and passive approaches to prevention are usually necessary. In public health sciences these observations are usually captured in the three E's of prevention: education, engineering, enactment. Our prevention program reviews have necessitated economics and evaluation be added as criteria for determining program effectiveness. Prevention requires attention to all five E's. However, this added complexity makes it even more challenging to know what constitutes "exemplary practice," what works, and how to invest time and money in prevention.

It is not difficult to examine the literature on injury prevention without concluding that it is mired in competing language and models. Although a considerable body of work has emerged, little is known about how programs meet their preventative goals. All sorts of interventions are called prevention programs. Some represent prevention by fiat, others repackage—but not materially alter—previously existing work, and still others fail to produce demonstrable outcomes. The case studies presented in this volume help to overcome some of these problems by providing a holistic view of traumatic injury prevention programs.

Nearly everything that involves people, from antipollution laws to legal limits on go-carts, can be seen as having implications for injury prevention, yet most of these relationships are vague and tenuous. In the face of this situation, prevention organizations are surely obligated to provide a clear justification for how their programs relate to important aspects of dealing with the problem of injury. It is precisely this justification that is lacking in many programs. Thus, the lack of holistic explanation of what works and what does not work in injury prevention is evident. At this point, we do not know enough about the multiplicity of functions that converge in the causes of injury. However, little prevention would be achieved if all our efforts were spent trying to elucidate etiology. Although some injuries are known to result from specific mechanical failures, these comprise only a small proportion of what constitutes a preventable injury. Since etiological theories do not provide specific enough information to direct programs, a descriptive focus on context may be more relevant to injury prevention. The idea that injury prevention needs a model of person–environment interaction is not new.

Haddon (1972) and others have argued that strategies of prevention should be founded on complex views of person–environment interaction. Interestingly, one may argue that much of the difficulty in developing genuine, valid injury prevention programs can be understood as a consequence of the lack of a complete portrayal of this complexity. A large proportion of prevention efforts have failed to demonstrate a connection to desired outcomes.

The problem with many injury efforts is that their explanations are vague. That is, they have little ability to articulate the connection between risk and protective factors. The cases reviewed in this book illustrate these factors and suggest some connections. An additional consideration points to a problem that is more insidious and far-reaching. In the absence of appreciating prevention programs in context, there is often a tacit assumption that specific etiological factors are known. This assumption manifests in the narrowness of goals that characterize a vast proportion of preventive efforts. Injury prevention needs to be conceptualized broadly enough that it can subsume a wide variety of specific scientific theories and the insights derived from research in a variety of disciplines. A broad conception of injury prevention overcomes these programming difficulties. Many programs provide services potentially relevant to prevention but with no demonstrated connection to injury prevention. Thinking contextually allows these undertakings to be considered as prevention resources. Furthermore, the place and potential of these resources can be understood in greater detail. This model is necessary before claims as to what constitutes prevention can be judged by an authoritative arbiter in terms of what is or is not a worthy program. Injury prevention necessitates conceptualizing personal and social change in terms of whole situations. Ultimately, this is a heuristically valuable way for designing and evaluating programs that avoid some of the pitfalls of narrow causal thinking described earlier. Risk and protective factors in injury need to be seen as interacting system elements, whole units and not as fixed attributes that are merely linked by cause and effect. Protective factors can be responses to risks, changes that follow active coping. Rather than risks acting on a passive individual, it is more beneficial for understanding prevention to account for active individuals responding on a continuum that may increase or decrease protection and vulnerability; for example, reducing exposure and adverse chain reactions, or increasing opportunities to gain information and skill.

An injury involves a complex person–context interaction. It is the nature of this interaction that is considered in efforts to assess what constitutes exemplary practice. As used here, the context includes terrestrial, energy, natural, artifactual environments, and an animated environment that is both personal and sociocultural. None of these environments alone are sufficient in themselves to describe and explain injury in a way that enables the evaluation of prevention programs. The demand for weaving all these components together is hampered by the idiosyncratic methods

and concepts of the various disciplines that are stakeholders in injury prevention. The shortcoming of most discipline-based research is that it usually begins with a reductionist account of causes of injury into parts. As noted above, however, injuries involve a fusion of components and are determined by multiple causes. The challenge is to ascertain how these components are organized and weighted in any prevention effort. In short, the focus of exemplary practice in injury prevention should be on the holistic nature of human change and the importance of time and timing in understanding human adaptation as part of a complex contextual system (Volpe, 1999; Volpe, 2012). Cohen and Swift (1999) describe this complexity as a "spectrum of prevention" and provide an outline for developing complex approaches to injury prevention. The spectrum has six interrelated levels: (1) strengthening individual knowledge and skills, (2) promoting community education, (3) educating providers, (4) fostering coalitions and networks, (5) changing organizational practices, and (6) influencing policy and legislation. Prevention efforts at all of these levels need to coalesce. Together, they help address the need to develop traumatic injury prevention efforts that are comprehensive and multifaceted.

1.2   Prevention as Change in Complex Systems

The traumatic injury prevention programs reviewed here illustrate that effective injury prevention programs and strategies are designed to bring about change. Further, these cases illustrate that although these preventative interventions usually begin at a particular entry point into a system, they need to address all sectors. Thus, the first common feature of best practice is the consideration and eventual involvement of relevant systems. These systems, in essence, own the conditions and transformative processes that contribute to the occurrence of injury. They need to address issues and come together to change conditions. A complex systems perspective on prevention process assumes that efforts to reduce injury involve interventions that change settings, situations, and the way people think and behave.

Personal and social factors interacting in the change process are often labeled as development. The nature of the interplay between the unfolding of individual lives, social structure, and culture is mostly unknown. Decades of research in this area has produced little or no consensus as to how macro and micro perspectives can be combined. There is a need to bring to the study of human development ideas and indicators that encompass social structural, social psychological (interpersonal), psychological, bio-physiological, and physical features of human existence and experience. Inherent in the interdisciplinary approach taken here is the assertion that human development is more than a function of the independent properties of the person and the environment. Instead, development is a consequence of both the person and the environment, a result of the joint functioning of individuals and their context. Context is an abstraction of the environment that includes objective circumstances and subjective definitions of situations accorded to events and activities. Development is, therefore, inextricably tied to context.

Conceptualization of this complexity can help to make explicit the many features and facets of the cases reviewed. That is, a holistic view is needed in which individual characteristics are defined in part by the system in which they operate. Portraying prevention as a planned intervention in human development involves exploring the emotional, cognitive, anatomic, physiological, ecologic, and behavioral change in living systems. The context of development contains both risks or challenges and protective factors or resources. Challenges catalyze change; resources support individual change. At different times and in different situations, what was once a challenge might become a resource and vice versa. The critical feature explaining development is the transaction between a person and his or her context. Through a process of interpreting, choosing, and manipulating their contexts people play a role in their development.

1.3 Context and the Life Space Study Framework

The complex systems that constitute an individual life space include both internal and external environments in which a person interacts and adapts. Contained in the life space are the resources and the challenges that become evident during the life course. Context may be pictured as a circle with four main divisions: sociocultural, interpersonal, ecological (physical environment), and internal states (see Fig. 1.1). This division into quadrants is arbitrary and serves primarily analytic purposes. In reality, the life space is a complex fusion of elements.

The Sociocultural quadrant consists of norms, values, and language. Interpersonal relationships involve actual interactions with others, the social basis for organizing experience (cognition) and the personal residues of relations with others. The Internal States dimension involves the genetic program, biochemical processes, and unconscious phenomena. The Physical Environment dimension contains both man-made and natural objects. Within this scheme, the change elements of each of the cases reviewed herein can be made explicit.

Evident in the four quadrants are four components underlying prevention as change/development: (1) the sociocultural opportunities available or the obstacles encountered as influenced by social class, ethnic membership, age, sex, personal contacts; social calamity (war, earthquake, and famine), economic adjustment, and major and minor social and technological change; (2) the sources of interpersonal support accessible to an individual; (3) what the physical environment offers in terms of stimulation (i.e., colors, textures, stairs, and walls), support, and security; and (4) the personal resources that an individual can command—his intelligence, appearance, strength, health, and temperament—investments of effort that the individual makes on his or her behalf. Although the content of systems is highly variable, we can begin to discern in the cases outlined common structural features of how change is brought about in the course of human development over the entire span of life.

Sociocultural

- Socio-economic status
- Language (Idiom)
- Norms and Values
- Reference Groups
- Family Composition
- Religion

Interpersonal

- Temperament
- Primary Relationships
- Reference Relationships (natural and professional helping networks)

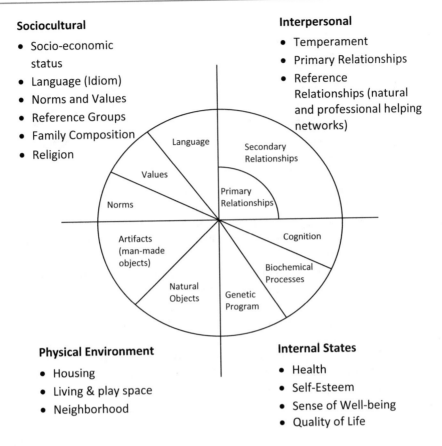

Physical Environment

- Housing
- Living & play space
- Neighborhood

Internal States

- Health
- Self-Esteem
- Sense of Well-being
- Quality of Life

Fig. 1.1 Four divisions of the life space

Compiling the casebook has provided an opportunity to reexamine what has been learned about programs from previous reviews (Volpe, 2012, 2013; Volpe & Lewko, 2009; Volpe, Lewko, & Batra, 2002) and to reconnect with promising programs that were in the process of being implemented or evaluated. Furthermore, it has been possible to follow up leads to new, innovative programs discovered during the later phases of the previous research. Thus, the casebook presents the results of an extensive worldwide investigation of both new and sustained program evaluations, the discovery of fresh and possibly missed prevention initiatives, and "raises the evidence bar" in program selection criteria by increasing attention to methodologically sound outcome evidence. The focus of this casebook is on the effective practices that emerge from meeting all nomination criteria and a high level of rigor in demonstrating outcome effectiveness.

1.4   Best Practices and Exemplary Programs

The cases selected as best practice for the casebook illustrate some of these issues and help to redress a loss in descriptive emphasis that resulted in attempts to further causal explanations of injury. Questions of why injuries occur have often taken precedence over how injuries occur. Both are important. The success of science can be related to explanations of why things occur that are solidly based on accurate descriptions of how they occur.

The term "best practice" has been employed in so many ways that it has become ambiguous. Currently, the term is a buzz word in such diverse practice fields as medicine, public health, nursing, urban planning, education, social work, and clinical psychology.

Best practice can be defined in a number of ways. Voluntary or mandated *standards* can be enunciated. A set of values can be set out as *principles* such as the Hippocratic Oath. The conditions necessary for an activity can be identified as *guidelines*. The Canadian Tri-Council Guidelines for Research Using Human Subjects have been widely adopted to ensure the safety and privacy of research subjects. Step-by-step practice *recipes* can be laid down as almost guaranteed ways to achieve results. Formulas laid out in lab and shop manuals are paint-by-number solutions for attaining best practice. Finally, when possible specific *outcomes* as ends sought in practice have been described and used as criteria in systematic reviews such as the Cochrane Collaboration.

The position taken here is similar but not the same as systematic reviews undertaken in pharmacology and medicine. In order to make the term "best practice" more explicit and useful in the area of injury prevention, it needs to be conceived in terms of best evidence. A best practice, a practice based on best evidence, is a way of doing business for both the individual clinical practice and the collective practice of prevention planning and policy-making. Both these undertakings seek improvement in decisions, problem-solving, and skills through inquiry and evaluation. Consequently, before proceeding it will be helpful to elaborate on what constitutes a best practice.

This approach began with the critical work of the British epidemiologist Archibald Cochrane. He observed that health care professionals, policymakers, and consumers were being inundated with huge amounts of information. In 1972 he asserted that a system of reviewing, evaluating, and disseminating this information was needed. He further contended that reviews of evidence should be systematic and based on the highest truth criteria such as random control trials. Cochrane became a tireless advocate of systematic reviews based on agreed-upon criteria that could provide substantial evidence of the effectiveness of practices.

In 1992, the United Kingdom National Health Service established the Cochrane Collaboration at Oxford University to provide the world health community with systematic reviews of medical and pharmacological studies. An international initiative produced by the Cochrane Library prepares and distributes the results of reviews throughout the world. The tying of the Library to the Collaboration has been the key to the success of this enterprise. The Collaboration involves a network of research groups, methods groups, libraries, and databases reflecting a sophisticated use of the World Wide Web. According to Cochrane, nothing is known about an area unless is has been systematically reviewed according to their criteria. Although the Cochrane Collaboration has grown rapidly, it remains a cordial, congenial, and collegial undertaking. By placing a premium on the importance of disseminating only rigorously evaluated information it has become one of the most significant examples of public knowledge building and evaluation and perhaps one of the first modern expressions of collective intelligence (Volpe, 2013).

Recognizing that the state of knowledge building in prevention science is not equal to what is known to work in medical sciences, the question must be asked: Does the rigor of the Cochrane approach outweigh its relevance in injury prevention and other areas not amenable to randomization and controlled experimentation? Further, it is reasonable to ask how likely is it that prevention programs that address the challenge of complexity are going to produce magic bullet cures and portable recipes for action. Fortunately, the Cochrane group and others from the social and behavioral sciences recognized that these important issues needed to be addressed in a way that preserves the rigor of systematic reviews and allows a wider variety of criteria to be used as the basis for determining best evidence. Because injury prevention requires a broad-based approach to evaluating program effectiveness, the Cochrane specifications making randomized control trials (RCTs) the gold standard for determining success is inappropriate at this stage in both the conceptual and the methodological development of prevention science. The norm in modern evaluation research is to combine evaluation methods.

This approach adheres to the notion of an experimenting society advanced by the late

Donald Campbell. Campbell argued that continual evaluation through a variety of appropriate methods offers the most promise of establishing a sound evidence base for intervention and prevention (Campbell & Russo, 1999). Consequently, another collaboration for the provision of systematic research reviews has evolved taking the name Campbell Collaboration. The work of this group is supported by the Cochrane Collaboration and intends to provide systematic reviews relevant to health, social and educational policies (Volpe et al., 2002). Extending this reasoning to injury prevention, it is evident that the random control trial should not be the most salient standard for evaluating evidence. The Campbell Collaboration has emerged from this recognition based on an appreciation of the role of multi-method research can play in establishing criteria in human service fields and prevention science. Operating along the same lines as the Cochrane Collaboration, the current casebook seeks to review the best evidence to help overcome human service turf wars, provide a reliable basis for intervention and prevention, and offer information for use in dealing with the political-economic aspects of advocacy.

1.5   The Concept of Evidence in Exemplary Programming of Practices

Dealing with what constitutes evidence, let alone best evidence, involves considering some of the thorny issues that divide disciplines and the variety of methods and truth criteria they employ (Sackett et al. 2000). Central to any consideration is attempting to answer the question: What does it mean to inform policy and practice through evaluation research? Without scrutinizing the relationship of research to practice, the question of best evidence becomes more of a political than rational enterprise. The complex relation of interdisciplinary and inter-professional research to practice is quickly glossed over, assumed to be self-evident, or believed in trust to be part of decision-making processes. Our aim in this casebook has been to advance the discussion of these issues and present programs that adhere to criteria of what constitutes the best evidence, while at the same time have a high probability of succeeding in reducing the incidence of injury in the complex real world.

The prevention of both injury and disease requires the systematic use of evidence-informed practices; injury prevention, however, must be handled differently than disease prevention—populations at risk cannot merely be inoculated against injury, nor does the mere existence of evidence provide a recipe for successful injury prevention. Instead, evidence in injury prevention enables practitioners to frame their decisions and actions using a knowledge base that increases the likelihood of effective practices being implemented.

Evidence-based practice in prevention science (EBPS) entails integrating the best available research with prevention expertise within a context of population characteristics, interpersonal relations, social structures, social determinants, cultural practices, personal preferences, beliefs, and choices. The purpose of EBPS is to promote effective prevention practice and enhance public health by applying empirically supported principles to the implementation and evaluation of prevention practices. "Best research evidence" refers to scientific results related to prevention strategies in laboratory and field settings as well as to practically relevant results of basic and applied research, social and behavioral science, and related fields. Evidence is derived from a mix of methods that includes but is not dependent on random control trials as the gold truth standard. It is important to recognize that the notion of what actually constitutes evidence-based practice is poorly understood. The generally agreed upon Institute of Medicine (IOM) definition is that it is the "integration of best research evidence with clinical expertise and patient values"; this requires elaboration when applied to the collective practice of public policy-making.

Use of evidence in this larger field requires distinguishing among what constitutes an actual best practice, an emerging practice that is promising, and an unproven practice with preliminary expectations that it can produce desired outcomes.

Evidence is important to practice because it provides a basis for change that is somewhat above politics. This is not to say that it is apolitical since turf and methodological wars do exist. However, the promise of evidence is the means to know what to do, how to do it, how to improve it, and what works. Understanding the nature of evidence involves recognizing the importance of hierarchies of evidence and establishing criteria for its selection, assessment, and prioritization. The effective implementation of evidence-based practices involves an understanding of what counts as a desired outcome. It also involves identifying which policy and practice questions can benefit from evidence and which cannot, because of their complexity and context. The central lesson that has emerged in the study of prevention best practices has been that merely pushing information out from researchers to practitioners is insufficient and ineffective. Strategies are needed that encourage a pull for information by end users.

Another important consideration is the careful employment of the terms evidence-informed and exemplary practice in contrast to often overused terms evidence-based practice and exemplary program. The notion of evidence employed here incorporates the definition provided by the Canadian Health Research Foundation (2000):

> Evidence is information that comes closest to the facts of a matter. The form it takes depends on context...The evidence base for a decision is the multiple forms of evidence combined to balance rigor with expedience—while privileging the former over the latter.

This view of the role of evidence is balanced and provides a more realistic and practical approach to the labeling of programs by describing them as exemplary as opposed to best practices. Documenting exemplary programs is a valuable source of knowledge because the cases provide alternative solutions that can improve decisions by providing policy-makers and practitioners with deeper insight into the many different aspects of traumatic injury prevention programming. The cases provided in this casebook are held up as examples, as sources of inspiration, planning can be based on what works in real-life practice. In gathering this information, we extensively went into the details of each practice. We focused on the ways that the practice has been adapted and applied as well as on the way the knowledge is transferred and disseminated. It is very important that information about these kinds of projects is made available worldwide so that other people can learn from their experiences. Calling programs "exemplary" suggests that they could be replicated, that useful ideas can be generated from them, and that they can contribute positively to both policy and practice.

In contrast, designating a program as an exemplary program implies that the programs surveyed were in a hierarchical competition. Moreover, the designation exemplary was also important because although our review process has been systematic and as comprehensive as possible, it cannot be seen as exhaustive. Because this review relied on nominations and published reports it is likely that some very good programs have been missed. Since they could have been included but were not, describing the ones that did get cased as the "best" seems inappropriate.

The aims of this book are to (1) survey the range of trauma prevention strategies and programs; (2) identify examples of effective, evidence-informed practice; (3) describe, analyze, and evaluate these in terms of their effectiveness; (4) develop and strengthen networks by mobilizing public support and encouraging the participation of stakeholders in traumatic injury prevention; (5) provide an easily accessible casebook of the world's exemplary evidence-informed trauma prevention efforts.

1.6 The Identification of Exemplary Programs

1.6.1 Overview Incidence and Literature Review Strategy

The purpose of the literature review was to support the evidence-informed practice, programs, and policies (strategies/interventions) by encouraging systematic assessment of reports of research, to see which ones can inform "effective practice" in the prevention of traumatic injuries. A review becomes a systematic review when research studies reach specific standards in terms of methodology, and the reviewer is explicit about how the studies were located and what exclusion and inclusion criteria were used.

The search strategy employed in this review involved multifaceted mining of every available literature source. Using previously developed procedures for finding and recording findings, the following sources were tapped (Volpe et al., 2002):

- Medline, PsycARTICLES, and other relevant bibliographic databases
- Cochrane controlled clinical trials register
- Foreign language literature
- "Gray literature" (unpublished or unindexed reports: theses, conference proceedings, internal reports, non-indexed journals, pharmaceutical industry files)Reference chaining from any articles found
- Personal approaches to experts in the field to find unpublished reports
- Hand searches of the relevant specialized journals

Literature was further selected based on its ability to provide information on (a) the risk and protective factors associated with traumatic injury; (b) investigations and evaluations on guidelines and interventions that focus on decreasing falls, road, traffic, and sports traumatic injury.

The current literature review also drew from secondary sources available through the University of Toronto Library online database, Scholars Portal with literature also accessed through Google™ and Google Scholar™. The sources derived from Scholars Portal and Google Scholar™ were academic and peer-reviewed literature, which provided an epidemiological context about safety culture in healthcare centers, as well as an overview of the systematic evaluations available for safety culture and prevention programs within healthcare settings. Searching on Google™ provided access to information about the prevention programs themselves from the

standpoint of the institutions implementing them and the organizations that supported them.

The establishment of the final grounds for the inclusion and exclusion of literature pertaining to risk and protective factors associated with traumatic injury were carried out in consultation with injury prevention experts. What follows is an appraisal format that has been proven useful in previous reviews that is applicable to both experimental (random control trial) and quasi-experimental research reports. Because of the importance of mixed-method research to health promotion, a similar protocol has been developed for survey, qualitative, synthetic (systematic), and meta-analytic investigations.

The appraisal process can be divided into three sections:

1. *Relevance*: Does the article deal with factors that contribute to understanding the risk and protective factors associated with falls? What is the contribution to prevention science?
2. *Soundness*: Are the conclusions justified by the description of the methodology and the findings?

   There are three sets of soundness screening questions:
   (a) Did the study address a clearly focused issue?
   (b) How was the sample selected?
     - Is it big enough (power calculation), and is it representative?
     - Was the assignment of subjects to treatments randomized?
     - Were all the subjects who entered the study properly accounted for at its conclusion?
     - Are there any differences between the two groups in terms of selection bias or confounding variables, which could explain the differences between them (e.g., age, sex, and social class)?
     - Were the groups similar at the start of the trial (i.e., in terms of age, sex and any confounding variables)?
     - Were the groups treated equally?
     - Were the subjects "blind to the treatment?

(c) What are the results?
  - How large was the treatment effect? (What outcomes were recorded and how the differences between the groups were expressed?)
  - How precise was the estimate of the treatment effects?
3. *Usefulness*: Can the finding be generalized?
  (a) Are the risk and protective factors similar to those present in the lives of those in Western societies?
  (b) Were all the relevant outcomes considered? (If any were neglected, does this affect the interpretation?)
  (c) Are the benefits worth the harms and costs?

1.6.2 Exemplary Programs Review Methodology

To gauge and identify exemplary programs, we employed a multiphase process. Information for the review was gathered by interviewing program representatives face-to-face, by telephone and the Internet. Case information was obtained from a variety of methods described in the following three phases. Phase 1 outlines the tangible steps taken to establish case selection and identify possible Exemplary Programs. Phase 2 describes the data gathering methods employed. Also included here is an outline of the case analysis framework based on a complex systems conceptual scheme of human development described as the Life Space Framework. Lastly, Phase 3 establishes the final set of criteria used to identify chosen programs as "Exemplary."

1.6.2.1 Phase 1: Steps to Identify Exemplary Programs

Investigation
Various search tools were utilized to provide a broad picture of traumatic injury prevention on a global level, which include a meta-search of the World Wide Web, academic literature reviews, nominations from consortium members and

partners, and legislative and regulatory information. Specifically, meta-searches on the web enabled us to access relevant worldwide information. A literature review of systematic databases (outlined above) provided a meta-analysis of effective traumatic injury prevention programs. National centers for rehabilitation and traumatic injury prevention research acted as information resources regarding traumatic injury prevention practices on national levels. Referrals were garnered through literature reviews and key informants. Based on past experiences in the evaluation of Exemplary Programs for other projects, we have learned that knowledge of unpublished, yet worthwhile, programs is often gained by networking with program personnel. Systematic reviews were also obtained from the relevant published and unpublished reports to uncover traumatic injury prevention programs/models on an international scale. Programs identified that fell within the identification standards (including efforts at all levels, such as legislative, environmental, community, and individual) were considered for nomination.

Nomination
The nomination step aimed to form a broad picture of programs that seem promising and deserving of further study. Key informant contacts were identified and/or established through program documents such as annual reports and evaluations requested so that further referral information could be obtained. Only programs that satisfied collaboratively agreed upon criteria were investigated and ultimately evaluated for the review. The following Nomination Criteria were suggested for use during the nomination stage of the project:

1. The credibility of source: a rating of the authority of the source in the field
2. Community reputation: a rating of the program's standing among members of the field
3. Frequency of referral: the number of times a specific program is nominated by different referral agents
4. Country and region: the geographical location of the program

5. Position and demonstrated experience: length and degree of experience of the program since its inception
6. Stakeholder participation: whether stakeholders have roles in the program

Selection

Documented information received from programs that have met the nomination criteria were further examined to determine if they met the selection criteria so as to help us to further develop a profile of what constitutes Exemplary Program. This set of criteria was created by the combined research knowledge and expertise of the research team and contacts established within the traumatic injury prevention field and included:

1. Replicability and adaptability to Western societies
2. Sufficient documented information
3. Innovative strategies
4. Open and cooperative participation in the case writing process

Criteria number 4 was crucial. Program designers, managers, and evaluators were destined in this participative and mostly appreciative evaluation to become key informants, people in the know about their programs. As proxies for their organizations, they were expected to elaborate on program background and operation and fill in any existing blanks in documents and evaluations. They also were expected to share their program knowledge with others interested in adapting and implementing a prevention program their work may have inspired.

1.6.2.2 Phase 2: Data Gathering Methods

Programs that have met the requirements of Phase 1 became candidates for more in-depth investigation. In Phase 2, we began by using a semi-structured questionnaire (primarily a telephone interview) that followed the BRIO Model (Background, Resources, Implementation, Outcome) in order to provide a consistent way of describing each case so that a comprehensive yet succinct understanding of the program's structure and operation could be made explicit. The second half of Phase 2 was to understand how the program fits into the Life Space Case Analysis Framework, using the Complex Systems Conceptual Scheme outlined below.

The BRIO Model

Background. According to the BRIO Model, exploring the background of a program is to uncover its history and the environment and events that have shaped the program development and implementation (e.g., legal mandates in a community, unique funding opportunities, community reactions to the program). Background inquiries aim to understand why the traumatic injury prevention program takes a particular form, and how, for example, relevant policies, legislation, and community needs have influenced the objectives of the program. Sample questions that probed the background of the nominated programs include:

1. What was the traumatic injury issue at the intervention site before program implementation?
2. Who initiated the program?
3. What were the original goals and objectives of the program?
4. What events surrounded the development of the program?
5. What were the community reactions to the program at the time of program development?
6. What were the reactions of program personnel at the time of development?
7. How do associated professionals and sponsors perceive the program?
8. Who (if any) are the chosen community partners?
9. What is evidence for program sustainability? Are the stages of implementation (exploration, installation, initial and full implementation, innovation, and sustainability) discernible in the current integrated and compensatory practices of the program?

All of the programs and strategies profiled were organized into the BRIO and Life Space case frameworks and classified according to the major areas of traumatic injury prevention.

Resources. The term *resources* calls for an investigation of the program design and resource allocation, particularly, how the program intends to achieve the articulated objectives. Financial resources and the strategies adopted to promote injury prevention strategies are critical inputs to the program that should be clarified. Knowledge of alternative implementation and prevention strategies is useful to gauge the fit of the chosen approach. The following are examples of questions that examine resources:

1. What injury prevention strategies are employed in the program?
2. What financial resources are committed to the program?
3. What kinds of resources are developed for and allocated to the program?

Implementation. When discussing program implementation, we refer to the operationalization of a program, comparing the intended program design with how the program is actually practiced. The Fixsen, Naoom, Blase, Friedman, and Wallace (2005) model was employed here to assess potential implementation drives such as the explicitness of fidelity features and potential for staff training/coaching. Moreover, the Fixsen stages of implementation (exploration, installation, initial implementation, and full implementation) were used as descriptors in the nominee's program history. In this detailing the review examined how and why a traumatic injury prevention or injury prevention program does or does not adhere to the original plans for program governance, administration, management, implementation, and practice. Questions probing implementation issues include:

1. Have checks on program process been made?
2. What evidence exists as to the relation between what was intended in the program's design and what exists today?

3. How and when are adjustments to the program made?
4. How is feedback structured and given to management and front-line service providers?

Outcome. To understand a program's outcome is to determine the impact of the program. This component asks how practitioners, participants, and observers judge the attainments of the program. Long- and short-term outcome measures of the program, including intended and unintended positive (e.g., improved awareness of safety standards in the workplace) and negative outcomes, are of interest. Examples of questions that explore the outcome of a program include:

1. How do practitioners, participants, and observers judge the attainments of the program?
2. What are the short-term and long-term outcomes of the program?
3. What were any unanticipated positive or negative outcomes of the program?
4. How does the program measure success or effectiveness?
5. How (if at all) does the program disseminate program information?

Life Space Case Study Analysis Framework

While the BRIO model structures the story of a program, the Life Space Study Framework discussed above (Volpe, 2012) provides the features for its analysis in terms of four interrelated components: interpersonal relations, intrapersonal (internal) states, the physical environment, and the sociocultural environment. This division into these features is arbitrary and serves primarily analytic purposes. In reality, the life space is a complex fusion of elements. The facilitation of traumatic injury prevention requires that multidimensional programs enable individuals as opposed to one-dimensional interventions that focus merely on adjustment or adequate functioning.

The four components capture complex system changes in human development: (1) the sources of interpersonal support accessible to an individual;

(2) the personal resources that an individual can command—intelligence, appearance, strength, health, and temperament—investments of effort that the individual makes on his or her own behalf; (3) what the physical environment offers in terms of stimulation, support, and security; and (4) the sociocultural opportunities available or the obstacles encountered as influenced by social class, ethnic membership, age, gender, personal contacts, social calamity, economic adjustment, and technological change. Although the content of systems is highly variable, the common structural features within each case show how change is brought about in the course of human development over the entire life span. In this framework, change is seen as a relationship between resource and challenges in the life space. Injury prevention efforts were depicted as a resource mobilized in the response to the challenge of trauma. Each complex system is different and varied in its approach but developed according to the needs of individuals or communities targeted in programmatic efforts.

All of the programs and strategies profiled using the BRIO Model were then organized into the Life Space Case Study Analysis Framework and classified according to the major areas of traumatic injury prevention. The Life Space Framework allowed us to understand what doing injury prevention means to stakeholders. This approach captures how a program addresses the resources and challenges associated with traumatic injury prevention (See BRIO and Life Space Table Summaries for each case).

1.6.2.3 Phase 3: Final Criteria for Determining an Exemplary Program

In this phase, actual "Exemplary Programs" were identified. The descriptive analysis of each nominated program employed a set of collaboratively generated Exemplary Program criteria derived from the previous reviews and from the team's professional experience, partners associated with the research initiative, published literature, and from successful practices and programs:

- Avowed Support of Traumatic Injury Prevention
  - How does the program prove its commitment to traumatic injury prevention?
  - Is the program committed to injury prevention at the primary and secondary levels (i.e., at the pre-event and event stages)?
- Multidisciplinary Framework and Multilevel Approaches
  - Does the program use a multidisciplinary framework or approach?
- Environmental and Behavioral Strategies
  - Does the program employ a combination of environmental and behavioral strategies?
  - Does it create new injury risks?
- Developmental Approaches, Flexibility, and Adaptability
  - Does the program incorporate a developmental perspective?
- Implementation and Outcome Evaluation
  - Is the program's methodology grounded in credible and appropriate sources?
  - Can the program be defined in terms of its implementation?
- Broad-Based Community Support and Capacity Building
  - Does the program have active community support?
- Cost-Effectiveness Analyses
  - Does the program employ a cost analysis?
  - Can it adopt one with a long-term perspective?
- Sustainability
  - How has attention to the long-term viability of the program been addressed?
  - How adequate are efforts to continue, maintain benefits, and build capacity?
- Contribution to Prevention Science
  - How does the program's evaluation research contribute to the refinement and elaboration of the conceptualization of injury prevention?

The review and casing of Exemplary Programs in the prevention of traumatic injury helped to establish useful connections between a complex systems perspective of prevention and to create a unique set of cases for advancing traumatic injury prevention.

1.7 Overview of Area Previews and Case Studies

The determination of what constitutes an exemplary or effective program involved the application of the series of selection criteria reviewed above. What follows are the multilevel case studies that resulted from the application of these criteria. Mixed methods were employed to assess the validity of program descriptions. All program stakeholders reviewed, and when necessary, revised accounts of their enterprise. Moreover, the programs that qualified as exemplary practices also incorporated at least three of the five E's (engineering, enactment, education, economics, and evaluation).

As discussed above, traumatic injury prevention is becoming more important as a goal in public health and in the public policy cycle. The case studies presented in this volume demonstrate that complex multilevel programs are vital to effective injury prevention. The programs reviewed in this casebook are among the exemplary programs in the world and are offered not as templates, but as opportunities for adaptation and improvement.

Within a complex systems approach, the main goal of this casebook is to illustrate how the prevention of traumatic injury can be effectively addressed through a variety of multifaceted, multilevel programs that are systematically presented as exemplars of effective prevention initiatives. A further goal has been to make explicit a case selection and investigation framework that increased the detail and depth of the case studies being offered as exemplars.

This volume is divided into four parts. Each part is preceded by a chapter that overviews the area of traumatic injury prevention addressed. Chapter 2 attends to the consequences of traumatic sports injury that often results in long-term disability and impedes educational, occupational, and personal fulfillment. Associated personal and social burdens are extended because sports injuries most frequently occur among children and young adults. These problems are compounded by the fact that athletes are at risk for multiple injuries. Chapter 12 considers how the significant financial burden to our healthcare system as well as the considerable social burden, given the interference with work and family, of falls-type injuries is increasingly being addressed by life-span-oriented, community-based interventions. Chapter 18 draws attention to the constant need to improve road safety because of the hazards associated with motor vehicle traffic and the seriousness of injuries resulting from collisions. The case studies in this part are among the leading road safety policies and implementation practices in the world. Finally, Chap. 27 examines unified and collaborative, community-wide approaches to traumatic injury prevention. These cases illustrate success in realizing the social and economic benefits of scaled-up prevention strategies.

References

Campbell, D. T., & Russo, M. J. (1999). *Social experimentation*. Thousand Oaks, CA: Sage.

Canadian Research Foundation. (2000). *Annual report*. Ottawa, Canada: Canadian Institutes of Health Research.

Cohen, L., & Swift, S. (1999). The spectrum of prevention: developing a comprehensive approach to injury prevention. *Injury Prevention, 5*, 203–207.

Fixsen, D., Naoom, S., Blase, K., Friedman, R., & Wallace, W. (2005). *Implementation research: A synthesis of the literature*. Tampa, FL: National Implementation Research Network (NIRN).

Haddon, W. (1972). A logical framework for categorizing highway safety phenomena and activity. *Journal of Trauma, 12*(30), 12–22.

Lewko, J., & Volpe, R. (2009). *Learning to work safely: A guide for managers and educators*. Charlotte, NC: Information Age.

Sackett, D. L., Straus, S. E., Richardson, W. S., Rosenberg, W., & Haynes, R. B. (2000). *Evidence-based medicine: How to practice and teach EBM* (2nd ed.). New York, NY: Churchill Livingstone.

Volpe, R. (1999). Knowledge from evaluation research. In Evans, P., Hurrell, P., Lewis, M., and Volpe, R. (Ed.). *Children and families at risk: New issues in integrating services* (pp. 149–167). Paris, France: Organization of Economic Cooperation and Development (OECD).

Volpe, R. (2012). *Injury prevention as change in complex systems*. Toronto, Canada: SMARTRISK Foundation.

Volpe, R. (2013). *Casebook of exemplary evidenced informed programs that foster community participation after brain injury*. Charlotte, NC: Information Age.

Volpe, R., & Lewko, J. (2009). *Science and sustainability in the prevention of serious injury*. Toronto, ON: Ontario Neurotrauma Foundation.

Volpe, R., Lewko, J., & Batra, A. (2002). *A Compendium of effective, evidence-based exemplary practices in the prevention of neurotrauma*. Toronto, Canada: University of Toronto Press.

Part I

Sports and Recreation-Related Traumatic Injury Prevention Programs

Overview of Sports and Recreation-Related Traumatic Injury Prevention Programs

Sabrina Amicone

Sports and recreation activities are intended to be pleasurable pastimes for individuals and communities, providing positive attributes such as improved physical endurance and health, as well as cognitive and psychosocial benefits, particularly for the youth. However, the beneficial purposes of these activities can disintegrate in an instant when the activity itself results in debilitating or life-altering harm and injury—especially when that injury involves the head or spinal cord.

In 2012, the US estimated number of hospital emergency department visits concerning treatment for sports and recreation-related injuries included 1,298,671 individuals (see Table 2.1; Neiss Data Highlights, United States Consumer Product Safety Commission, 2012). The activities with the highest prevalence of traumatic brain injuries include basketball, football, operating all-terrain vehicles (ATV), bicycling, and playground activities. Injuries and deaths associated with sports and recreation activities correlate with age and gender. For example, between the years 2001 and 2005, 70% of sports and recreation-related traumatic brain injuries and emergency department visits were male. The greatest rates for both males and females occurred among youth aged 10 to 14 years, followed by those aged 15–19 years

(see Table 2.2; Gilchrist, Thomas, Wald, & Langlois, 2007).

Similar results were observed internationally. In Australia, for example, sports injury hospitalizations were observed at greater rates among younger individuals—65% of injuries were accumulated by individuals under the age of 35 years. Additionally, more than three quarters of those admitted into the hospital for sports-related injury in 2011 and 2012 were men (see Table 2.3; Kreisfeld, Harrison, & Pointer, 2014). In 2005, the cost of sport injuries for the Australian community was roughly $2 billion (Australian dollars) with 27% of people injured requiring an average of 11 days off work (Medibank Private, 2006).

In Europe, there are approximately 7000 fatalities per year from injuries associated with sports activities (EuroSafe, 2006). Annually, almost six billion individuals are treated in hospitals for sports-related injuries with 10% requiring one full day or more of hospitalization. Furthermore, "team ball" sports account for roughly 40% of all hospital-treated sport injuries with European football (soccer) encompassing 74% of the injuries. The injury risk in team ball sports is moderately high compared to other types of sports due to its common one-on-one encounters between players. The injury rank-order per specific team ball sport is football (74%), basketball (8%), volleyball (7%), and handball (3%). According to European Union (EU) records, a majority of the

S. Amicone (✉)
University of Toronto, Toronto, ON, Canada

© Springer Nature Switzerland AG 2020
R. Volpe (ed.), *Casebook of Traumatic Injury Prevention*,
https://doi.org/10.1007/978-3-030-27419-1_2

Table 2.1 Estimated number of injuries involving sport or recreational equipment in the United States treated in ER Departments for the year 2012

Sports and recreation activities	Estimated number of injuries	ER visits (treat and release)	Hospitalization
ATV, snowmobile	226,549	198,477	28,040
Skateboards	114,120	110,565	3539
Exercise and equipment	459,978	427,989	31,844
Playgrounds	271,475	257,776	13,683
Totals	1,298,671	994,807	77,106

Note: Table was created using data from National Electronic Injury Surveillance System (NEISS), by United States Consumer Product Safety Commission, 2012
ER emergency room

Table 2.2 Estimated annual number of injuries due to sports and recreation activities based on data collected between the years 2001 and 2005 in the United States

Age, years	ER visits	Traumatic brain injuries
0–4	158,876	14,406
5–9	529,481	36,756
10–14	1,084,041	60,272
15–19	879,184	61,851
Gender	Male	1,810,260
	Female	840,838

Note: Table was created using data from "Nonfatal Traumatic Brain Injuries from Sports and Recreation Activities—United States, 2001–2005", by J. Gilchrist, K. E. Thomas, M. Wald, & J. Langlois, 2007, Morbidity and Mortality Weekly Report, 56(29)
ER emergency room

Table 2.3 Incidences of sports injury hospitalizations in Australia for the years 2011–2012

Sport type	Number of cases of hospitalization
Wheeled motor sports	2737
Australian football	3186
Rugby	2621
Roller sports	1632
Soccer	2962
Total	36,237

Note: Table was created using data from Australian Sports Injury Hospitalisations 2011–12 [INJCAT 168], by R. Kreisfeld, J. E. Harrison, & S. Pointer, 2014, Canberra, AU: Australian Institute of Health and Welfare

sports-related injuries are a result of participating in nonorganized, or individually organized, sports activities (EuroSafe, 2006). A comprehensive and comparable estimate of the financial burden sports-related injuries have on European communities was not available. However, in practice, indicators of economic burden can be estimated by observing the average cost of a one day in-hospital treatment and considerations of relative severity of injuries. As developed by the EUROCOST project, such a calculation leads to an estimated direct medical cost of at least $2.4 billion annually to the European community (Bauer et al., 2004).

In Canada, injuries related to sports and recreation activities resulted in 263 deaths and 115,724 emergency room visits in the year 2010 alone. Playground injuries were considerably more likely to result in partial or permanent disability whereas activities involving snowmobiles or ATVs had greater incidences of death (see Table 2.4; Parachute, 2015). The full economic burden of sports and recreation-related injuries and deaths to Canadian citizens must include direct costs—such as health care costs from injuries—and indirect costs—such as injury costs associated with social productivity, hospitalization, disability, and premature death. Thus, when calculating both the direct and indirect costs, in 2010 Canadians spent an estimated $883 million on sports and recreation-related injuries (see Table 2.5; Parachute, 2015).

As the epidemiology across several nations demonstrates, injuries related to sports and recreational activities are pervasive and occur at alarming proportions. The cost of these injuries not only affects an individual's physical health and productivity, but further produces significant financial burden to the individual, community, and the nation as a whole. Nevertheless, aside from the financial cost injuries generate for communities, an individual's life and healthy functioning is invaluable. In recent years, neu-

Table 2.4 Canadian epidemiology of sports and recreation-related injuries for the year 2010

	Deaths	Hospitalization	ER visits	Permanent disability	
				Partial	Total
Struck by/against sports equipment	<5	664	68,355	518	39
ATV, snowmobile	190	4311	21,107	1043	88
Skates, boards, blades, skis	68	3771	23,106	1022	90
Playgrounds	<5	194	3156	8882	812
Total	263[a]	8940	115,724	11,465	1029

Note: Table was created using data from *The Cost of Injury in Canada*, by Parachute, 2015, Toronto, Canada: Author. Copyrighted 2015 by Parachute
[a]Approximate

Table 2.5 Canadian economic burden of sports and recreation-related injuries for the year 2010

	Total costs	Direct costs	Indirect costs
Struck by/against sports equipment	$187 million	$97 million	$90 million
ATV, snowmobile	$262 million	$245 million	$507 million
Skates, boards, blades skis	$295 million	$221 million	$516 million
Playgrounds	$139 million	$100 million	$239 million
Total	$883 million		

Note: Table was created using data from The Cost of Injury in Canada, by Parachute, 2015, Toronto, Canada: Author. Copyrighted 2015 by Parachute

rotrauma such as traumatic brain injuries (TBI) and spinal cord injuries (SCI), resulting from sports and recreational activities has gained scientific and public interest as a proliferating and prevalent health concern. The United States experiences roughly 1.6–3.8 million cases of sports and recreation-related TBIs annually with 75% of cases presenting as "mild" (Centers for Disease Control and Prevention [CDC], 2017b; Langlois, Rutland-Brown, & Wald, 2006). Concussions, for example, are considered by many medical professionals to be a mild Traumatic Brain Injury (mTBI); however, research has indicated that brain damage from multiple concussions over a long-term period can result in cumulative deficits (CDC, 2017b). Furthermore, second-impact syndrome (repeated mTBIs over a very short time) may lead to brain swelling and/or death (CDC, 2017b). This can be exacerbated as many individuals with mTBIs do not receive medical attention either in a hospital emergency department or by a general practitioner (Prince & Bruhns, 2017).

The consequences of head injury or TBI, whether mild or severe, can alter an individual's cognitive, physical, and emotional functioning (CDC, 2017b). Developing children and adolescents are particularly vulnerable to injuries related to sports and recreation given that an estimated 38 million US youth participate in organized sports each year (National Council of Youth Sports, 2001). Spinal Cord Injury (SCI) is also a relevant risk factor when participating in sports and recreational activities and often results in permanent debilitating outcomes. It has been estimated that worldwide 7–18% of SCIs are acquired from sports and recreational activities (World Health Organization [WHO] & International Spinal Cord Society [ISCS], 2013). An SCI can occur from high or low elevation falls/stumbles/jumps from playground equipment, horseback riding, skiing, snowboarding, diving, bicycling; or from contact sports such as football, soccer, or rugby. Recreational vehicles such as ATVs are also a high culprit of fatal injuries, head injuries, and SCIs (WHO & ISCS, 2013).

2.1 Section Chapters

This section reviews case studies that demonstrate exemplary practice in injury and neurotrauma prevention programs associated with sports and recreational activities. The commonality of the programs lies in their integration of evidence-informed environmental and behavioral strategies to interventions. Research indicates that behaviorally based educational interventions are effective due to their more nuanced approach to injury prevention—recognizing the range of complex determinants and mechanisms of behavior and carefully applying theories and research from behavioral sciences (Gielen & Sleet, 2003; Thompson, Sleet, & Sacks, 2002). The programs in this section utilize community participation, program evaluations, as well as multidisciplinary approaches in their construction, organization, and execution. They are respectable models that provide cohesive components and frameworks necessary for successful injury prevention outcomes in sports and recreation-related programs. The programs in this section are divided into two categories: (1) Organized Team Sports—Injury Prevention Initiatives, which, for the purpose of this review, will include contact sports performed between competing teams and are part of an organization or institution (e.g., sports clubs/schools); and (2) Individual Sports and/or Recreational Activities— Injury Prevention Initiatives, which, for the purpose of this review, will include activities that involve individual participation and are performed for either recreational and/or competitive sport purposes.

2.1.1 Organized Team Sports

The Heads Up: Concussions in High School Sports Program (Chap. 3) is a nationwide initiative established by the Centers for Disease Control and Prevention (CDC), which aims to reduce the risks of concussions and other severe head injuries for youth athletes. Heads Up targets schools as central distributors for concussion/ head-injury awareness and prevention by educating stakeholders such as school professionals, coaches, sports officials, parents, health care professionals and athletes of all high school sports. The CDC's Heads Up program has joined with the National Federation of State High School Association (NFHS) in its efforts to educate and improve awareness and management

of concussion through a free online training course for stakeholders of high school sports. The online training course, along with other free resources—such as online videos, online customizable information fact sheets/posters, mobile phone helmet safety apps, PSAs, and podcasts—are publicly available on the CDC website. These resources and toolkits are designed and tailored to educate each stakeholder of all high school sports with the purpose of assisting in the implementation of safety protocols for young athletes. The online resources additionally promote and educate the importance of safety play positions, procedures for potential concussion assessment, appropriate practices to ensure athletes safely return to play after injury; and, for applicable sports, proper helmet use (CDC, 2017a). The Heads Up: Concussion in High School Sports initiative is a nationwide success that encompasses multiple evidence-informed components, and, thus, prevails as an exemplary practice in sports and recreation-related injury prevention programs.

Ice hockey is a popular team sport, particularly, for North American adults and youth. Hockey players are at risk of serious injury resulting from collisions that may occur at high speeds (Lemair & Pearsall, 2007). The Play It Cool Program (Chap. 4) was established to prevent serious injuries in ice hockey and was based on four fundamental properties. First, this program was accessed via the Internet and required a facilitator to monitor and coach participants. Secondly, the program insisted upon continuous and active coach participation. Third, it demanded asynchronous delivery and utilized a variety of technological tools that are accessible and flexible for coach participation. Finally, the program initiated a community of practitioners, whereby coaches could interact and facilitate a learning and training environment. Initially, the Play It Cool program was well received by participating stakeholders; however, the lack of support from hockey's governing bodies created barriers, which ultimately resulted in difficulties for sustainability as an organized program (W. Montelpare, personal communication, November 3, 2017). Nonetheless, the modules and curriculum, which are the key components of the program, continue to be successfully utilized or adopted as exemplary guides in continuing education courses for coaches, parents, educators, and health care professionals in ice hockey, as well as other contact sports. Furthermore, the research conducted for the Play It Cool program has led to an unfolding of other research (W. Montelpare, personal communication, November 3, 2017). For instance, a current research focus is on head injury evaluation and appropriate rehabilitation supporting children's safe return to play (W. Montelpare, personal communication, November 3, 2017). Regardless of sustainability difficulties of the program, Play It Cool contains key exemplary elements that can be implemented into various sports-related injury prevention initiatives.

Likewise, rugby, which is the national sport of New Zealand (NZ), has gained injury prevention attention due to its rigorous tackles and contact plays. It became essential for NZ to recognize the epidemic of severe injuries, such as SCIs, that the sport was inflicting on athletes; therefore, the New Zealand Rugby Union and Accident Compensation Corporation of New Zealand (ACC) developed the RugbySmart Injury Prevention Program (Chap. 5). The program's purposes are to prevent injuries for players where possible, reduce impact of an injury with treatment as a standard requirement, and provide support for best possible recovery results (New Zealand Rugby Union [NZRU], 2017). It accomplishes these goals by implementing six specific modules, which include Educating Players, Health Provider Engagement, First Aid in Rugby (FAIR), Respect and Responsibility, Rugby Specific Warm-ups, and Coach and Referee Education (NZRU, 2017). The RugbySmart initiative is delivered through their website (www.rugbysmart.co.nz) and uses the six modules to provide athletes, coaches, and referees the knowledge and guidelines necessary to maintain the physical health of athletes. Further, it reinforces safety techniques and positioning with videos and information pages. With rugby becoming increasingly popular globally, particularly with North American young

adults and youth, an injury prevention program such as RugbySmart provides well-established foundations necessary for intensive contact sports, marking the program as an exemplary practice.

Another team sport that is internationally popular is soccer (or what many non-North American countries refer to as "football"). According to a survey conducted by Fédération Internationale de Football Association (FIFA) in 2001, there are more than 240 million people worldwide who play soccer regularly; and five million referees, assistant referees and officials directly involved in the game. A direct blow from a soccer ball or a loose kick can cause serious injuries including fractures, bruising, concussion, and even death (McGrath & Ozanne-Smith, 1997). Data from the United States estimates that over a 10-year period there were 28,000 injuries classified as either a skull fracture or internal head injury from soccer (Delaney, 2001). Additionally, research has indicated an increase in head and spinal cord injuries from soccer due to the voluntary use of head and ball impact, as well as player-to-player contact (Pickett, Streight, Simpson, & Brison, 2005). The literature suggests that the proportion of total head, spine and trunk area injuries is approximately 4–22% in adults and 9–26% in youth (McGrath & Ozanne-Smith, 1997). The Injury Prevention Program SafeClub (Chap. 6) was developed in New South Wales to assist community soccer clubs to adopt accessible and useful risk management practices. The program aims to make soccer safe through inclusive procedures that analyze and manage injury risks (Fuller & Drawer, 2001). The program consists of three training sessions of two hours per session. It utilizes adult-based learning principles centered on methods in which information is provided to participants and the information is tailored to all learning types. Additionally, adult-based learning principles give participants a chance to practice what they may have gained during SafeClub training sessions (K. Abbott, personal communication, January 23, 2008). Due to lack of funding and difficulties in achieving participation from soccer clubs, SafeClub was not sustained (M. Zappia, personal communication, December 4, 2017). With soccer club administrators and managers working on a volunteer basis, resistance was met in putting forward training for SafeClub since it was not mandatory (M. Zappia, personal communication, December 4, 2017). Moreover, the reluctance of sporting associations to mandate the program was also a barrier the program encountered (M. Zappia, personal communication, December 4, 2017). Regardless of the challenges to sustainability for the SafeClub program, its foundation in research and framework are acknowledged as exemplary practices.

2.1.2 Individual Sports and/or Recreational Activities

Snowboarding and skiing can be an individual, leisurely activity or a competitive sport. Regardless of the purpose for participating in these activities, snowboarding and skiing can result in severe injuries when proper equipment is not utilized. The It Ain't Brain Surgery Initiative (Chap. 7) was an injury prevention program that changed the culture and attitudes in snowboarding and skiing communities by making helmet use mainstream, thus minimizing the risks of head and spinal cord injury. Head and spinal cord injuries make up a significant portion of all injuries among skiers and snowboarders. According to a literature review by Levy and Smith (2000), among skiers and snowboarders, head injuries account for 3–15% of injuries while spinal cord injuries account for 1–13% of all reported injuries. Many studies that have analyzed injuries of skiers and snowboarders have found head injuries to be the leading cause of death in this group (Levy, Hawkes, Hemminger, & Knight, 2002; Myles, Mohtadi, & Schnittker, 1992). According to the United States Consumer Product Safety Commission (United States Consumer Product Safety Commission, 1999), helmet use by skiers and snowboarders could reduce 44% of head injuries among adults and 53% of head injuries in children. In another literature review on effectiveness of helmets by Ackery, Hagel, Provvidenza, and Tator (2007),

it was discovered that helmets reduced head injuries by 22–60%. Therefore, an injury prevention program in this area should have a focus on helmet use and include mechanisms to increase helmet use. The It Ain't Brain Surgery program, which was initiated in Denver, Colorado, was found to be an effective program in increasing helmet use and reducing the rates of brain injuries among skiers and snowboarders. The program utilized evidence-informed research to promote as well as implement its initiative while maintaining financial and public support from important collaborators and stakeholders. Furthermore, the program was a catalyst in making helmets a typical piece of equipment for snowboarders and skiers nationwide, thus, resulting in the discontinuation of the program as its intentions to promote mainstream helmet use in these sports was successfully accomplished. The It Ain't Brain Surgery Initiative is an exemplary practice as it demonstrates procedures and supports necessary to change behaviors in helmet use for sports and recreation-associated activates.

Riding and Road Safety Test Program. Another activity that can be either a recreational activity or competitive sport is horseback riding. The Riding and Road Safety Test Program (Chap. 8), developed by the British Horse Society in the United Kingdom (UK), aims is to educate recreational and/or professional horseback riders in safety techniques and awareness through theoretical, as well as practical lessons to reduce the risks of serious injuries while riding or handling a horse. In the United States alone, up to 30 million Americans ride in a given year (Carlton Reckling & Webb, 1996; Dekker et al., 2004). According to Silver (2002), horse-riding-related injuries are expected due to the dangerous combination of the rider's head being situated up to 13 ft from the ground and the horse traveling at high speeds of up to 65 km/h. Additionally, riding on public roads, which is common in the UK, adds another dimension of risk to recreational riders (Silver, 2002). As a result of the dangers associated with riding on public roads, approximately 3000 horse-related road traffic accidents occur each year in the UK (Road Safety

Congress, 2007). Northey (2003) found evidence indicating that significant brain damage can result from falls of as low as 23 in. Even equestrian sport professionals with considerable riding experience are at risk for head injuries, despite wearing helmets during competition and performances (Fleming, Crompton, & Simpson, 2001). The British Horse Society's Riding and Road Safety Test was designed to prevent collisions between ridden horses and vehicles. The program has a history of more than 30 years of educating horseback riders in road safety with the explicit goal of minimizing the risk of injuries, particularly when riding on roads. In 2017, the name of the program was changed to the Road Safe Award and some additions to the program were implemented, for instance, a broadening of its subject area, a broadening of riding environments, and a broadening of diverse riding conditions (British Horse Society, 2017). These current additions to the program have further benefited an already successful program. Moreover, the fundamentals, framework, and support of stakeholders of this program earn recognition as an exemplary program in the area of sports and recreation-related injury prevention.

The 4-H Community ATV Safety Program (Chap. 9), which was initiated in Alaska and then expanded nationwide in the United States, educates youth and adult users of All-Terrain Vehicles (ATVs) in reducing the risks of serious injuries through workshops, courses, camping programs, mass media, and community ATV clubs. ATV use has increased dramatically from roughly 4.2 million in the year 2000 to seven million in 2004 (Helmkamp, Furbee, Coben, & Tadros, 2008). ATVs are most frequently used for labor or recreational purposes; however, despite their popularity they can cause serious injuries. Approximately 25–35% of ATV-related injuries in children involve the brain and/or the spinal cord (Brandenburg, Brown, Archer, & Brandt Jr, 2007). By researching the manner and pattern of ATV crashes, Brandenburg et al. (2007) have identified the risk factors associated with ATV-related injuries. Analyzing the circumstances of 193 people seen initially at the emergency of a Level II Trauma center in Tulsa, Oklahoma,

ranging from age 2 to 71 years, Brandenburg et al. (2007) found that adults were more likely than children to be hurt from a rollover at 72% and 51% respectively, and that for adults, the rollover mostly happened traveling uphill when the ATV rolled backward, whereas children mostly experienced injury from right-sided rollovers on flat or uneven ground, usually riding alone. Helmets were worn by only 20% of patients, and children were more likely to ride ATV with passengers. The three patients who died in this study were all children who had injury to the torso and the brain from collisions. Furthermore, 48% of this study group sustained a brain injury. The 4-H Community ATV Safety program provides education and hands-on training to young riders and the adults who supervise them through safety curriculum and resources at 4-H community sites dispersed throughout most states in America. Training workshops are offered throughout the year at different locations to train youth–adult teams to design a customized locally based and sustainable ATV safety program. The efforts in enhancing ATV safety in the United States by the 4-H Community ATV Safety program is recognized as an initiative that possesses the elements and foundations that can be utilized as exemplary practice for sports and recreation-related injury prevention.

Bicycling is not only a pleasurable recreational activity, but also a mode of transportation or many youth and adults. The Bicycle Transportation Alliance's Bicycle Safety and Awareness Program (BSAP; Chap. 10) was formed in Portland, Oregon, a city considered one of the major bicycle-friendly cities in the United States (City of Portland, 1998; Ross, 2008). Designed for children in fourth through seventh grade, this primary prevention program addresses a variety of issues relevant to children's bicycle safety, such as negotiating traffic, independent travel, and helmet use (United States Department of Transportation, 2002). Bicycling presents traffic safety and injury risks; a concomitant degree of skill and cognitive ability is required in the navigation of a bicycle (Safe Kids Canada, 2007). Children between the ages of 5 and 15 years represent a particularly vulnerable segment of the population, having the highest rate of injury per million cycling outings (Rivara & Aitken, 1998). According to Safe Kids Connecticut (2005), cyclists under the age of 14 years are at five times higher risk for injuries compared to older riders and fatality rates were greatest for ages 10–15 years, followed by ages 5–9 years. Bicycling is a common activity for children and many community-based programs exist to teach them how to cycle safely and responsibly (Rivera & Metrik, 1998; United States Department of Transportation, 2002). However, there are many methodological difficulties inherent in the evaluation of community-based childhood injury prevention programs and the interpretation of a program's effectiveness (Klassen, MacKay, Moher, Walker, & Jones, 2000; Towner & Dowswell, 2002). The Bicycle Transportation Alliance's Bicycle Safety and Awareness Program (BSAP) has addressed many of the issues inherent in evaluating community-based health prevention programs in the area of child injury while delivering a multifaceted school-based program. The more acclaimed bicycle safety programs for youth have incorporated features such as traffic safety education, promotion of helmet use, safety guidelines, and experiential training with an on-bike focus into a comprehensive package (Rivera & Metrik, 1998). Comprehensive program components include a focus on environmental, legislative, and behavioral factors. The BSAP is one particular comprehensive program that holistically addresses multiple factors related to safety making it an exemplary practice in injury prevention. In recent years, the Bicycle Transportation Alliance has changed its name to The Street Trust and the program name Bicycle Safety and Awareness Program (BSAP) has changed to the Bicycle Safety Program (BSP). Despite the name changes, the program continues to operate under its original format and continues to be supported by the Oregon Department of Transportation.

The National Program for Playground Safety (NPPS; Chap. 11) initiative is dedicated to ensuring that playground equipment is constructed and maintained at a high level of quality that will minimize the risks of injury for children. The propor-

tion of falls occurring in the home seems to decline as children grow older; however, the number of falls occurring in educational, sports, and recreation settings increases with age (Public Health Agency of Canada, 1998). Children between the ages of 5 and 9 years have the highest number of playground injuries (Brown, 1997). Injuries to the head or face have accounted for 49% of injuries to children between the ages of 0 and 4 years, while older children between the ages of 5 and 14 years are vulnerable to fractures to the arm and hand (National Program for Playground Safety, 2001). Proper maintenance of the playground is an important aspect of playground safety as children can be seriously injured when they are inadequately maintained. The NPPS estimates that nearly 30% of playground injuries can be attributed to poor maintenance (Thompson & Hudson, 2002). There are a number of factors that contribute to childhood injuries on playgrounds, which includes inadequate surfacing materials, inappropriate height of equipment, lack of maintenance, lack of adult supervision, and lack of age-appropriate playground equipment. Attention to proper implementation of these elements for playgrounds is necessary in order to ensure a decrease in playground injuries. A program such as the National Program for Playground Safety is a dynamic initiative that focuses on the different aspects of playground safety. The NPPS model includes a blueprint of action steps at the national, state, and local levels. The NPPS provides major goals for playground safety and these goals target the major areas that contribute to reducing playground injuries rendering the program as an exemplary practice in recreational injury prevention.

2.2 For What Follows

It is vital for communities to implement, promote, and fund prevention programs that minimize the risks of serious injuries in order to reduce the negative health and economic consequence for its citizens. Each of these programs fits the constructs for exemplary practice, providing frameworks for formulating initiatives that prevent the occurrences of injuries associated with sports and recreational activities. Subsequently, in this section, each individual program will be reviewed and discussed with greater depth and examination of their conceptualization, resource development, implementation, and evaluations.

References

Ackery, A., Hagel, B. E., Provvidenza, C., & Tator, C. H. (2007). An international review of head and spinal cord injuries in alpine skiing and snowboarding. *Injury Prevention, 13*, 368–375.

Bauer, B., Kejs, T. M. A., Larsen, F. C., Petridou, E., McCarthy, T., Pitidis, A. et al. (2004). *Final report: A surveillance based assessment of medical costs of injury in Europe: phase 2*. Retrieved from https://moodle.adaptland.it/pluginfile.php/8246/mod_resource/content/0/surveillance_based_assessment_phase_2_2004.pdf

Brandenburg, M. A., Brown, S. J., Archer, P., & Brandt Jr., E. N. (2007). All-terrain vehicle crash factors and associated injuries in patients presenting to a regional trauma center. *Trauma, 63*(5), 994–999.

British Horse Society. (2017). Ride Safe Award. Retrieved November 18, 2018, from https://pathways.bhs.org.uk/ride-safe-award/.

Brown, J. (1997, November). A comparison of injuries on various types of playground equipment. *The Canadian Hospitals Injury Reporting and Prevention Program News, 12*(7).

Carlton Reckling, W., & Webb, J. K. (1996). Equestrian sports. In R. G. Watkins (Ed.), *The spine in sports* (pp. 527–539). St. Louis, MO: Mosby.

Centers for Disease Control and Prevention. (2017a). *Heads up to school sports*. Retrieved December 15, 2017, from https://www.cdc.gov/headsup/highschoolsports/index.html.

Centers for Disease Control and Prevention. (2017b). *Traumatic brain injury & concussion*. Retrieved December 11, 2017, from https://www.cdc.gov/traumaticbraininjury/.

City of Portland. (1998). *Bicycle master plan*. Portland, OR: Office of Transportation.

Dekker, R., Van Der Sluis, C. K., Kootstra, J., Groothoff, J. W., Eisma, W. H., & Ten Duis, H. J. (2004). Long-term outcome of equestrian injuries in children. *Disability and Rehabilitation, 26*(2), 91–96.

Delaney, J. S. (2001). Comparative review of US consumer product safety board data for soccer, ice hockey and American football from 1990 to 1999. *British Journal of Sports Medicine, 35*, 367–377.

EuroSafe. (2006). *European association for injury prevention and safety promotion*. http://www.eurosafe.eu.com/csi/eurosafe2006.nsf/wwwVwContent/BF89D11DC5D636DEC1257AA40079ED0D?opendocument&context=546FDA82B09D2691C12571AE0049DB2B.

Fédération Internationale de Football Association. (2001). *FIFA survey: Approximately 250 million footballers worldwide*. http://www.fifa.com/aboutfifa/news/y=2001/m=4/news=fifa-survey-approximately-250-million-footballers-worldwide-88048.html.

Fleming, P. R., Crompton, J. L., & Simpson, D. A. (2001). Neuro-ophthalmological sequelae of horse-related accidents. *Clinical and Experimental Ophthalmology, 29*, 208–212.

Fuller, S., & Drawer, C. W. (2001). Propensity for osteoarthritis and lower limb joint pain in retired professional soccer players. *British Journal of Sports Medicine, 35*(6), 402–408.

Gielen, A. C., & Sleet, D. (2003). Application of behavior-change theories and methods to injury prevention. *Epidemiologic Reviews, 25*(1), 65–76.

Gilchrist, J., Thomas, K. E., Wald, M., & Langlois, J. (2007). Nonfatal traumatic brain injuries from sports and recreation activities – United States, 2001–2005. *Morbidity and Mortality Weekly Report, 56*(29), 733–737.

Hardy, S. (2007). *Encouraging education in road safety*. Paper presented at the Road Safety Congress.

Helmkamp, J. C., Furbee, P. M., Coben, J. H., & Tadros, A. (2008). All-terrain vehicle-related hospitalizations in the united states, 2000–2004. *American Journal of Preventive Medicine, 34*(1), 39–45.

Klassen, T. P., MacKay, J. M., Moher, D., Walker, A., & Jones, A. L. (2000). Community-based injury prevention interventions. *The Future of Children, 10*(1), 83–110.

Kreisfeld, R., Harrison, J. E., & Pointer, S. (2014). *Australian sports injury hospitalisations 2011–12 [INJCAT 168]*. Canberra, ACT: Australian Institute of Health and Wellness.

Langlois, J. A., Rutland-Brown, W., & Wald, M. M. (2006). The epidemiology and impact of traumatic brain injury a brief overview. *Journal of Head Trauma Rehabilitation, 21*(5), 375–378.

Lemair, M., & Pearsall, D. (2007). Evaluation of impact attenuation of facial protectors in ice hockey helmets. *Sports Engineering, 10*(2), 65–74.

Levy, A. S., Hawkes, A. P., Hemminger, L. M., & Knight, S. (2002). An analysis of head injuries among skiers and snowboarders. *Journal of Trauma and Acute Care Surgery, 53*, 695–704.

Levy, A. S., & Smith, R. H. (2000). Neurologic injuries in skiers and snowboarders. *Seminars in Neurology, 20*, 233–245.

McGrath, A., & Ozanne-Smith, J. (1997). *Heading injuries out of soccer [Report no. 125]*. Melbourne, ACT: Monash University, Accident Research Centre.

Medibank Private. (2006). *Safe sports report*. Retrieved from http://www.theage.com.au/ed_docs/sport.pdf.

Myles, S. T., Mohtadi, N. G., & Schnittker, J. (1992). Injuries to the nervous system and spine in downhill skiing. *Canadian Journal of Surgery, 35*, 643–648.

National Council of Youth Sports. (2001). *National council of youth sports market research: NCYS membership survey*. Retrieved from http://www.ncys.org/pdfs/2001/200-participation-survey.pdf.

National Program for Playground Safety. (2001). Playground-related statistics. http://www.uni.edu/playground/resources/statistics.html

New Zealand Rugby Union. (2017). *Objectives*. Retrieved November 24, 2017, from https://www.rugbysmart.co.nz/objectives.

Northey, G. (2003). Equestrian injuries in New Zealand, 1993–2001: Knowledge and experience. *The New Zealand Medical Journal, 116*, 1182), 1–1182), 8.

Parachute. (2015). *The cost of injury in Canada*. Toronto, ON: Author.

Pickett, W., Streight, S., Simpson, K., & Brison, R. J. (2005). Head injuries in youth soccer players presenting to the emergency department. *British Journal of Sports Medicine, 39*(4), 226.

Prince, C., & Bruhns, M. E. (2017). Evaluation and treatment of mild traumatic brain injury: The role of neuropsychology. *Brain Sciences, 7*(8), 105.

Public Health Agency of Canada. (1998). *For the safety of Canadian children and youth*. Retrieved from http://www.phac-aspc.gc.ca/publicat/fsccy-psjc/ch7/index.htm.

Rivara, F. P., & Aitken, M. (1998). Prevention of injuries to children and adolescents. *Advances in Pediatrics, 45*, 37–72.

Rivera, F. P., & Metrik, B. S. (1998). *Training programs for bicycle safety*. Seattle, WA: Harborview Injury Prevention Research Center.

Ross, W. (2008, July 28). Pedal vs. Metal. *Newsweek*.

Safe Kids Canada. (2007). *Ride safe: Overview of injuries*. Retrieved from May 20, 2008, from http://www.sickkids.ca/SKCForParents/section.asp?s=Safety+Information+by+Topic&sID=10774&ss=Wheeled+Activities&ssID=11341&sss=Ride+Safe%3A+Overview+of+Injuries&sssID=12980.

Safe Kids Connecticut. (2005). *Bicycle injury fact sheet*. Hartford, CT: Author.

Silver, J. R. (2002). Spinal injuries resulting from horse riding accidents. *Spinal Cord, 40*, 264–271.

Thompson, D., & Hudson, S. (2002). *National action plan for the prevention of playground injuries*. Cedar Falls, IA: National Program for Playground Safety.

Thompson, N. J., Sleet, D., & Sacks, J. J. (2002). Increasing the use of bicycle helmets: Lessons from behavioral science. *Patient Education and Counseling, 46*(3), 191–197.

Towner, E., & Dowswell, T. (2002). Community-based childhood injury prevention interventions: What works? *Health Promotion International, 17*(3), 273–284.

United States Consumer Product Safety Commission. (1999). *CPSC staff recommends use of helmets for skiers, snowboarders to prevent head injuries*. Retrieved from http://cpsc.gov/cpscpub/prerel/prhtml99/99046.html.

United States Consumer Product Safety Commission. (2012). *National electronic injury surveillance system* (NEISS). Retrieved from https://www.cpsc.gov/s3fspublic/blk_media_2012NeissDataHighlights.pdf.

United States Department of Transportation. (2002). *Good practices guide for bicycle safety education*. Washington, DC: Author.

World Health Organization, & International Spinal Cord Society. (2013). *International perspectives on spinal cord injury*. Geneva: World Health Organization.

Heads Up: Concussion in High School Sports

Helen Looker

The purpose of the Heads Up: Concussion in High School Sports (https://www.cdc.gov/HeadsUp/) program is to assist, educate, and train coaches, parents, teachers, health care providers, and athletes in preventing or minimizing the risk of concussions and other head injuries for youth athletes participating in school sports.

3.1 Background

The Centers for Disease Control and Prevention (CDC) was given a specific mandate "under the Children Health Act of 2000 to implement a national Traumatic Brain Injury (TBI) education and awareness campaign" (Mitchko et al., 2007, p. 99). The CDC first targeted the medical community, developing a toolkit with the intent of helping health care providers move toward better clinical management of Mild Traumatic Brain Injury (MTBI), thereby improving patient outcomes. Between 2003 and 2007, more than 200,000 toolkits were distributed to health care providers nationwide. Building on the success of this initial step and positive feedback from health care providers, CDC went on to produce another toolkit targeting athletic coaches in high schools; the toolkit was named Heads Up: Concussion in High School Sports (Centers for Disease Control and Prevention

[CDC], 2007a). Heads Up represents the first time a federal agency has developed a toolkit for high school coaches (K. Sarmiento, personal communication, June 6, 2008). Development of the toolkit involved the application of mixed methods research and review of the literature, and materials were also produced in Spanish.

Beginning with an environmental scan in March 2003 of pre-existing published materials covering the topic of concussion, CDC found that coaches were in need of materials tailored to the occurrence of concussions in sport in order to promote prevention, recognition, and effective management of such injuries. An expert panel was convened in April 2003. Due to the extensive resources necessitated by the program, a pilot study was conducted to refine development before a national launch. High school coaches were surveyed by telephone, and focus groups were used. With input from these sources, focus groups consisting of high school coaches in Virginia, Texas, and California and others consisting of students from Maryland and Virginia high schools were used to assess the initial design and content of multimedia toolkit materials. The toolkit was a vehicle to convey knowledge to coaches and heighten awareness of concussion, to provide coaches with the means and motivation to educate others, and to help coaches build up their own skill and capacity to prevent and manage concussions sustained by the athletes they worked with (Mitchko et al., 2007).

H. Looker (✉)
University of Toronto, Toronto, ON, Canada

© Springer Nature Switzerland AG 2020
R. Volpe (ed.), *Casebook of Traumatic Injury Prevention*,
https://doi.org/10.1007/978-3-030-27419-1_3

3.2 Resources

Although CDC is well known and respected in medical, academic, and research communities worldwide, the organization is not so familiar to the layperson. Collaboration with organizations, particularly the National Federation of State High School Associations (NFSHS) was, therefore, pivotal to CDC's capacity to not only reach, but also gain acceptance and cooperation from athletic coaches to utilize materials (K. Sarmiento, personal communication, June 6, 2008). Altogether, 14 organizations from leading sports and medical organizations at state and national levels contributed to promotion and dissemination of the Heads Up toolkit. These partners were acknowledged within material text and also the packaging box for the materials (Mitchko et al., 2007). CDC used a thorough review of the literature to help prepare materials for the educational program strategically referencing key articles on concussions in all of the materials developed that would be of relevance to coaches in high schools. The toolkit met intended goals by providing factual information on risk factors for concussion, incidence rates, the current definition of concussion, who is most at risk for concussion, and how to recognize a concussion. The toolkit also was designed to deliver clear, essential advice on concussion management, prevention strategies known to be effective, and supportive, practical ideas for coaches' role communicating with athletes, family members, and officials within the school system. The resources provided included:

- Letter of introduction from CDC.
- Concussion guide in brochure format for coaches.
- Coach's wallet quick reference card on concussion.
- Coach's clipboard sticker bearing concussion facts and place to write emergency contacts.
- Fact sheets for parents and athletes: English and Spanish versions.
- Posters for training rooms.
- Educational DVD/video of concussion feature produced by News Hour, PBS.
- CD-ROM of resources to download and journal articles.

3.3 Implementation

3.3.1 The Pilot Study

Information from four sources, namely, literature reviews, the expert panel, focus groups, and a telephone-based survey of 497 high school coaches drawn from five states helped to formulate the initial toolkit for the Heads Up program. Toolkits were mailed, followed by a postcard requesting participation in a telephone survey. The pilot study probed personal perceptions and appraisal of materials by coaches and to what extent they used the materials in the toolkit and if there was future intent to use the materials (Centers for Disease Control and Prevention [CDC], 2007b).

3.3.2 Pilot Study Outcome

The high school coaches who received the toolkits approved of them and 94% were satisfied with the details provided with few revisions that had to be made (Mitchko et al., 2007). One-third of the coaches reported having no access to materials relevant to the prevention and management of concussions and greater than two-thirds of coaches were aware of past concussion injuries in athletes at their schools (Mitchko et al., 2007).

3.3.3 First Focus Groups

Every effort was made to reduce bias by ensuring balanced representation in coaches participating in the two telephone focus groups. The groups consisted of male and female coaches from varied socioeconomic backgrounds, coming from private and public schools in urban and suburban areas, coaching girls' and boys' sports. Twenty-nine coaches participated in the focus groups to assess the toolkit concept put forward by the expert panel. Coaches had concerns about the ambiguous nature of concussions and difficulty perceiving symptoms. Coaches were receptive to educational material that could be shared with athletes and administrators and reported counseling athletes on headgear, but no formal channels were in place to maintain awareness of concussion injury. Coaches agreed that critical medical decisions ought to be made by trainers or health professionals. While admitting the need for information, coaches wanted the toolkit to provide essential information with clarity (Mitchko et al., 2007).

3.4 Outcome

3.4.1 The National Launch

In planning the national launch of the Heads Up toolkit in September 2005, CDC asked the US Surgeon General, Vice Admiral Richard H. Carmona, M.D., M.P.H., F.A.C.S. to be a leading spokesperson during promotional campaigns. The Surgeon General and Dr. Ileana Arias, the Director of CDC's National Center for Injury Prevention and Control discussed the toolkit in radio interviews, broadcasted nationally to an audience in excess of three million. Opportunities were sought in every possible media to raise awareness about concussion. For efficiency and expediency, "hundreds of media outlets" were contacted by e-mail (Mitchko et al., 2007 p. 102). The uppermost 25 news markets in the United States in regional and national newspapers and magazines with niche and general readerships were the focus of over 100 calls made to get publicity for the Heads Up toolkit. The CDC put out a press release on their website and made the toolkit available as a download (Mitchko et al., 2007).

CDC learned from members of the expert panel and collaborative partner organizations that knowledge transfer must follow a hierarchical path from athletic directors to the target audience of coaches. Initial mailings for the Heads Up toolkit were sent to the principals and athletic directors of high schools in order to reach coaches. Early partnering of diverse organizations facilitated an iterative process for review and improvement of materials and greater commitment to the CDC project, especially in promotion and dissemination of the toolkit. In turn, organizations were regularly updated on the project and were involved in review of the multimedia materials. Within three months of launching Heads Up: Concussion in High School Sports across the United States, over 20,000 toolkits were ordered and sent out, and the website for the toolkit had more than 19,000 hits (CDC, 2007a).

3.4.2 Evaluation Study

CDC contracted Constella Health Sciences in 2005 to perform an evaluation of the toolkit 1 year after the national launch in September 2005. CDC was particularly concerned with the toolkit's impact, usefulness, and sustainability as a TBI resource. Answers to questions on the following topics were the deliverables to CDC:

- Environment—What barriers and resources affect how coaches respond to concussions?
- Materials—How have coaches used the toolkit materials?
- Knowledge—What did coaches learn from the toolkit?
- Attitudes—How has the toolkit changed coaches' attitudes toward the severity of concussions?
- Behavior—How did coaches use the toolkit to educate others?
- Skills—How did the toolkit change the ways in which coaches prevented or managed concussions? (CDC, 2007a).

CDC surveyed 1009 coaches from the 13,199 coaches that were eligible resulting in a 45% response rate, netting 333 qualified respondents (CDC, 2007a). A survey instrument gathered data quantitatively, and qualitative data was gathered through a sampling of the survey respondents to answer the research questions forming the basis of the evaluation study. CDC contacted coaches of high impact and low impact sports through publicly listed telephone numbers and e-mail addresses for participation in focus groups by telephone conferencing arrangements in April–May 2007 (CDC, 2007a).

3.4.3   Evaluation Outcome

Evaluation of the toolkit demonstrated positive changes in high school coaches' knowledge, attitudes, behavior, and skills related to concussion prevention and management.

- Fifty percentage of coaches reported viewing concussions more seriously after using the toolkit.
- Sixty-eight percentage of coaches reported using the toolkit to educate others about concussions, including athletes, athlete's parents and other coaches.
- Thirty-four percentage of coaches reported that the toolkit increased their knowledge about how to prevent and manage concussions.
- Thirty-eight percentage of coaches reported making changes in how they dealt with concussions, including placing more emphasis on training techniques and safety equipment that minimize the risk of concussion.

The focus groups of coaches averaged four people, 78% male representing 13 sports in 12 states. Sports coached included: baseball, softball, track & field, fencing, football; ice hockey, gymnastics, lacrosse, rugby, for boys; basketball, soccer, tennis, for girls & boys; volleyball for girls (CDC, 2007a). The most popular sports were boys' football at 41%, followed by basketball for boys at 13% and soccer for girls at 11%. States of origin for participant coaches were: Colorado, Georgia, Illinois, Kansas, Massachusetts, Minnesota, Missouri, New Jersey, New York, Pennsylvania, Virginia, and Wisconsin (CDC, 2007a, p. 5). Just over half of the coaches had at least 10 years of experience (53%), taught mostly within the public-school system (78%), at schools with less than 1000 enrolled students that were nonurban (43% suburban schools and 38% rural schools). From subjective survey responses, coaches indicated that 62% of their athletes had parents

with middle incomes. Athletes and coaches from high schools were randomly selected for focus groups to test the preliminary toolkit. The cross section of sports represented included wrestling, baseball, volleyball, soccer, basketball, and football (CDC, 2007a).

Coaches responding to the survey indicated an awareness of a club or school policy for sports-related concussion (60%), but discussing this topic within focus groups revealed that while clubs and schools probably have injury policies in place covering concussion management, there were few policies addressing sports-related concussion specifically (CDC, 2007a). Coaches reported limitations in concussion prevention due to their exclusion in policymaking plans or initiatives. Notwithstanding this power differential, the majority of coaches were fully cognizant of their responsibility for due diligence concerning the impact of concussion education, prevention, and management for athletes they worked with especially as coaches do not have the added support of a medical professional at the sideline of game play. The attitude of athletes and their parents can make concussion management for coaches difficult, so having a fact sheet handout for parents eliminates the need for persuasion to treat concussions seriously (CDC, 2007a).

The materials from the toolkit considered most useful by coaches were primarily the booklet, closely followed by the wallet card that has space for important contact numbers, a summarized action plan reminder, and lists of subjective and objective signs and symptoms of concussion. The video and fact sheets for athletes were also popular with coaches, 59% and 57% respectively. Toolkit materials were commended for being succinct and easily comprehended. Although many coaches were very experienced, over one-third found something new to them in the concussion toolkit. Some coaches were "high implementers," meaning that they applied use of at least four items from the toolkit and due to their initiative and early adoption, "were almost twice as likely to have learned something new than low implementers" who applied use of three or less items from the toolkit (CDC, 2007a,

p. 12). For those coaches who were already well informed about concussions, there was praise for the quality of information and its presentation. Certain views previously held by half of the coaches who responded to the survey not only changed, but also influenced behavior so that they educated others and stressed the importance of safety equipment and training techniques to play safely. Figure 3.1 shows the reach of the toolkit materials, which encouraged coaches to share educational information. Behavior modification was greater in high implementers of the toolkit, compared to low implementers. The following are quotes from individuals after the implementation of the Heads Up program:

- I spend more time on the correct way to head the ball in soccer."
- "I teach Heads Up Hockey! when you check an opponent or if you are checked, you need to hit the boards with anything but your head!"
- "We are more cautious when hitting and playing tags on players."
- "I spend more time talking about proper tackling and take down techniques and talk about proper fitted equipment, helmet and head gear" (CDC, 2007a).

In documenting the process of the project to develop materials for a comprehensive health-education campaign with national reach, CDC hopes that health educators will learn from their approach and use it as a model for raising awareness on health issues among desired

audiences (Mitchko et al., 2007). Sustainability of the toolkit seems assured as coaches found the toolkit relevant and practical, favoring ongoing use of the booklet, fact sheets for parents and athletes, and the wallet card. Given the opportunity to discuss concussion implications for youth in high schools, ideas arose from participants in focus groups for new audiences that would benefit from enhanced knowledge about concussions: "Youth league coaches, summer recreation coaches, parochial school coaches, health teachers, school nurses, physical education teachers, athletic trainers, athletic directors, and elementary school monitors" (CDC, 2007a, p. 17). CDC has acted on these suggestions as high school nurses and staff have expressed interest in the toolkit, and a new initiative is underway directed toward teachers and parents to impart general information about concussions (K. Sarmiento, personal communication, June 6, 2008).

3.4.4   Analysis

In terms of access to the resource of expertise, CDC is ideally positioned to garner support for projects from experts in many fields of endeavor throughout the United States. Staff at CDC are also highly trained and knowledgeable specialists who may have considerable experience and are able to draw on the expertise of other CDC staff and departments. As an entity, the CDC also has well-defined and practiced methodologies to

Fig. 3.1 Education about concussions from the toolkit shared by coaches with others (CDC, 2007a)

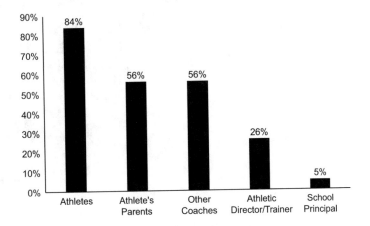

implement projects on a national scale. CDC's process of designing and delivering comprehensive health education on TBI in sports throughout high schools in the United States can be likened to a "complex adaptive nested system" (see Fig. 3.2; Cooper & Greyer, 2008). The beginning consisted of an environmental scan, review of the literature, and forming of an expert panel. Phase I was the early formulation of the Heads Up toolkit, Phase 2 was pretesting of proposed materials, Phase 3 was the pilot testing of the toolkit, and Phase 4 was the full-scale national launch and then evaluation of the materials. CDC's approach reflects a framework of complexity as there was constant adaptation to new information arising from the process of developing, testing, and assessing the Heads Up toolkit (K. Sarmiento, personal communication, June 6, 2008). Using a mix of quantitative and qualitative methods to triangulate the emergent findings from pretesting, surveys, and focus group work is also indicative of a complex systematic way to deliver health education as it represents adaptability and receptiveness for uncertainty (Cooper & Greyer, 2008).

Selecting people in health-related professions as spokespersons gave the Heads Up program a high-profile status readily attracting media attention. Focus group discussions of environmental barriers to appropriate concussion management also raised the issue of inadequate health insurance, which may be a significant problem for families in the United States. Health coverage may also be an issue in Alberta, Canada, too, where physician fees are covered but fees for care provided by other health professionals, are not covered (CDC, 2007a; Rose, Emery, & Meeuwisse, 2008). Job security for working parents may also be a concern where young people need to convalesce at home but need to be under supervised care by an adult. Environmental barriers such as health care coverage, falling into social and political domains, are not easily changed to facilitate injury prevention. Figure 3.3 shows that the annual rate of nonfatal TBIs needing treatment at emergency departments for males and females is highest in the school years of students' lives when students spend most of their waking hours at school and in social activities like sports. Injury prevention and management of concussion, therefore, is very much a social responsibility requiring sustained commitment by multiple stakeholders influencing the healthy development and quality of life for

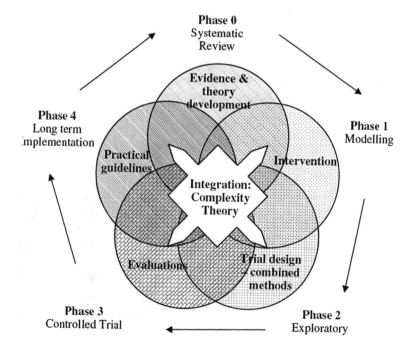

Fig. 3.2 Logic model of a 'complex adaptive nested system' (Cooper & Greyer, 2008)

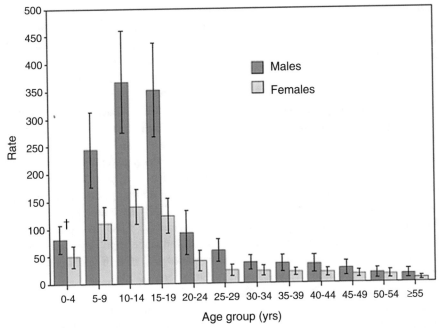

* Per 100,000 population.
† 95% confidence interval.

Fig. 3.3 Estimated annual rate (per 100,00) of nonfatal, sports and recreation-related traumatic brain injuries treated in emergency departments, by age group and sex. National Electronic Injury Surveillance System, All Injury Program, United States, 2001–2005 (CDC, 2007b)

youth in sports (Emery, Hagel, & Morrongiello, 2006). Beyond fulfillment of their obligation to devise an effective national campaign to raise awareness of concussion, however, the CDC team that developed the Heads Up toolkit continue to monitor feedback, new literature, and seek new outlets for disseminating valuable information on concussion (K. Sarmiento, personal communication, June 6, 2008).

3.5 Conclusion

The CDC Heads Up: Concussion in High School Sports program has succeeded in educating high school coaches nationwide with information about concussion and providing them with tools to share that knowledge. The use of Internet technology now provides easy access to an online concussion training course video for high school and youth sport coaches, as well as health care clinicians. Additionally, mobile apps, podcasts,

and social media platforms have also been implemented in recent years for coaches, youth athletes, and parents creating convenient access to concussion information in order to maximize ongoing outreach and accessibility to the toolkit while minimizing future costs. Sustainability is assured from the proactive dissemination of toolkit materials by coaches, as determined from the evaluation study. Motivated by the positive response to the Heads Up: Concussion in High School Sports the program has been replicated in a similar format for a younger demographic, also at risk for concussive injuries; the program is Heads Up: Concussion in Youth Sports.

With the momentum of these initial Heads Up programs growing, the CDC continued to expand its programs to promote education and prevention of concussions/head injuries, which are tailored to specific stakeholders and include Heads Up to Parents, Heads Up to Schools, and Heads Up to Health care Providers. Currently, the CDC's Heads Up website is packed with resources, materials, information, and training tools/course that have been developed to assist each specific stakeholder, including the youth sports athletes themselves, in having a greater awareness and knowledge about concussions and head injuries, and how to minimize the risks (CDC, 2017). Furthermore, the CDC's Heads Up program has not only grown to be a nationwide success but has further been adopted by youth sports programs North America to prevent concussions and head injuries.

Acceptance of injury in sports as "an inherent part of the game" is an "archaic notion" that the CDC Heads Up: Concussion in High School Sports program has sought to change and has done so through a diligent process of collaboration, responsive communications, and producing a relevant, user-friendly toolkit (Weaver, Marshall, & Miller, 2002). Concussion in high school athletes is important not only because of costs, complications, disability, and the vulnerability of the immature brain, but also because most individuals participating in high

contact sports or sports where collisions occur are under 19 years of age (Buzzini & Guskiewicz, 2006). Colloquial expressions describing concussions, used frequently in the media such as "ding" or "he had his bell rung" are ingrained in journalistic style and not easily eradicated (Buzzini & Guskiewicz,, 2006). Youth participating in sport and social activities outside of organized sports at schools have likely sustained many underreported concussions with unappreciated consequences. In a hierarchy of responsibility for sport-related injury prevention where CDC occupies the highest level of responsibility, CDC has effectively leveraged their influence and expertise to initiate a psychological shift in thinking about concussion (Emery et al., 2006).

Acknowledgements The author would like to express sincere appreciation to the key informant for this case study: Kelly Sarmiento of the National Center for Injury Prevention & Control, Centers for Disease Control in Atlanta, GA, USA—whose consultation made this project possible.

BRIO Model: Heads Up—Concussion in High School Sports

Group Served: The program targets high school sports coaches.

Goal: The program faims to educate and train coaches to recognize and minimize the risk of concussions and other head injuries in youth sports athletes.

Background	Resources	Implementation	Outcome
In 1984, 'second impact syndrome' characterized highlighting the risks of multiple concussions in a short time period MTBI toolkit developed for health care providers following duty to implement national awareness and educational campaign for TBI after passing of the Children's Health Act of 2000 Successful campaign disseminated 200,000 toolkits led to multimedia toolkit for high school athletic coaches	Environmental scan in March 2003 Literature reviews April 2003 Expert Panel convened Focus groups of high school students from two states and high school coaches from three states Telephone survey of coaches Partnership with the National Federation of State High School Associations Evaluation Study	Pilot Study with coaches in five states Comprehensive sports-related materials on concussion developed and pretested Toolkit launched nationally September 2005 US Surgeon General, Vice Admiral Richard H. Carmona, M.D., M.P.H., F.A.C.S. a key spokesperson promoting the toolkit	Target group identified Approach to concussion recognition and management improved Awareness of concussion as a serious injury achieved 20,000 toolkits distributed across the United States within 3 months of launch Internet downloads add to sustainability Materials made accessible via the CDC website Outreach through the media by email, telephone contacting editors and reporters Radio interviews discussing the toolkit.

Life Space Model: Heads Up—Concussions in High School Sports

Sociocultural: civilization/community	Interpersonal: primary and secondary relationships	Physical environments: where we live	Internal states: biochemical/genetic and means of coping
Raising awareness that any concussion is a serious injury and that adolescents are more vulnerable than adults Multiple media strategy to communicate a health-related message nationally to educate targeted audiences about concussion and its management Toolkit available in English and Spanish	Professional networks leveraged to convene an expert panel to determine best approach and development of toolkit Attitudinal change in perception of concussion by athletes, parents, coaches Behavioral change by coaches in prevention education and management approach to concussion	20,000 Toolkits distributed in the national launch Widespread, long-term dissemination of materials through the Internet Awareness of concussion as a risk in low contact and high contact sports	Coaches acquired new skills and knowledge to recognize concussions Empowerment of coaches to educate athletes and their parents about the severity of concussion Coaches influenced to reinforce and emphasize injury prevention education

References

Buzzini, S. R., & Guskiewicz, K. M. (2006). Sport-related concussion in the young athlete. *Current Opinion in Pediatrics, 18*, 376–382.

Centers for Disease Control and Prevention. (2007a). *Heads Up, Concussion in High School Sports. Follow-up evaluation of a concussion toolkit for high school coaches. Final report*. Atlanta, GA: CDC.

Centers for Disease Control and Prevention. (2007b). *Morbidity and mortality weekly report*. Atlanta, GA: CDC. Retrieved July 27, 2007, from http://www.cdc.gov/mmwr/preview/mmwrhtml/mm5629a2.htm

Centers for Disease Control and Prevention. (2017). *Heads up*. Retrieved from https://www.cdc.gov/headsup/index.html.

Cooper, H., & Greyer, R. (2008). Using 'complexity' for improving educational research in health care. *Social Science & Medicine, 67*, 177–182.

Emery, C., Hagel, B., & Morrongiello, B. (2006). Injury prevention in child and adolescent sport: Whose responsibility is it? *Clinical Journal of Sport Medicine, 16*(6), 514–521.

Mitchko, J., Huitric, M., Sarmiento, K., Hayes, G., Pruzan, M., & Sawyer, R. (2007). CDC's approach to educating coaches about sports-related concussion. *American Journal of Health Education, 38*(2), 99–103.

Rose, M. S., Emery, C. A., & Meeuwisse, W. H. (2008). Sociodemographic predictors of sport injury in adolescents. *Medicine and Science in Sports and Exercise, 40*(3), 444–450.

Weaver, N. L., Marshall, S. W., & Miller, M. D. (2002). Preventing sports injuries: Opportunities for intervention in youth athletics. *Patient Education and Counseling, 46*, 199–204.

Play It Cool: Hockey Safety

4

Daria Smeh

The purpose of the Play It Cool program is to minimize the risk of head and spine injuries for youth ice hockey players through educating hockey coaches on injury prevention practices, which they would implement and teach to their players.

4.1 Background

Play It Cool was created in 2001 by the Canadian Spinal Research Organization (CSRO) and Mitron Sports. CSRO created the program to respond to the need for a safe ice hockey tool that could be available to prevent spinal injuries in hockey. However, following preliminary evaluation of the program, Dr. John Lewko, from the Ontario Neurotrauma Foundation (ONF) and Barry Munro of the CSRO, observed a lack of stakeholder (i.e., coaches) buy-in for the program. In response, the ONF advertised a Request for Application of Proposals in 2004 to have a new approach developed for the Play It Cool program (W. Montelpare, personal communication, September 21, 2008).

One of the applications submitted was from a team of researchers from Lakehead University, Brock University, York University, the University of Toronto, Queens University, and the University of Waterloo, which was successfully awarded the application. Dr. William Montelpare, professor at the School of Kinesiology from Lakehead University headed the team; he organized the initial evaluation of the existing program and redeveloped the program as a result of discussions with several key informants (W. Montelpare, personal communication, September 21, 2008). In general, the evaluation of the old program revealed that discussants felt the program had merit, but because it was delivered on a small CD in a pocket-sized notebook, most individuals would not take the time to review the contents of the CD or to read or implement any of the materials (W. Montelpare, personal communication, January 9, 2008).

According to Montelpare's evaluation (personal communication, September 21, 2008), the previous program was a passive approach to coach education and facilitation. Thus, although multimedia was utilized, there was a lack of a tool to facilitate stakeholders (or users of the program). As a result, coaches were not engaged, and the program was not used frequently (W. Montelpare, personal communication, September 21, 2008).

In response, the program was modified into a facilitated online delivery system comprised of multimedia tools that delivers content asynchronously over the web (W. Montelpare, personal communication, September 21, 2008). Delivery included regularly scheduled teleconferences and asynchronous web-based discussion boards.

D. Smeh (✉)
LoyalTeam Environmental, Toronto, ON, Canada

© Springer Nature Switzerland AG 2020
R. Volpe (ed.), *Casebook of Traumatic Injury Prevention*,
https://doi.org/10.1007/978-3-030-27419-1_4

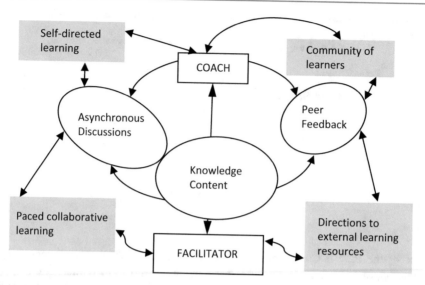

Fig. 4.1 The structure and philosophy of Play It Cool. (Reprinted from *Using Facilitated Online Curriculum Delivery for Coach Preparation in Teaching Safety and* *Injury prevention in Ice Hockey* [PowerPoint] 2008. Presented at the Safe Hockey Summit, Thunder Bay, Canada)

The curriculum was developed to inform participants about behaviors and actions that can cause an injury, giving coaches specific examples of drills, games, and strategies that provide players with alternative choices or considerations during game situations, which specifically intended to reduce and prevent injuries (W. Montelpare, personal communication, September 21, 2008) (Fig. 4.1).

Play It Cool is based on a set of seven ice hockey skills. In order to translate these skills into a training program, the researchers decided to build upon the success of the Public Health Agency of Canada's SKILLS program. The program formally known as the Skills Enhancement for Public Health is delivered using an online course module to public health practitioners across Canada (W. Montelpare, personal communication, September 21, 2008).

The first step to developing the program plan for the Play It Cool project was for researchers to decide how to best deliver the Play it Cool program, both technologically and pedagogically. Technologically, online-facilitated delivery over the Internet was chosen because it was perceived to be accessible to participants and a method that would more easily engage them. Pedagogically, the development team aimed to minimize how

academically based their approach was. As a result, the research group chose to use an upstream approach to program development— that is choosing a prevention approach versus a treatment approach (W. Montelpare, personal communication, January 9, 2009).

The grade or level of the materials covered in the modules, the web-log pages, and the discussion board text were devised from an early stage to be at a level to ensure that even the novice coach could comprehend and apply the terminology, injury prevention messages, and methods to develop skills. They aimed to choose content that was useful, usable, and effectively communicated in its delivery (W. Montelpare, personal communication, January 9, 2009).

Over the years, the program was modified as a result of feedback from the CSRO and ONF, who provided the use of their stakeholder network and resources since the time of Play It Cool's development. Since then, feedback has been also sought from all Hockey Federations in Ontario, who at the administrative level have complete buy-in into the program. Coaches also provided insight into the delivery of the prevention strategy; they assisted in the theory and module development. From their initial involvement, it has been difficult to ascertain complete coach buy-in. Coach buy-in has grown over the years, but it has been met with some resistance. As a result, attendance and participation has tended to be sporadic.

4.1.1 Target Population

The Play It Cool Program was created to deliver a message that the principles of safe hockey could be taught and learned by participants of all ages (e.g., 9–90). However, the actual target population of the Play It Cool program is comprised of coaches that are directly linked to, or working with, children in the developmental ages (8–16). Therefore, the content of the program was designed to target these coaches (W. Montelpare, personal communication, September 21, 2008).

The program is being delivered to coaches that coach minor age players. More specifically, the program is being applied with Adam (ages 9–10), Peewee (ages 11–12), Bantam (ages 13–14) and Midget (ages 15–17) players. For research purposes, the target sample for one study is being extracted from coaches who coach Bantam age boys in Ontario; two cohorts are being drawn, one from Toronto (17 teams) and one from Thunder Bay (17 teams) (W. Montelpare, personal communication, September 21, 2008).

All coaches are welcome to take part in the Play It Cool program, as there are no exclusionary criteria. Coaches, male and female, of all economic status, are welcome to participate (W. Montelpare, personal communication, September 21, 2008). However, although there has been an expression of interest to participate, there are currently no cohorts of exclusively women coaches. This is a major focus of the next steps in coach recruitment (W. Montelpare, personal communication, January 9, 2009).

4.1.2 A Review of the Prevention Strategies

The online-facilitate delivery of the prevention strategies in the Play It Cool program are presented in seven modules, which are held over an 8-week period (3 weeks of delivery, 1-week break, 4 weeks delivery). The online format includes hyperlinked text, videos, animation, sound effects, discussion boards, questionnaires, and blogs. The site is password protected, thereby allowing for monitoring participant attendance and completion rates. Each module or "competency" can be completed in 35–60 min (W. Montelpare, personal communication, September 21, 2008).

Originally the modules or competencies were referred to as "skills." However, evaluation of the original program concluded that teaching coaches how to teach skills is a passive approach that is not adopted easily by participants. Competencies speak to an active approach that engages participants and makes them responsible to learn the information and apply it. The aim from its inception was to create a method of delivery for Play It Cool that is usable and that can be applied in many different ways by coaches and players (W. Montelpare, personal communication, September 21, 2008). The competencies modules include:

1. Ethics and sportsmanship.
2. Skating skills.
3. Principles of play.
4. Awareness of the playing area.
5. Teaching techniques and building an optimum environment.
6. Teaching checking as a skill.
7. Controlling risk as a coach (Safe Hockey Summit, 2008).

In its application, however, it tends to be difficult to assess the level of skills each player has after the coach has applied the information in the modules. However, the role of the coach and the development of the coach are mainstays of the program by creating awareness about the risk factors in ice hockey, and ultimately having players utilize what they have been taught. The coaches must be competent in their knowledge and their ability to impart that knowledge (W. Montelpare, personal communication, September 21, 2008).

Overall coach education should include modules covering the risks associated with youth and hockey participation (Cowie-Bonne, 2000). However, research has shown that education programs lack a focus on these risks. Research by Cowie-Bonne (2000) showed that all coaches who participated in her study had extensive hockey knowledge and experience; however, they lacked knowledge about the developmental stages of childhood and youth. They also lacked knowledge about motivational needs and instructive skills to impart knowledge to these age groups.

Coaches who participate in the Play It Cool program are encouraged to create their own profile by completing a questionnaire that describes their coaching background, their confidence as a coach, and their intention to teach safe hockey behaviors. To encourage dialogue in the program specifically related to essential topics within the modules and about individual coaching experience, coaches are designated into groups ranging from 8 to 12 individuals based on the level they coach and their coach experience level. The research group has specifically arranged for coaches with different experience levels to be in a single group. Where available, there has been a mixing of male and female participants as well as a mixing of coaches that coach both male and female teams (W. Montelpare, personal communication, September 21, 2008).

4.1.3 Goals and Objectives of the Play It Cool program

One of the main goals of the Play It Cool program is to create a safer game of ice hockey by changing the culture of ice hockey through an enhancement of coach education. Another main goal is to make the Play It Cool program a part of the ice hockey long-term athlete development system in Canada, the United States, and throughout the world (W. Montelpare, personal communication, January 9, 2008).

Implicitly, there are several goals that are all under the umbrella of changing the culture of hockey in Canada. These implicit goals include:

- Provide awareness of safer behaviors in hockey to coaches, players, parents.

- Modify the way in which administrative bodies (e.g., leagues, hockey federations, Hockey Canada) perceive injury and safety.
- Better inform the culture of hockey in a way that encourages respect and fair play.
- Reach the stakeholders in hockey right now because it is an opportunistic time to prepare stakeholders in the way they change the culture of hockey (W. Montelpare, personal communication, September 21, 2008).

To achieve these goals, Montelpare is using the stage-gate model. The stage-gate model is used to break down the elements of the project into specific stages (personal communication, September 21, 2008). Each time a stage is achieved (i.e., arriving at the gate) the researchers evaluate (informally) what has been accomplished; that is, they assess the strengths, weaknesses, opportunities, and threats (SWOT) before progressing to the next stage (W. Montelpare, personal communication, January 9, 2008).

The Play it Cool program is structured in its content to improve the ability of coaches who can demonstrate a particular level of knowledge and skills related to the delivery of safe hockey behaviors for minor hockey players.

One suggested goal for Play It Cool is to complete evaluations on a continuous basis to ensure up to date evaluation results. Evaluations should be conducted on short- and long-term goals as they will speak to the achievement of short- and long-term outcomes. A comparison can then be made to expected outcomes, and timely modifications can continue to be made.

4.2 Resources

4.2.1 Stakeholders and Collaborators

The main stakeholders for the Play It Cool Program are coaches, parents, and players. The program primarily communicates with coaches and uses coaches as a vehicle to communicate with players.

There is increasing expectation that coaches are aware of an athlete's complete psychological and social development, which broadens outside of the coaching environment (Borrie & Knowles, 1998). Amateur coaches are assuming a progressively more central role in youth development in general; therefore, training or certification programs developed for coach education definitely require a positive improvement for coaches (Gilbert & Trudel, 1999). One of the most relevant challenges to offering athletic programs is to ensure the presence of well-prepared coaches, defined as coaches who know the sport, are great teachers, comprehend and use regulations to manage risk, cater their approaches to the players they coach, are superior communicators, and can understand parents and their demands. As untrained educators, and with reduced resources, there is a critical need for innovative coach-education programs (Stewart, 2006).

Success in shorter programs, such as New Zealand's RugbySmart and Australia's SafeClub (See Smeh & Singla, 2008 for complete overview), has shown that targeting coaches is an efficient way to reach all players; it is also strategic, as coaches possess "connections to the players as well as having knowledge and passion for the game" (S. Gianotti, personal communication, July 17, 2007). This is based on research performed in the 1990s where coaches were identified by rugby players as fulfilling a key role in demonstrating and providing injury-prevention-related messages to players (Simpson et al., 1994). Both of these programs offer 1-day workshops that include multimedia and the use of a facilitator. Following the implementation of RugbySmart and the mandatory attendance of coaches and referees, serious injuries to the neck, spine and back were reduced by 13%.

Stakeholders also include the decision-makers from minor league hockey; that is, agencies and governing bodies that create regulations for the sport, including Hockey Canada and the Ontario Hockey Federation. The aim of the engaging stakeholders is to use their input to direct the research derived from Play It Cool programming and adequately inform decision-making. Members of the research group have at least 10 years of past research collaboration with Hockey Canada, the implementers of the Play It Cool Program, and are able to have a grassroots understanding—from the stakeholder's perspective—of what happens when a child sustains an injury. This acts as a foundation from where the research and development of the Play It Cool Program can mature. Research like this is not being used to create rules and regulations necessarily, but it is being used to strengthen evidence-informed decision-making in ice hockey. The first Hockey Summit was held in August 2008, where all potential stakeholders were invited to participate and collaborate on raising awareness and engaging members of the hockey community (coaches, players, referees, families of players, spectators, etc.) (W. Montelpare, personal communication, October 24, 2008).

Hockey researchers and ice hockey teams in the United States are also stakeholders. In 2005, a relationship was established with the University of North Carolina. The Head Impact Telemetry System (HITS) was developed and researched by academics at the UNC in collaboration with Lakehead University and the University of Toronto. UNC recruited 30 coaches from Massachusetts hockey leagues to complete the Play It Cool Program modules. W. Montelpare (personal communication, November 11, 2008) notes that attendance has been problematic in implementing the program in the United States. Although coaches sign up for the program and tend to complete the first module, their rates of attendance decrease significantly thereafter (no attendance rates were provided, but they were notable by observation).

In Summer 2008, the Mayo Clinic researchers and coach participants from Rochester, Minnesota approached Dr. Montelpare about implementing the Play It Cool program. They were scheduled to launch the program in 2009 (W. Montelpare, personal communication, November 11, 2008). The Play It Cool research team and their counterparts at the Mayo Clinic and UNC should aim to continue to address the issue of attendance dropouts; this is particularly important because Montelpare has noted strong commitment and interest from the cohort in Massachusetts.

Hockey experts verify the information that is presented on the website. The Play It Cool program is hosted by the Wellnet Group, which provides an interface for the website, but provides no input on the content of the program. The CSRO also supports the program by providing incentives for coaches to participate. They acquired signed jerseys, which are then distributed to coaches. The coaches would then fund-raise for their team by auctioning them off, or they would award them to coaches who participated in Play It Cool (W. Montelpare, personal communication, November 14, 2008).

At initial development, the response from stakeholders through discussion and use of the Play It Cool Program website was overwhelmingly positive. Overall, the target population encountered connectivity problems at the time of development. Logging in was an issue, as was the need for a high bandwidth connection—the program was easily amended to meet this need. An ongoing issue is the attendance to the Play It Cool program (W. Montelpare, personal communication, November 14, 2008).

There is also a lack of incentives to participate, particularly considering coaches volunteer their time to coach (W. Montelpare, personal communication, October 24, 2008). W. Montelpare (personal communication, October 24, 2008) found that if participants complete the second week, they are likely to complete the entire program. Those who complete the program comment on its quality. There is particular satisfaction expressed about the online tools, the blog, discussion board, coach-to-coach interaction, and the method to provide and receive feedback from the facilitator.

According to W. Montelpare (personal communication, October 24, 2008), there are three main aspects that would make stakeholder participation more salient and consistent. First, it is important that decision-makers for hockey leagues in Canada make it mandatory for stakeholders to attend the classes. If sport governing bodies find value in the program and stakeholders are required to participate, then leagues will have coaches who are prepared to coach and reduce the risk of injury.

W. Montelpare (personal communication, October 29, 2009) also believes that from a sound risk management perspective, coaches cannot coach without completing the program. It is Hockey Canada who would need to mandate the program as their standard and regulation governing coaching bodies and leagues. It can be argued that initially, if the program is mandated as a coach certification requirement, there may be a reduced number of coaches, or drop-off of a number of coaches, who may not want to take the course. But W. Montelpare (personal communication, November 21, 2008) argues that because incentives will be offered and will expand to include a younger generation of coaches who are well-trained, coach populations will increase.

Montelpare and the Play It Cool research team are taking a leading role in developing, implementing, and evaluating the program. Now, Montelpare (personal communication, October 24, 2008) argues decision-makers need to take a leading role and the provincial government needs to support these decision-makers to ensure support for the program. Essentially, however, a plan needs to be devised to liaise and negotiate making Play It Cool a mandatory program. It is imperative that a guided approach to facilitating active support from decision-makers is put in place as it will increase their support for the program. A plan will also enable the Play It Cool developers to provide a salient, thorough, and adequate justification for mandating Play It Cool. It will also make it easier for decision-makers in hockey to approve the program.

Initial financial, informational, and human resources for the Play It Cool Program were provided by CSRO and the Mitron Hockey Systems. Following the application for proposals won by Montelpare and his team, the CSRO and the ONF allocated funding for designing and implementing the program. A breakdown of funding, which is solely derived from grant applications, is provided in Table 4.1 (W. Montelpare, personal communication, October 29, 2008).

The funding has been used to buy helmets for the HITS. It has also been used to develop a computer program that enables them to understand the true exposure of injuries. A program was also

Table 4.1   Funding for Play It Cool

Year	Amount ($)	Purpose
2001–2003	Funded by CSRO & Mitron Systems in its previous iteration	
2004	200,000	Redesign and first evaluation
2005	–	
2006	237,000	Play It Cool Program; HITS design
2007–2008	100,000	Play It Cool Program, HITS implementation

Note: W. Montelpare, personal communication, October 29, 2008

designed that could be run on computer tablets. This program enables researchers to sit up in the stands and monitor game playing time, observe contacts between players and the surfaces and record injuries (W. Montelpare, personal communication, October 29, 2008).

Montelpare employed 20 undergraduate students at Lakehead University to conduct research and evaluation on the components of Play It Cool. He also hired ten graduate students from his university, and several of his colleagues' graduate students completed the projects as well. The Play It Cool Program is being implemented by five staff members from Lakehead University, in addition to the team that works out of all of the universities. The HITS system, because of the collaboration with the United States, is being implemented by 11 people in both countries. Most of the work is completed at Lakehead University, and when required, Montelpare travels for presentations on the Play It Cool Program or to discuss possible implementation (W. Montelpare, personal communication, October 29, 2008).

Funding allocated would be used for enhancing real knowledge around injury prevention and management. Overall, W. Montelpare (personal communication, October 29, 2008) posits that more funding is required to hire more staff because hockey injury is a complex problem. To house this staff, he also argues that more space is required, which is why he is proposing a Center of Excellence. The space and human resources would enhance knowledge production capabilities.

According to W. Montelpare (personal communication, October 29, 2008), proper infrastructure is required to conduct thorough research and coordinate research efforts more effectively. Research and implementation of the Play It Cool

Program requires longer-term commitments by employees and researchers. He suggests that a Center of Excellence be constructed to optimize the Play It Cool program and enhance research efforts about the program. Although infrastructure is needed to enhance the research knowledge and base of Play It Cool, initially, research should be completed to assess where exactly there is a need for further research. The research projects being undertaken will properly define where resources should be and are to be best allocated. These research projects will be discussed in the Outcomes section of this chapter.

Stakeholders (such as hockey federations, hockey coaches, and the medical community) can be vital in offering feedback and support to enhance research into the target populations. The developers of the Play It Cool program have already established a vital and strong relationship with coaches. Since they consistently and continuously provide their time and feedback about the program through the online mechanisms (e.g., email, Play It Cool Program website), a stronger focus on where research and capacity building will take place is becoming apparent. Pertinent information that is being gathered from these mechanisms, particularly as a result of the commitment by Montelpare and his team, will enable Play It Cool as a program and the evaluations being undertaken to provide insight into the impact of Play It Cool (W. Montelpare, personal communication, October 29, 2008).

W. Montelpare (personal communication, October 29, 2008) hopes the program matures into a graduated certification program. Graduated certification would break the Play It Cool Program down and expand it to five levels (Table 4.2).

Table 4.2 Proposed Graduated Certification Program for Play It Cool

Level	Duration (weeks)	Description
I	5	Introduction to safe hockey–proper technique, introduction to risk management of player injury
II	4	Running a practice, injury management, managing games
III	6	On ice demonstrations
IV	4	Advanced level coach development
V	TBD	Training for provincial team coaches

Note: W. Montelpare, personal communication, October 29, 2008

For example, to coach the Rep level, coaches would be required to complete up to Level III, while house league coaches would need to complete up to Level II. Ultimately, the parents of players would only allow their children to be coached by certified coaches.

An assessment of the current structure of the coach education system has informed the need to create a graduated certification. However, the completion of additional evaluations being undertaken is required to determine the final appropriate structure of the course. The structure should also continue to be informed by stakeholder feedback.

4.3 Implementation

Play It Cool can be cited for a number of successes. The design of the website has been particularly successful and well received by stakeholders—Montelpare has collected substantial structured feedback from focus groups to attest to the support for the programs content and detail. In fact, as a result of seeking this feedback continuously, the site has been modified four times and Montelpare insists that being flexible to modifying it and keeping the content and style up to date is essential. Stakeholders have expressed extreme satisfaction in addition of pictures, videos, and the discussion board (W. Montelpare, personal communication, October 31, 2008).

The research teams have tried to make the curriculum a comprehensive, consolidated, and well-established conglomeration of information. The information is devised to be thought provoking, and both generic and specific to hockey so

that all audience can relate to the material. Although it is based and informed by scientific, academic research, it is made to be nonthreatening or non-overwhelming for users and uses technology that is readily accessible to participants. That is, the environment is designed to be encouraging and nurturing. According to Montelpare, (personal communication, October 31, 2008), the Play It Cool program provides asynchronous delivery, which ultimately creates both a community of practice, as well as a community of practitioners.

Coach recruitment is one practice that has been suggested to be effective but has not achieved optimal participation rates. Recruitment has been particularly effective in Massachusetts. Further, Montelpare and his team have approached coaches one on one, league administrators, coach conveners (i.e., oversees about a dozen coaches in a division), and hockey organizations (e.g., the Greater Toronto Hockey League, which includes a number of neighborhood-based leagues, e.g., Etobicoke League). With the coaches, they approach them either during or after a game and pitch the program, further exchanging emails and phone numbers with the coaches (W. Montelpare, personal communication, October 31, 2008).

Although they expressed enthusiasm and tremendous support for the program verbally, there has been a lack of follow-up to participate by coaches. Montelpare and his team ensure that frequent contact is made to try to ensure they are committed to attending; however, response has been weak. W. Montelpare (personal communication, October 31, 2008) feels they have exhausted their efforts in trying to recruit coaches, but they are still willing to try.

Ultimately, he posits that convincing stakeholders that participation is important has to come from the governing bodies. If the program is mandated by the governing bodies, it will become "second nature" and valued as an opportunity for career development by coaches. According to W. Montelpare (personal communication, October 31, 2008), the Play It Cool Program is an emerging practice that, once its importance is understood, people will comprehend the value it adds to sport coaching. Although it is clear that many efforts have been taken to encourage governing bodies to recognize the program formally, a plan to enable better buy-in from organizations who would adopt Play It Cool is required. Further brainstorming is required to generate ideas for, and to ensure buy-in both amongst the Play It Cool team and with the governing bodies.

W. Montelpare (personal communication, October 31, 2008) notes that their ability to liaise in the research community has been quite effective. They have established strong relationships with partners in the United States, including the University of North Carolina and the Mayo Clinic. The strong interest by these international organizations in hosting the program, as well as running it independently, with the guidance of Canadian researchers, is noted as a successful collaboration with many potential benefits (e.g., expanding reach, enhancing research practice and evaluation). It is vital that such linkages were established as it enhances the research and knowledge base regarding the various aspects that are effective about the program. Montelpare (personal communication, October 31, 2008) recognizes the importance of such collaboration and makes specific efforts to nurture such relationships (e.g., visiting for presentation, facilitating the launch/implementation of different program components).

The Play It Cool program has also successfully been able to heighten the awareness about the risks of injuries in ice hockey. By enhancing coach education and teaching individuals how to prevent and manage injuries, better injury monitoring is possible. The focus groups demonstrated the increase in awareness.

According to W. Montelpare (personal communication, October 31, 2008), injury outcome is an incorrect marker to be using because it is a rare event relative to exposure to risk of injury. As such, research is being conducted at Lakehead University by examining game films recorded during actual games. The aim of this research is to effectively observe the behaviors of children and understand what practices will most effectively curb those behaviors. Each level must be approached individually because depending on the type of league, the level of contact made, and the nature of play, different injuries will be present. A better understanding of injury in ice hockey is being developed. However, the results from this research are still yet to be completed. Its release is slated for Spring/Summer 2009.

Tator, Provvidenza, Lapczak, Carson, and Raymond (2004) state that "accurate, ongoing and consistent data collection is an important aspect of injury prevention" (p. 466). Ultimately, in order for risk management approaches to function optimally in a sport, coaches, players, and administrators should be involved in collecting injury data, and work to identify the associated risks of participation (Finch & Hennessy, 2000).

Another potential effective practice is to staff someone for injury surveillance. The system must ensure people are accountable, and therefore, reporting to an objective party will likely guarantee that they report to someone. Play It Cool is working toward accountability in hockey leagues through injury reporting, but self-reporting remains challenging for all sports. To compensate, Play It Cool is examining risk exposure through documentation of injuries through game film. As mentioned earlier, the role of the facilitator has shown to be imperative and is listed as an effective practice that will develop over the continuous implementation of the curriculum. It is important to encourage injury reporting as well.

4.3.1 Methods for Evaluation

A coach's successful participation and completion of the program is evaluated if each module of the course has been completed in full. There is online attendance taking and the assignments are required to be submitted at the end of each session. Coaches are reminded to attend the sessions via email so as to ensure follow through (W. Montelpare, personal communication, November 21, 2008).

As mentioned earlier, an analysis of game video is also being undertaken to understand the type of risks and the timing of when risk is most likely to occur. Researchers are also working toward monitoring random behaviors through the recordings. Monitoring the type and number of penalties also allows them to assess the cause of and risk of injury. Since coaches are required to complete coach profiles and conduct self-efficacy testing when they participate in the Play It Cool Program, the researchers will be able to assess a positive or negative change in their "stages of change" score (W. Montelpare, personal communication, November 21, 2008).

Focus groups with coaches are paramount in making appropriate assessments of the style and content of the program. It guarantees that the program appeals to and is valued by the target audience. Feedback has been continuously and consistently sought and the changes in the program have already reflected the results in this evaluation tool. Feedback has also been sought from professionals and collaborators. For example, Andrew Link of the Mayo Clinic said:

- Overall the content was very helpful from a coaching perspective, especially for any coach who is new to coaching or new to a level of coaching.
- I helped out with the High School team here, and much of the content didn't apply so much to that audience because they were not new to coaching. But there are many great takeaway lessons and reminders.
- The people in our group that did finish the program all agreed that it had good content and that they learned a lot. There were some criticisms as far as the structure. The opening sign-up questionnaire needs to be modified because the questions have a lot of double negatives and are awkwardly phrased.

- Another suggestion was to just have one message board for everyone, since everyone looked at everyone's message board anyway.
- Another suggestion was not to have the 3 or so minute introduction to every module, but rather to just get to the goal or point of the module.
- Further, more relevant visuals that correlate to the lessons in the modules would improve the program. Oftentimes the images were repeated or else just seemed like pictures to fill the space.

Similarly, Dr. Walter Epp, an Associate Professor in the department of Education at Lakehead University said,

- The website really looks fantastic—very professional—and seems to incorporate ease of access with relevant and well-organized content. The coach's handbook is a great resource and the blogs and message boards provide plenty of opportunity for interaction.
- The feedback commentary is certainly very instructive. Listening to people who have gone through it is very interesting. It seemed that what the coaches wanted was coaching strategies—they seemed more interested in drills and strategies than safety—safety was kind of a value-added feature to well-organized coaching.
- I don't think it is bad as it gives participants flexibility—It probably couldn't work synchronously given the schedules—the synchronous method can even tend to be contrived–but they do work well sometimes. If there is, there should be a 3 asynchronous–1 synchronous asynchronous ration for balance.
- There should also be a consideration about time—these coaches are too busy for this time-consuming process-burn out.
- I haven't seen any of the data surrounding the organization and delivery or effectiveness of the course—this would be useful to understanding the effectiveness of the program.

Feedback seems to be positive, and the Play It Cool team seems to be aware of the weaknesses highlighted by Link. Therefore, communication between stakeholders is clearly strong and ongoing.

Since the Play It Cool approach is to change the culture of hockey, parental feedback will also be sought in the next round of evaluations. In these evaluations, they seek to understand what kind of community is developed as a result of participation, the capacity for idea sharing, the ability and value of learning from others (W. Montelpare, personal communication, November 21, 2008). The results of the feedback from coaches and research pending for release on Play It Cool should be released and applied effectively prior to major development on the parental component.

4.3.2 Improving the Play It Cool Program

The Play It Cool program can be enhanced if: (1) it is mandated by hockey governing bodies, (2) it matures into a graduated certification program, and (3) it involves a definable and consistent outcome for coaches and parents (W. Montelpare, personal communication, November 21, 2008).

Montelpare (personal communication, November 21, 2008) also suggests a more active role from the Minister of Health Promotion. He hopes that a task force can be created that works specifically with hockey issues in Canada. It is key to understand the relationship that has already been established between the hockey community and the Ministry of Health staff and the programming that already exists to address ice hockey injury, risk, and safety (W. Montelpare, personal communication, November 21, 2008). This requires an organized and strategic approach in the political realm. The development team will be more prepared to address this goal when evaluation results are released. The evidence-informed results derived from multifactorial evaluations of Play It Cool will give implementers, researchers, and politicians a better understanding of the value of the program, its strengths, and its weaknesses.

The program is inclusive of all groups who are interested in participating in the Play It Cool Program. In the past, girls' hockey coaches have participated in the program and were provided a female facilitator as per their request. The developers of the program had an Olympian from the Canadian women's hockey team facilitate the curriculum online. Although hockey tends to be considered a sport for men, the Play It Cool program encourages the Ontario Women's Hockey Association (OWHA) to take part (W. Montelpare, personal communication, November 21, 2008). According to Montelpare (personal communication, November 21, 2008) the OWHA, although limited in their involvement, expressed strong support for the program in the 2008 Hockey Summit and have expressed an interest to participate in the program because they believe in the concept of it.

Overall, it is important that the lines of communication are open between those who develop and implement the Play It Cool Program, and the hockey federations who govern the leagues. The program needs to cater to the needs of the consumer. As such, the program needs to be less geared toward researchers and scientists, and more user-friendly to the target population (W. Montelpare, personal communication, November 14, 2008). The content must be modified to fulfill this need, which is why it is suggested that the graduated certification may be more appropriate—that is, it will make it more sensitive to the time constraints of volunteer coaches and it should cover material, in content and in presentation, which is relevant to the user depending on the level. Once again, however, the length of each level must reflect the feedback and needs of coaches.

W. Montelpare (personal communication, November 21, 2008) contends that this is their aim, and modification is welcome and ongoing. Communication should also be fostered, en mass, at the grassroots with the coaches; parents should also be consulted so as to redefine the culture of hockey adequately (W. Montelpare, personal communication, November 21, 2008). Table 4.3 provides an overview of the program needs for Play It Cool. According to Montelpare (personal communication, November 21, 2008), these

Table 4.3 Program needs and status

Program need	Status
Continue developing the graphic arts story (designed for kids) (i.e., hockey comic book)	Ongoing
Acquire a stable stream of funding that is sustainable and continuous	Ongoing
Ensure coach buy-in and time commitment from coaches	Ongoing
Promote a communal and consolidated approach to promote safe approaches to hockey among all	Ongoing
Create incentives to participate (e.g., sign jerseys and sweat shirts, free ice time credit)	Ongoing and planning
Develop the coach material into a full year curriculum with national coaching certification designation so as to advance coach learning capacity	Proposed
Mandate the program from the league level	Proposed
Establish a Center of Excellence	Proposed
Foster political will for the program, e.g., involvement from health minister	Proposed
Inform and involve parents using course modules (with goal of having parents be able to identify, monitor, and diagnose possible injury, even when their child returns home after a game, e.g., concussion)	In planning

activities are either ongoing, in program planning, or in the proposed stage.

Montelpare (personal communication, November 21, 2008) says his team is open to collaboration, so they are willing to foster any efforts to achieve these goals. He also believes responsibility is shared and divided among all stakeholders from the administrative level (e.g., ONF, CSRO, Hockey Canada) to the program level (e.g., Play It Cool development team) to the grassroots level (e.g., coaches, referees, parents, and players). Overall, he argues that better infrastructure is needed to better delegate roles and account for responsibilities. He suggests a board of directors and an advisory council be established, who can work under the Centre of Excellence (W. Montelpare, personal communication, November 21, 2008).

4.4 Outcome

Pilot studying is still ongoing as the Play It Cool Program is still completing evaluations for their first assessments. Stakeholders are participating in the research projects to provide insight and outcome results into the impact the Play It Cool Program has on the target population (Table 4.4).

Additional evaluations include:

- Measuring implicit bias.
- Parental attitudes.
- Neck strength.
- Coach Assessment.
- mTBI and Return to Play,
- Electroencephalography (EEG) response.
- Balance testing.
- Aerobic and anaerobic testing.
- Children's attitudes as ice hockey players.

Future research by the Play It Cool team includes the development of a comprehensive event reporting system that would include both the reporting of injuries as well as the reporting of fights, violent events, etc. (W. Montelpare, personal communication, 9 January 2009). Challenges in program planning and implementation, as well as evaluation, have arisen since Play It Cool's redevelopment. Montelpare (personal communication, November 24, 2008) noted that these challenges have informed a better program, as well as an improvement in the manner in which the program planning and evaluation is approached. Challenges of particular importance have been:

- Commitment to completing the modules, course drop-out rate is too high.
- Lack of incentives to complete the program.

Table 4.4 Evaluation tools to assess components of Play It Cool

Evaluation tool	Description	Status
Injury Surveillance[a]	Uses an online survey (http://sprout.lakeheadu.ca/~hockey) and is based on the Hockey Canada Injury Insurance forms Collect information about general injuries as well as concussion-specific injuries for all player participants in each participating cohort measure A major problem in this data collection has been the truthful and timely reporting of injury events. A recommendation of our research is that a clear, concise, and accurate definition of injuries be established for all participants	Ongoing Due for completion Spring/Summer 2008
Attention Network Test (ANT)[a]	Neurocognition surveillance test related to head impact for minor league players. The test partitions test response scores into alerting, orienting, and executing functions of cognition	Evaluation intends to compare the results of these measures against the Connors test and the ImPACT test results Ongoing Due for completion Spring/Summer 2008
Connors Test[a] (Cognition testing)	Neurocognition surveillance test related to head impact for minor league players. The specific features of the Connors test include that it is a standardized test of memory and cognition Evaluation will provide important information about cognitive deficits which are directly related to concussive events	Ongoing Due for completion Spring/Summer 2008
ImPACT[a]	Neurocognition surveillance test related to head impact for minor league players ImPACT is currently accepted in the field of sports injury, but cannot be considered as a gold standard test, despite its widespread use There are major shortcomings in the vigilance of participants taking the test and therefore the extent to which these measures truly assess cognition may be questioned	Ongoing Due for completion Spring/Summer 2008
Exposure Measures	Helps to describe the actual risk of players to injury as a result of time on a task. The measure can be used to identify coaching behaviors relative to distribution of playing time across a team, and to assist in developing training programs relative to players as a result of number of shifts, time per shift, and by period of play	Montelpare, W. J., Baker, J., Faught, B., Corey, P., MacKay, M., Lavoie, N., Nystrom, M. (2007) Development of A Computing Utility To Measure Time-On-Task In Injury Research Studies, *International Journal of Sports Science and Engineering*, 1(3):183–187. (Refereed)
Head Impact Telemetry System (HITS)	Hockey helmets (CSA approved) were equipped with six linear accelerometers and a wireless system that transmitted data to a receiver interfaced with a computer Head impacts sustained at 27 home games during the 2006–2007 season were measured using the Head Impact Telemetry System (HITS). Nine games were recorded using a field videography system to capture player collisions. A HITS profile was determined, which included the number of impacts (>10 g) by player, the total number of impacts, the average number of impacts per game, and the mean linear acceleration value for all impacts per player	Based on these results, ten taped trials for the players sustaining greater than 250 total impacts over the season were qualitatively analyzed. They captured 2753 head impacts over the season, with the average number of impacts per player per game ranging from 3 to 16 with a mean linear acceleration of 15.8 g (SD = 13.76) While specific players may be predisposed to head impacts of a greater frequency and magnitude because of their style of play, these characteristics can be changed to reduce risk of potential injury Ongoing Due for completion Spring/Summer 2008
Blood biomarkers	Assesses the efficacy of using S100b as a method for evaluating post-concussion effects	Due for completion April 1, 2008

(continued)

Table 4.4 (continued)

Evaluation tool	Description	Status
Module preparation	Rewritten modules and spent 10 months distributing them to coaches in the state of Massachusetts and in the city of Rochester Minnesota	Collecting exit surveys from coaches as well as others who have participated in delivery of the modules Due for completion March 1, 2009
Heart rate variability	Assesses the rhythmicity of the r-r waves of the electrocardiogram based on frequency domain analyses (Fast Fourier Transforms using SAS based on data recorded at rest and during exercise). The analysis enables us to separate parasympathetic and sympathetic nervous system activities in each subject, and to compare the measures across time	Due for completion March 30, 2009
Computer programming for data collection	Using html and x-html with PHP and MySQL to produce a web-based approach to data input. Analysis generally relies on SAS functions to provide accurate and efficient output of our data sets	Ongoing
Game film analysis		Due for completion April 4, 2009

ª There seems to be a general lack of enthusiasm to complete these tests. Subjects report boredom with the repetitive nature of the tests as a major inhibitor to their willingness to participate

- Continuous training of facilitators to keep them up-to-date on the knowledge they have and information they provide to the coaches.
- Length of the program.

4.4.1 Short- and Long-Term Outcomes

From the goals, as well as the evaluations listed above, Montelpare (personal communication, November 24, 2008) has specifically chosen two primary expected short-term outcomes and four primary expected long-term outcomes for the program. These expected outcomes are listed in Table 4.5.

The program has already merited some unanticipated positive and negative outcomes to date. A positive outcome includes the enthusiasm by participants and players' parents as well as the rapidity of uptake of the program. A negative outcome has been the lack of buy-in from the sport governing bodies. Although there has been extreme enthusiasm over the program, it was assumed that all stakeholders would jump at the chance to participate in a free program that has been already established and oriented specifically to audiences serious about hockey. Overall, W. Montelpare

Table 4.5 Short-term and long-term outcomes

Short-term outcomes	Long-term outcomes
Curb the dropout rate: Have 60 coaches in the next season complete the program. Currently, 30 have been recruited; however, about one-third have dropped out of the program Also, a long-term expected outcome	Establish Center of Excellence. The institution would act as a broker for the program. It would allow for monitoring, managing, and act as a central repository for all of the information that is being created for Play It Cool. The institution would allow for accountability and sustainability of the program
Continue to understand the bench-top science Advance knowledge around attention tests, helmets, heart rate variability, etc. The aim is to understand the behavioral characteristics that predispose someone to neurotrauma Also, a long-term expected outcome	Create a guideline strategy for Return to Play The purpose is to understand injury, try to prevent it, and when it cannot be prevented, to manage the injury based on the individual characteristics of the individual
	Expanding stakeholder reach Involving parents, referees, hockey federations en masse Mandating the program and evaluating the effect of mandating it

(personal communication, November 24, 2008) says that they assumed stakeholders, such as hockey governing bodies, would want to push the program and make it more popular and widespread so as to expand the reach.

4.5 Conclusion

Ultimately, Play It Cool's methodological approach will likely lead to interesting as well as effective outcomes. The program components are clearly well thought out, meticulously devised, and energetically implemented. Program developers, particularly Montelpare, are passionate and well informed. The team and Montelpare are clearly the program champions of Play It Cool. The dedication and commitment by a well-prepared and enthusiastic program champion is imperative. It is important that the team continues to solicit feedback from stakeholders, as they have done in the past.

Montelpare has tried numerous ways to engage the target population and continues to dedicate time to diversifying this strategy. However, his intention to modify the length of the course, as well as the structure of the course (i.e., to a certification program), seems to speak to the needs of the target population. Finally, the role of the decision-makers seems vital to Play It Cool's success and their role in hockey injury prevention should be reexamined and reapproached.

However, at the time of writing this, several key elements still needed to mature – namely, those evaluations listed in the outcomes section.

The results from these evaluations would provide better insight into the role that the government can assume in prioritizing hockey injury and in funding hockey injury prevention programs. These evaluations would also provide incentives for further funding and development of the program, as well as the consideration for a Center of Excellence.

There is a good foundation for data collection in Canada; however, more effective monitoring and recording of injury should continue. Moreover, more thorough and comprehensive preventative interventions are required. The review of the literature determined that evaluation of preventative interventions is a knowledge gap in the ice hockey literature. Therefore, the release of evaluation data from Play It Cool will be one of the first programs to fill this knowledge gap.

Ultimately, outcomes will be derived from a continuous participatory, research process and consultative process. Montelpare (personal communication, November 24, 2008) contends that as the work and their teams mature in their work, they will have a better informational infrastructure to work from. This foundation will make the program implementation more efficient and effective. Evaluation results will also provide a foundation for improved programming.

Acknowledgments The author would like to express sincere appreciation to the key informants for this case study: William J. Montelpare of the University of Prince Edward Island in Charlottetown, PEI, Canada and Andrew Link of the Mayo Clinic Sports Medicine Center in Minneapolis, MN, USA—whose consultation made this project possible.

Brio Model: Play It Cool—Hockey Injury Prevention Program

Group Served: Children in the developmental ages (8–16).

Goal: To reduce injuries and exposure to risk of injury in youth ice hockey.

Background	Resources	Implementation	Outcome
Play It Cool was created in 2001 by the Canadian Spinal Research Organization (CSRO) and Mitron Sports to respond to the need for a safe ice hockey tool that could be available to prevent spinal injuries in hockey Following evaluation of the program, Dr. John Lewko, from the Ontario Neurotrauma Foundation (ONF) and Barry Munro of the CSRO, observed a lack of stakeholder (i.e., coaches) buy-in for the program The program was modified into a facilitated online delivery system comprised of multimedia tools that delivers content asynchronously over the web Delivery includes regularly scheduled teleconferences and asynchronous web-based discussion boards Play It Cool is based as a set of seven ice hockey competencies The program is continuously modified as a result of feedback from the stakeholder network The target population of the program is comprised of coaches that are directly working with children in the developmental ages (8–16)	The CSRO and the ONF allocated funding for designing and implementing the program Dr. Montelpare employed 20 undergraduate students at Lakehead University to conduct research and evaluation on the components of Play It Cool The developers of the Play It Cool program have already established a vital and strong relationship with coaches The development team consistently and continuously provide their time and feedback about the program	The design of the website has been particularly successful and well received by stakeholders The research teams have tried to make the curriculum a comprehensive, consolidated, and well-established conglomeration of information The program has successfully been able to heighten the awareness about the risks of injuries in ice hockey Overall, it is important that the lines of communication are open between those who develop and implement the Play It Cool Program and the hockey federations who govern the leagues Need to be more sensitive to the time constraints of volunteer coaches and the program should continue to cover material, in content and presentation, which is relevant to users, depending on the level Coach recruitment is one practice that has been suggested to be effective but has not achieved optimal participation rates Although they expressed enthusiasm and tremendous support for the program verbally, there has been a lack of follow-up to participate by coaches	Pilot studying is still ongoing as the Play It Cool Program is still completing evaluations for their first assessments Stakeholders participating in the research projects to provide insight and outcome results into the impact the program has on the target population A positive outcome includes the enthusiasm by participants and players' parents as well as the rapidity of uptake of the program A negative outcome has been the lack of buy in from the sport governing bodies Challenges of particular importance have been: – Commitment to completing the modules, course drop-out rate is too high – Lack of incentives to complete the program – Continuous training of facilitators to keep them up to date on the knowledge they have and information they provide to the coaches – Length of the program Research results are required to be released to make a definite conclusion as to the program's impact on reducing injuries and exposure to risk of injury

Life Space Model: Play It Cool—Hockey Injury Prevention Program

Sociocultural: civilization/community	Interpersonal: primary and secondary relationships	Physical environments: where we live	Internal states: biochemical/genetic and means of coping
Facilitated online delivery system comprised of multimedia tools that delivers content asynchronously over the web Program presented in seven modules (http://bolt.lakeheadu.ca/~playcool/), which are held over an 8-week period (3 weeks of delivery, 1 week break, 4 weeks delivery). The online format includes hyperlinked text, videos, animation, sound effects, discussion boards, questionnaires and blogs	The actual target population of the Play It Cool program is comprised of coaches that are directly linked to or working with children in the developmental ages (8–16). Therefore, the content of the program was designed to target these coaches	Teaching coaches how to teach skills in a passive approach that is not adopted easily by participants Competencies speak to an active approach that engages participants and makes them responsible to learn the information and apply it The aim of the program was to create awareness and a usable program that can be applied in many different ways by coaches and players	Empowerment of coaches by training in proper technique and physical conditioning, among other aspects Risk management and assessment utilized to increase safety practices in ice hockey

References

Borrie, A., & Knowles, Z. (1998). Reflective coaching. *Insight, 1*, 1–4.

Cowie-Bonne, J. A. (2000). *Participeant-centred sport: An evaluation of community hockey coaches and the Coach Level Training Course.* Master's thesis, University of Toronto. Retrieved from http://hdl.handle.net/1807/13638.

Finch, C. F., & Hennessy, M. (2000). The safety practices of sporting clubs/centres in the city of Hume. *Journal of Science and Medicine in Sport, 3*(1), 9–16.

Gilbert, W. D., & Trudel, P. (1999). Framing the construction of coaching knowledge in experiential learning theory. *Sociology of Sport On-line, 2*, 1.

Safe Hockey Summit. (2008). *Using facilitated online curriculum delivery for coach preparation in teaching safety and injury prevention in ice hockey* [PowerPoint]. Presented at the Safe Hockey Summit, Thunder Bay, ON.

Simpson, J., Chalmers, D. J., Waller, A. E., Bird, Y. N., Quarrie, K. L., Gerrard, D. F., et al. (1994). *Tackling rugby injury: Recommendations for reducing injury to rugby union players in New Zealand.* Dunedin, New Zealand: Injury Prevention Research Unit & Human Performance Centre, University of Otago.

Smeh, D. T., & Singla, D. (2008). RugbySmart – Prevention of spinal and head injuries in rugby in New Zealand. In R. Volpe (Ed.), *Evidence-based best practices in the prevention of severe sports injuries.* Toronto, Ontario, Canada: Ontario Neurotrauma Foundation; Life Span Adaptation Projects, University of Toronto.

Stewart, C. (2006). Coach education online: The Montana model. *Journal of Physical Education, Recreation & Dance, 77*(4), 34–36.

Tator, C. H., Provvidenza, C. F., Lapczak, L., Carson, J., & Raymond, D. (2004). Spinal injuries in Canadian ice hockey: Documentation of injuries sustained from 1943- 1999. *Canadian Journal of Neurological Sciences, 31*(4), 460–466.

RugbySmart

5

Daria Smeh and Daisy Radha Singla

RugbySmart is a program that prevents injuries for amateur and professional athletes of rugby through educational courses, workshops, videos, training, and other instructive materials for coaches, referees, and athletes.

5.1 Background

Studies from countries where rugby is a popular sport have demonstrated that the number of spinal-cord-related injuries increased dramatically during the 1970s and 1980s (Quarrie, Cantu, & Chalmers, 2002). At the time of this report, Rugby News—the world's most popular rugby magazine (Paul, n.d.)—reported that half of the current 8000 adolescents aged 13 years who participate in rugby today would not be playing in 5 years, citing injury or fear of injury as the reason they would drop out (Paul, n.d.).

According to the Accident Compensation Corporation (ACC), the most prevalent unintentional injuries in the New Zealand Rugby Union (NZRU) are soft-tissue injuries, which occur slightly more often than fractures and dislocations (ACC, 2006). Meanwhile, 63% of all injuries are deemed moderate-to-serious injury, which comprise any injury that requires five or more days of absence from employment (ACC, 2006). The ACC is New Zealand's nationwide, governmental program that provides personal injury coverage for all New Zealand's citizens, residents, and temporary visitors (S. Gianotti, personal communication, July 16, 2007).

With respect to sport, the ACC is committed to collecting accurate statistics on the incidence of injury in rugby and reducing both the number and severity of injuries to sports participants, with a strong focus on rugby (S. Gianotti, personal communication, July 16, 2007). To reduce injury, the ACC examines the statistics to understand the injury site—the location and/or contact point where the injury occurs (S. Gianotti, personal communication, July 16, 2007). Serious injuries are defined as when a player is prevented from participating in rugby practices or games for 21 days or more (Quarrie & Hopkins, n.d.). Moderate-to-severe injuries in rugby account for 72% of the overall costs attributed to rugby sports claims (see Table 5.1; S. Gianotti, personal communication, July 16, 2007).

In relation to the North American context, a retrospective study showed that between 1978 and 2004 rugby injury patterns in the United States were similar to New Zealand, overall, in terms of injury site but differed by age and sex (Fig. 5.1). Figure 5.2 illustrates that among

D. Smeh (✉)
LoyalTeam Environmental, Toronto, ON, Canada

D. R. Singla
Sinai Health System, University of Toronto, Toronto, ON, Canada
e-mail: daisy.singla@utoronto.ca

© Springer Nature Switzerland AG 2020
R. Volpe (ed.), *Casebook of Traumatic Injury Prevention*,
https://doi.org/10.1007/978-3-030-27419-1_5

Canadian adults and children, 24% and 27%, respectively, sustain head, face, or neck injuries. Overall, in Canada between 5% and 25% of rugby injuries are head injuries, including concussions (B.C. Injury Research and Prevention

Table 5.1 Moderate-to-serious injuries sustained in rugby

Injury site	% of total moderate-to-serious injuries
Knee	24.5
Shoulder	18.8
Ankle	10.3
Leg (between ankle and knee)	6.4
Neck and spine	4.8

Note: Quarrie, Gianotti, Hopkins, and Hume (2007)

Unit, n.d.). Of the head injuries, 44% are concussions (Yard & Comstock, 2006).

Similar to American and Canadian statistics, males outnumber females exponentially in regard to injury rates in New Zealand. Furthermore, younger rugby players internationally are more likely to suffer injury due to participation in rugby. For example, US rugby players 18 years of age or younger were significantly more likely to be diagnosed with concussions than those older than 18 years (Yard & Comstock, 2006). Corresponding to these statistics, the incidence of injury increases with age for New Zealand rugby players. For example, players aged 16 and over are twice as likely to encounter an injury compared to those 16 and under (Quarrie, n.d.).

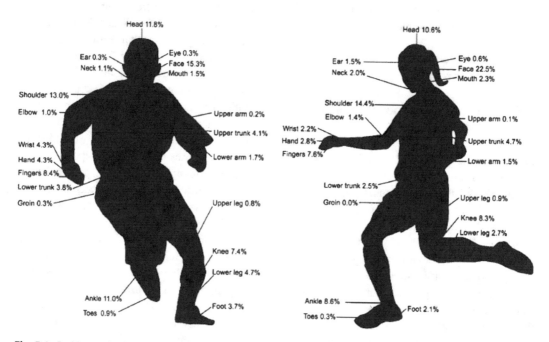

Fig. 5.1 Incidence of Injury in US Rugby, 1978–2004 (Yard & Comstock, 2006)

Fig. 5.2 Incidence of injury in Canadian Rugby (B.C. Injury Research and Prevention Unit, n.d.)

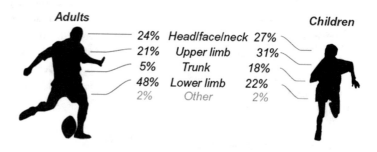

Due to the popularity of rugby and the physical nature of the game, rugby in New Zealand results in a far higher number of injury compensation claims than other sports. As displayed in Fig. 5.3, new claims in moderate-to-serious rugby injuries amount to 3500 per year—by contrast, soccer, which ranks second in injury claims after rugby, resulted in 1800 new moderate-to-serious claims per year (S. Gianotti, personal communication, July 16, 2007).

Due to the high incidence of injury, it follows that rugby also represents the largest cost to New Zealand's ACC injury financial compensation Scheme (ACC, 2006), whereby one serious claim can amount to NZ$5–14 million (approximately C$4–11 million). According to Armour, Clatworthy, Bean, Wells, and Clarke (1997), "one tetraplegic is worth a thousand sprained ankles" (p. 114). For example, a previously educated 20-year-old tetraplegic has a one in five chance of being employed in his or her lifetime, while costs for his or her care totals NZ$2–3 million dollars during a lifetime. Essentially, a large number of claims for moderate-to-serious injuries in a particular sport can be inferred as a great cost for the ACC (see Fig. 5.3).

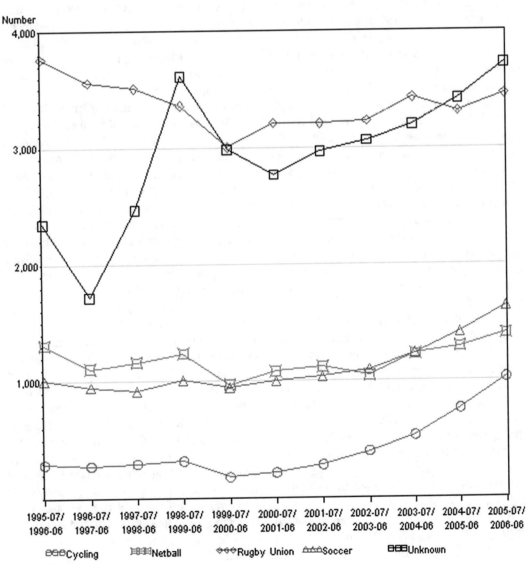

Fig. 5.3 Number of new claims: Comparison between sports covered (ACC, 2006)

5.1.1 Neurotraumatic Injuries

Medical researchers have identified a significant increase in the frequency of spinal injuries among rugby union players in many countries. Furthermore, injuries to the cervical spine are among the "most tragic occurring (from) rugby participation" (Quarrie et al., 2002, p. 634). While the correlation between rugby participation and injuries has been reviewed for over a century, Quarrie et al. (2002) give an example of a rugby injury documented in 1869 that read "... in the course of a severe scrimmage a young gentleman named Lomax got down, with his head bend under his chest, and in this position was trampled on by many of the players. He was picked up insensible, and, with the exception of short intervals of consciousness, he has remained so until the present time ... If he survives (which is still doubtful!), it is feared he will be a cripple for life" (p. 32). The focus on spinal-cord-related injuries has "received greater attention in the medical community over the past 30 years" as they occur more frequently than any other type of rugby injury in documented rugby history (Quarrie et al., 2002, p. 634). Once again, reports of the frequency and type of catastrophic spinal injuries due to rugby were documented and heavily publicized during the 1970s and 1980s, including epidemiological studies of rugby injury (Dalley, Laing, Rowberry, & Caird, 1982; Quarrie et al., 2007).

In 1993, the University of Otago conducted a study with 356 rugby players from Dunedin regarding rugby injury, risk factors in the game, and the effects of injury on performance (Simpson et al., 1994). Aiming to identify risk and protective factors associated with rugby injury, this analysis led to a 5-year prospective cohort study called the Rugby Injury and Performance Project (RIPP). By 1999, the RIPP represented a groundbreaking, comprehensive approach whose design permitted the evaluation of both intrinsic and extrinsic injury risks for players (see Fig. 5.4).

Utilizing a panel consisting of members of the NZRU, ACC, and the Injury Prevention Research Unit (IPRU), these members applied RIPP's results along with health promotion and injury prevention principles to develop strategies specifically for rugby. During this developmental phase between 1993 and 1999, a series of potential interventions were cultivated and discussed among the ACC, NZRU, and IPRU, and tested by the IPRU at the University of Otago.

Yet research conducted in 1996 by Armour et al. regarding the dramatic increase and ongoing consequences of spinal cord injury in rugby and an alarming 18 rugby-related spinal cord injuries in 1995 alone elicited the national body of New Zealand and New Zealand Rugby Union to propose strategies to address the rate of spinal cord injuries (S. Gianotti, personal communication, July 18, 2007). The strong support elicited by the government as a result of the findings from Armour et al.'s (1997) research provided the foundation from which to develop preliminary strategies (i.e., compulsory workshops) preceding the development and implementation of RugbySmart. At that time, the ACC provided financial support for the workshops; they financed TV advertisements that demonstrated high-profile players doing physical conditioning (i.e., warm-up and cool-down stretches before rugby matches). Due to the fact that these initiatives were fragmented and did not comprise a formal strategy that focused on encompassing the entire epidemiology of rugby injuries, more work was required to formalize a well-targeted strategy (K. Quarrie, personal communication, July 18, 2007).

The ACC had not only decided to play a major role in funding and establishing RugbySmart in 1999, but efforts toward specific game-focused initiatives began in 2002 when Simon S. Gianotti was appointed Program Manager for Sport & Recreation at the ACC. Gianotti began working with Kenneth Quarrie who was previously hired in 2000 as the Rugby Injury Prevention Manager at the NZRU. Overall, Gianotti recognizes the important roles he and Quarrie played in the development of RugbySmart; however, Gianotti attributes progress toward forming RugbySmart as the result of a "national body wanting to do something about [the increasing number of] injuries—both spinal and otherwise—among rugby players" (K. Gianotti, personal communication, July 16, 2007).

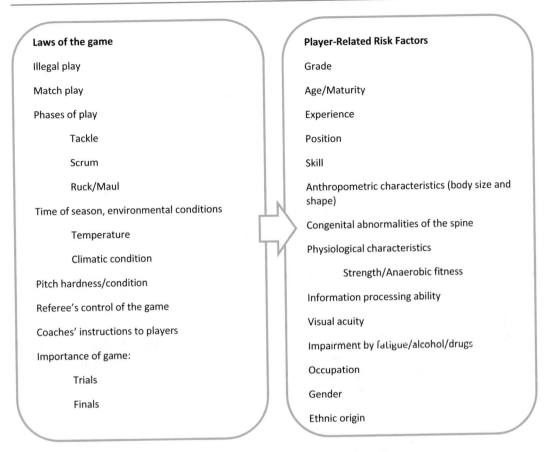

Laws of the game

Illegal play

Match play

Phases of play

Tackle

Scrum

Ruck/Maul

Time of season, environmental conditions

Temperature

Climatic condition

Pitch hardness/condition

Referee's control of the game

Coaches' instructions to players

Importance of game:

Trials

Finals

Player-Related Risk Factors

Grade

Age/Maturity

Experience

Position

Skill

Anthropometric characteristics (body size and shape)

Congenital abnormalities of the spine

Physiological characteristics

Strength/Anaerobic fitness

Information processing ability

Visual acuity

Impairment by fatigue/alcohol/drugs

Occupation

Gender

Ethnic origin

Fig. 5.4 Extrinsic and intrinsic-related risk factors of injury in rugby (Quarrie, n.d.)

Among many definitions, RugbySmart has been described as "a multifaceted injury prevention program" and "vehicle for delivering information on injury prevention to rugby coaches, referees, and players in New Zealand" (Quarrie et al., 2007, p. 1151). Taking into consideration and prioritizing the need to attend to the large number of spinal cord injuries, "a major goal of the NZRU and ACC in establishing RugbySmart was to eliminate spinal injuries within the context of a contact sport" (Quarrie et al., 2007, p. 1151). Over time, the program has developed successfully as new information about risks in rugby participation has emerged starting with an understanding of the biophysical nature of injury in rugby.

RugbySmart was developed from van Mechelen's Sequence of Prevention Model (see Fig. 5.5; Quarrie et al., 2007). The model is comprised of four steps, which means establishing the size of the injury problem (i.e., with surveillance), recognizing risk factors and causes of the injuries sustained in the activity (e.g., rugby plays in scrums), implementing prevention initiatives, and continuing injury monitoring (i.e. designed to assess the beneficial effect in reducing the injury burden with changes implemented; Quarrie et al., 2007).

According to Gianotti (personal communication, July 18, 2007), the most crucial step to the success of any injury prevention program is adhering to the final step of Van Mechelen's model: that is, evaluating prevention strategies. Referred to as a "cycling process," necessary modifications are made according to continual monitoring of not only the number of injuries but also the knowledge, attitudes, and behaviors of RugbySmart itself (S. Gianotti, personal communication,

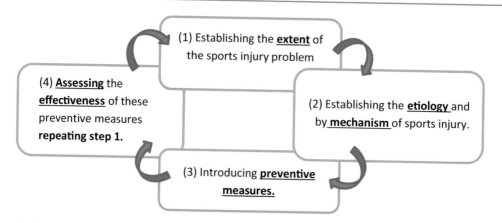

Fig. 5.5 Van Mechelen's Sequence of Prevention Model (Chalmers, 2002; Van Mechelen, Hlobil, & Kemper, 1992)

July 18, 2007). However, it is important to note that if the other steps of the cycle have not been attended to, injury prevention cannot be possible (K. Quarrie, personal communication, January 16, 2008).

In 1999–2000 and in accordance with ACC's general injury prevention program known as SportSmart, NZRU adapted its framework of a 10-point Action Plan to rugby after initial meetings with ACC regarding the content of an injury prevention program. The framework was developed with key informants from the rugby sport community throughout New Zealand including Sports Medicine New Zealand, Sport Science New Zealand, the Hillary Commission (now SPARC), national sporting organizations, and sport scientists (ACC, n.d.-a).

ACC's large financial investment into RugbySmart was supported by the promise made by the NZRU to ensure compulsory attendance for coaches in RugbySmart workshops. To enforce compulsory attendance, an NZRU Board directive was given to all NZRU affiliates in 2000, which required all coaches of all levels to attend the RugbySmart workshops. Ultimately, this guaranteed delivery mechanism resulted in two major advantages for Rugby Smart:

1. It fostered strong collaboration between ACC and NZRU, which plays a major role in the sustainability of RugbySmart.
2. Due to its compulsory nature, studies show that RugbySmart workshop attendance

reaches close to 100% for both coaches and referees in New Zealand (S. Gianotti, personal communication, July 16, 2007).

Therefore, while the formal development of RugbySmart began in 2000 at the NZRU, the injury prevention program of RugbySmart was delivered for the first time in 2001 in conjunction with both the ACC and the NZRU.

Due to the ubiquitous presence of rugby in New Zealand, the target population of RugbySmart was established as, and currently is, the entire rugby-playing base of New Zealand. The program includes both males and females, and the Pacific Island, Maori and European populations. Specifically, RugbySmart targets all players aged 16–44 years old because this is the primary population who participate in rugby in New Zealand. Furthermore, this age group constitutes 83% of all rugby injuries and consequently 86% of ACC rugby claim costs (S. Gianotti, personal communication, July 16, 2007).

Furthermore, RugbySmart targets coaches and referees, as they are the primary communicators with the players on and off the field. There are 140,000 rugby players in all of New Zealand's rugby leagues, while there are approximately 8000 coaches and 2000 referees. Thus, reaching all coaches and referees is seemingly more feasible due to their smaller population. It is also quite strategic to target coaches as they possess "connections to the players as well as knowledge and passion for the game" (S. Gianotti, personal communication, July 17, 2007). The notion to target coaches is based on research performed in the 1990s, whereby rugby players identified coaches as fulfilling a key role in demonstrating and providing injury prevention-related messages to players (Simpson et al., 1994). Meanwhile, referees play a key role in controlling the pace of the game—a notion often responsible behind the occurrence of rugby injuries (S. Gianotti, personal communication, July 17, 2007). For example, RugbySmart demonstrates to referees what they need to be doing to control the scrimmage and observe sign of injury, thereby preventing dangerous tackles that cause serious injury.

The attempt to engage coaches and referees met with some resistance during the initial delivery of RugbySmart. Veteran coaches with more coaching experience particularly demonstrated resistance (S. Gianotti, personal communication, July 22, 2007). While this early resistance has since been eroded, its impact cannot be underestimated. For example, due to this initial resistance by coaches, ACC deemed the duration of RugbySmart as a pilot program for only 2 years.

Another factor that reduced coach resistance to RugbySmart is the adherence Step 4 of Van Mechelen's Sequence of Prevention Model, which stresses the need to continually evaluate the delivery of the RugbySmart products (S. Gianotti, personal communication, July 22, 2007). Since implementation, and as a result of annual evaluation, RugbySmart products continue to provide a fresh perspective on the program's delivery of injury prevention (K. Quarrie, personal communication, July 16, 2008). For example, in 2002, coach education in RugbySmart courses was deemed inadequate because coaches assumed education tools were overly safety-oriented. Consequently, through the input of ACC, NZRU, and those delivering and participating in RugbySmart sessions, RugbySmart was modified to communicate key messages in a language more meaningful to rugby coaches, referees, and players. Eventually, participants came to understand RugbySmart's primary focus that the "winning technique is also the correct technique…

[through] player strategies as oppose to safety strategies" (S. Gianotti, personal communication, July 16, 2007). Furthermore, RugbySmart has pledged a long-term commitment to respond to any resistance toward the RugbySmart program (S. Gianotti, personal communication, July 16, 2007; K. Quarrie, personal communication, January 16, 2008).

Consequently, evidence from the initial pilot program demonstrated a number of success factors, such as an increased interest from coaches to learn better techniques, a reduction in the incidence of serious injury, and a reduced number of serious injury claims of RugbySmart within the first 3 years of implementation. As a result, RugbySmart will enter its ninth year of implementation in 2008.

Ultimately, the delivery of RugbySmart has followed similar protocols since its original development, including the use of a DVD that is presented to all coaches and referees across the nation during a one-hour compulsory workshop and the instatement of Rugby Development Officers (RDO) who are responsible for ensuring attendance of coaches and referees to the workshops. They are also responsible to engage in discussions during the workshops and are allowed to distribute the DVDs to the coaches and the referees for them to take home or show to the players on their teams. The NZRU also provided a series of articles about injury prevention via 'GamePlan RUGBY' magazine, which is distributed free of charge to all coaches two or three times per year.

Consequently, results from epidemiological studies have demonstrated that the number of injuries—specifically those of spinal injuries causing permanent disability—due to participation in the rugby union in New Zealand have decreased and are significantly lower than projected statistics since the implementation of RugbySmart (Quarrie et al., 2007). The outcomes of the program provide sound support for educational programs like RugbySmart to be continued in New Zealand and to become a viable option for injury prevention in other nations where the popularity of rugby is also increasing across ages, genders, and abilities.

5.2 Resources

5.2.1 Financial Resources

The stakeholders who initially supported the establishment of RugbySmart are generally the same as those that currently support the program. These stakeholders include the: (1) government via the nationally funded ACC by financing the programs and staff for RugbySmart; (2) NZRU through financing for staff (i.e., Rugby Injury Prevention Manager Kenneth Quarrie; secretarial support in the ACC office including letter writing and other administrative tasks) and devoted RDOs; and (3) the research and medical community with whom ACC has a strong relationship and whose expertise is readily available. For example, to establish the concussion management program, feedback was sought from the clinicians who work with rugby players and with brain injury as well as the medical research experts from the University of Pittsburgh concussion program. The leading role of the initiation, development, and delivery of RugbySmart injury prevention strategies is equally attributed to ACC and NZRU (S. Gianotti, personal communication, July 22, 2007).

Since safety strategies in rugby began in 2001, the ACC has steadily increased its contribution of funding. Since the inception of RugbySmart, the ACC has provided NZ$1.3 million to the development and implementation of RugbySmart strategies and human resources (Table 5.2). The ACC and NZRU have a contract in which ACC provides funds for RugbySmart to the NZRU, whereby NZRU manages these funds (K. Quarrie, personal communication, January 16, 2008). Funds spent on the strategy include development

of RugbySmart DVDs, posters, booklets, and Sideline Concussion Cards. Furthermore, the funding from the ACC provides financial support to each provincial rugby union to assist with costs associated with conducting seminars and presentations. No cost is incurred on rent or office equipment as both the ACC and the NZRU allow the staff of RugbySmart to operate out of their buildings. Savings in this capacity, as well as steadily increased funding, translate into the ability to allocate funding to improve RugbySmart products. For example, while the duration of the initial RugbySmart video lasted 18 min in 2001, the DVD in 2007 is 40 min (S. Gianotti, personal communication, July 22, 2007). The length of the video is informed by the demand by the coaches and players for more and better rugby techniques.

Funding has been allocated from the ACC to employ a Program Manager for Sport and Recreation, as well as two additional sports-related injury prevention employees (S. Gianotti, personal communication, July 25, 2007). The NZRU have ensured funds for an Injury Prevention Manager, secretarial staff within the High-Performance Team, as well as access to resources from community rugby teams (K. Quarrie, personal communication, July 25, 2007). The two injury prevention employees are responsible for ensuring that regular meetings are held for all stakeholders. These meetings are held frequently, and the two representatives are readily available for consultation to both senior management at their own organizations and to the outside community. The costs of travel and accommodations for conferences and tournaments are supported by the NZRU because the program has an excellent reputation in sport injury prevention (S. Gianotti, personal communication, July 25, 2007).

The financial resources are attained and allocated annually by completing a business case and an operational plan, which demonstrate how RugbySmart can be implemented, as well as demonstrating Key Process Indicators (KPIs). To present their case, Gianotti and Quarrie meet key stakeholders from government to re-justify funding and confirm the goal to commit long

Table 5.2 ACC funding for RugbySmart

Year	Amount
2001	$200,000
2002	$200,000
2003	$200,000
2004	$250,000
2005	$250,000
2006	$300,000
Total	1.3 million

term to the betterment of injury prevention within the NZRU (S. Gianotti, personal communication, July 22, 2007). ACC is statutorily required to attempt to prevent injuries in New Zealand (K. Quarrie, personal communication, January 16, 2008). Furthermore, ACC is supported by taxpayers' levies or taxes, which cover injury insurance, and of which a portion is distributed to ACC to work on programs for injury prevention. New Zealand Rugby Union also receives income from sponsors and broadcasters, which is then used to fund and support injury prevention programs such as RugbySmart (K. Quarrie, personal communication, July 25, 2007).

At the time of this case study, both Quarrie and Gianotti agreed that there is no difficulty in accessing necessary financial and human resources. They indicated that increasing funding is not required for RugbySmart as program needs are met annually with the funding that is issued. Furthermore, they both feel that they are in a position to ask for additional funding if they think something is lacking in the program; if they were able to access more funding, they would allocated it toward filming the RugbySmart video (S. Gianotti, personal communication, July 22, 2007) and more publicity and advertising (K. Quarrie, personal communication, July 25, 2007).

5.2.2 Human Resources

At the game level, the NZRU is particularly responsible for organizing a meeting for all rugby professionals located in each province in New Zealand's franchise areas with the aim of deriving feedback on the delivery of RugbySmart programs. Specifically, they use a peer support system in which they pair amateur coaches with experienced professional coaches. At the administrative level, NZRU chief executives meet to discuss the relationship between sub-organizations within the NZRU, including the department that deals with RugbySmart. Along policy lines, during the development of strategies for RIPP in the late 1990s, the NZRU made a policy change to enforce the compulsory nature of the workshops. This policy was enforced for RugbySmart (S. Gianotti, personal communication, July 25, 2007).

Meanwhile, the medical and physiotherapy communities contribute directly and indirectly: the professional teams have their own physicians and physiotherapists. Yet, as the ACC and the NZRU have formed strong relationships with these experts, they act as key informants and stakeholders who can be consulted at any time for advice concerning RugbySmart protocols as well as to provide feedback for the implementation of the program (S. Gianotti, personal communication, July 25, 2007). At the grassroots level, people are "quite passionate" and so they are vocal about any concerns regarding local rugby members with injured spinal cords; while the media and the academic community support RugbySmart by bringing attention to the need for injury prevention strategies through news or journal articles (S. Gianotti, personal communication, July 25, 2007).

RDOs have been involved since the inception of RugbySmart and are responsible for facilitating the compulsory workshops; a resource book has been prepared, which includes a great deal of information about injury prevention, injury statistics, and presentation materials outlining specific expectations of RugbySmart sessions (K. Quarrie, personal communication, July 25, 2007).

Overall, the stakeholders of RugbySmart are arranged within a reasonably flexible, nonhierarchical structure where any stakeholder can be engaged "without hesitation or formalities" (S. Gianotti, personal communication, July 25, 2007). According to S. Gianotti (personal communication, July 22, 2007), geographical proximity between the ACC and the NZRU contributes to the flexibility. The offices for the ACC and the NZRU are a mere 10-min walk from one another. Being in the same city is highly beneficial because they are able to engage more frequently and readily for face-to-face communication, and further, it enables more immediate implementation of any new developments of RugbySmart (S. Gianotti, personal communication, July 22, 2007).

5.3   Implementation

The implementation of RugbySmart is based on removing injury as a barrier, so players can increase their participation in sport as well as in other physical activities. The aim of implementation is also to improve the health of players and reduce health costs associated with injuries. The primary method of implementation for RugbySmart continues to be the utilizing of the strategic connection between coaches, referees, and players and providing them with educational resources. Ultimately, the strategies implemented in RugbySmart were developed based on promoting a combination of single approaches relevant to improving technique in the game of rugby; RugbySmart has become a multifaceted approach to injury prevention (S. Gianotti, personal communication, July 18, 2007).

By 2007, RugbySmart continued to operate under the principles of the Ten-Point Action Plan of the SportSmart program. As previously mentioned, SportSmart is the ACC's general injury prevention program. SportSmart aims to optimize peak performance while simultaneously preventing injury. From the Ten-Point Action Plan, RugbySmart utilizes strategies to address injury prevention at three stages: primary, secondary, and tertiary prevention. Primary prevention prevents injury from happening on the rugby field; secondary prevention reduces the impacts of injury during the game; and tertiary prevents reinjury primarily by ensuring that players are fully recovered before returning to play (S. Gianotti, personal communication, July 18, 2007). In order to discuss the Ten Point Action Plan in relation to the three stages of injury prevention, each point is highlighted by the title as it appears in the Plan, as well as its numbers in sequence within the plan (indicated within brackets).

5.3.1   Primary Prevention

RugbySmart begins with the player profile (1), whereby the players are screened to assess technical skill, playing grade/level, physical conditioning, and predisposition to injury. Players complete a health questionnaire and undergo a physical assessment with their coaches. To measure player improvements and the effectiveness of training, RugbySmart encourages coaches to do follow-up screenings with their players throughout the season (New Zealand Rugby Union [NZRU] & ACC, 2004). The process of screening enables monitoring of a player over the course of the season, so as to predict the long-term health of the player and the propensity for injury.

Players are encouraged to prevent injuries at the primary level by warming up, cooling down, and stretching (2). The aim of the cool down and stretch is to increase the rate of recovery for players so that they are physically and mentally equipped to play games throughout the season. The warm-up includes aerobic exercise, dynamic stretching, and position-specific stretches; the cool down and stretch includes aerobic exercise, static stretching, and recovery (i.e., rehydration) (NZRU & ACC, 2004). Stretching information is provided in the form of a wallet card, which is distributed electronically to coaches. Since the coach is responsible for printing the information out and distributing it to the players, any barriers or issues regarding printing costs and distribution are practically nonexistent for the ACC, as this cost is shared by the NZRU (S. Gianotti, personal communication, July 18, 2007).

Two other main components of primary prevention in RugbySmart include physical conditioning (3) and technique management (4). Physical conditioning requires coaches to progressively introduce impact activities to build 'rugby fitness' or 'match fitness'… and progressively increase … training as players improve their conditioning levels (NZRU & ACC, 2004). Physical conditioning is addressed in four key phases: off-season (November to January; general preparation); pre-season (February–March; specific preparation); in-season (April–August; maintenance); and transition (September–October; recovery). Although the focus of the training changes based on the phase, the overall objective is to assess whether a player is (continually) fit to play rugby throughout the year (NZRU

Table 5.3 Technique recommended by RugbySmart

Smother tackles	Scrum—pre-engagement	Scrum—engagement
Not recommended for younger or less experienced players Build your players skills progressively—players should not attempt the smother tackle unless they have mastered the basic tackle technique The same steps apply as for any tackle except that contact is made between the waist and chest The arms should be wrapped around the ball-carrier's arms preventing the release of the ball	Prepare for engagement on the ref's call "crouch and hold" Front rows are safe distance apart—crouched and bound Feet, hips, and shoulders are all square Bend at the knees and hips Shoulders above hips at all times Head up, chin off chest Back straight—spine in line Eyes focused on the target area Weight off the heels and on the balls of your feet If not in the correct position or feel unsafe shout: "Not ready, ref" Never look away from your opponent once in the crouch position Engage only on the ref's call: "engage"	Drive from a low position up Loose-head binds onto the middle of the opposing tight-head's lower back Tight-head binds onto the middle of the opposing loose-head's lower back Binding should be firm and held until the scrum is completed

Note: RugbySmart (2007)

& ACC, 2006). For example, for scrum machine safety, modifications are made based on observations made during team trainings. RugbySmart revised previous trainings on scrum machines from a couple of hundred scrum machines trainings per week, to no more than 50 per week. The aim of this modification was to reduce the incidence of the degeneration of the spine (S. Gianotti, personal communication, July 18, 2007).

Physical conditioning techniques, such as scrum drills, are introduced to players by the coaches and RDOs in the 40-minute RugbySmart DVD. For all techniques on physical conditioning instructed in the DVD, coaches are responsible for encouraging players to browse the website to access more detailed information about how to ensure training is planned and position specific (S. Gianotti, personal communication, July 18, 2007).

A notable number of spine injuries also occur from improper techniques (S. Gianotti, personal communication, July 17, 2007). Technique management requires coaches in all playing levels of rugby to demonstrate how the correct technique in the contact phases of the game reduces mild to serious rugby injuries, while simultaneously showing how it ensures optimal player performance and wins games (S. Gianotti, personal communication, July 18, 2007). Safe and correct technique instruction is provided on the DVD for

tackling, smother tackles, taking the ball into contact, pre-engagement scrums, and engagement scrums (Table 5.3).

Coaches, referees, and players are all required to understand how to correctly undertake a tackle and properly take the ball into contact and to innately understand the scrum (i.e., the way in which to restart play and gain control of a game). More specifically, coaches are expected to make sure that players avoid contact situations that are not appropriate for a specific age or level of experience (NZRU & ACC, 2004). In fact, a lack of knowledge about technique strategies has been linked to many injuries in the amateur game (e.g., the person being tackled is more severely injured than the person doing the tackling). Thus, making changes to the professional rugby techniques that are applied at the amateur level is vital as the amateur game is less technique savvy and more widely played (S. Gianotti, personal communication, July 17, 2007).

Meanwhile, referees are expected to communicate with players during, for example, scrum-engagement to ensure that players are sufficiently experienced and strong enough to play the strategic positions of the scrum. Referees are also required to listen actively when the player instructs them "not ready, Ref" so they can reposition themselves in the scrum (NZRU & ACC, 2004).

5.3.2 Secondary Prevention

RugbySmart values fair play (5), where players are instructed to play with respect, dignity, and discipline within their own teams as well as with the opposition. It follows that if the game gets out of control, play can become reckless and dangerous—increasing the potential for injury. Therefore, foul play is not tolerated, and the decisions of the referees are supported and respected (NZRU & ACC, 2006).

RugbySmart emphasizes the use of protective and correct equipment (6), for example, mouth guards or footwear. With regard to mouth guards, there has been an increase of self-reported use by players from 67% to 93% between 1993 and 2003, respectively (Quarrie, Gianotti, Chalmers, & Hopkins, 2005). Consequently, dental injury claims have reduced 43% between 1995 and 2003 following the compulsory use of mouth guards in New Zealand (Quarrie et al., 2005). For protective equipment, the program tries to ensure that the proper footwear is worn for practices and games. Although the NZRU is not sponsored by Adidas as they are not allowed to endorse a merchandise provider, an Adidas representative does demonstrate to players the proper footwear for the rugby field. The NZRU and the ACC approve the type of footwear demonstrated so as to ensure quality assurance (S. Gianotti, personal communication, July 18, 2007). Therefore, RugbySmart reduces the risk of sustaining mild-to-serious injury in play and in practice that results from poor gripping and fitting of footwear. RugbySmart encourages rehydration and proper nutrition (7).

5.3.3 Tertiary Prevention

Injury reporting (8) involves identifying and reporting the injury and is also considered both a primary and secondary prevention method. Players are expected to report injury and modify or avoid training so as to reduce the risk of reinjury (e.g., reduce or avoid scrum machine at practice; S. Gianotti, personal communication, July 18, 2007). Meanwhile, for injury reporting the responsibility lies with the player and the team in general—it follows that if a player is injured, he is encouraged to inform the coach; if a player is seriously injured, the coach is required to inform the Provincial Union using the serious injury report form (NZRU & ACC, 2004).

Environment (9) refers to ensuring safe indoor and outdoor surfaces for play, adequate sport equipment is used, as well as monitoring weather conditions. Meanwhile, injury management (10) utilizes the information from injury reporting to develop two strategies: the sideline concussion card, and instructions in injury management techniques provided on the DVD to players, referees, and coaches (such as getting injured players off the field to seek treatment and using techniques derived from CPR methods). CPR techniques strongly suggest to coaches, referees, and players to stop the game completely and adequately address situations where players have potentially sustained serious neck and concussion injuries. More specifically, coaches, referees, and players are explicitly instructed not to move someone with a serious neck injury unless they stop breathing; in this case, the injured player must be rolled over. They are also instructed not to move a player who has been concussed. If they want or need to continue the game, then the referee is allowed to hold the game so as wait until the player has been removed from the field, or they can move the game to another field nearby (S. Gianotti, personal communication, July 18, 2007).

Overall, injury management is emerging as the key tertiary injury prevention strategy within RugbySmart. At this time, the main tertiary prevention strategy in the program is to try to encourage the player to stay out of the game until he or she is physically fit to return to play (K. Quarrie, personal communication, July 23, 2007). According to Gianotti (personal communication, July 18, 2007), the NZRU and the ACC are changing the ethos of the game regarding issues of playing after injury while reinjured: coaches need to understand that it is effective to rotate the squad, to manage injuries of their players, and to not put pressure on players to come back to play too early. To iterate this effectively, the RugbySmart DVD in 2007 had a player from the New Zealand's professional league, the All Blacks, discuss the implications of returning to the game too quickly. He discusses how he was reinjured because he returned to play unfit, which resulted in him being reinjured and removed from play for a year so as to recover. Overall, by avoiding play, however, the team is ensuring that the player will be able to continue later in the season, or in the subsequent season in top condition (S. Gianotti, personal communication, July 18, 2007).

5.3.4 Examples of the Prevention Methods for Brain and Spinal Cord Injury

RugbySmart sideline concussion card. To identify and prevent severe brain injury at the amateur level, RugbySmart distributes the Sideline Concussion Card—it is an affordable and convenient card that is distributed to players from amateur to professional levels of rugby (at the professional level, ImPACT System or the COG Sports System is available). The concussion card is credit card sized (Campbell, n.d.) and fits in the palm of the hand. It asks 12 medical and amnesia questions (S. Gianotti, personal communication, July 16, 2007) and is introduced to rugby players in the RugbySmart DVD and also by the RDOs in the RugbySmart sessions.

The aim of the concussion card is simply to manage the symptoms of a concussion so as to reduce the severity of injury and the likelihood of reinjury (S. Gianotti, personal communication, July 16, 2007). The questions highlight the signs and symptoms of a concussion and provide a protocol on how to follow up 48 hours after a suspected trauma to the brain or a concussion has occurred. According to Gianotti (personal communication, July 18, 2007), "if any of the 12 orientation, concentration, and memory questions is answered incorrectly, further medical evaluation is recommended before the player can return to the game" (Campbell, n.d., p. 11). Should a concussion or head trauma be diagnosed, the NZRU has a mandatory three-week period for which players must rest; to return to the training or play, the player must receive medical clearance and be symptom free (Campbell, n.d.).

Back straight—spine in line. The aim of the Back Straight—Spine in Line technique is to reduce the risk of spinal injuries during a scrimmage. In the RugbySmart DVD, explicit instruction is provided on how to get the back straight and spine in line. The DVD suggests players get a mirror to examine their posture as they are on all fours; if they see a curvature of the back, they tilt their pelvis in so that their back is completely straight. The player is then suggested to stand up, bend forward at the waist, and take the same position, with the pelvis tilted forward so that the back is completely straight (NZRU & ACC, 2007).

Head up, chin off chest. Head up, Chin off Chest instructs players not to tilt their head too far up while in the scrum position. In the DVD, the player is instructed to wear a pair of sunglasses as they crouch and hold so that they are just able to look just above the sunglasses as they are in the crouch and hold scrum position. The position is verified to be the correct technique when the player stands in a normal, upright position and is able to face forward as he or she would naturally in everyday life. The position will prevent the head from dropping and being turned to the side in contact situations (NZRU & ACC, 2007).

Pelvic tilt. The Pelvic Tilt instructs players to put their forefinger and thumb on their hips bending at the knees slightly, so the legs are partly relaxed. The players are subsequently instructed to push their pelvis forward and back to demonstrate the way in which the pelvis can rotate forward and back. The players are then instructed to practice the wrong technique, crouching while shifting their pelvis forward. They are shown how this restricts their mobility downward. They are subsequently instructed to push their pelvis back and to crouch and hold, which enables the player to be in the perfect scrum position (NZRU & ACC, 2007).

Back Straight—Spine in Line, Head up, Chin off Chest, and the Pelvic Tilt are all techniques instructions for the scrum pre-engagement (i.e., means of restarting play and gaining control of a game). In the scrum pre-engagement, players prepare for engagement on the referee's call "crouch and hold" and engage only on the referee's call: "engage." All of these changes have been directly linked to a fundamental change in the game—increased control by the referees in the game—and have reflected positively in the reduced rates of injury (NZRU & ACC, 2007).

5.3.5 Effective Strategies for Implementation

Strong and open communication between all of the stakeholders involved in the program was identified as one of the most effective strategies used to implement the prevention techniques of RugbySmart. In fact, to facilitate communication, relationship building is imperative (Bourgeois, Noce, Smeh, & Morton, 2006). According to Gianotti (personal communication, July 24, 2007), strong and open communication has led to the development of better products (e.g., DVD, compulsory sessions, concussion cards, stretching cards) due to the fact that the ACC and the NZRU understand who the target audience is, what is important to them, and how to communicate the correct techniques and strategies to them. Creating two-way communication with an open dialogue, where the input of the stakeholders is valued, means that the program is relating meaningfully to the target population. Once the stakeholders invest meaning into the program, they are more likely to adapt or change their behavior (S. Gianotti, personal communication, July 24, 2007).

The compulsory nature of the seminars is another one of the most effective strategies used in RugbySmart. The sessions are attended by almost 100% of coaches and referees thereby demonstrating their effective employment (K. Quarrie, personal communication, July 24, 2007). Ultimately, this implies that if 100% of coaches are attending the session, then the reach to the players is immense because the link to the players is the coach (K. Quarrie, personal communication, July 17, 2007). If coaches do not attend the RugbySmart seminar they are required to withdraw from competition by the NZRU until they have completed the requirements of RugbySmart. Meanwhile, referees are also penalized for not attending the compulsory sessions, by not being assigned matches to referee (K. Quarrie, personal communication, July 24, 2007). To encourage attendance to the compulsory sessions, the information presented at the sessions has also been designed so that implementation is relatively easy to execute and useful to the target audience (K. Quarrie, personal communication, July 24, 2007).

RugbySmart mainly focuses on being interactive and understandable in practical terms for all cultures and genders (S. Gianotti, personal communication, July 24, 2007). A diversity of people from different ethnic backgrounds appear in the video, and some of the RDOs are able to communicate in languages other than English. Some educational materials are available in Maori, Samoan, and Tonga (i.e., the concussion card) and the wording found in all of the material tends to stay away from highly complex scientific, biomechanical, and statistical language. Further, since there is no specific ethnicity or culture group that needs more focus in the program (K. Quarrie, personal communication, July 24, 2007), RugbySmart does not modify the DVD or the compulsory courses for any particular ethnic group (S. Gianotti, personal communication, July 24, 2007).

5.3.6 Effective Strategies for Preventing Injuries

The techniques provided in RugbySmart have been deemed effective in preventing injuries from occurring in rugby. Some aspects of the injury management section have also been effective to prevent injuries, for example, strategies that deal with soft tissue injury severity and concussions, and mouth guards (S. Gianotti, personal communication, July 24, 2007).

The content of the materials devised for the physical conditioning, technique, and injury management aspects of RugbySmart have been specifically designed to enhance player performance and safety. More specifically, RugbySmart materials and workshops encourage coaches, referees, and players to understand the manner in which spinal injuries can occur when loading the body into various positions (K. Quarrie, personal communication, July 24, 2007). For example, the correct scrummaging techniques have been notably successful because they specifically show how the spine must be positioned in order not to injure the spinal cord (S. Gianotti, personal communication, July 24, 2007). A second example comes from injury management: the strategy follows that coaches and players understand that reinjury is not a smart sport strategy; rather, a winning strategy is not to let the player return too early to train and to play (K. Quarrie, personal communication, July 24, 2007).

Gianotti (personal communication, July 24, 2007) indicates that RugbySmart is continually evolving so as to continuously enhance the implementation of the program strategies as well as to further ensure injuries are being prevented. The ACC and the NZRU examine claim data in the short, medium, and long term to determine the most prevalent nature, severity, and cause of injury. In 2007, based on examination into past entitlement claims data, the ACC and the NZRU decided to focus specifically on safe and effective tackles for the 2008 RugbySmart program (S. Gianotti, personal communication, July 24, 2007). The NZRU undertook a large-scale prospective study of risk factors for tackle injuries among professional rugby players from 2003 to 2005. The information yielded by this study will play a part in developing injury prevention strategies that focus specifically on the tackle. They also decided to focus on tackles because they found out through surveying that most coaches were unaware that tackles were the cause of the greatest number of serious spinal injuries in rugby in the last 10 years (K. Quarrie, personal communication, January 16, 2008). The ACC and the NZRU intend to work with coaches to redesign the tackle strategy so that it is useful to win games, while simultaneously effective to prevent spinal injury. Once the strategy has been included into the RugbySmart DVD, and the technique is applied in the game, the results of the strategy's effectiveness will be measurable almost immediately because injuries are tracked as they occur

and interaction with coaches is done readily throughout the season (S. Gianotti, personal communication, July 24, 2007).

The main obstacle to implementing the strategy is resistance from the coaches to participate in the compulsory nature of the program (S. Gianotti, personal communication, July 24, 2007). Quarrie (personal communication, July 24, 2007) understands the rigidity in making the seminar compulsory and then requesting that stakeholders volunteer their time to participate. But he notes that the compulsory requirement reflects how important the issue of injuries is and how seriously the NZRU and the ACC take the issue of player safety and player welfare in rugby. Further, in response to such resistance, the ACC and the NZRU try to reinforce the perception and understanding that RugbySmart adds value to the game of rugby and maintains the ethos of the game (i.e., to win and to ensure player safety; S. Gianotti, personal communication, July 24, 2007).

Overall, the obstacles remain the same, but they change in degree of importance to the stakeholders and in the initiatives the ACC and the NZRU employ in addressing them (S. Gianotti, personal communication, July 24, 2007). For example, to incorporate change, the NZRU and the ACC typically examine the injury statistics of the game and watch for emerging trends. They also look for outside examples of exemplary practice in other contact sports and use feedback from the coaches and the RDOs (S. Gianotti, personal communication, July 24, 2007; K. Quarrie, personal communication, July 24, 2007).

The structured (e.g., questionnaires and meetings for RDOs, coaches, and referees) and unstructured (e.g., anecdotal when ACC or NZRU staff go to the games) feedback from coaches, referees, and players is valued and considered utmost in the decision making and planning process at the amateur level because of its large size (S. Gianotti, personal communication, July 24, 2007; K. Quarrie, personal communication, July 24, 2007). All of these stakeholders, however, are considered experts who help to make optimal decisions for RugbySmart (S. Gianotti, personal communication, July 24, 2007).

The final decision to employ changes that are suggested from the feedback is executed by Quarrie and Gianotti, who meet every 2 weeks and consider their partnership an equal 50/50 split (S. Gianotti, personal communication, July 24, 2007; K. Quarrie, personal communication, July 24, 2007). For coaches, players, and referees, the strategies are redeployed when RugbySmart is released the next season; while within the ACC and the NZRU, the changes in the program are presented in the case operational and financial plans. Ultimately, the changes made to the product are aimed at reflecting added value to the product (S. Gianotti, personal communication, July 24, 2007), in which no large bureaucracies or politics impact the decision making to improve the program (K. Quarrie, personal communication, July 24, 2007). Should any bureaucracies, politics or even disagreements come up, both Gianotti and Quarrie speak to one another to resolve the issue. If the issue is too large for Gianotti and Quarrie to contend with, it is outlined in their contracts that they are able to speak to people at higher levels of their respective organizations (S. Gianotti, personal communication, July 25, 2007; K. Quarrie, personal communication, July 24, 2007).

Other checks made regarding the RugbySmart strategies include RDOs taking attendance at the workshops to ensure that coaches have attended the compulsory workshops (K. Quarrie, personal communication, July 24, 2007). To check the rate of attendance in each region, the number of coaches who attend the workshop is cross-checked and stored in a database with the number of teams in each region; attendance is further cross-checked anecdotally when Gianotti or Quarrie attend games on weekends and discuss procedures with RDOs or coaches (S. Gianotti, personal communication, July 25, 2007). The NZRU and the ACC take attendance to RugbySmart's compulsory sessions very seriously. In fact, if a serious injury occurred to a player in one of the provincial union teams where the coach of the team had not met RugbySmart, the provincial union would be under scrutiny as to why the injury took place. Further, in terms of accountability of the RDOs, as New Zealand is a

relatively small country, if coaches were going to these sessions and found that RDOs were not doing their job well, the NZRU and the ACC claim they would likely be informed (K. Quarrie, personal communication, July 24, 2007).

According to Gianotti (personal communication, July 25, 2007), for effective implementation early preparation is imperative, which is why modifications are designed within a year prior to the start of the new season, and employed at the beginning of each new rugby year (i.e., plans for the 2008 season are made starting in July 2007; S. Gianotti, personal communication, July 25, 2007; K. Quarrie, personal communication, July 24, 2007). In fact, Gianotti (personal communication, July 25, 2007) contends that "if you're not ready by the start of the season, you might as well give up, go home and do it next year. There's no point introducing something three-quarters of the way through the season or halfway through the season." To date, there have been several adjustments made to RugbySmart's implementation based on past internal and external evaluations. For example, the frequency of requalification for coaches in certain leagues (S. Gianotti, personal communication, July 25, 2007).

5.4   Outcome

Quarrie (personal communication, July 25, 2007) states that an explicit goal of RugbySmart is "to produce an evidence-based best practiced product that speaks to coaches and referees in language that they understand and that they identify with [so] to try and make sure they [the stakeholders] know [and]…apply the information that's being provided [to them]". Since the conception of RugbySmart, there have been reductions in rugby-related injury claims every year. In fact, in 2005 the number of claims reduced by 4% compared to statistics in 2004 (NZRU & ACC, 2006); and in 2006 compared to 2005, claims were further reduced by 5.5% (S. Gianotti, personal communication, July 24, 2007). By bodily location of injury, neck/spine and back have decreased by 13%; knee, ankles, and lower legs have decreased by 4%; shoulders have decreased by 7%, and dental claims have decreased by 7% (NZRU & ACC, 2006) since the implementation of RugbySmart in 2001 (see Fig. 5.6).

From 2001 to 2005, there were five recorded spinal injuries in New Zealand rugby, while the predicted number based on previous experience with rugby injuries was 18.9. Further, between 2001 and 2005, there was one scrum-related spinal injury versus the nine predicted to occur. Table 5.4 further demonstrates that scrum-related injuries were recorded as 0 for 4 of the 5 years between 2001 and 2005 (highlighted in bold).

For tackles, rucks, and mauls, there were seven reported injuries, lower compared with a predicted 9 (Quarrie et al., 2007).

In the long term, scrum-related serious injuries have also decreased significantly. According to Quarrie et al. (2007), there were 77 scrum-related injuries between 1976 and 2005, and 35 permanently disabling scrum-related spinal injuries (Quarrie et al., 2007). Of these totals only one occurred between 2001 and 2005 (see Fig. 5.7). The rationale for studying the injuries from the past 30 years was to ensure that the

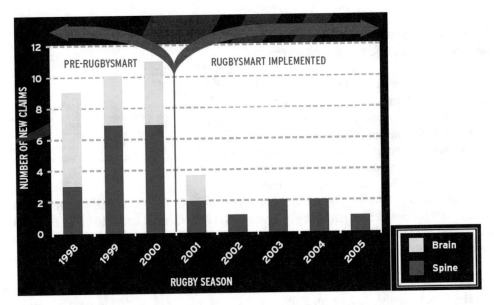

Fig. 5.6 Number of serious injuries in rugby as illustrated by ACC claims, 1998–2005 (NZRU & ACC, 2006)

Table 5.4 Player numbers and injury rates per year, 1996–2006

Year	No. of players (thousand)	Change from previous years (%)	Scrum injuries	Other injuries	Injury rate (per 100,000 players per year)
1996	NA	NA	3	1	NA
1997	NA	NA	0	1	NA
1998	122	NA	0	2	1.6
1999	130	6	4	1	3.9
2000	129	−1	2	3	3.9
2001	120	−7	0	2	1.7
2002	122	1	0	1	0.8
2003	121	−1	0	2	1.7
2004	129	6	1	1	1.6
2005	138	6	0	1	0.7

Note: Quarrie et al. (2007)

Fig. 5.7 Permanently disabling spinal injuries in the NZRU, scrum, other, and total, 1976–2005 (ACC, n.d.-b)

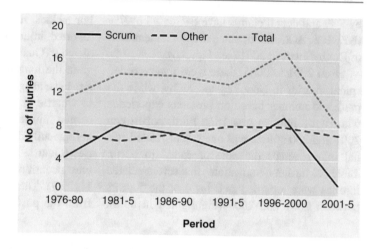

outcomes of RugbySmart were "not a fluke or coincidental" (S. Gianotti, personal communication, July 16, 2007).

The country of New Zealand has a system that comprehensively collects nationwide injury data, which has allowed researchers to conclude the effectiveness and communicate the new law on scrum engagement through RugbySmart. Results show that among the moderate-to-serious claims between 2002 and 2006, there were only three injuries that occurred following the amateur season, while two injuries had people taking greater than 2 months to seek ACC treatment. At the end of the first year, analysis shows that the new law change seems to have had the intended impact on scrum-related head and neck injuries (Gianotti, Hume, Hopkins, Harawira, & Truman, 2008).

One strategy that has shown particularly positive outcomes at the community level is the sideline concussion card. Research into claim statistics has shown that there has been a 24% decrease in moderate-to-serious head injury claims in the first year, which was maintained in the second year. More specifically, there has even been a decrease in the number of days between having been injured and going to seek treatment (median 6 days vs. median 3 days; S. Gianotti, personal communication, July 16, 2007). Overall, the Concussion Management Education Program (CMEP) including the sideline concussion card, as well as the RugbySmart educational video resulted in cost savings of US$690,690 (actual) to US$3,354,780 (forecast). In fact, "the 2-year

Table 5.5 Changes in behavior pre and post RugbySmart

Behavior	Response		
	1997, %	1998, %	2005, %
Spending time on training tackle techniques		56	86
Safe tackle in play		41	68
Safe scrum in play	73%		93

Note: S. Gianotti, personal communication, July 16, 2007

cost of CMEP was US$54,810 returning US$12.60 (actual) and US$61.21 (forecast) for every $US1 invested (ROI)" (Gianotti & Hume, 2007, p. 4).

In 2005, the NZRU and the ACC also conducted a self-assessed behavior survey among 473 players in all NZRU leagues (no more than four players were surveyed from one team) to compare with a survey conducted in 1997 and 1998. The questions were asked as the players got off of the field to ensure that the answers would be as situational as possible (Table 5.5).

According to Gianotti (personal communication, July 16, 2007), between 1997 and 2005 claims made to the ACC from the NZRU have decreased and there has been a change in behavior in roughly more than the 20% magnitude (see Fig. 5.8; S. Gianotti, personal communication, July 16, 2007).

To evaluate the effectiveness of a strategy, a 5-year prospective study was conducted to formally evaluate the program in 2006–2007, a self-assessed survey of players was conducted in 2005,

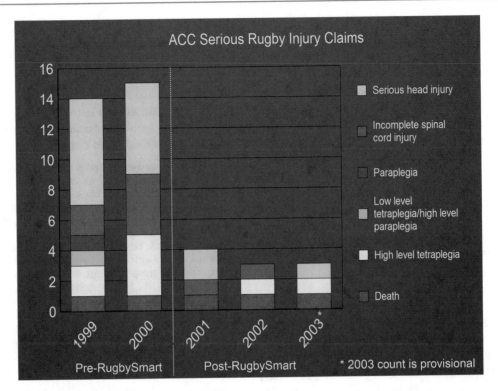

Fig. 5.8 ACC serious rugby injury claims (ACC, n.d.b)

which was a survey already conducted in 1997 and 1998; and the NZRU and the ACC have coaches complete a quiz at the end of the compulsory sessions so as to evaluate the knowledge gained from the DVD and other materials, and to also understand how to improve the program. This quiz has been employed annually since 2004 (S. Gianotti, personal communication, July 25, 2007).

For internal evaluation, the ACC provides monthly progress reports to their management. The progress reports describe the corporate target that RugbySmart aimed to achieve and are sent for evaluation to the minister and a board of executives. To improve the quality of data in evaluations, the NZRU and the ACC encourage players, coaches, and referees to make claims with the ACC where statistics realistically reflect the program's target population (S. Gianotti, personal communication, July 25, 2007).

So that the outcomes reflect the strategies of RugbySmart positively, the NZRU and the ACC rely heavily on stakeholders to provide anecdotal evidence of what they are actually experiencing because they are practitioners and the producers at the community level. For example, 1 year the grips were demonstrated in a slightly incorrect manner in the DVD, which the coaches and players identified as unrealistic to the game. Stakeholder role is formalized and valued because they are brought in to provide input on the contents of the DVD. They are also the main actors for the DVD (S. Gianotti, personal communication, July 25, 2007). RDOs are also crucial evaluators of the program because they act as mediators between the NZRU leagues and the administration at the NZRU and the ACC (K. Quarrie, personal communication, July 25, 2007).

The accountability of the program implementers and all of the stakeholders is reflected in the strong relationship between the NZRU and the ACC, the use of insurance claims data (which are collected monthly), the number of serious injuries (collected monthly at hospitals and by provincial unions), feedback provided from the RDOs, general stakeholder contentment with the program, financial records compiled the ACC and provided to auditors, and approval from management at the NZRU and the ACC (S. Gianotti, personal communication, July 25, 2007; K. Quarrie, personal communication, July 24, 2007). By dividing the responsibility to evaluate the program, RugbySmart has been able to achieve both its long- and short-term goals, including reducing serious injuries, developing a strong relationship between the NZRU and the ACC (S. Gianotti, personal communication, July 25, 2007), and improving accuracy in the public perception of the risk of injury and attitude toward playing with and treating the injury (K. Quarrie, personal communication, July 25, 2007). The short-term goals that have been achieved are the success in the information and program strategies that are produced annually and monthly changes in the rate of injuries and the changes in behaviors (S. Gianotti, personal communication, July 25, 2007; K. Quarrie, personal communication, July 25, 2007).

Openness to set new goals is particularly important to RugbySmart due to the unanticipated positive and negative outcomes that may arise as the program is being implemented and redesigned and as changes are being made to the game as a whole. For example, historically, the rules of rugby have changed, which resulted in changes to game structures and match activities. As a result of these changes, there was an increase in the risk of scrum-related spinal injuries. In response to a change such as this, they made sure the DVD and materials addressed the causes of these injuries. Moreover, on the whole, the NZRU and the ACC try to ensure that they are prepared for whatever positive or negative outcomes may arise from any change; where they are not prepared, they try to learn from the outcomes and redevelop the approach taken in RugbySmart (K. Quarrie, personal communication, July 25, 2007).

Quarrie and Gianotti (personal communication, July 25, 2007) contend that to achieve this goal and to adequately apply the lessons learned from implementation, they create open lines for stakeholders to communicate, are innovative in the design of RugbySmart strategies, and, foremost, are active listeners to what their stakehold-

ers are trying to communicate. Further, according to Gianotti (personal communication, personal communication, July 25, 2007) without the strong support of a national body, this goal could not be achieved, and they would not be facilitated to make improvements and learn from past judgments. Quarrie (personal communication, July 25, 2007) concurs and states that:

> …there are advantages for sports to have internal drivers for injury prevention, who can promote the messages that injury prevention is the corollary of great performance, not the other way around. It's very important for the sport to own the issues, if you try and impose upon a sport, injury prevention programs that are seen as being something of an external agency, or if the language is not the language used by the participants, these things will not be as successful…So the sports need to understand clearly what the benefits are, and they need to believe in those benefits. [They need to invest the] time to take on-board and change behaviors because otherwise these behaviors won't change [and] they don't see that the benefits [of change] outweigh the costs [of not changing].

Ultimately, strategies that enhance the implementation of RugbySmart and the prevention of injuries in the sport are initiatives that add value to the sport of rugby and respond to the needs and expectations of the stakeholders. The strategies employed in RugbySmart to reduce mild-to-severe injuries have been and will continue to improve the techniques for players, which will ultimately win games for both players and coaches (S. Gianotti, personal communication, July 24, 2007). According to Gianotti (personal communication, July 24, 2007), it is "really (about) understanding what your client wants, and working out what you want, and then coming up with something magical in the middle to meet the two."

The RugbySmart program continues to grow and sustain success in its initiative to prevent and treat injuries for rugby players through expanding education and training for coaches and referees, as well as health care providers, athletes, and parents. Through a recent expansion to its program objectives as outlines on its website, RugbySmart has defined three objectives that are fundamental to the program with six specific modules to execute its objectives (NZRU, n.d.; see Fig. 5.9).

The Three Objectives that Underpin the Program:

1. Injuries are prevented where possible
2. Treatment for injury is of a required standard to minimize the immediate impact to the individual; and
3. Recovery is supported to ensure the best long-term outcome possible

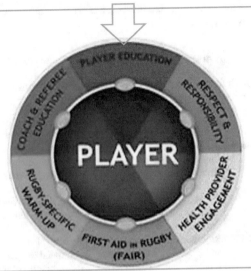

1. Player Education: providing players with skills and techniques to keep them and their team meats safe
2. Health Provider Engagement: tools and decision-making aids to allow health providers to manage concussion and other sport related injuries more effectively.
3. First Aid in Rugby (Fair): First aid education for the rugby community that equips individuals with the skills to better manage injured athletes safely.
4. Respect and Responsibility: Tailored program with a focus on respectful relationships, including consent, sexual assault and violence prevention
5. Rugby Specific Warm-Up: Research based injury prevention program based around a warm up routine for training and playing rugby.
6. Coach and Referee Education: This represents the current RugbySmart program that ACC invests in a detailed addendum to this established module to include the Blue Card initiative forms part of this document.

Fig. 5.9 The objectives that underpin the program (NZRU, n.d.)

The RugbySmart program continues to grow and expand with the persistent support of the ACC, who announced in 2016 that they will invest $7 million over the next 4 years into the program to enhance education in injury prevention and treatment for rugby players (ACC, 2016).

Acknowledgments The authors would like to express sincere appreciation to the key informants for this case study: Simon M. Gianotti of the Accident Compensation Corporation in Wellington, New Zealand and Kenneth Quarrie of the New Zealand Rugby Union in Wellington, New Zealand—whose consultation made this project possible.

BRIO Model: RugbySmart

Group Served: Amateur to professional rugby players 16–44, coaches and referees.

Goal: To prevent injuries to the head and spine from tackle, scrummage, ruck, and maul techniques.

Background	Resources	Implementation	Outcome
Over 140,000 players in amateur and professional leagues across New Zealand 63% of all injuries are deemed moderate-to-serious injury, which comprise any injury that requires 5 or more days of absence from employment NZRU was so concerned about data emerging about serious injuries in rugby; they made it compulsory for all coaches to attend nationwide safety seminars by 1996 Five years after this compulsory initiative and a review of the injury incidence statistics, RugbySmart was developed The aim of RugbySmart was to optimize the role coaches, players and referees can play to reduce injuries	The ACC has provided NZ$ 1.3 million to the development and implementation of RugbySmart strategies and human resources The ACC and NZRU have a contract in which ACC provides funds for RugbySmart to the NZRU and NZRU manages these funds The NZRU made a policy change to enforce the compulsory nature of the workshops The NZRU made a policy change to enforce the compulsory nature of the workshops RDOs have been involved since the inception. Their role is to facilitate the workshops using a resource book; this includes a great deal of information about injury prevention and statistics and to present materials about expectations of RugbySmart sessions	The strategies implemented into RugbySmart were developed based on promoting a combination of single approaches relevant to improving the technique in the game of rugby, which has become a multifactorial approach By 2007, RugbySmart continued to operate under the principles of the Ten-Point Action Plan of the SportSmart program, which aims to optimize peak performance, while simultaneously preventing injury E.g. Technique management requires coaches in all playing levels to demonstrate how the correct technique in the contact phases of the game reduces mild-to-serious rugby injuries, while simultaneously showing how it ensures optimal player performance and wins games	By bodily location of injury, neck/spine and back have decreased 13%; knee, ankles, and lower legs have decreased by 4%; shoulders have decreased by 7% and dental claims have decreased by 7% since the implementation of RugbySmart in 2001 From 2001 to 2005, there were five recorded spinal injuries in New Zealand rugby, while the predicted number based on previous experience with rugby injuries was 18.9 Research into claim statistics have shown that there has been a 24% decrease in moderate-to-serious head injury claims in the first year, which was maintained in the second year

Life Space Model: Rugby Smart

Sociocultural: civilization/community	Interpersonal: primary and secondary relationships	Physical environments: where we live	Internal states: biochemical/genetic and means of coping
Awareness Raising through DVD materials Use of rugby community and league to promote safe techniques in rugby practices and games Contractual obligation to adhere to the safe techniques promoted by RugbySmart Multi-faceted strategy that includes rugby players, coaches, referees, community health practitioners, media, and national-level government	Relationship between New Zealand Rugby Union and Accident Compensation Corporation to increase knowledge and improve techniques to prevent and target injuries in rugby Relationship between coaches, players, and referees to divide responsibility for the implementation of the 10-point action plan of RugbySmart	Contact sport Detailed assessment to adequately address the high-risk nature of tackles, mauls, scrums, and rucks Evaluation of the characteristics of the rugby culture and biomechanics of rugby to implement appropriate preventative measures Adoption of the 10-point action plan	Empowerment of coaches, players and referees by training in proper technique and physical conditioning, among other aspects Strengthening relationships among key stakeholders in the game to enhance communication and prevent injury in rugby

References

Accident Compensation Corporation. (2006). Accident Compensation Corporation injury statistics 2006 (First Edition). Section 20: Sports claims. Retrieved July 17, 2007, from http://www.acc.co.nz/about-acc/acc-injury-statistics-2006/SS_WIM2_063081.

Accident Compensation Corporation. (2016). New Zealand rugby team up with ACC to expand player safety focus. Retrieved November 18, 2017, from https://www.acc.co.nz/about-us/newsmedia/latestnews/rugby-expand-safety-focus/.

Accident Compensation Corporation. (n.d.-a). How did ACC SportSmart start? Retrieved November 8, 2007, from http://www.acc.co.nz/injury-prevention/sport-safety/what-is-acc-sportsmart/WCM000589.

Accident Compensation Corporation. (n.d.-b). Sideline concussion check cards, ACC SportSmart resources. Retrieved November 11, 2007, from http://www.acc.co.nz/injury-prevention/sport-safety/resources/index.htm.

Armour, K. S., Clatworthy, B. J., Bean, A. R., Wells, J. E., & Clarke, A. M. (1997). Spinal injuries in New Zealand rugby union and rugby league: a twenty year survey. New Zealand Medical Journal, 110, 462–465.

B.C. Injury Research and Prevention Unit. (n.d.). Rugby injuries, safe risks and practices. Vancouver, BC: B.C. Injury Research and Prevention Unit.

Bourgeois, R., Noce, M., Smeh, D., & Morton, T. (2006). Sustainability of community-based health interventions: A literature review. Unpublished manuscript, University of Toronto, Toronto, ON.

Campbell, D. (n.d.). Head cases. Big Issue, 1, 10–13.

Chalmers, D. J. (2002). Injury prevention in sport: not yet part of the game? Injury Prevention, 8(4), 22–25.

Dalley, D. R., Laing, D. R., Rowberry, J. M., & Caird, M. J. (1982). Rugby injuries: an epidemiological survey, Christchurch, 1980. New Zealand Journal of Sports Medicine, 10, 5–17.

Gianotti, S., & Hume, P. A. (2007). Concussion side line management intervention for rugby union leads to reduced concussion claims. NeuroRehabilitation, 22, 1–9.

Gianotti, S., Hume, P. A., Hopkins, W. G., Harawira, J., & Truman, R. (2008). Interim evaluation of the effect of a new scrum law on neck and back injuries in rugby union. British Journal of Sports Medicine, 42, 427–430.

New Zealand Rugby Union. (n.d.). Objectives. Retrieved November 18, 2017, from https://www.rugbysmart.co.nz/objectives.

New Zealand Rugby Union & Accident Compensation Corporation. (2004). RugbySmart guide. Wellington: Authors.

New Zealand Rugby Union & Accident Compensation Corporation. (2006). RugbySmart guide. Wellington: Authors.

New Zealand Rugby Union & Accident Compensation Corporation. (2007). RugbySmart DVD. Wellington: Authors.

Paul, G. (n.d.). Risky business. Rugby News, 10–13.

Quarrie, K., & Hopkins, W. (n.d.). Player management for team success. Gameplan Rugby, 25–31.

Quarrie, K.L. (n.d.). GamePlan.

Quarrie, K. L., Cantu, R. C., & Chalmers, D. J. (2002). Rugby union injuries to the cervical spine and spinal cord. Sports Medicine, 32, 633–653.

Quarrie, K. L., Gianotti, S. M., Chalmers, D. J., & Hopkins, W. G. (2005). An evaluation of mouthguard requirements and dental injures in New Zealand Rugby union. British Journal of Sports Medicine, 39, 650–654.

Quarrie, K. L., Gianotti, S. M., Hopkins, W. G., & Hume, P. A. (2007). Effect of nationwide injury prevention programme on serious spinal injuries in New Zealand rugby union: Ecological study. *British Medical Journal, 2*, 334–1150.

Simpson, J., Chalmers, D., Waller, A., Bird, Y., Quarrie, K., Gerrard, D., et al. (1994). *Tackling Rugby injury: Recommendations for reducing injury to rugby union players in New Zealand. A proposal prepared for the Accident Rehabilitation and Compensation Insurance Corporation and the New Zealand Rugby Football Union*. Dunedin: Injury Prevention Research Unit and Human Performance Centre, University of Otago.

Van Mechelen, W., Hlobil, H., & Kemper, H. C. (1992). Incidence, severity, etiology and prevention of sports injuries: A review of concepts. *Sports Medicine, 14*, 82–99.

Yard, E. E., & Comstock, R. D. (2006). Injuries sustained by rugby players presenting to United States emergency departments, 1978–2004. *Journal of Athletic Training, 41*(3), 325–331.

SafeClub: An Effective Soccer Injury Prevention Program

6

Daisy Radha Singla

SafeClub is an injury prevention program designed for the soccer community to promote risk management techniques in soccer practices and games, which utilizes multifaceted strategies that incorporates soccer club administrators.

6.1 Background

6.1.1 History and Development

YouthSafe (ca. 1982, formerly SpineSafe) began as an injury prevention program solely devoted to preventing spinal cord injury. SpineSafe disseminated injury prevention information by employing an individual who was experiencing a spine injury to conduct information sessions about how to prevent spinal cord injury. These informational sessions were presented to youth in school settings. The implementation of SpineSafe continued until 1999 when the organization examined injury prevention evidence. As a result, YouthSafe, what was once considered a branch of SpineSafe, became SafeClub. Furthermore, while spinal cord injury remains a focus of both YouthSafe and SafeClub, both YouthSafe and SafeClub decided to focus on primary prevention of all

D. R. Singla (✉)
Sinai Health System, University of Toronto, Toronto, ON, Canada
e-mail: daisy.singla@utoronto.ca

injuries (K. Abbott, personal communication, January 23, 2008).

The program SafeClub was devised in 2001 by Alex Donaldson, former Health Promotion Officer at Northern Sydney Health Promotion Service. The foundation of the program began with research into sports safety techniques among 150 community clubs across four codes (i.e., sports): rugby league, rugby union, netball, and soccer. This research concluded that few community sports clubs implemented organized risk management techniques, and soccer community clubs were the most likely to implement the least number of sports safety-related activities (Abbott & Donaldson, 2004). A joint venture between YouthSafe and Northern Sidney Central Coast Health (NSCCH), SafeClub was subsequently founded as a private organization in 2002.

Consultations with local community sports clubs were undertaken by YouthSafe. These consultations involved communicating with sports administrators, players, and coaches to request information including current sports safety activities and resources, those lacking in demand and those activities required to support community sports clubs (K. Abbott, personal communication, January 23, 2008). According to Abbott, feedback determined that "it was obvious that giving information on a specific topic wasn't going to be relevant to a vast majority of these clubs." Thus, SafeClub was devised specifically to provide a systematic execution in managing

© Springer Nature Switzerland AG 2020
R. Volpe (ed.), *Casebook of Traumatic Injury Prevention*,
https://doi.org/10.1007/978-3-030-27419-1_6

soccer injuries regardless of their given location (K. Abbott, personal communication, January 23, 2008). To do this, they aimed to (1) identify injury priorities and (2) reduce injury risks. Consequently, a flexible and accessible 5-stage strategy of risk management was created.

6.1.2 SafeClub Risk Management Strategy and Its Implementation

According to Drawer and Fuller (2001), short-term injury management strategies are limited by a lack of financial resources; those resources available tend to be allocated toward club administration and team maintenance. This includes funding provided for the treatment and rehabilitation of injured players. However, a risk management approach has long-term benefits, as it supports the adequate allocation of sufficient resources toward injury prevention strategies (Drawer & Fuller, 2001). The 5-stage risk management model used for SafeClub was devised by Harvey, Finch, and McGrath (1997) and informed by risk management strategies in the financial legal and occupational health and safety sectors (see Fig. 6.1; Abbott & Donaldson, 2004; Abbott, Klarenaar, Donaldson, & Sherker, 2007a). It aims to achieve long-term benefits in soccer injury prevention.

Risks need to be accurately estimated and evaluated with a specific set of criteria, accepted by the general population of that sport. The responsibility for risks and minimizing risks associated with injuries and reinjuries can be identified; further, strategies for addressing these risks can be executed (Drawer & Fuller, 2001). As a result, shared responsibility, SafeClub distributes the role of implementation and risk management among all stakeholders. Specifically, SafeClub targets community sports club administrators to demystify the risk management strategy, attempting to assist community sports clubs to improve their sports safety activities.

Primary prevention in soccer benefits from the risk management concept because it is flexible and adaptable to reducing safety risks in individual clubs (Abbott, Klarenaar, Donaldson, & Sherker, 2007b). For example, NSHP found that among all sports, safety priorities of sports clubs varied significantly across a variety of factors including club size, geographic locations, facilities, the availability of human resources, and spectator characteristics (Abbott et al., 2007b). In response to this diversity, risk management provides an organized framework to identify and subsequently decrease the injury risks that are identified (Abbott et al., 2007b).

6.1.3 Pilot Study

In 2003, the implementation of the SafeClub risk management pilot study was conducted. This study included the participation of administrators

Fig. 6.1 Five-stage risk management model (Abbott & Klarenaar, 2007)

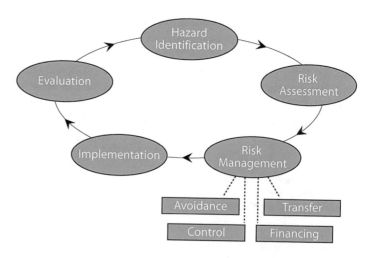

from four community soccer clubs, aiming to assist these clubs in developing and implementing a comprehensive sports safety plan based on a risk management training package. Prior to the first training session, participants completed a questionnaire to provide baseline information regarding the sports safety policies and practices implemented in their club. During training, participants were introduced to the five stages of risk management through a weekly five-session training and educational program. Participants were also introduced to injury prevention concepts. They also identified issues faced by their club and were encouraged to develop practical, evidence-informed intervention strategies to manage safety risks. Participants were then asked to complete exercises between sessions and consult with other representatives from their club. In the final session, participants were given the opportunity to develop an individualistic and comprehensive written safety plan to implement and monitor at their club.

Adult learning principles were developed based on these sessions, and a review session was held six weeks after the final training session (Abbott & Donaldson, 2004). As a result of constructive participant feedback provided at the end of each training session in the pilot study, the program was changed from five to three sessions and from 1 to 2 weeks apart between sessions. In addition, the session was changed from the beginning of the soccer season to the middle of the soccer season due to time constraints of club administrators early in the season. The content was modified to ensure that risk management-related skills were well developed and easy to understand (K. Abbott, personal communication, January 2008).

It is important to note that during the pilot study, the researchers at NSHP found that the phrase "risk management" alone make community clubs "anxious" (Abbott et al., 2007a). In response, SafeClub attempts to demystify risk management misperceptions by making the concepts and ideas applicable to the soccer community. Through a "practical, problem-centered" approach of the learning strategies, the implementers are able to "capitalize on participants'

knowledge and experience" (J. Nethery, personal communication, November 26, 2008). Furthermore, when community sports administrators are able to saliently identify, assess, and manage their specific safety risks, they are able to understand risk management beyond the legal and insurance perspective (J. Nethery, personal communication, November 26, 2008).

6.1.4 Goals and Implementation Strategies

The stated goal of SafeClub has always been to assist community clubs to reduce injury risks through the use of risk management (K. Abbott, personal communication, January 23, 2008). The goals of this strategy also include increasing the awareness, knowledge, and skills of community soccer administrators in addressing the safety and injury issues relevant to the individual club's needs (Abbott & Donaldson, 2004). Implicit goals of SafeClub also run parallel with the worldwide obesity epidemic. According to Abbott (personal communication, January 23, 2008), there is a fear that injury will cause a decrease in participation in physical activity. In turn, by introducing SafeClub and encouraging safer sports technique, SafeClub implicitly encourages parents and participants to increase their physical activity through safe sport (K. Abbott, personal communication, January 23, 2008).

6.2 Resources

Since its inception, SafeClub has targeted sports administrators (usually club secretaries and/or directors). Sports administrators were chosen as SafeClub's target population as they act like key facilitators (or antagonists) for sports safety activities (K. Abbott, personal communication, January 23, 2008). The role of this key population in relation to SafeClub is to attend SafeClub training sessions and augment their knowledge in risk management in soccer. These stakeholders are volunteers 99% of the time (personal communication, K. Abbott, January 23, 2008). SafeClub developers have chosen an individualized approach catering to club administrator habits and needs, rather than promote a prescribed set of irrelevant safety activities that may be generalized for the soccer community (Abbott et al., 2007b). In addition, the notion that these 99% of these stakeholders are volunteers is crucial to SafeClub's approach in developing a program addressing barriers of time, resource, and acquiring sports safety knowledge.

At the time of SafeClub's development, principal stakeholders of SafeClub include New South Wales Injuries Committee, Soccer New South Wales, and injury prevention professionals (K. Abbott, personal communication, January 23, 2008). Soccer New South Wales (NSW) is the governing body for soccer associations in New South Wales and a member of the national governing body, Soccer Federation Australia (SFA) (Soccer NSW, 2008). Their role as a stakeholder was to identify four affiliated community soccer associations in the Greater Sydney area for the pilot study. Soccer NSW participated in SafeClub

because of increasing pressure to use risk management strategies despite a lack of knowledge on how to support clubs at a systematic level (K. Abbott, personal communication, January 23, 2008). In turn, 101 soccer clubs were contacted to participate in the 2-year SafeClub evaluation. This involved attending three SafeClub training sessions and completing process evaluations at the start of the 2005 season (baseline), at the end of the 2005 season (post-season), and mid-2006 (12-month follow-up; Abbott et al., 2007b). During each evaluation, participating clubs completed the 72-item modified Sports Safety Audit Tool (SSAT; see Fig. 6.2, Tables 6.1 and 6.2).

New South Wales Injuries Committee (NSWIC) is an insurance body, established in 1978 by the New South Wales government (NSWIC, 2008). NSWIC is constantly facing the challenge to reduce sports injury-related claims due to sporting injuries. Due to this priority, NSWIC partially funded SafeClub's 2-year evaluation through the Research and Injury Prevention Scheme (K. Abbott, personal communication, January 23, 2008; Abbott et al., 2007a). Their

SECTION 1 – DEMOGRAPHICS

D1. What is your main position at your club *(tick one box)*

☐ President   ☐ Secretary   ☐ Treasurer   ☐ Other.............................

D2. Is your Club incorporated?   ☐ Yes   ☐ No

D3. Approximately how many players are registered with your club this year?

Age	Total players	12 and under	13-18 yrs	19-34 years	35 + years
No. players					

D4. How many teams are registered with your club this year?

D5. How many members form your club's committee?

D6. Does your club employ a paid administrator?   ☐ Yes   ☐ No
If Yes, approximately how many PAID hours does the employee work each week?

D7. What is your club's approximate annual budget? $

D8. In what year was your club established?

Fig. 6.2 Section 1 of the Sports Safety Audit Tool (Abbott et al., 2007b)

Table 6.1 Section 2 of the Sports Safety Audit Tool

Does your club have…	Yes ✓	No ✓
A documented sports safety or risk management policy to demonstrate club commitment and address broad aspects of safety and injury prevention?	Y	N
A current documented sports safety plan (outlining planned club safety activities). If yes, does it include:	Y	N
(a) Current safety priorities?	Y	N
(b) Individual responsibilities?	Y	N
(c) Time frames?	Y	N
(d) Review processes?	Y	N
A documented policy on: Emergency action in the event of severe injury?	Y	N
The management of head injuries?	Y	N
Pre-participation health screening for players (e.g., gathering information about pre-existing medical conditions or injuries)?	Y	N
A blood rule	Y	N
An infectious diseases policy—other than blood rule?	Y	N
Sun protection?	Y	N
Qualifications of referees attending competition?	Y	N
Qualifications of coaches for club teams?	Y	N
Attendance of qualified first aiders/sports trainers at competition?	Y	N
Attendance of qualified first aiders/sports trainers at training?	Y	N
Safety inspection of home ground facilities (e.g., club rooms, change rooms, showers, etc.)?	Y	N
Safety inspection of playing surfaces before competition?	Y	N
Safety inspection of playing surfaces before training?	Y	N
Wearing/use of protective equipment during competition?	Y	N
Wearing or use of protective equipment during training?	Y	N
Participation of players at competition or training under the influence of alcohol?	Y	N
Drugs in sport?	Y	N
A code of conduct/fair play policy for players?	Y	N
A code of conduct on the acceptable behavior of people attending competitions (e.g., coaches, officials, spectators)?	Y	N
Modified rules for juniors?	Y	N
Child protection?	Y	N
Issues related to pregnant players?	Y	N
Adverse weather and safe conduct of play?	Y	N
Do you have any other specific documented safety policies? If yes, please list:	Y	N

Note: Section 2 includes the sports safety policy. The questions seek to identify club's policy on a range of safety issues. For the purposes of this questionnaire, a "policy" is defined as a specified plan, strategy, guiding principle, or statement of procedure. Certain club's policies may have been developed at club or association level (Abbott et al., 2007b)

relationship formally began in 2004 and was ongoing at this time of this report (J. Nethery, personal communication, November 26, 2008).

During the initial stages of the program's development, SafeClub collaborators included the Injury Risk Management Research Centre (IRMRC)—an independent research center of the University of New South Wales—New South Wales Safe Communities, and Northern Sydney Central Coast Health. In addition, New South Wales Health represents both a partner and collaborator of SafeClub and YouthSafe. While NSW Safe Communities served as an initial collaborator in providing funding for initial SafeClub pilot and program development, this funding and parallel collaboration has since been terminated.

New South Wales Health and NSW Research Unit can be noted as current collaborators of SafeClub (K. Abbott, personal communication, January 28, 2008). Injury prevention professionals

Table 6.2 Section 3 of the Sports Safety Audit Tool

			Yes ✓	No ✓
1. This question asks about what type of injury records your club keeps				
Does your club keep a record of:	Games	Training		
(a) Injuries that result in an insurance claim	☐	☐	Y	N
(b) Injuries that require attendance to hospital	☐	☐	Y	N
(c) Injuries that require attending a medical practitioner or health professional	☐	☐	Y	N
(d) Injuries which result in missing a match	☐	☐	Y	N
(e) Injuries that require first aid	☐	☐	Y	N
(f) Others: please indicate			Y	N
2. Apart from injury records, what other sources of injury risk information does your club collect?				
(a) Injuries research (from the Internet or the library)			Y	N
(b) Soccer NSW/Football Federation Australia.			Y	N
(c) Safety audits conducted by club representatives			Y	N
(d) Others: please indicate			Y	N
3. If injury records and injury risk information is collected, has your club reviewed this information in the last 12 months?			Y	N
4. If injury records and injury risk information is collected, has the information been used to identify safety priorities in the last 12 months?			Y	N
5. Has your club informed the following groups about club safety activities in the last 12 months?				
(a) Players?			Y	N
(b) Coaches?			Y	N
(c) Committee members?			Y	N
(d) Referees and other game officials?			Y	N
6. Does your club have a specific safety budget? If yes, approximately what proportion of your overall budget is allocated to safety?			Y	N
7. Does your club have a committee or coordinator specifically responsible for safety?			Y	N
8. If your club has a current sports safety plan, has it been acted upon? ☐ N/A			Y	N
9. What safety activities has your club undertaken in the past 12 months?			Y	N
10. Is sports safety a regular agenda item at your clubs committee meetings?			Y	N
11. Have the following groups been consulted about injury risks in the last 12 months?				
(a) Players			Y	N
(b) Coaches			Y	N
(c) Committee members			Y	N
(d) Referees and other game officials			Y	N
12. Have the sports safety policies and plans of your club been reviewed in the last 12 months?			Y	N

Note: Section 3 includes the Sports Safety Infrastructure (Abbott et al., 2007b)

also represent a SafeClub stakeholder. Professionals such as doctors, chiropractors, and academics play an important role in research and development of SafeClub (K. Abbott, personal communication, January 23, 2008). YouthSafe and Northern Sydney Central Coast Health (NSCCH) share equal ownership of SafeClub intellectual property. Consequently, the two organizations share the role in delivering and implementing SafeClub strategies (K. Abbott, personal communication, January 28, 2008).

Northern Sydney Safe Communities continues to support SafeClub through the promotion and generation of interest among club administrators toward SafeClub. They endorse SafeClub through newsletters, bulletin boards, and word of mouth. Club administrators using SafeClub promote its use, particularly those who have won awards at the Sporting Injuries Festival Safety Awards for their use of risk management techniques (K. Abbott, personal communication, January 28, 2008).

The collaboration between YouthSafe and IRMRC was created after the results of the pilot program were presented. While the evaluation demonstrated promising results, the IRMRC was asked to assist the SafeClub team to perform a more intensive evaluation of the strategy because of their focus on evidence-based responses to injury (Injury Risk Management Research Centre [IRMRC], 2008). The IRMRC was granted the funding to complete a 2-year evaluation of the SafeClub risk management program (S. Sherker, personal communication, February 10, 2008).

SafeClub also collaborates with and is accountable by the YouthSafe Board of Committee Members during an annual action planning meeting. During the initial pilot program and 2-year evaluations of SafeClub, the SafeClub committee provided quarterly reports to funders and met to discuss the progress of SafeClub development (K. Abbott, personal communication, January 30, 2008).

6.2.1 Perception of Stakeholders

During the time of development, the reaction of stakeholders was not considered to be "overwhelmingly positive" due to the lack of certainty that SafeClub could guarantee success (K. Abbott, personal communication, January 23, 2008). However, through participation in SafeClub sessions, club administrators expressed a positive perception of the program

and provided positive feedback regarding the risk management strategy during the pilot study. Overall, positive perceptions around the program developed following the 2-year evaluation as SafeClub was able to demonstrate successful and sustainable results. As a result, stakeholders have expressed extreme satisfaction with the program.

SafeClub, as an injury prevention program, is in demand across soccer clubs in Australia (K. Abbott, personal communication, January 28, 2008). According to Nethery (personal communication, November 26, 2008), YouthSafe Project Officer, SafeClub is being implemented all over NSW. They are collaborating to introduce SafeClub sessions to clubs in Football NSW, and they have an accreditation scheme planned for 2010. Accreditation provides incentives for participation, and possible incentives include discounts on insurance premiums and providing equipment from sponsors. Incentives are available to any community club members who complete SafeClub training. This scheme is believed to enhance the credibility of the program, encouraging participants to want to attend and complete its required duration (J. Nethery, personal communication, November 27, 2008). Ultimately, in order for risk management approaches to function optimally in sport, coaches, players, and administrators should be involved in collecting injury data and work to identify the associated risks of participation (Finch & Hennessy, 2000). SafeClub educates clubs on how to identify the risks, and the community clubs work as a team to collect the data to address these injury-related risks.

In the past year, soccer associations from Sydney completed SafeClub training, and they are in discussion with different sports (e.g., rugby league and AFL bodies) with the intention of future collaboration. Based on the increasing demand of SafeClub, the position of a SafeClub Project Coordinator has recently been created. However more funding is required to address this demand and promote SafeClub on a larger scale (K. Abbott, personal communication, January 28, 2008).

6.2.2 Financial Resources

As mentioned above, New South Wales Safe Communities assisted in providing a financial grant toward the initial development of SafeClub and its pilot program. Following the success of the SafeClub pilot study, New South Wales Sporting Injuries Committee (NSWSIC) partially funded SafeClub's intensive 2-year evaluation. Initial financial support was provided by both New South Wales Safe Communities and NSWSIC, who provided external funding for evaluations.

After the completion of the pilot and 2-year evaluation, both New South Wales Safe Communities and NSWSIC no longer provide financial support. YouthSafe and Northern Sydney Central Coastal Health continue to support and pay for all financial costs incurred by SafeClub (K. Abbott, personal communication, January 28, 2008). YouthSafe is partially funded by New South Wales Road and Traffic Authorities, a governmental department, and partially by New South Wales Health. These funds are used to support staff salaries and administrative costs. Due to spending surpassing the initial proposed budget and earned grant monies, YouthSafe and NSCCH supplemented all extra costs.

Administrative costs to implement SafeClub (e.g., computers, telephone, and stationary) total to AUD$89,000 per year. The cost for the implementation of a SafeClub program delivered to 10–12 community clubs over three sessions is approximately AUD$1650 /session, which includes trainer fees, manuals, and materials (K. Abbott, personal communication, January 28, 2008). It is important to note that the more clubs attending a SafeClub training session, the cheaper it is to implement the program (K. Abbott, personal communication, January 28, 2008).

Overall resources are lacking to finance and offer SafeClub to community sports clubs on a sponsorship basis. Consequently, SafeClub is encouraging organizations such as Football NSW to collaborate with their insurance bodies to potentially receive funding. The objective of establishing reliable sponsorship is to ensure that attendance from community clubs would not reduce due to funding (K. Abbott, personal communication, January 28, 2008).

6.3 Implementation

Using adult-based learning principles adapted from work and safety organizations (K. Abbott, personal communication, January 23, 2008), the program consists of three training sessions of 2 h per session. Adult-based learning principles are centered on the way the information is provided to participants and is based on the concept of delivering the information to appeal to all learning types. Furthermore, adult-based learning principles give participants a chance to practice what they may have gained during SafeClub training sessions (K. Abbott, personal communication, January 23, 2008). For example, between sessions, participants are asked to implement their self-created strategies created during the training and to provide feedback on the potential effects of these ideas. The training helps community sports clubs to identify and prioritize individualistic safety issues through the utilization of a risk management approach. At the conclusion of the training, participants are expected to establish an individualistic, working, and sustainable Sports Safety Manual and Action Plan that they, themselves, have designed specifically for their sports club (Abbott & Klarenaar, 2007).

6.3.1 Effective Practices

SafeClub considers the wide variety of barriers affecting club administrators (K. Abbott, personal communication, January 30, 2008). As community sports clubs in Australia rely almost entirely on their volunteer base of club administrators (Abbott & Klarenaar, 2007), there is a limited amount of time and resources. There is also a lack of knowledge regarding risk management safety techniques and, as mentioned above, apprehension to utilize them (Abbott et al., 2007a). However, SafeClub is "easy to do and interactive, which uses humor," and identifiable scenarios risk management is presented as a simple, interactive adaptable concept (K. Abbott, personal communication, January 30, 2008). The use of humor through video clips depicting the simplicity of risk management allows participants to enjoy SafeClub sessions. Furthermore, SafeClub presents risk management as a strategy in which participants are already engaging. For example, at the beginning of their first SafeClub session, participants are shown a brief video clip demonstrating the simplicity of risk management techniques through a common situation experienced by soccer club administrators. In addition to an explanation of risk management, proper initiatives are introduced to address these common safety issues (K. Abbott, personal communication, January 30, 2008).

Overall, the unique and flexible approach of risk management is the foundation to preventing injuries from occurring. Risk management is a different way to approaching safety in allowing club administrators—rather than a safety expert—to identify their own safety risks and priorities. This self-created list of individualized priorities by club administrators is fundamental in preventing injuries because it fosters interest, understanding, and consequent action toward safety practices in community sports clubs (K. Abbott, personal communication, January 30, 2008).

Furthermore, the interactive component between club administrators in generating safe practices is also heralded as an essential component by SafeClub participants. In interacting with other club administrators through a workshop format, participants' anxieties are assuaged in witnessing others encountering similar obstacles (K. Abbott, personal communication, January 30, 2008).

SafeClub prevention strategies account for cultural and diversity issues through its flexible approach. While SafeClub targets community clubs, this approach can be applied to any organization, sport, and level of play. Its interactive process in teaching an approach of risk management rather than providing information sessions on

safety is appealing and axiomatic to a wide range of socioeconomic groups. It is expected, however, that club administrators are literate to comprehend SafeClub training resources (K. Abbott, personal communication, January 30, 2008).

The key factor in facilitating the implementation of SafeClub risk management strategies is the devotion of volunteering club administrators to their individual soccer clubs. This passion translates into a willingness to devote the time and effort necessary not only to have a functioning soccer club but also to create an environment which facilitates communication. K. Abbott (personal communication, January 30, 2008) states that "club administrators are not doing it because they get paid or because they have to, they're doing it because they love it." Consequently, club administrators are willing to attend SafeClub training sessions knowing that it may potentially improve their sports club.

6.3.2 Actors in Decision Making and Planning

Committees involved in decision making and planning are YouthSafe and NSCCH. Heading those organizations are Kristy Abbott and Jane Nethery of YouthSafe and Paul Klarenaar of NSCCH. Managers and administrators from both committees are involved on major decisions (e.g., funding, progress reports of the program). Furthermore, feedback from club administrators at SafeClub training sessions is considered when these decisions are made. In addition, governmental departments such as the Department of Recreation—a group not currently involved in SafeClub decision making and planning—are suggested to be involved in promoting and sponsoring community sports clubs to attend SafeClub training sessions (K. Abbott, personal communication, January 30, 2008).

Communication with stakeholders is regular and conducted through meetings, telephone calls, or emails. Final decisions regarding SafeClub program administration, development, and implementation are executed through a joint discussion between YouthSafe and NSCCH. Working relationships and communication systems are frequent and positive, which fosters the ease of modifications necessary in the program and its implementation. In the event of a dispute, YouthSafe and NSCCH have established a dispute resolution process; this process has yet to be utilized. Sherker (personal communication, February 10, 2008) highlights the benefits of individuals of different disciplines contributing various strengths to the development and outcomes of the SafeClub program. Furthermore, the relationship between IRMRC, YouthSafe, and NCHSS is noted as a "very harmonious interaction," with the shared goal of SafeClub's optimal development and success (S. Sherker, personal communication, February 10, 2008).

6.3.3 Barriers to Implementation

Obstacles in implementing SafeClub include limited time and financial resources fundamental to completing this program. More specifically, in order to make this program more widely available, more trainers conducting more SafeClub training sessions occurring simultaneously are necessary. However, while the SafeClub committee realizes there is a more cost-effective method of delivering safety practices via mail, they prefer the interactive, face-to-face approach utilized in SafeClub training sessions to ensure participants are actively participating and applying the knowledge and strategies gained (K. Abbott, personal communication, January 30, 2008).

6.3.4 Enhancing SafeClub

SafeClub is in the process of developing a "train the trainer" program. Trainers will be expected to have relevant qualifications (e.g., Certificate 4) and experience in adult education and/or relevant tertiary qualifications (e.g., education, physiotherapy, sports science, etc.). Other practices include gaining support from relevant governing bodies. Promotion could be an endorsement

through the provision of financial support for community clubs to attend SafeClub training. In addition, continuing education tools that targets community soccer clubs who have previously completed SafeClub training would be essential, for example, devising a website where club administrators can register their club information and provide informative feedback. It is also important to better understand the barriers encountered by club administrators at the grassroots level (K. Abbott, personal communication, January 30, 2008).

6.3.5 Ongoing Evaluation

Evaluations of SafeClub are regular and are conducted through process evaluations. Here, SafeClub participants are asked to complete a feedback evaluation form (see Table 6.3), which includes Likert questions that rate program aspects from 1 to 5, as well as open-ended questions. Questions investigate the perceptions of course content, the program facilitators, and materials available for use (see Tables 6.4 and 6.5).

At the conclusion of each training program, a report is produced which includes feedback received from participants. This information is provided to key stakeholders and collaborators (K. Abbott, personal communication, January 30, 2008). The feedback is then used to improve and develop the SafeClub program. One principle modification to date was the duration of SafeClub sessions. Taking into account the time constraints of club administrators and coaches, sessions were modified from three sessions of 2 h each to two sessions at 3 h each. Therefore, modifications are continuously made to the program using stakeholder consultation as a mechanism for decision making; the aim is to enhance its quality in theory and application.

Further funding is expected so as to examine the relationship between SafeClub training sessions and injury outcomes (K. Abbott, personal communication, January 30, 2008). Implementers encourage participating clubs to collect and analyze injury/incident data from their own clubs.

Table 6.3 SafeClub training—evaluation questionnaire

	Strongly disagree	Disagree	Neutral	Agree	Strongly agree
Course content					
The content of the SafeClub course is relevant to my club	1	2	3	4	5
The course lived up to my expectations	1	2	3	4	5
The activities in this course gave me sufficient practice and feedback	1	2	3	4	5
The difficulty level of this course is appropriate	1	2	3	4	5
The pace of this course is appropriate	1	2	3	4	5
I will be able to use what I learned in this course	1	2	3	4	5
Course facilitators					
The trainers were well prepared	1	2	3	4	5
The trainers were helpful	1	2	3	4	5
Course materials					
The audiovisual display is an important aspect of this course	1	2	3	4	5
The Participant Workbook assisted my learning	1	2	3	4	5
The SafeClub CD-ROM will be useful to my club	1	2	3	4	5
The Safety Manual (folder) will be useful to my club	1	2	3	4	5
Any comments on the above:					
What action do you intend to take as a result of attending this course?					
Improvements					
How would you improve the course—tick all that apply: ☐ Provide better information before the course ☐ Increase content covered in the course ☐ Improve course organization ☐ Make the course more difficult ☐ Speed up the pace of the course ☐ Shorten the time for the course	☐ Reduce content covered in the course ☐ Make course activities more stimulating ☐ Make the course less difficult ☐ Slow down the pace of the course ☐ Allot more time for the course				
What other improvements would you recommend in this course?					
What did you like least about this course?					
What did you like most about this course?					
What further information or support do you think your club needs in order to successfully implement the ideas introduced in this course?					

Note: Instructions for the evaluation. Please take a few minutes to give us your feedback on the SafeClub course. Your input will be used to further improve and develop the SafeClub program. Please circle your response to each item. Rate the course on a scale of 1–5 where 1 = strongly disagree and 5 = strongly agree (Abbott et al., 2007b)

They are to use the results from this data to inform their own policies and procedures.

As an increasing number of clubs are trained in SafeClub, there is a greater opportunity to examine more data in a study to examine this issue. Plans for this evaluation are were put on hold at this time as it requires adequate time and money to complete (J. Nethery, personal communication, November 26, 2008).

To improve the design of SafeClub evaluation methodologies, a significant adjustment included the modification of Donaldson's original SSAT. Specifically, a more sensitive tool to measure change in safety policy and infrastructure over a short period of time was required. While the original SSAT provided a score of one point to each policy the community club reported, modification was necessary to weigh certain policies more significantly than others (S. Sherker, personal communication, February 10, 2008). Thus, items that were considered fundamental as well as wide-reaching management practices that were

Table 6.4 Summary of 34 participating SafeClub community sports responding to statements related to various aspects of training

	Strongly disagree	Disagree	Neutral	Agree	Strongly agree
Course content					
The content of the SafeClub course is relevant to my club	0	0	0	8	26
The course lived up to my expectations	0	0	3	18	13
The activities in this course gave me sufficient practice and feedback	0	0	1	18	15
The difficulty level of this course is appropriate	0	0	3	18	13
The pace of this course is appropriate	0	1	2	16	15
I will be able to use what I learned in this course	0	0	0	7	27
Course facilitators					
The trainers were well prepared	0	0	0	6	28
The trainers were helpful	0	0	1	4	29
Course materials					
The audiovisual display is an important aspect of this course	0	0	1	22	10
The Participant Workbook assisted my learning	0	0	1	15	18
The SafeClub CD-ROM will be useful to my club	0	0	2	13	19
The Safety Manual (folder) will be useful to my club	0	0	3	9	22

Note: Abbott et al. (2007a)

Table 6.5 Summary of participating SafeClub community sports response to statements related to various aspects of training

	Strongly disagree	Disagree	Neutral	Agree	Strongly agree
Course content					
The content of the SafeClub course is relevant to my club	0	0	0	5	7
The course lived up to my expectations	0	0	0	4	7
The activities in this course gave me sufficient practice and feedback	0	0	0	9	4
The difficulty level of this course is appropriate	0	0	1	9	3
The pace of this course is appropriate	0	1	4	7	1
I will be able to use what I learned in this course	0	0	0	3	9
Course facilitators					
The trainers were well prepared	0	0	0	2	11
The trainers were helpful	0	0	0	2	11
Course materials					
The audiovisual display is an important aspect of this course	0	0	0	5	7
The Participant Workbook assisted my learning	0	0	0	4	7
The SafeClub CD-ROM will be useful to my club	0	0	0	2	11
The Safety Manual (folder) will be useful to my club	0	0	1	1	11

Note: YouthSafe (2008)

identified through research were scored more highly than specific, individual items considered less important to overall sports safety (Abbott et al., 2007a). For example, more points are scored to a club adopting a policy to check environmental concerns (such as the quality of turf and the risk of tripping hazards) versus a sun-smart policy where players were expected to apply sunscreen prior to participating in soccer matches (S. Sherker, personal communication, February 10, 2008).

6.4   Outcome

The evaluation of SafeClub, based on stakeholder responses, illustrated "overwhelmingly positive feedback" (K. Abbott, personal communication, January 23, 2008). Participants felt the content of the training was relevant and suggested that SafeClub should be made widely available (Abbott & Donaldson, 2004). Abbott (personal communication, January 28, 2008) states that there was "an excellent initiative to raise the awareness of safety within all clubs. The content provided a thoughtful and good coverage of safety topics and a strong basis for Club Policy," according to one SafeClub participant.

According to Finch (2006), sports injury prevention programs should measure player/club recruitment rates, as well as evaluate the uptake of the initiatives being evaluated, including reasons for its use or nonuse. SafeClub records this data, and they also encourage individual soccer clubs to report the factors fostering its implementation (including policy changes, injury data collection, etc.)

SafeClub was piloted and presented, in modified form, as a workshop at a national scientific conference prior to their 2-year intensive evaluation. This evaluation measured the impact of SafeClub on sports safety activities of participating community soccer clubs in Sydney, Australia. Response rates included 32 of a possible 50 intervention clubs (64% response rate) and 44 of a possible 51 (86% response rate) control groups enrolled in this study. After completing the SSAT three times (early 2005 season, baseline; end 2005 season, post-season; and mid-2006 season, 12-month follow-up), clubs were ranked on policy, infrastructure, and safety scores. These policy items included documented risk management policy, sports safety plans, documented policies, and current sports safety plans, while infrastructure items include record of injuries, safety budget, safety coordinator, and safety being a regular agenda item. Safety scores were allocated under both policy items and infrastructure items. The maximum possible safety score was 65, with top scores of 24 for policy and 41 for infrastructure. Participating clubs were represented by club administrators, in which presidents and secretaries were preferred representatives (Figs. 6.3 and 6.4; K. Abbott, personal communication, January 23, 2008; Abbott et al., 2007b).

An increase in safety scores immediately after training is expected as the information gained from SafeClub training is fresh in the minds of club administrators. However, unlike many injury

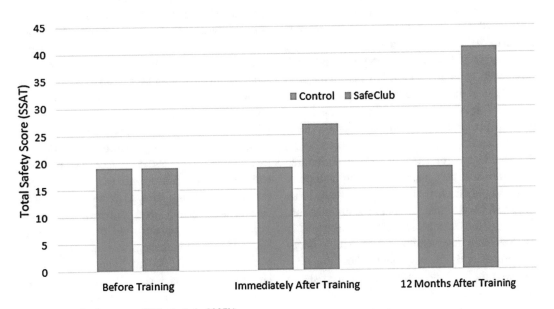

Fig. 6.3 Total safety score (Abbott et al., 2007b)

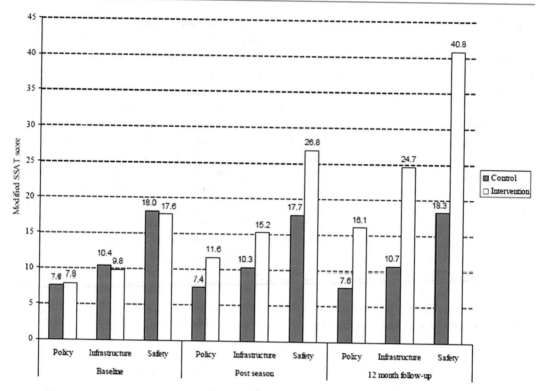

Fig. 6.4 Mean policy, infrastructure, and overall safety scores for control and intervention clubs at baseline, post-season, and 12-month follow-up (YouthSafe, 2007)

prevention programs, which fail to demonstrate long-term effects, SafeClub has managed to maintain rising scores even 12 months after community clubs attended SafeClub training sessions. Sherker (personal communication, February 10, 2008) found these results strongly encouraging and something "very rare in all her experience in injury prevention research." It is hypothesized that the successful and sustainable results of SafeClub are based on the modifications made to infrastructure that is a requirement for community clubs. For example, creating an allocated budget for safety or a safety committee enables further permanent changes to club practices and policies that allow improvements to be sustained (S. Sherker, personal communication, February 10, 2008). Most notably, more clubs in the SafeClub intervention group had a documented safety/risk management policy (Fig. 6.5), reviewed their injury records and injury risks in the previous 12 months (Fig. 6.6), and had created a safety committee or coordinator (Fig. 6.7)

compared to control groups who hadn't received SafeClub training.

The results of the SafeClub 2-year evaluation suggest that SafeClub achieved its aim in assisting community soccer clubs to improve their sports activities. As participating clubs have made changes, they have been improved in quality, increased in quality, and sustained over time. Most impressive was SafeClub ability to enable clubs to lay solid foundations for good risk management practices, including establishing core infrastructure (e.g., appointing a safety committee or coordinator), putting key processes in place (e.g., regularly reviewing injury risk records and information to review plans, having safety as a committee meeting agenda item, acting upon and reviewing safety plans in a timely manner), and writing and regularly reviewing comprehensive safety policies and plans (Abbott et al., 2007a). Injury risks are regularly reviewed through consult with sporting bodies on injury risks. Injury risks have been identified so as to properly understand specific concerns

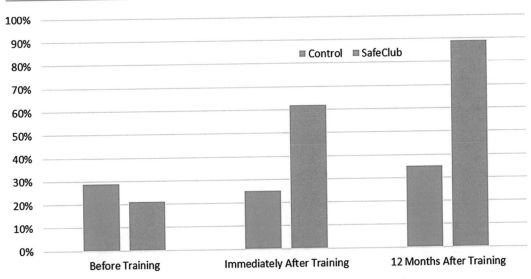

Fig. 6.5 Percentage of community soccer clubs with a sports safety/risk management policy. The total safety score is the total score a club receives as measured by the Sports Safety Audit Tool. Clubs that received the SafeClub training improved their safety scores while the group that didn't receive SafeClub showed no improvement. These results were sustained immediately after the training and 12 months following the SafeClub training (Abbott et al., 2007b)

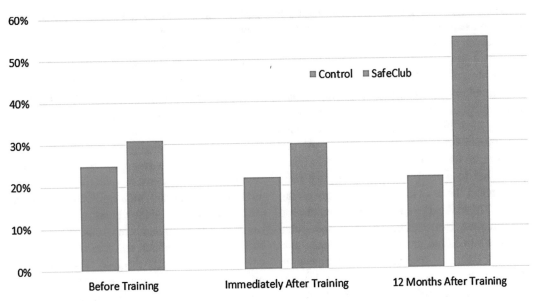

Fig. 6.6 Percentage of community soccer clubs who reviewed their club injury records and risks (Abbott et al., 2007b)

which are addressed during the SafeClub session. For example, goalposts have been identified as a significant injury risk in soccer. Football NSW in particular has made strong efforts to minimize this risk; these risks are also explored through SafeClub training (J. Nethery, personal communication, November 26, 2008). According to Dickinson (2003), goalposts should not be made of a timber frame; rather aluminum, steel tubing, a combination of both materials, or polyvinyl chloride (PVC) plastic tubing should be used. Further, "homemade" goal posts should not be used. The document advises that goal posts must be tested to ensure strength in the structure (Dickinson, 2003).

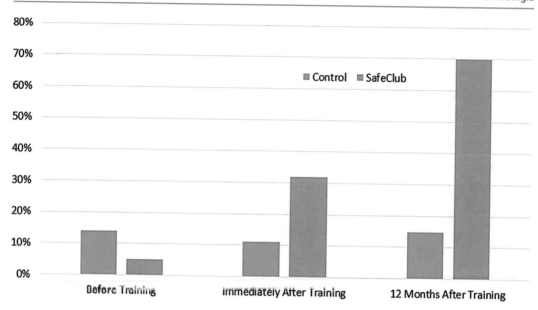

Fig. 6.7 Percentage of community soccer clubs with a safety committee or coordinator (Abbott et al., 2007b)

According to Michelle Hanley, Risk Manager and State Member Protection Officer of Football NSW, sports require a program like SafeClub in place. The program allows feedback to be given so that the program can be improved. Football NSW monitors injury rates through injury data collected by insurance claims; individual associations also collect it from their clubs. This allows an internal monitoring system. At this time a more formal reporting system was being considered to collect and monitor injury rates that connect the associations with the governing bodies. They intend to collect data to understand real outcomes. However, because only one course has been run so far, the idea has only been proposed. Hanley (personal communication, December 15, 2008) suggests that the leagues themselves have difficulty retaining their own volunteers due to their workload; therefore, their ability to collect data is limited.

Overall, Hanley (personal communication, December 15, 2008) posits that the overall awareness of risk management and injury prevention is more obvious since the SafeClub course. In fact, some associations have begun to review and amend processes and policies for next season. In addition to this, a strong relationship has been fostered with YouthSafe; their supportive nature

prior to and following the course was particularly useful. Most important is their respect for their participants and how they value feedback. Hanley (personal communication, December 15, 2008) states that YouthSafe has listened to any comments the associations have provided about the course and their appropriate suitability to the sport of soccer. Football NSW feedback changed the course from three separate sessions to a two-session course; however they would prefer the course is run over one session. YouthSafe has advised them that the initiative is more effective with two sessions—with a break in between the sessions. Their comments regarding the structure and suggestions about the improvements and adjustment were well received. Football NSW intends to improve SafeClub at the individual association level and then promote more collaboration among the associations in 2010.

Hanley (personal communication, December 15, 2008) strongly believes that SafeClub has and will continue to increase awareness and change the mind-set of being safe and proactive toward risk management injury prevention. With this mentality change will follow a revisit of the policies and more active monitoring (e.g., ground inspection checklists before games). This is possible as SafeClub is "very practical, easy to use and you can make it personal so you can kick start risk management (catered to) your association" (M. Hanley, personal communication, December 15, 2008).

Injury risk and incidence were of particular concern to the clubs, and modifications to this aspect have been particularly successful. At baseline (i.e., prior to SafeClub), only 16% of clubs that received SafeClub training had a head injury policy; immediately after SafeClub training, 33% created a policy; and at the 12-month follow-up period, 52% of clubs reported sustaining this policy (K. Abbott, personal communication, January 23, 2008; Abbott et al., 2007b).

Another success has been in the value of the workshop format. Community clubs have particularly expressed keen satisfaction with the incorporation of adult-based learning principles in an interactive environment; it is the reason they most enjoy attending SafeClub training (K. Abbott, personal communication, February 2, 2008).

In recognition for their efforts and success, SafeClub was awarded Best Risk of Compliance Education and Training Program at the 2006 Australian Risk Management Awards and had won a Gold Award at the 2006 NSW Sports Safety Awards. Furthermore, individual community soccer clubs that participated in SafeClub training received gold and bronze awards at the 2005 NSW Sports Safety Awards for their risk management-based safety programs (K. Abbott, personal communication, February 2, 2008; see Box 6.1).

Box 6.1 Rationale for NSW Sporting Injuries Committee Award Selection

YouthSafe has won two key NSW Sports Safety Awards for its SafeClub program. In 2006, YouthSafe with Northern Sydney Central Coast Health successfully won gold in the regional category for the SafeClub project. In 2007, YouthSafe, in partnership with the University of New South Wales, successfully won silver in the research category of the awards.

In 2006, the NSW Sporting Injuries Committee recognized the practical nature of SafeClub in assisting and educating sporting volunteers by taking them through their safety concerns and showing them how to develop their own comprehensive risk management plans that are tailored to their needs. The end result of the program is a user-friendly risk management plan which the organization can easily implement and update as they have developed it themselves. In comparison to other risk management training courses, SafeClub is interactive, enjoyable, and practical and more importantly produce results.

In regard to the Research Award in 2007, the SafeClub Research Project conducted by the University of New South Wales was titled "Can risk management training improve the safety activities of community soccer clubs?" The objective of this research was to evaluate whether participation in the SafeClub risk management program improved the safety activities of the community sports clubs involved in the controlled trial. At baseline there was no significant difference in the safety scores of intervention and control clubs. At postseason, intervention clubs achieved significantly higher safety scores than control clubs. Moreover, the improvement in the safety scores was even greater at the 12-month follow-up. These results suggest that SafeClub effectively assists clubs to improve their sports safety activities particularly the foundations and processes for good risk management practice in a sustainable way. Further, this is the first evaluation of a risk management sports program in reviewed literature.

Note: S. Jenkins, personal communication (December 14, 2008).

As a result of the success, YouthSafe, NSCCH, and IRMRC aim to examine the effect of SafeClub training on the reduction of injury incidence in community sports clubs. This implication will require the development of a satisfactory proposal and methodology as well as securing funding to implement this project (S. Sherker, personal communication, February 10, 2008).

6.4.1 Lessons Learned: Improving SafeClub

SafeClub's development and maturation is the product of the application of the lessons learned from its design and implementation. Abbot (personal communication, February 2, 2008) notes the importance of understanding your target audience through extensive consultation process conducted prior to implementing an injury prevention program. By understanding community sports clubs at a grassroots level during the developmental stages, they were able to create a salient, engaging, and relevant program catering to a diverse audience. She also notes the significance of evaluation which is the importance of developing process "checks" ensuring continuous growth and refinement in the program (K. Abbott, personal communication, February 2, 2008).

Evaluation in the form of systematic research is not only reported as necessary but an "ethical responsibility" among the implementers of any research program. The evaluations of SafeClub have and will continue to appropriately identify the program's weaknesses from an objective outside perspective. This will allow the developers of SafeClub to make necessary modifications and demonstrate an accurate level of success that will build confidence among the program users (S. Sherker, personal communication, February 10, 2008).

Acknowledgments The author would like to express sincere appreciation to the key informant for this case study: Kristy Abbot of Youthsafe in Putney, NSW, Australia—whose consultation made this project possible.

BRIO Model: SafeClub

Group Served: Community-level soccer clubs.

Goal: To prevent head, spine, and other injuries for soccer players.

Background	Resources	Implementation	Outcome
An increased interest in examining head and spinal cord injuries in soccer Early consultations by YouthSafe and Northern Sydney Central Coastal Health (NSCCH) confirmed gaining interest-specific information was considered valuable by most communities SafeClub was founded in 2002 Pilot study in 2003 aimed to assist clubs to develop and implement an in-depth sports safety plan based on a risk management training SafeClub is a training program based on a 5-stage risk management model aimed to assist community clubs to reduce injury risk	During development, principal stakeholders included New South Wales Injuries Committee, Soccer New South Wales, and injury prevention professionals YouthSafe and NSCCH currently share equal ownership of SafeClub intellectual property, as well as the role in delivering and implementing SafeClub strategies IRMRC performed intensive evaluation of SafeClub after its initial pilot program	Uses adult-based learning principles adapted from work and safety organizations The program consists of three training sessions of 2 h per session Practices most effective include consideration of the wide variety of barriers affecting club administrators Demonstrates that risk management is simple Implementation is facilitated by the devotion of volunteering club administrators to their individual soccer club Continual evaluation made on the implementation of SafeClub occurs regularly using process evaluations	Success in SafeClub has been and will remain a measure of increased safety activities among community sports clubs as a result of SafeClub training The 2-year evaluation of SafeClub examines changes in sports safety activities and changes that clubs make The results of the SafeClub evaluation suggest that SafeClub achieved its aim in assisting community soccer clubs to improve their sports activities Effectiveness of SafeClub training did possess one of the unanticipated positive outcomes, which is in the long-term, sustainable results produced

Life-Space Model: SafeClub

Sociocultural: civilization/community	Interpersonal: primary and secondary relationships	Physical environments: where we live	Internal states: biochemical/genetic and means of coping
Awareness raising through video clips at SafeClub information/ training sessions Use of soccer community to promote risk management techniques in soccer practices and games Multifaceted strategy that includes soccer club administrators	Relationship between YouthSafe, Northern Sidney Central Coast Health (NSCCH), and IRMRC to increase knowledge and improve techniques to prevent and target injuries in soccer Relationship between club administrators and SafeClub trainers through contractual obligation to adhere to the safety techniques promoted by SafeClub Relationship between club administrators, players, coaches, and referees to adhere to SafeClub contracts established during SafeClub training	Endurance sport Contact between players Contact between player and soccer ball because head is voluntarily used to control and advance the ball Risk management encourages club administrators to consider and modify the physical environment (soccer field and surroundings) as a means to increase safety practices in soccer Adoption of individualized action plans created by club administrators	Risk management as a means to increase safety practices in soccer Empowerment of club administrators and in turn coaches, players, and referees through risk management training Strengthening relationships among key stakeholders in the game to enhance communication and prevent injury in soccer

References

Abbott, K. & Donaldson, A. (2004). *Development and piloting of the SafeClub training course for administrators of community sports clubs. Project summary report.* YouthSafe & NSCCH.

Abbott, K. & Klarenaar, P. (2007). *Risk management for sports injury prevention: Can it work in community sports clubs?* YouthSafe & NSCCH. Retrieved from www.youthsafe.org.

Abbott, K., Klarenaar, P., Donaldson, A., & Sherker, S. (2007a). *Safeclub: sports safety for community sports clubs. Evaluation report.* Youthsafe & Northern Sydney Central Coast Health.

Abbott, K., Klarenaar, P., Donaldson, A., & Sherker, S. (2007b). Evaluating SafeClub: Can risk management training improve the safety activities of community soccer clubs. *British Journal of Sports Medicine, 42*(6), 460–465.

Dickinson, N. (2003). *Goal post safety, grassroots soccer – Precautions and measures for fixed and portable goalposts.* Standard issue 1 – August 2003, Policy Document 03/01, NSW.

Drawer, S., & Fuller, C. W. (2001). Evaluating the level of injury in English professional football using a risk based assessment process. *British Journal of Sports Medicine, 35*(6), 402–408.

Finch, C. F. (2006). A new framework for research leading to sports injury prevention. *Journal of Science and Medicine in Sport, 9*, 3–9.

Finch, C. F., & Hennessy, M. (2000). The safety practices of sporting clubs/centres in the city of Hume. *Journal of Science and Medicine in Sport, 3*(1), 9–16.

Harvey, D. M., Finch, C., & McGrath, A. (1997). Sport safety plans: Managing the risks of sport injuries. *The Sport Educator, 10*(2), 12–15.

Injury Risk Management Research Centre. (2008). *About the IRMRC.* Retrieved February 24, 2008, from http://www.irmrc.unsw.edu.au/About/objectives.asp.

New South Wales Injuries Committee. (2008). *NSW Sporting Injuries Committee.* Retrieved February 24, 2008, from http://www.sportinginjuries.nsw.gov.au/about_us.asp.

Soccer New South Wales. (2008). *About us*, Retrieved February 24, 2008, from http://www.soccernsw.com.au/index.php?id=10.

YouthSafe. (2007). *NSW health awards entry template 2007*, NSW Health.

YouthSafe. (2008). *Evaluation football NSW Association.* SafeClub training- evaluation questionnaire results.

It Ain't Brain Surgery: A Prevention Program for Snowboarders and Skiers

Negar Ahmadi

The purpose of the It Ain't Brain Surgery program is to educate and promote to snowboarders and skiers the importance of wearing a helmet while engaging in these activities in order to prevent or minimize the risk of head/brain injuries.

7.1   Background

The program It Ain't Brain Surgery was initiated by Dr. A. Stewart Levy, a neurosurgeon at St. Anthony Central Hospital, a Level 1 Trauma Center in Denver, Colorado. This institution receives about one third of all patients in Colorado with traumatic brain injury (TBI) due to skiing or snowboarding (Levy, Hawkes, & Rossie, 2007). Levy, Hawkes, Hemminger, and Knight (2002) performed an analysis of the demographics and types of injuries in patients treated at this trauma center from 1982 to 1998, the time period before the start of the program. According to this analysis (Levy et al., 2002), 1214 patients were admitted to the trauma center between 1982 and 1998 with injuries related to skiing and snowboarding. Of those patients, 350 (28.9%) were identified to have TBI. Although this figure tends to be higher than those reported in the literature, Levy et al. (2002) have concluded that this is perhaps due to the nature of this trauma center receiving more

patients with severe brain injuries than other institutions in the area. Furthermore, there were 16 deaths of the total 1214 patients referred for injuries from skiing or snowboarding. Among those who died, brain injury was identified as the main cause of death among the majority ($n = 14$, 87.5%). The demographics of the 350 patients with traumatic brain injuries from skiing or snowboarding accidents treated at this trauma center between 1982 and 1998 are further summarized in the Table 7.1 (Levy et al., 2002).

The mechanism of injury among those with TBI was as follows: 47% collision with a stationary object (tree, rock, or other), 37% falls, and 13% collision with another skier (Levy et al., 2002). Therefore, the majority of skiing and snowboarding brain injuries treated at this institution are found to be the result of direct-impact collisions (falls or collision with stationary object). In 1998, the It Ain't Brain Surgery program was initiated targeting the skiers and snowboarders at Colorado ski resorts. This program was the first community-based program aimed at increasing helmet awareness and helmet use among skiers and snowboarders.

Currently, the It Ain't Brain Surgery program is composed of the following three components: social marketing campaign, helmet loaner program, and distribution of helmets to ski patrollers and instructors. The three components of the program are each unique in nature, and yet they all convey the same message to the public. All three

N. Ahmadi (✉)
McMaster University, Hamilton, ON, Canada

© Springer Nature Switzerland AG 2020
R. Volpe (ed.), *Casebook of Traumatic Injury Prevention*,
https://doi.org/10.1007/978-3-030-27419-1_7

Table 7.1 Demographics of the 350 patients with traumatic brain injuries from skiing or snowboarding treated at a Level 1 trauma center in Denver

Demographic	%
Gender	
Male	77.7
Female	22.3
Age	
<10	3.1
10–15	11.7
16–25	46.9
26–35	17.1
36–45	8.9
46–55	6.3
56–65	4.0
65+	2.0
Sport	
Ski	82.6
Snowboard	17.4

Note: Reprinted from "An Analysis of Head Injuries Among Skiers and Snowboarders", by A. S. Levy, A. P. Hawkes, L. M. Hemminger, & S. Knight, 2002, Journal of Trauma, 53

components of the program were designed by Dr. Levy himself in an effort to incorporate various elements into an injury prevention model geared towards increasing helmet use and reducing brain injuries resulting from skiing or snowboarding.

7.1.1 Social Marketing Campaign

The social marketing campaign involved a series of interviews and presentations in various formats including newspapers, magazines, and television targeting a wide audience. According to Levy et al. (2007), the messages conveyed in these interviews and presentations were that:

1. TBI can occur in skiing/snowboarding.
2. The most common cause of TBI in skiing/snowboarding is hitting a stationary object such as a tree.
3. TBI is the leading cause of death and serious injury among skiers and snowboarders.
4. Many TBIs can be prevented by wearing a helmet.
5. Free loaner helmets are available at Christy Sports.

Table 7.2, adopted from Levy et al. (2007), shows a representative sample of interviews or articles published as part of the social marketing campaign component of the program.

Furthermore, a logo (Fig. 7.1) was created for the program and was displayed on all the helmets used for the program. In order to increase awareness of the program as well as the importance of wearing helmets when skiing or snowboarding, brochures and posters were made and displayed within the community and throughout the stores participating in the program. An example of a brochure used for the program is shown in Fig. 7.2.

7.1.2 Helmet Loaner Program

The helmet loaner program was the most important component of the program, and it involved the cooperation of Christy Sports, a local ski and snowboarding equipment retailer. Christy Sports has several retail outlets across Colorado, and it offers ski and snowboarding equipment rentals for all ages. As part of the helmet loaner program, the participating Christy Sports stores offered a free loaner helmet (provided to them by the program) to anyone who rented ski or snowboarding equipment. The helmet loaner program was initiated during the 1998–1999 ski season only as a pilot study. However, during the following three seasons, the program was expanded to 24 more Christy Sports locations across Colorado. The program was further expanded to some of the Christy Sports locations in Utah as well as other rental programs including a rental facility at a YMCA camp and a Young Life Christian Center (Levy et al., 2007).

The third component of the program involved distribution of helmets to ski patrollers and instructors providing the ski patrollers and ski instructors at several ski resorts with free helmets and encouraging them to wear their helmets on the slopes while working. The purpose of this component was to have the ski patrollers and instructors act as role models on the hills in order to increase helmet use among skiers and snowboarders. To further emphasize the effectiveness

Table 7.2 A representative sample of interviews or articles published as part of the social marketing campaign component of the It Ain't Brain Surgery program

Type of publication	Approximate circulation/viewers
National newspaper	
"Helmets cut risk for skiers, boarders," USA Today (Ruibal, 2001)	5 million
Los Angeles and Denver newspapers	
"Taking the kids: Even the hardheaded need ski helmets," Los Angeles Times (Ogintz, 2002)	1 million
"Doctor says making helmet decision isn't, well, brain surgery," Rocky Mountain News (Denver; Melani, 2002)	300,000[c]
"Ski safety's a matter of brains: Denver neurosurgeon maintains helmets offer vital protection to those on the slopes," Rocky Mountain News (Denver) (Frazier, 2001)	300,000[c]
"It's a no-brainer: Doctor crusades for helmet use on slopes," Rocky Mountain News (Denver) (Stedman, 2000)	300,000[c]
"Doctors push ski helmets," The Denver Post (Schrader, 1999)	300,000[d]
Denver television	
Channel 9 News. Interview with A. Stewart Levy, February 2002	110,000[e]
Channel 7 News. Interview with A. Stewart Levy, January 2001	78,000[e]
Channel 9 News. Interview with A. Stewart Levy, January 2001	110,000[e]
Channel 2 News. Interview with A. Stewart Levy, May 2000	25,000[e]
Local newspapers in ski resort areas	
"Helmets on slopes—A healthy trend," Sky-Hi News/Daily Tribune (Bonville, 2003)	3650[f]
"Brain buckets: The great helmet debate," Vail Trail (Boyd, 2002)	16,500[f]
"Free ski helmet program is larger," Winter Park Manifest/Daily Tribune (Williamson, 2000)	NA
"A heady debate," The Daily Camera (Kauder, 2000)	34,000[g]
"Doctors expanding ski helmet promotion," Summit Daily News(1999)	NA 34,000[g]
"Local shops, doctors, and hospital provide helmets," Winter Park Manifest/Daily Tribune (Williamson, 1998)	NA
Ski magazines	
"A heady debate," Ski magazine (Katagi, 2000)	450,000[h]
"Neurosurgeons buy 1250 helmets for free rentals," Wintersport Business Magazine (Mazzante, 2002)	NA
Press release	
"Skiers and snowboarders need to exercise caution on the slopes" (Congress of Neurological Surgeons, 1999)	NA

Note: Reprinted from "Helmets for Skiers and Snowboarders: An Injury Prevention Program", by A. S. Levy, A. P. Hawkes, and G. V. Rossie, 2007, *Health Promotion Practice, 8*, 260

NA not available

[a]USA Today Media Kit. (2003). USA Today. Retrieved October 10, 2003, from http://www.usatoday.com/media_kit/pressroom/pr_ justfacts_usatoday.htm

[b]Los Angeles Times reports March circulation. (2003, May 5). Los Angeles Times. Retrieved October 20, 2003, from http://www.latimes .com/services/newspaper/mediacenter/la-mediacenter-2w003- 0505abc.html

[c]Profile of our businesses: Newspaper. (2003). Rocky Mountain News (Denver). Retrieved October 10, 2003, from http://www.scripps .com/corporateoverview/businesses/newspaper/denverhtml

[d]100 largest U.S. newspapers. (2001). Retrieved October 20, 2003, from http://www.freep.com/jobspage/links/top100_99.htm

[e]Top 50 Market Profiles: No. 18—Denver. (2003). Mediaweek. Retrieved October 10, 2003, from http://www.mediaweek.com/ mediaweek/top50/denver.jxp

[f]American Newspaper Representatives, Inc. (2003). Colorado. Retrieved October 10, 2003, from http://www.anrinc.net/Newspaper %20Database/CO.htm

[g]Top 50 Boulder and Broomfield County employers: No. 43. (2003). Boulder, CO: Boulder Publishing LLC. Retrieved October 10, 2003, from http://www.dailycamera.com/bdc/business/article/ 0,1713,BDC_2400_1950749,00.html

[h]Katagi, K. (2000, October). A heady debate. Ski magazine. Kauder, C. (2000, March 13). A heady debate. The Daily Camera, pp. 1B, 8B

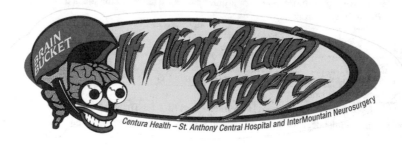

Fig. 7.1 The program's logo, displayed on all helmets used for the program

of helmets, annual information sessions were offered to ski patrollers and instructors to educate them about the effectiveness of wearing helmets while skiing or snowboarding. Moreover, the program funds were used to purchase helmets for the ski patrol and race course personnel during the 2002 Winter Olympics in Salt Lake City.

The following Table 7.3, adopted from Levy et al. (2007), summarizes the three components of the program.

7.1.3 Helmet Program for Ski Schools

During the 2000–2001 ski season, a helmet loaner program was initiated by Dr. Levy at a ski school rental facility at the Winter Park Children's Center. Through the program, all children enrolled in ski school were offered free loaner helmets for the days they participated in ski school. During the following seasons, this program was expanded, and more helmets were donated to the ski schools. When the program first started, it was optional for the children to use the free helmets. However, throughout the following ski seasons, wearing a helmet while in the ski school became a default option unless the parents indicated that they did not want their children to wear the helmets. This further increased helmet use as well as helmet acceptance among the children in ski schools.

Box 7.1 Helmet Saving Lives
Denver Haslem, a 27-year-old, is alive today because of a helmet. In 2003, he had a collision with a tree while skiing when he suffered several internal injuries, broken bones, and bruises. However, despite his severe injuries, he only suffered a mild brain injury and was able to recover completely thanks to his helmet. When asked about his experience, he said: "I owe my life to a helmet" (Colorado Mines Prepares for Ski-a-thon, 2008). Denver started wearing a ski helmet 1–2 years prior to his accident, as a result of his participation in the ski-a-thon organized by his fraternity and Dr. Leo. Since his accidence, Denver has continued to be involved with the It Ain't Brain Surgery program and has participated in the ski-a-thon every year, working tirelessly to raise awareness about the program and about slope safety and helmet use.

7.2 Resources

7.2.1 Stakeholders

Christy Sports. As one of the key stakeholders, Christy Sports played an important role in advocating the It Ain't Brain Surgery program. When this

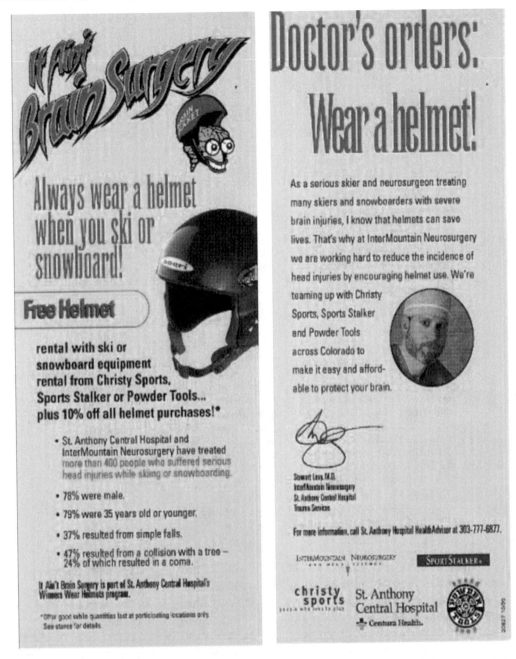

Fig. 7.2 Brochures for the program distributed throughout the community. (Reprinted from "Always Wear a Helmet when you Ski or Snowboard [Brochure]" by It Ain't Brain Surgery, n.d., Denver, CO: St. Anthony Central Hospital)

program was initiated, helmets for skiing and snowboarding were just being introduced to the public as new equipment. Therefore, participating in a program where helmets were provided to customers at no additional cost to the stores seemed appealing to the stores as it allowed them to assess the financial benefits of selling or renting helmets to customers. The participating stores gained business by promoting the program which attracted customers to their stores and increased helmet sales.

Table 7.3 Summary of the three components of the It Ain't Brain Injury program (Levy et al., 2007)

Component	Description	Purpose	Evaluation
Marketing campaign	Interviews with and presentations along with stickers (to place helmets), posters, and informational brochures, which were then distributed in target communities and in participating stores. Message was as follows: (a) TBI can occur in skiing/snowboarding, (b) most common cause of TBI in skiing/snowboarding is hitting a stationary object such as a tree, (c) TBI is the leading cause of death and serious injury among skiers/ snowboarders, and (d) many TBI can be prevented by wearing a helmet	Increase public awareness and knowledge about (1) ski- and snowboard-related TBI and (2) the helmet loaner program. Influence skiing public's beliefs about helmets	Observations of public's helmet use on the slopes
Helmet loaner program	Developed in cooperation with Christy Sports: anyone renting ski or snowboard equipment from any of the participating stores was offered a free loaner helmet to use for the duration of the rental period	Reducing barriers to wearing a helmet by making loaner helmets available at no cost and (2) influencing skiing public's belief about helmets	(1) Comparison of helmet acceptance among renters at study stores to helmet acceptance among renters at nonparticipating stores. (2) To determine acceptability of helmets, a survey was administered to a convenience sample of customers returning rental equipment to one of the study stores during the pilot season
Instructors and patrollers	(a) Ski patrollers and ski instructors were given helmets and encouraged to wear a helmet while working on the slopes and (b) were educated about TBI and the effectiveness of helmets at their annual fall "refresher courses" and after caring for patients with a significant TBI	(1) Have ski industry professionals set an example for the skiing public and (2) influence skiing public's beliefs about helmets	Observation of patrollers' and instructors' helmet use on the slopes

Note: Adapted from "Helmets for Skiers and Snowboarders: An Injury Prevention Program", by A. S. Levy, A. P. Hawkes, and G. V. Rossie, 2007, *Health Promotion Practice, 8*, 259

St. Anthony Hospital. As a Level I Trauma Center, the mission of the hospital includes the promotion of public health and injury prevention. Therefore, supporting the program provided the opportunity for St. Anthony Hospital to maintain its mission. The program was supported by the Trauma Services Department at St. Anthony Hospital, where involvement with education and research is also a criterion that needs to be fulfilled. Therefore, for both St. Anthony Hospital, as a whole, and for the Trauma Services Department specifically, supporting the It Ain't Brain Surgery program provided the opportunity to promote public health and safety while fulfilling their mission.

Ski Resorts. The ski resorts are one of the stakeholders of the program by agreeing to let ski school participation in the helmet program and also promoting helmet use among their ski instructors and patrollers.

Hence, the implementation and development of the program involved several stakeholders. Some of the issues faced at the time of development and implementation involved the cooperation of the different stakeholders. For instance, obtaining the approval of the ski resorts to allow ski schools to participate in the helmet loaner program was one of the issues that was faced at the time of implementation. Moreover, maintaining the cooperation of Christy Sports after the program was initiated was also a challenge. One way to overcome these challenges was to convince the stakeholders of the effectiveness of helmets in reducing brain injuries among skiers and snowboarders. Therefore, several presentations and information seminars were delivered by Dr. Levy to both the ski resorts and the potential participating stores. The presentations included the scientific literature on the effectiveness of helmets and promoted the program as an effective way to increase helmet use among skiers and snowboarders.

7.2.2 Collaborators

Christy Sports. One of the main collaborators of the It Ain't Brain Surgery was Christy Sports by expanding the program to more than 30 stores in Colorado and later in Utah. Having informational brochures and posters all over the stores as well as training the staff about the helmet program contributed significantly to the implementation of the program. Additionally, Christy Sports advertised the program widely and paid for a comprehensive public awareness campaign one season. Yet, the main role that the participating Christy Sports played was in running the helmet loaner program in their stores and offering free helmets to customers as part of their rental package. The collaboration began in the 1998–1999 ski season when the pilot project was initiated and further continued until the 2006–2007 season. However, during the 2007–2008 season, Christy Sports was no longer willing to offer the free helmet loaner program as the program was seen as a lost potential revenue stream since more people started wearing helmets. This lack of further collaboration restricted the helmet loaner program to the smaller rental stores and ski schools. Nonetheless, for the period of their collaboration, Christy Sports did play an important role in promoting the program and increasing helmet use among skiers and snowboarders.

Media. The media contributed significantly to the success of the program by taking part in the social marketing campaign. The message advocated by the program regarding helmet use was spread through newspaper, magazine, and television reaching a wide range of audience. In other words, various forms of publications were used to educate the public about the importance of wearing helmets when skiing or snowboarding and further inform them about the It Ain't Brain Injury program. Therefore, the close collaboration with the media helped spread the message and possibly contributed to the popularity of the program.

In addition to the collaborators who were involved at the beginning of the initiative, a few other individuals became involved throughout the following years and their collaborations helped the implementation of the program. One such collaborator was an anesthesiologist, Dr. Paul Leo, who became interested in the program and contributed to the maintenance of the program. At the time the program was initiated, Dr. Leo was involved with a fraternity organization devoted to running a ski-a-thon fundraising event, to raise money for various causes. However, after the involvement of Dr. Leo with the program, the ski-a-thon incorporated the theme of helmet use among skiers and snowboarders at their events and also donated the money raised from the ski-a-thon to buy helmets for the program.

The funding for the It Ain't Brain Surgery program came from a variety of sources and was allocated solely to the purchasing of helmets for the program. The marketing costs—including logo design and production of stickers, brochures, etc.—as well as the administration of the program, were covered entirely by volunteer efforts and "in kind" donations. The helmets for the pilot program were purchased by Dr. Levy's practice at InterMountain Neurosurgery (Levy et al., 2007) and were used for 1 year (1998–1999) in the participating stores, then donated to the National Sports Center for the Disabled. For the following 3 years, the program was funded primarily through grants from the St. Anthony Health Foundation. However, other sources of funding were used and included donations from InterMountain Neurosurgery, Centura Trauma Services at St. Anthony Central Hospital, and private individuals, as well as funds raised via the Beta Phi Ski-a-thon.

Christy Sports, as the store advocating the program, also provided support by providing helmets at wholesale cost, providing the labor hours to administer the program, advertising the program at their store, and paying for a comprehensive public awareness campaign during one season. A few helmet manufacturers—Boeri, Leedon, and Giro—further provided helmets for the program below wholesale price. Furthermore, every dollar raised through all sources was used to purchase helmets. The marketing costs for publishing the logo, stickers, brochures, and posters were covered by Dr. Levy's primary hospital. The brochures were made available for the public throughout the community as well as the participating Christy Sports locations. The stickers were put on the helmets used for the program, and the posters were displayed in the participating stores to promote the program. The administration of the entire program was further done by volunteers and gift-in-kind labor. Currently, the program is mainly administered in ski schools, and the primary source of funding for the program comes from fundraising events used to buy helmets of different sizes for the ski schools (S. Levy, personal communication, April 22, 2008).

In terms of the personnel administering the program, the participation of the store managers of Christy Sports was one of the key factors in the success of this program. The store managers were informed about the program by the area manager (who was involved with the program since its initiation). The store managers in turn educated the store personnel and the rental technicians. The rental technicians were instructed to inform the customers about the helmet loaner program and offer them the loaner helmet at the time of the equipment rental. As one of the components of the program was aimed at having ski industry professionals set an example for the public, the cooperation of such professionals was certainly helpful for the success of the program. The ski patrollers and ski instructors were given helmets and were encouraged to wear them while working on the slopes. Furthermore, the ski patrollers and instructors were educated about the

significance of head injuries and the effectiveness of helmets in preventing them. The education sessions for the ski patrollers took place during their annual fall "refresher courses" and "debriefing" follow-up sessions (Levy et al., 2007).

7.2.3 Inputs to the Prevention Model

The program has undergone some changes since it was first implemented. Firstly, the program expanded to more locations and even to a few other states in the United States. One other change that happened during the 2007–2008 season was that Christy Sports was no longer willing to participate in the program. Therefore, the program became limited to smaller rental stores and ski schools. This change came about as Christy Sports saw the free helmet loaner program as a potential loss of revenue, since they found more people wearing helmets and therefore more people were willing to pay to buy or rent their helmets. Furthermore, certain changes have taken place in terms of funding the program.

As the program gained more popularity, more people became involved with the program and participated in organizing fundraising events to raise public awareness and also raise money to buy more helmets. Another important development was the initiation of the ski school program where helmets are offered at no extra cost to the children. This change came in place to further expand the program among children and make helmets an integrated part of skiing or snowboarding. The first phase of the ski school program started in the 2000–2001 season when 500 helmets were donated to the Winter Park Children's Center. Later, in the 2002–2003 season, another 500 helmets were donated to the ski school program. Since then, fundraising events (such as ski-a-thons) have contributed significantly to the ski school program in terms of providing the funds to purchase helmets for other ski schools in Colorado.

Nonetheless, after the initiation of the program, the ski-a-thons, which are annual fundraising events, became devoted to the It Ain't Brain Surgery program. It was first agreed that 20% of the total money raised during the fundraising events would go towards the It Ain't Brain Surgery program. However, throughout the following years, this proportion was raised to 50%, and currently 100% of the funds raised by the Beta Phi ski-a-thon go towards supporting the It Ain't Brain Surgery program. The money provided by the fundraising is in fact used to purchase helmets for the ski school program. The fundraising events also create public awareness of the program and the effectiveness of helmets in preventing brain injuries among skiers and snowboarders.

7.3   Implementation

7.3.1   Effective Practices

The It Ain't Brain Surgery program utilizes several effective practices in implementing the program. One such practice is educating the public about the significance of TBI and informing them about the loaner helmets offered by the program. This effort was made through a broad social marketing campaign and by using various means of publications (e.g., newspapers, magazines, and television) to deliver the message advocated by the program. In addition, including the helmets with the rental packages implicitly conveyed the message that a helmet is a necessary piece of equipment when skiing or snowboarding (Levy et al., 2007). Yet, offering the helmets at no extra cost to customers was perhaps the most effective practice in implementing the program. In fact, this practice follows the health benefit model which states that outweighing the costs by the benefits encourages people to act (Levy et al., 2007). In the model used in this program, the benefit of having protection against brain injuries by wearing a helmet easily outweighs the cost of wearing a helmet, since they were provided free of charge to renters at participating stores (as otherwise, some might not want to wear a helmet when skiing or snowboarding). Therefore, more

people are willing to participate in the program and wear helmets.

In addition, several other factors facilitated the implementation of this program. One important factor was the cooperation of Christy Sports as a large corporation with multiple retail outlets which served to enhance the popularity and far-reaching scope of the program. On the other hand, the nature of the program made it appealing to the stores, as it offered marketing advantages for them as well. The program not only attracted more people seeking rental equipment to the participating stores, but it might have played a role in increasing helmet sales in the participating stores as people in these stores became more familiar with the risk of brain injuries and the effectiveness of helmets in preventing these injuries. Moreover, the timing of the initiation of the program was a significant factor in how it succeeded later on. The program was initiated immediately after the high-profile and highly publicized fatalities of Michael Kennedy and Sonny Bono. According to Dr. Levy (personal communication, April 22, 2008), these events preceding the initiation of the program helped with the implementation and the success of the program, by focusing the attention of the media, and thus the public, on the topic of brain injuries and the potential benefit of helmets on the slopes.

Nonetheless, there were some obstacles to implementing the program. One such obstacle was persuading the ski patrollers and instructors to wear helmets to serve as role models for the other skiers and snowboarders on the hills. Efforts were made to buy helmets for ski patrollers and instructors and also to educate them about the effectiveness of helmets in reducing brain injuries. However, the results later showed that these efforts were not as effective as had been hoped, as only a small proportion of ski patrollers and instructors were found to be wearing helmets on the hills even a few years after the program was initiated. One other obstacle to implementing the program was that despite all efforts, still some customers did not accept the loaner helmet as part of their rental package. Therefore, further strategies are needed to increase enrollment in the program. Finally, one other obstacle was that the program did not become self-sustaining and the financial needs of the program are currently mainly met by means of fundraising (Levy et al., 2007).

After a few years, the program was transferred to ski schools and some smaller rental shops, as Christy Sports no longer wished to participate. In fact, running the program in the ski schools was a success as assessments showed that it resulted in the majority of children wearing helmets. When this program was transferred to the ski schools, some changes were made as helmets were provided to all the children as a default option unless their parents explicitly indicated that they did not want their children wearing one (S. Levy, personal communication, April 22, 2008).

7.3.2 Actors in Decision Making and Planning

Among those currently involved with the decision making and planning of the program, Dr. Levy is the one mainly responsible for running the program. However, there are other individuals involved with the program particularly in terms of supporting the program financially. For instance, Dr. Leo, an anesthesiologist who is also involved with organizing the Beta Phi ski-a-thon, became interested in the program and has been organizing the annual ski-a-thon to support the It Ain't Brain Surgery program. The ski schools are also now involved with the program as they are offering the loaner helmets to children at their ski schools. Furthermore, the volunteers involved with the fundraising are also currently involved with the program. Nevertheless, there are individuals who are not currently involved with the program, but their involvement could contribute to achieving greater success. For instance, according to Dr. Levy (personal communication, April 22, 2008), ski resorts, individual ski patrollers, and ski instructors and the National Ski Patrol are among those individuals or groups whose involvement with the program could contribute significantly to the success of the program.

7.4 Outcome

7.4.1 Evaluation Method

The evaluation of the It Ain't Brain Surgery program has multiple components. One component of the evaluation was assessing the effect of the program on helmet acceptance among skiers and snowboarders. Helmet acceptance was measured objectively by calculating the percentage of the total number of helmet days per rental days as well as subjectively by self-reports completed by customers at rental stores. To further investigate the effect of the program on helmet acceptance, researchers compared helmet acceptance among customers at the participating stores to those in nonparticipating stores. During the pilot project 1998–1999 season, rental data from the three stores participating in the program were compared to those of four nonparticipating stores at the same ski resort. However, during the 2000–2001 and 2001–2002 seasons, when the program spread to more stores, the control group consisted of 30 nonparticipating stores in corresponding locations across the state. Researchers calculated the percentage of the total number of helmet days as an objective measure of helmet acceptance by dividing the total number of helmet days per season by the total number of rental days for the season and multiplying it by 100.

Furthermore, to assess people's subjective feeling towards wearing helmets, a survey was administered to 117 skiers and snowboarders returning their rental equipment to one of the participating stores. The survey included questions about the frequency of wearing the helmets as well as the likelihood of buying a helmet in the future. Another component of the outcome research of the It Ain't Brain Surgery program involved an observational study of the general skiing and snowboarding population to assess proportion of skiers or snowboarders wearing helmets. These observational studies simply involved observers counting the number of skiers and snowboarders wearing helmets on the hills. Observations were done at various resorts in the lift areas as skiers and snowboarders loaded into chairlifts. Moreover, the degree of helmet acceptance and helmet use was assessed among ski patrollers and instructors who participated in the program.

7.4.2 Result

The results of the evaluation of the program showed positive effects of the program in enhancing both helmet acceptance and helmet use where the program was implemented. The results of the evaluation are summarized in an article by Levy et al. (2007). The results show helmet acceptance rates of customers renting equipment from both participating and nonparticipating stores. For instance, in the pilot season only 1.38% of customers renting snowboarding and skiing equipment from the nonparticipating stores paid the extra cost of renting a helmet. However, within the same time period, about 13.8% of those who rented equipment from the participating stores accepted the free loaner helmets as part of their rental package. Furthermore, helmet acceptance kept increasing significantly throughout the following years the program was implemented. Therefore, the program was proven to be effective in increasing helmet acceptance among skiers and snowboarders. Levy et al. (2007) also reported that overall the stores participating in the program sold 5 times more helmets than the control stores. Therefore, one could assume that the program increased people's awareness of the effectiveness of helmets in reducing brain injuries such that more people were willing to buy helmets.

The results of the survey completed by customers returning their equipment to one of the participating stores showed that firstly, 83% of those who rented equipment from the participating stores did participate in the program. In other words, more than 80% of people renting ski and snowboarding equipment, who completed the survey, also accepted the loaner helmet that was offered to them through the program. However, the results of the study showed that snowboarders had a significantly higher rate of helmet acceptance and were more likely to rent a loaner helmet than skiers. Secondly, of those who accepted the loaner helmet, 91.1% of skiers and 85.7% of

snowboarders indicated that they wore their helmets all day. From the results it appears that once customers rented helmets, they were very much likely to wear them. Putting the program logo as stickers on the loaner helmets might have played a role in emphasizing the importance of wearing the helmets at all times and consequently resulted in the high degree of self-reported compliance observed among those participating in the program.

The results of the survey also showed that out of all skiers and snowboarders ($n = 97$) who accepted a helmet, 86.6% said that they would buy a helmet in the future. As previously mentioned, assessing the sales records during the pilot program also showed that the participating stores sold five times more helmets than the nonparticipating stores. Interestingly, Levy et al. (2007) in their report state that even among those who did not participate in the loaner program (i.e., did not accept a loaner helmet), almost half reported that they would likely buy a helmet in the future. Therefore, it appears as though the raised awareness about the effect of helmets in reducing brain injuries had long-term outcomes as it encouraged more people to consider buying their own helmet.

Furthermore, the results of the observational study of skiers and snowboarders loading into chairlifts showed that during the 4-year period of the study (1998–2002), helmet use increased significantly (Levy et al., 2007). Figure 7.3 adopted from Levy et al. (2007) shows the mean percentage of skiers and snowboarders who were observed to be wearing helmets on the hills in Colorado. The results showed that the snowboarders were significantly more likely to wear helmets than skiers. This is yet another important positive effect of the program as previous studies have shown that snowboarders have a higher risk of acquiring brain injuries (Hackam, Kreller, & Pearl, 1999; Hagel, Goulet, Platt, & Pless, 2004; Levy et al., 2002; Nakaguchi et al., 1999). Therefore, the program was successful in increasing helmet use particularly where most serious injuries are happening.

With regard to the third component of the program which involved providing helmets for

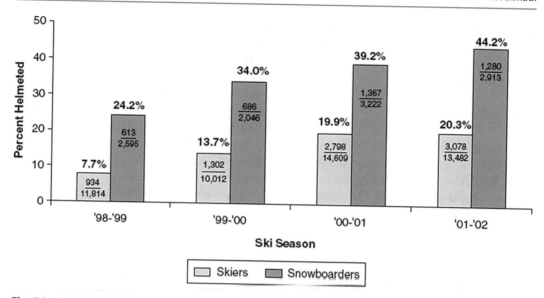

Fig. 7.3 Mean percentage of skiers and snowboarders who wore helmets on the hills from 1998 to 1999 ski season to 2001–2002 season. (Reprinted from "Helmets for Skiers and Snowboarders: An Injury Prevention Program", by A. S. Levy, A. P. Hawkes, and G. V. Rossie, 2007, *Health Promotion Practice, 8,* 263)

ski patrollers and instructors, evaluation was done in terms of assessing the proportion of ski patrollers and instructors who actually wore their helmets on the hills. The results showed that during the 2001–2002 season, only 9.5% of ski patrollers and 12% of ski instructors were found to be wearing helmets on the slopes in Colorado. When asked about their lack of motivation in wearing the helmets they were given, ski patrollers and instructors claimed that they did not believe the helmets could reduce the risk of brain injuries among skiers and snowboarders and, in fact, indicated that they believed that helmets could lead to more risk-taking behaviors in skiers and snowboarders. However, this belief is contrary to what the research in this area has shown. Unfortunately, this aspect of the program did not show the desired effect. Improvements to this component could possibly include a more comprehensive educational and awareness campaign mainly targeting ski patrollers and instructors.

Overall, the evaluation of the program shows that it was at least partly responsible for the increased awareness of the importance of helmets in preventing brain injuries among skiers and snowboarders. Furthermore, it appears that increasing numbers of skiers and snowboarders started wearing helmets or even buying helmets during the course of the program. In fact, several studies investigating the rate of helmet use across different regions have reported a significantly greater helmet use in Colorado where the It Ain't Brain Surgery program was first initiated (Andersen et al., 2004; Buller et al., 2003). Therefore, it is clear that the program was fairly successful in accomplishing the initial goals and objectives.

7.4.3 Effect of the Program on Brain Injury Rates

Assessing the direct effect of the program on incidence of brain injuries is rather more complex. According to Dr. Levy (personal communication, April 22, 2008), over the years the program was running, there were over 400,000 helmet loaner days. Studies have shown that the rate of brain injury in skiers and snowboarders is around 0.25 per 1000 skier-days and helmets can reduce the risk of a brain injury by 50–75% in skiers and snowboarders. Therefore, one can estimate that the many helmets loaned out throughout the program prevented approximately 100 brain injuries (S. Levy, personal communication, April 22, 2008). Furthermore,

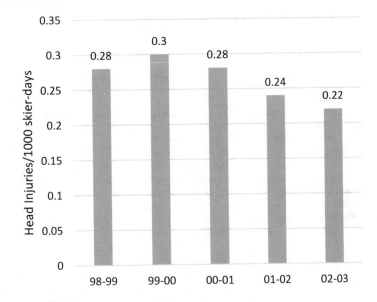

Fig. 7.4 Skier and snowboarder brain injury trends during study period (1998–2003). (Reprinted from a PowerPoint presentation by Levy (2004))

no skier or snowboarder sustained a brain injury while wearing a helmet provided through the loaner program. Additionally, the injury rates before and after the program were assessed at one of the resorts where the program was active, as means of assessing the influence of the program on injury rates. Figure 7.4 summarizes the brain injury rates during the program from 1998 to 2003 (Levy, 2004).

Therefore, as shown in the figure, brain injury rates were reduced during the years following the initiation of the program. In summary, the evaluation of the It Ain't Brain Surgery program shows that the program was successful in increasing helmet acceptance and helmet use among skiers and snowboarders. More importantly, it was found to be successful in reducing the incidence of brain injuries among skiers and snowboarders.

7.5 Conclusion

Skiing and snowboarding are among some of the most popular winter sports. Nonetheless, the injury rates among those participating in these sports are also shown to be significant. In particular, brain injuries constitute a significant portion of serious injuries among skiers and snowboarders and are found to be on the rise. Research studies have shown that helmets are effective in reducing brain injuries among skiers and snowboarders. Therefore, an effective injury prevention model should focus on helmets as the primary mechanism of injury prevention. The program It Ain't Brain Surgery, initiated in Colorado by a neurosurgeon, Dr. Levy, has a focus on helmet use and has unique features that make it an exemplary practice in preventing brain injuries among skiers and snowboarders. This program is composed of three components, with the main one being the helmet loaner program. The program involved the close collaboration of different bodies such as the media, the ski rental stores, as well as the ski schools. The evaluations of the program showed that it succeeded in increasing helmet acceptance and helmet use among skiers and snowboarders. Furthermore, the evaluation showed that the rates of brain injuries decreased in the study area during the years following the implementation of the program. Therefore, the It Ain't Brain Injury program can be identified as an exemplary practice program in reducing brain injuries among skiers and snowboarders.

Acknowledgments The author would like to express sincere appreciation to the key informants for this case study: A. Stewart Levy of St. Anthony Hospital and Centura Health in Lakewood, CO, USA—whose consultation made this project possible.

BRIO Model: It Ain't Brain Surgery

Group Served: All snowboarders and skiers.

Goal: To promote the use of helmets to snowboarders and skiers for the prevention on head/brain injuries.

Background	Resources	Implementation	Outcome
Injuries happen frequently among skiers and snowboarders; brain injuries constitute about 20–30% of all injuries and are the leading cause of death in this group. Helmets are shown to be effective tools in reducing brain injuries; however they are not widely used among skiers and snowboarders In 1998 in response to the increasing number of brain injuries, the It Ain't Brain Surgery program was initiated by a neurosurgeon in Denver, Colorado The aim of the program was to increase helmet use among skiers and snowboarders The program included three parts: marketing campaign, helmet loaner program, and educating instructors and patrollers	The program has been funded through various sources: grants from the St. Anthony Health Foundation, InterMountain Neurosurgery, Centura Trauma Services at St. Anthony Central Hospital, private individuals, and fundraising events Funds were mainly used to purchase helmets which were offered at no extra cost to skiers and snowboarders renting equipment at participating Christy Sports stores Extensive media coverage on effectiveness of helmets in reducing head injuries and promotion of the program was launched	The program included a multidisciplinary approach to injury prevention and incorporated the health benefit model (i.e., benefit of wearing helmet outweighs the cost) The program also provides marketing advantage for the participating stores by attracting more customers to the stores since helmets are provided for free The program is now expanded to other ski rental stores and ski schools Currently, at the ski schools, helmets are provided to all the children as a default option unless their parents explicitly indicate that they do not want their children to wear a helmet	The program was successful in increasing the rates of helmet rentals at the participating sites The surveys conducted at the participating sites revealed high helmet acceptance rates as well as high degrees of self-reported compliance Observational studies showed that a significantly greater number of skiers and snowboarders in locations where the program was implemented were wearing helmets The program decreased the rates of brain injuries over the years despite the increase in participation

Life-Space Model: It Ain't Brain Surgery

Sociocultural: civilization/community	Interpersonal: primary and secondary relationships	Physical environments: where we live	Internal states: biochemical/genetic and means of coping
Awareness raising through extensive mass media coverage on effectiveness of helmets and the program itself Involvement of Christy Sports as an environment to run the helmet loaner component of the program Participation of the community in fundraising events to contribute to the program financially and raise awareness Multifaceted strategy that includes snowboarders, skiers, instructors, health professionals, and researchers	Close relationship between Christy Sports and initiators of the program to promote helmet use and run helmet loaner program Relationship with the funding bodies such as helmet manufacturers and St. Anthony Hospital to allow for the program to run Close cooperation with ski schools in order to allow for the implementation of the program in the ski schools	Detailed assessment of the mechanism of injury among skiers and snowboarders Evaluation of the effectiveness of helmets in reducing brain injuries in this group Involvement of the local stores in the implementation of the program	Training the ski instructors and patrollers in risks associated with this sport and promotion of helmet use by offering them free helmets Training the staff at the participating stores about the risk of injury and importance of wearing helmets Expansion of the program to other ski resorts and ski schools

References

Andersen, P. A., Buller, D. B., Scott, M. D., Walkosz, B. J., Voeks, J. H., Cutter, G. R., et al. (2004). Prevalence and diffusion of helmet use at ski areas in Western North America in 2001–02. *Injury Prevention, 10*, 358–362.

Buller, D. B., Andersen, P. A., Walkosz, B. J., Scott, M. D., Cutter, G. R., Dignan, M. B., et al. (2003). The prevalence and predictors of helmet use by skiers and snowboarders at ski areas in western North America in 2001. *Journal of Trauma, 55*(5), 939–945.

Colorado Mines Prepares for Ski-a-thon. (2008). Retrieved from http://www.betathetapi.org/index.php?option=com_content&task=view&id=729&Itemid=223.

Hackam, D. J., Kreller, M., & Pearl, R. H. (1999). Snow-related recreational injuries in children: Assessment of morbidity and management strategies. *Journal of Pediatric Surgery, 34*, 65–68.

Hagel, B. E., Goulet, C., Platt, R. W., & Pless, I. B. (2004). Injuries among skiers and snowboarders in Quebec. *Epidemiology, 15*, 279–286.

Levy, A. S. (2004). Power point presentation.

Levy, A. S., Hawkes, A. P., Hemminger, L. M., & Knight, S. (2002). An analysis of head injuries among skiers and snowboarders. *Journal of Trauma, 53*(4), 695–704.

Levy, A. S., Hawkes, A. P., & Rossie, G. V. (2007). Helmets for skiers and snowboarders: An injury prevention program. *Health Promotion Practices, 8*(3), 257–265.

Nakaguchi, H., Fujimaki, T., Ueki, K., Takahashi, M., Yoshida, H., & Kirino, T. (1999). Snowboard head injury: Prospective study in Chino, Nagano, for two seasons from 1995 to 1997. *Journal of Trauma, 46*(6), 1066–1069.

Riding and Road Safety Test

Helen Looker and Julia Forgie

The purpose of the British Horse Society's (BHS) Riding and Road Safety Test is to prevent injuries by educating horseback riders in reducing the risks of accidents when riding on roads and in general riding activities.

8.1 Background

Accurately determining the incidences of horse-riding accidents is difficult since injured riders may not always consult a doctor. Furthermore, even if an injury is reported to a doctor, there may be no formal record made of the incident. Accidents involving horses reported to the British Horse Society (BHS) number approximately eight per day, of which over one third may consist of head injuries (British Horse Society [BHS], 2007; Silver, 2002). In 1992, the UK Office of Population Census reported 12 equestrian-related fatalities (Carlton Reckling, & Webb, 1996). Similarly, through voluntary, self-reported data collected by the British Horse Society, 11 riders were killed and 39 injured in 117 accidents in 2002 (BHS, 2007). This representation, however, likely does not reflect an accurate number of horse-related accidents on roads since there are currently no compulsory recording systems in place (BHS, 2007).

Regarding riding-related injury statistics in the United States, the National Electronic Injury Surveillance System (NEISS) found that in 1997, 58,647 people attended a hospital with horse-related injuries and in 1998, this figure had risen to 64,693 (Silver, 2002). Furthermore, from 2001 to 2003, an estimated 102,904 Americans were treated for horse-related injuries, of whom approximately 19% were children and youth aged 14 years or younger (Thomas, Annest, Gilchrist, & Bixby-Hammett, 2006). While overall, females have a higher rate of injury than males due to differences in rates of participation, sex-specific injury fluctuates across age groups (see Fig. 8.1).

Due to the elevation of the rider's body and head above the ground, the predominance of head injuries in the spectrum of injuries sustained by horse riders is not surprising. An Australian study examining 18 fatal horse-related injuries, for example, found that 13 of the deaths were the result of head injury (Pounder, 1984). Similarly, a Canadian study found that 22 of 38 horse-related fatalities were the result of head injury (Aronson & Tough, 1993). A recent study conducted in the United Kingdom describing the demographics and nature of injuries occurring on or around horses found that "isolated head injuries constituted 45 (17.3%) of the patients" in the study, 53.3% of which "had a cerebral injury" (Moss, Wan, & Whitlock, 2002, p. 413; see Fig. 8.2).

H. Looker (✉) · J. Forgie
University of Toronto, Toronto, ON, Canada

© Springer Nature Switzerland AG 2020
R. Volpe (ed.), *Casebook of Traumatic Injury Prevention*,
https://doi.org/10.1007/978-3-030-27419-1_8

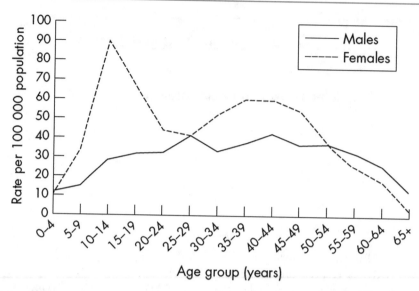

Fig. 8.1 National annual rates of nonfatal horse-related injuries treated in emergency departments, by sex and age group—USA, 2001–2003. (Reprinted from "Non-Fatal Horse Related Injuries Treated in Emergency Departments in the United States, 2001–2003", by K. E. Thomas, J. L. Annest, J. Gilchrist, and D. M. Bixby-Hammet, 2006, British Journal of Sports Medicine, 40, p. 620. Copyright 2006 British Journal of Sports Medicine)

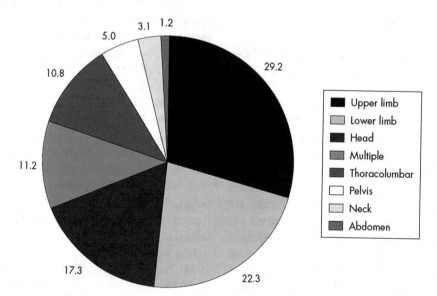

Fig. 8.2 Anatomical distribution of injuries in percentages. ("A Changing Pattern Of Injuries To Horse Riders" by P. S. Moss, A. Wan, and M. R. Whitlock, 2002, *Journal of Emergency Medicine, 19*, p. 413. Copyright 2002 by the Emergency Medicine Journal)

Given the popularity of horseback riding and the frequency of severe injury, specifically head and spinal cord injury, there is a critical need for efficient means of injury prevention (Firth, 1985). The BHS's Riding and Road Safety Test aims to prevent injuries and educate riders about reduc-ing the risk of accidents in general riding activities (hacking) and also when riding on roads.

Drivers are required by law to understand the behavior of all road users and pass a test before they venture alone; for the moment, equestrians do not have to comply by passing a similar test in order to use roads, and it is, therefore, even more important that they are encouraged to take responsibility for their own safety and learn the correct way to approach riding on today's busy roads (Hardy, 2007).

The BHS Riding and Road Safety Test seeks to fill the void created by the lack of requisite training and accreditation of equestrians who ride both on and off road.

The BHS continues to develop their Riding and Road Safety Test and has offered the test on a voluntary basis since 1976 (Hardy, 2007; Sheila Hardy, personal communication, August 21, 2007; Kerry, 1993). Peter Cannon was the BHS safety officer when the program began (Kerry, 1993). The program was initially designed to target the entire horse-riding population, "all people, from all walks of life—not just wealthy horse owners" (S. Hardy, personal communication, November 2, 2007). The test has always been and will continue to be a test made available to anyone interested because according to S. Hardy (personal communication, November 2, 2007), "road safety applies to everyone and should be open to everyone." Candidates may be aged from 12 to 70 years to be eligible to take the test. Candidates over the age of 70 may take the test but must take out their own insurance before doing so, and riders under the age of 12 may take the test through The Pony Club, "an international voluntary youth organization" (D. Kerry, personal communication, April 21, 2008; The Pony Club, n.d.).

The Riding and Road Safety Test is comprised of three distinct components. The first component is a written examination involving a series of multiple-choice questions (Fig. 8.3). The second component consists of a simulated road route in a fenced off area, while the final component consists of a practical exam that takes place on the road. The Riding and Road Safety Test utilizes many effective injury prevention strategies such as the use of helmets, knowledge of horse behavior, knowledge of road and traffic regulations, well-conducted lessons by a trained instructor, rider education, and the use of protective equipment and clothing (BHS, 2007).

Over its 30-year life span, the Riding and Road Safety Test content has changed very little, and the only significant changes made following internal evaluations by BHS have been to improve the standard of training. When the program began, the BHS was subdivided into many departments including British Eventing, British Dressage, British Horse Driving Trials, Vaulting, Endurance, and The Pony Club. Each department used to handle their own safety measures; the Riding and Road Safety Test was operated by the Safety Department which was much smaller than it is now. In 1997, impasse and organizational division led to the separation of The Pony Club and establishment of the current-day British Horse Society, in which some departments were amalgamated and others diffused, resulting in the establishment of the Safety Department as it is currently structured. Subsequently, the administration for the Riding and Road Safety Test began increasing in scale (S. Hardy, personal communication, January 7, 2008) (Fig. 8.4).

In 1999, training for the test was reviewed resulting in greater effectiveness, and in 2001, the training program was completely redeveloped for purposes of standardization, which vastly improved the quality of training systemically. Prior to 2001, the British Horse Society was subdivided into 13 geographical regions, and each designated individual within each region was responsible for conducting their own training sessions. According to S. Hardy (personal communication, January 7, 2008), "some did a very good job, others did a very poor job," so standards varied greatly from one region to the next. Today, one team of trainers (six individuals) trains each group of trainers in order to maintain fidelity in standards. Concomitantly, the core teaching is the same for all 1000 approved trainers (S. Hardy, personal communication, January 7, 2008).

8.2   Resources

The British Horse Society has retained registered charity status and receives its funding for the Riding and Road Safety Test almost exclusively through the test's licensing fees, which are £32

Our Ref: SAFETY / SAFETY / THEORY TEST QUESTIONS / QP1 MAR2001

British Horse Society
Riding & Road Safety Test
Question Paper 1

Candidate Name: .... Tabard Number: ....

Venue: .... Date: ....

Mark out of 10: ....

Marking Examiner: ....

1. Identify the road sign your examiner is holding

   Answer: ....

2. Why is there a tack and turnout inspection at the beginning *at* every Road Safety Test?
   a) To see who has the cleanest tack
   b) To ensure the rider's clothing and horse's tack are in a safe and satisfactory condition for riding
   c) So the Examiner can assess the horse

3. When riding along the highway, in which hand should you carry your whip?
   a) It depends whether you're left handed or right handed
   b) The left hand
   c) The right hand

4. When riding your horse/pony on the roads, are you required to obey all traffic signs and police signals?
   a) Only those which relate to horse riders
   b) Yes
   c) No, they do not relate to horse riders

5. On a very windy day, what exceptional hazards should be looked for?
   a) Fast cars
   b) Paper bags and litter being blown across roads and flapping in hedges
   c) Holes in the road

Road Safety Congress 2007

Page 1 of 10

Fig. 8.3 Sample of questions in the theory component of the Riding and Road Safety Test. (Reprinted from *Encouraging Education in Road Safety,* by S. Hardy, 2007, Paper presented at the Road Safety Congress)

6. If you have to lead a horse, to which side of the road should you keep?
   a) Left
   b) Right
   c) On the pavement

7. What is the maximum number of riders recommended to form a group on the road?
   a) 6
   b) 8
   c) 10

8. What is the ABC of Emergency Aid?
   a) Airway. Breathing. Circulation
   b) Access. Blood. Circulation
   c) Airway. Blood. Cardio

9. What is the sequence of lights at a pelican crossing?
   a) Red, amber, green, amber
   b) Red, red and amber, green, amber
   c) Red, flashing amber, green, amber

10. Which of the following describes the sign for NO ENTRY?
   a) Horizontal red bar on a white disc
   b) Horizontal white bar on a red disc
   c) Horizontal white bar on a blue disc

Comments:

Road Safety Congress 2007 **Page 2 of 10**

Fig. 8.3 (Continued)

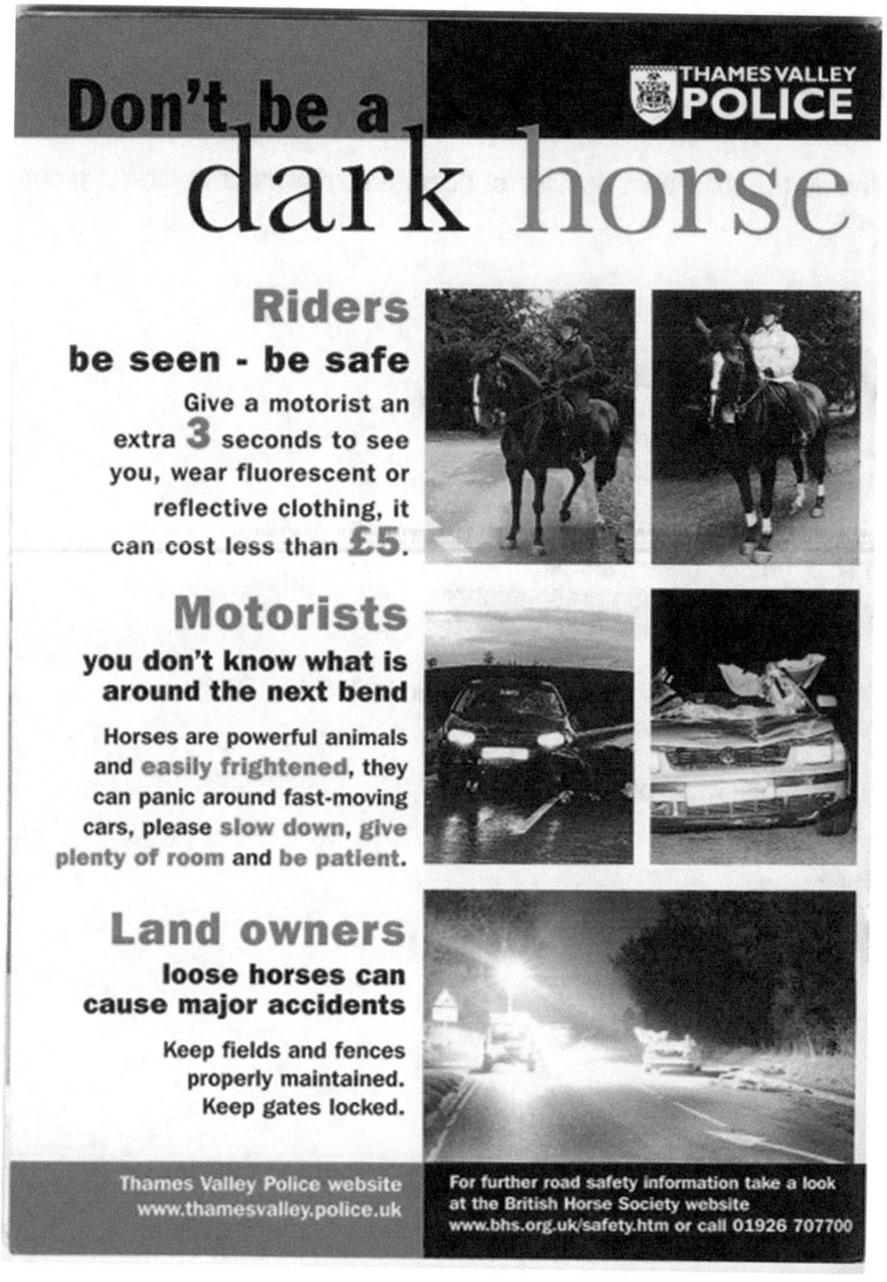

Fig. 8.4 Advertisement for the British Horse Society's "Don't be a dark horse" campaign in collaboration with the Thames Valley Mounted Police. (Reprinted from *Riding and Roadcraft* (11th ed.), by the British Horse Society, 2003, Addington, U.K.: Kenilworth Press)

for BHS members and £42 for nonmembers (S. Hardy, personal communication, January 7, 2008; BHS, 2007). Since trainers who help prepare candidates for taking the test are independent of the British Horse Society (yet certified to train, under BHS regulations), the Safety Department receives no profit from training fees and, as such, must be financially self-sufficient in attaining adequate revenue to run the program. The Riding and Road Safety Test is often supported by private riding organizations, and to encourage members to complete the test, some private clubs subsidize the cost of the licensing fees and/or training sessions (S. Hardy, personal communication, January 7, 2008).

The British Horse Society often receives private donations that help to subsidize the cost of running the organization. S. Hardy (personal communication, January 7, 2008), however, states that the Safety Department is rarely the recipient of private donations, since "donors usually prefer to give to more flamboyant departments." This further supports the notion that the Safety Department must rely on its own incoming resources to sustain itself. The road safety budget comes mostly from licensing and training fees with the remainder coming from rare donations, some government funding, and a very small portion of the BHS membership dues. This budget covers staff salary expenses, training days, and test administration costs. Not only must the Safety Department be self-sustaining financially, but also surplus income must be earned to help fund other BHS departments. Safety Department operations are undoubtedly sustainable over the long term, so long as demand for licensing remains constant which it has, over time (S. Hardy, personal communication, January 7, 2008).

BHS and its Safety Department have successfully collaborated with many corporate and community partners in financing, supporting, and promoting the Riding and Road Safety Test. Over the years, the BHS Safety Department has maintained a close relationship with the British Department for Transport. In 2001, the Department for Transport donated approximately £8000 to the Safety Department to produce a theory training manual and program for Riding and Road Safety trainers. A few years later, the Department for Transport gave an £18,000 grant to the Safety Department for the creation of their Road Safety CD-ROM (S. Hardy, personal communication, January 7, 2008).

BHS has also collaborated with other community partners and is fortunate to have a member of the Thames Valley Mounted Police sitting as a member of their Riding and Road Safety

Committee. The Thames Valley Mounted Police has also worked with the Safety Department in promoting their "Don't be a dark horse" campaign (Thames Valley Police Fig. 8.4), in which riders are encouraged to wear high-visibility riding clothing (high viz) to improve riding safety (BHS, 2003; S. Hardy, personal communication, January 7, 2008).

In addition to their involvement on the "Don't be a dark horse" campaign (Thames Valley Police Fig. 8.4), the Thames Valley Mounted Police have also donated to the Safety Department from the sale of unclaimed lost property. At this time, the Thames Valley Mounted Police gave a donation of £500 to the Safety Department's Riding and Road (S. Hardy, personal communication, January 7, 2008).

The BHS Safety Department has also worked in collaboration with V-Bandz, a company that sells and manufactures high-visibility riding gear. According to Hardy, Fiona Kennedy, who leads the company, is a great supporter of the BHS Riding and Road Safety Program and gives a substantial discount on products to those who have passed the test. V-Bandz has also donated equipment to the British Horse Society and was involved in the development of the CD-ROM to promote the use of high-viz clothing (S. Hardy, personal communication, January 7, 2008).

BHS has partnered with the South Essex Insurance Brokers so that qualifying BHS members may receive complimentary riding liability and accident insurance (Fig. 8.5; BHS, 2003; S. Hardy, personal communication, January 7, 2008).

8.2.1 High-Visibility Clothing

Campaigns to reduce equestrian injury on the roads in the United Kingdom have stressed visibility of horse and rider; "Be seen – be safe," for example, is a themed slogan from the "Don't be a dark horse" campaign (Thames Valley Police Fig. 8.4) from the Thames Valley Police force (Thames Valley Police, n.d.). Another message of the "Don't be a dark horse" campaign (Thames Valley Police Fig. 8.4) advises that reflective clothing costing as little as £5 would give a

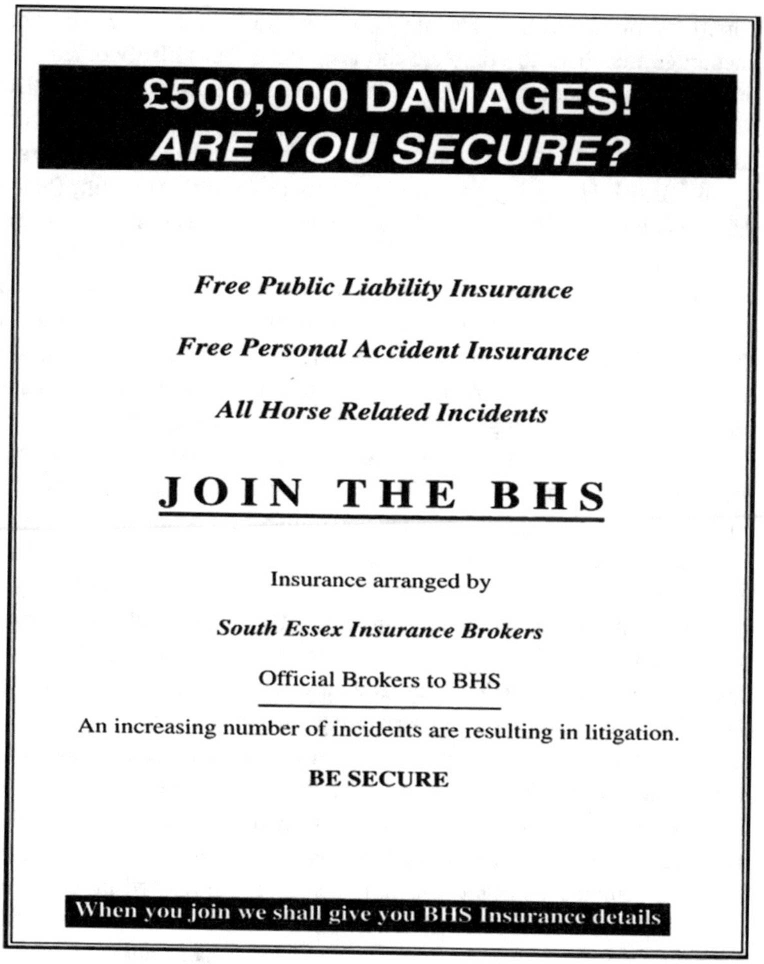

Fig. 8.5 South Essex Insurance Brokers advertisement featuring complimentary riding liability and accident insurance provided to qualifying BHS members. (Reprinted from *Riding and Roadcraft* (11th ed), by the British Horse Society, 2003, Addington, U.K.: Kenilworth Press)

£500,000 DAMAGES!
ARE YOU SECURE?

Free Public Liability Insurance

Free Personal Accident Insurance

All Horse Related Incidents

JOIN THE BHS

Insurance arranged by

South Essex Insurance Brokers

Official Brokers to BHS

An increasing number of incidents are resulting in litigation.

BE SECURE

When you join we shall give you BHS Insurance details

three-second lead to a motorist's awareness of a horse and rider ahead (Thames Valley Police, n.d.). The need or the expectation that riders maximize their visibility when using roads has directly impacted personal injury claims against drivers. Riders are encouraged to wear clothing and accessories on themselves and their horses just as motorists must use headlights with functioning rear and brake lights when driving at night (D. Kerry, personal communication, April 21, 2008). A horse might wear leg bands and/or a neck belt made with Scotchlite™ which is reflective at 1000 ft; this would be adequate for an attentive driver to notice a horse on a road as the stopping distance for a vehicle traveling at 70 mph is 315 ft (Be Reflective, n.d.; Department for Transport, 2007). In a 1988 study from Helen Muir and Chris Edwards at Cranfield University,

England, it was found that even though drivers reduced speed when passing a horse, an additional 6 km/h reduction occurred if the rider had reflective clothing, but speed was reduced to 43 km/h from the average 77 km/h when the ridden horse was equipped with reflective leg bands to make it as conspicuous as the rider (Clarkson, 2006; Kerry, 1993).

8.3 Implementation

BHS administration is centralized at its headquarters in Stoneleigh Park, Kenilworth, Warwickshire. The BHS has 400 examiners throughout the United Kingdom and 1000 trainers, some of whom also act as examiners to deliver the Riding and Road Safety Test (D. Kerry, personal communication, April 21, 2008). Also, since 1961, more than 900 riding school establishments in the United Kingdom, Ireland, Belgium, Spain, Italy, the United States, Hong Kong, Singapore, Dubai, and Malaysia became accredited under the BHS approvals scheme where annual surprise inspections check operating standards, animal welfare, quality of instruction, and safety standards (BHS, 2003). In the 13 geographic regions in the United Kingdom where BHS is represented, local authority road safety associations include one member from the region, one road safety officer from the local council, two mounted police officers, and one trustee of the BHS; all of the safety advisory committees consist of volunteer members (D. Kerry, personal communication, April 21, 2008).

A key strategy to the success of the Road Safety Test was to achieve inclusion status within the national Highway Code which dictates the rules of the road for anyone who wishes to qualify for a driver's license. Hardy and the Safety Department work closely with the Department for Transport to promote safety for riders and their horses on British roads. This collaboration has resulted in a set of questions becoming a part of the exam for prospective drivers where "learner" drivers are tested for perception of road hazards (S. Hardy, personal communication, August 21, 2007). To screen for medical contraindication, a prospective candidate must complete a medical questionnaire as part of the application process to take the Riding and Road Safety Test (BHS, 2003). The longevity of the program stems from selective use of experts and professionals such as road safety officers, to guide and complement volunteer involvement (D. Kerry, personal communication, March 10, 2008). Active and dynamic partnering of community and national stakeholders also demonstrates an approach to injury prevention that seeks to unite efforts for mutually desirable goals and share the responsibility of reducing injury and death.

The actual Riding and Road Safety Test has three segments:

1. Theory: Knowledge of the "Highway Code" applicable to England, Wales, and Scotland, or the "Rules of the Road" applicable to Northern Ireland, is tested by a written response to ten questions. Oral testing may be arranged at the discretion of the BHS. An 80% pass leads to part 2 and test papers must be handed to examiners and retained by BHS.

2. Simulated road route: This may be indoor or outdoor. An area is set up to test a rider's reactions to potential road hazards both visual and auditory in nature. Riders must have the horse trot between the simulated road hazards. At the beginning of the test, a tack and turnout inspection is conducted to ensure both horse and rider are safely prepared for riding. According to Finch and Watt (1996), "Attention to tack (or saddlery) is one of the major means of primary prevention" (p. 20). An 80% pass mark allows progress to the final test.

3. The road route: Candidates must wear the numbered tabards issued which are fluorescent or reflective and the horse is fitted with leg bands. A predesignated route is explained to the candidate on test day. A candidate may walk along the planned course before performing the test on horseback. A candidate's ability to deal with traffic and other hazards is tested. Candidates must show trot by the horse and use hand signals in application of the Highway Code. Successful candidates are awarded a certificate with a serial number and a badge (Hardy, 2007).

Two examiners are present to assess candidates, and the examiners are obliged by law to report any cases of suspected neglect or abuse in young candidates who take the Riding and Road Safety Test; guidelines from the British Equestrian Federation apply in addition to legislation for child protection and duty of care. A separate training course is given to educate examiners about child welfare, and volunteers are subject to a criminal record check before working for BHS (D. Kerry, personal communication, April 21, 2008; BHS, 2007). At the end of a testing session, the two examiners must leave together (D. Kerry, personal communication, April 21, 2008).

8.4   Outcome

Internal monitoring and evaluation of the Riding and Road Safety Test and associated functions by the BHS Safety Department has corrected the regional disparities in the education of trainers by using a core team to educate qualified trainers to a unified standard. Hardy attends and oversees all of the training sessions personally. BHS reports that the average number of individuals taking the Riding and Road Safety Test at this time exceeds 4000 annually. In testament to the effectiveness of the test relative to primary injury prevention, while the number of vehicles on the roads in the United Kingdom and the number of horse riders both increased over the last three decades, the number of accidents involving riders, horses, and motor vehicles has definitely declined according to data collected by the BHS Safety Department and mirrored in statistics published by the Department for Transport (DfT) in the United Kingdom. No other initiatives have been specifically designed to prevent equestrian injury involving vehicles. The Test has overwhelming government support, and statistics from the DfT reflect a declining trend in the number of reported road accidents resulting in personal injury where at least one ridden horse was involved. As shown on the BHS and DfT website for the years 2003–2006, these accidents numbered 153, 138, 136, and 123, respectively (BHS, 2007; Department for Transport, 2007).

Table 8.1 shows the history of recorded accidents where the 16–19 age group had the most casualties per 100,000 people in that demographic. Accurate injury data collection is not a straightforward matter as prevailing regulations for reporting accidents actually hinder the collection of consistently meaningful data, thereby obscuring the true impact of equestrian-related injury and death. Although it took 15 years of lobbying to get ridden horses as a category on the accident reporting form known as the STATS 19 coding form used by the police, it was left as an option to police forces as to whether or not they would use that section of the STATS 19 form (D. Kerry, personal communication, March 10, 2008; Western Morning News, 1998). D. Kerry suggested that understaffing, a focus on maintaining a community profile, and using resources for terrorist-related problems are current priorities for police attention rather than achieving full compliance on STATS 19 reporting amendments (personal communication, March 10, 2008).

In recent years, the BHS has added to its website a feature for riders to report any incidences of accidents or injuries they may have experienced while riding a horse on roads or in general riding (BHS, 2017c). The result of this self-reporting for riders to the BHS website has assisted the BHS in gathering a better understanding of incidents involving rider accidents and injuries (BHS, 2017c). As a result of gathering such information, the BHS has discovered an increase of occurrences involving rider- and vehicle-related injuries, as well as general riding injuries (BHS, 2017c). The BHS attributes the discovery of this increase to the fact that with adding a reporting system to their website, riders now have a better or easier resource for sharing their incidences of accidents or injuries; thus, the reason for the increase of incidences in recent years is evident (BHS, 2017c). In realizing this increase, it provoked the BHS in 2016 to launch

Table 8.1 Horse rider casualties by age, United Kingdom 1999–2002

Year	Age of casualty							
	0–11	12–15	16–19	20–24	25–39	40–59	60 and over	Total
1999	10	18	22	23	57	43	2	181
2000	10	28	19	13	37	34	5	149
2001	7	14	14	15	47	34	4	137
2002	6	14	18	14	49	31	3	143
Population (in 100,000 s)	83.7	29.7	28.8	35.1	125.8	151.6	120.1	575.1

Note: Reprinted from *Consultation Draft Equestrian Strategy*, by Redcar and Cleveland Borough Council, 2005, Yorkshire, U.K.: Redcar

an additional road safety campaign called the "Dead? Or Dead Slow?" to encourage and teach drivers of vehicles to pass horses safely on the road by reducing speed to 15 mph, avoiding any loud noises/honking of the vehicle, passing wide, and driving away slowly (BHS, 2017b). Furthermore, the BHS website provides drivers of vehicles with a video on how to safely pass a horse on the roadways (BHS, 2017b).

8.4.1 Exemplary Practice

The criteria for a program to be judged as "exemplary practice" depend on meeting at least three of the four "E"s rubric, namely: education, economics, enactment, and engineering (Volpe, Lewko, & Batra, 2002). Exemplary practices must also be sustainable, so the rubric is supplemented by considerations of evaluation and empowerment since these features are embedded within funding and the human resources associated with the success and sustainability of the program. Qualifying in each "E" category briefly outlined below, the BHS Riding and Road Safety Test is clearly an exemplary practice:

8.4.1.1 Education
Educating riders to ride safely, in particular on roadways, is the primary method of achieving injury prevention goals at BHS. Research conducted by the Department for Transport has identified education as the essential component in strategies to reduce road-related casualties (Department for Transportation, 2007). Advice on safety equipment for both horse and rider equates to secondary injury prevention. Knowledge and guidance are made available in print and video media briefly outlined below.

- BHS Riding and Roadcraft Manual: This aide, a well-illustrated handbook which is updated as necessary, is now in its 11th edition. The handbook orients an absolute beginner who has not ridden on public roads as to how to be prepared, weather considerations, Highway Code regulations, and "Roadcraft" which advises proper behavior for horse and rider,

especially at locations requiring special attention such as roundabouts. Alternative riding scenarios and practical advice about how to deal with accidents are also covered, ending with an overview of the BHS Riding and Road Safety Test including a sampler of theory questions which form one of the three components of the test. The manual also gives some first aid advice focusing on attention to airway/breathing, checking for bleeding, and the need for cardiopulmonary resuscitation; this represents tertiary injury prevention. The manual gives a candidate a thorough point-by-point description of the test objectives, overall organization, and regulations. The illustrations in the manual all show riders and horses wearing helmets and high-visibility accessories.

- The Highway Code: A government publication intended for all types of road users. Rules are formulated to reduce road accidents resulting in any form of casualty.
- BHS Road Safety Training CD-ROM: 2008 will be the third year this interactive award-winning tool has been available for trainers who prepare people to ride on roads. The CD-ROM ensures standardized delivery of educational components to benefit trainers, examiners, and individuals taking the Riding and Road Safety Test. The BHS augments the Riding and Road Safety Test with the official Highway Code produced by the Department for Transport since riders must recognize road signs and comprehend rules and regulations applicable to all road users.

For equestrian enthusiasts, passing the BHS Riding and Road Safety Test is essential for vocational and professional training. One of the professional pathways is the BHS coaching degree that BHS developed in partnership with University College Worcester (American Medical Equestrian Association News, 2000). Initially, this degree will supplement qualifications held by BHS instructors, but will evolve to include an academic education in sport science (American Medical Equestrian Association News, 2000). It is anticipated that degree credentialed coaches could apply their knowledge to elevate national performance standards to improve results in equestrian sport competition (American Medical Equestrian Association News, 2000). Numerous colleges and a few universities offer students equine qualifications or equine degree courses; approved institutions are listed on the website with hyperlinks to websites (BHS, 2007). BHS education for equestrians has made headway in the United States with exemplary representation at the Grand Cypress School, Florida (BHS, 2003).

8.4.1.2 Economics

The road test is affordable. Since professional or leisure-related equestrian pursuits may carry high risks of injury, trust in trainers and tour guides is a priceless commodity for riding establishments. The British Equestrian Trade Association (BETA) reports from the BETA 2005/2006 National Equestrian Survey that £732 million is spent on lessons annually, while £35 million is spent specifically on riding lessons (BHS, 2007). Starting in 2006, the South Essex Insurance Brokers has sponsored the Young Instructor of the Year competition to promote the development of teaching skills to people working to become coaches and instructors in the equestrian sport and leisure industry (Western Mail and Echo, 2007).

8.4.1.3 Enactment

The BHS has made the test a prerequisite for other certifications such as becoming a qualified trainer, the stage two BHS exam, and becoming a certified trek leader and assistant trek leader. Abiding by the Highway Code when using roads is expected by the Department for Transport, but is not a mandatory provision, so including the road regulations applicable to drivers ensures that riders obey similar practices when riding on roads shared with motorists. For mounted police officers, passing the BHS Riding and Road Safety Test is mandatory (S. Hardy, personal communication, November 2, 2007). The Police Training Committee was chaired by Sgt. Lesley Taylor of the Nottinghamshire Mounted Police Force who is also a member of the BHS Safety Advisory Committee.

8.4.1.4 Engineering

As with any exemplary practice in injury prevention, the application of multiple strategies directly and indirectly related to a program contributes to a culture of safety and serves to reduce the incidence and severity of injury. The BHS Safety Committee complements the Riding and Road Safety Test with promotion of helmets and high-visibility clothing for riders and horses. Peripherally, the BHS is also active in the assessment of road surfacing materials that may add considerable risk to equestrian road users. Due to incidents and concerns for horses slipping on roads, Keith Grant of Devon County council brought the concerns to the County Surveyors' Society (CSS) Soils and Material Design and Specification Group. The CSS formed a task group which collaborated with BHS to produce a guidance note for highway authorities in the United Kingdom outlining the issues for horses and riders associated with resurfaced roads that are too smooth due to the properties of a finishing film for newly paved roads designed to bind the road surfacing materials (CSS/BHS ENG 03/05). Just as slips, trips, and falls are causes of serious injury in many environments to people, so are hard, slippery road surfaces the cause of potential injury for both a rider and their horse (Finch & Watt, 1996). A survey conducted by CSS revealed that although 70% of highway authorities received complaints about slips by horses on roads, neither design changes nor surfacing procedures were modified in response to the complaints. In a questionnaire available to the membership on the BHS website to generate data on this particular source of injury, BHS asks the rider/informant if the Riding and Road Safety Test has been passed (CSS/BHS ENG 03/05). The guidelines produced by Grant for proper construction of Stone Mastic Asphalt surface finishes have now been adopted by local authorities nationwide (BHS, 2007). Similar to vehicle maintenance as a prerequisite to safe driving, BHS advises riders to ensure that their horses' hooves and shoes are well maintained by a farrier (CSS/BHS ENG 03/05).

8.4.1.5 Evaluation

The Riding and Road Safety Test and preparation for it, recommended as a minimum of eight 1-h lessons, is an educational program designed to modify the behavior of riders positively in aspects of riding associated with heightened risk of injury. In itself, the Riding and Road Safety Test evaluates the skills of each rider and their preparedness for risk management on the roadways for themselves and the horse they ride. Following rigorous evaluation, the organization and administration of the test have received accreditation by the Qualifications and Curriculum Authority (QCA) which regulates numerous academic and professional external qualifications for England and liaises with similar organizations in Wales and Northern Ireland (Qualifications and Curriculum Authority [QCA], 2006). Abiding by national standards and regulations helps BHS improve procedures associated with testing, examinations, and certificate granting, adding higher status to the certificates earned (QCA, 2006). The QCA monitored the BHS following accreditation reporting findings, observations, and accreditation conditions to BHS in a report. Systematic monitoring by the QCA has enabled the BHS to improve quality and control to meet the stringent statutory regulations of the national authority. Both the QCA post-accreditation monitoring report and the BHS action plan have been posted over the Internet.

In 2007, BHS was awarded a prestigious Prince Michael International Road Safety Award (PMIRSA) in the category of public education for production of their interactive CD-ROM which is useful to candidates, examiners, and trainers and complements the BHS Riding and Roadcraft Manual together with the Highway Code. The award recognized the complete training program for Riding and Road Safety. PMIRSA considers innovation, achievement, commitment, replicability, sustainability, and quality of research to evaluate and judge nominations for awards (Prince Michael International Road Safety Award [PMIRSA], n.d.). The organization RoadSafe organizes the PMIRSAs and is partnered with the Department for Transport and other organizations (RoadSafe, 2008).

8.4.1.6 Empowerment

The BHS Riding and Road Safety Test is the only initiative of its kind to empower riders to protect themselves and their horses from injury. Equestrian knowledge, combined with learning rights and responsibilities as road users, results in the application of defensive riding behaviors to share roadways and avoid traffic accidents with motor vehicle users. Through social and professional networks of those involved with the BHS organization, and particularly the development of the BHS Riding and Road Safety Test, many riders in other countries have benefited from both the safety culture and technical skills acquired in preparation for the BHS test; David Kerry has been instrumental in promotion of the test abroad (D. Kerry, personal communication, April 21, 2008).

While fully cognizant of the safety issues inherent in shared use of roads with motorists, BHS strives to maintain and offer alternatives for leisure riding. A new and innovative service recently launched in September 2007 called EMAGIN (Equestrian Mapping and Geographical Information Network) uses an in-house geographical information system (GIS), Ordnance Survey maps, and extra supplemental data and incorporates the popular "Where to Ride" public service to find nearby off-road riding routes and BHS services and approved centers (BHS, 2003).

After the success of its 2016 launch of "Dead? Or Dead Slow?" campaign, and the awareness in increases of incidences in accidents and injuries while riding a horse, the BHS made modifications to its Riding and Road Safety Test (BHS, 2017b, 2017e). In 2017, the Riding and Road Safety Test was replaced with the Ride Safe Award, which continues to provide riders with safety education, but covers a much broader subject area (BHS, 2017a). Its aim is to equip riders with the skills needed to ride safely and confidently not only on roadways, but in all environments and conditions (BHS, 2017d). Furthermore, the award is designed for riders with any level of ability and is also supported by the Department of Transportation (BHS, 2017a). The Ride Safe Award teaches practical examples, tips, and guidance on how to stay safe, how to effectively use hand signals on the road, how to safely dismount the horse, and how to keep control of your horse (BHS, 2017d). Riders who take the Ride Safe Award will undergo a 3-h long practical assessment to evaluate their learning outcomes on their ability to identify the rules in the Highway Code specific to horse riders, ability to know how to ride outside safely, and ability to ride a horse in an enclosed area and out on roadways (BHS, 2017b).

8.4.1.7 Analysis

The BHS has invested time and effort in the right places to complement equestrian skills with defensive riding techniques for use on roadways and instill the responsibility of knowing the Highway Code. The relationship forged with the Department for Transport ensures that riders are included when it comes to public safety messages and reminders that horses and riders will be encountered on many traffic routes as legitimate users. While many equestrian riders are also drivers, there are numerous drivers who have never ridden a horse and are likely not to be mindful of horseback riders without safety messages in the Highway Code (D. Kerry, personal communication, 2008). As many injuries are sustained by young, female riders who may not be drivers, this also underscores the importance and relevance of the Highway Code to all equestrian users (D. Kerry, personal communication, April 21, 2008).

With examination centers at international locations, such as the United States, Hong Kong, Singapore, Dubai, Malaysia, Belgium, Italy, and Spain, the BHS is well placed to be a valuable source of injury data and to respond to feedback so that education can be modified to improve safety for horses and riders and advocate for prevailing or emerging safety issues. The Riding and Road Safety Test may even be a model to base a program for cyclists who need to ride on roads but are particularly vulnerable to injury in traffic.

The BHS has made great progress in producing training programs that address all the needs of riders, from beginners to international experts who compete in dressage or jumping events, and these courses may be taught at unaccredited establishments. Although accredited instructors are recommended, this flexibility means that the Riding and Road Safety Test and other examinations are available to more consumers, so this arrangement serves to maximize injury prevention. To promote a culture of safety, BHS also mandates the wearing of appropriate footwear and a riding helmet that meet BHS safety standards for all candidates taking the road test. Information on helmets and other protective equipment needs to be showcased more prominently on the website, however, as knowing which helmets meet standards recommended by BHS is not obvious. The helmet standards mentioned in the 11th edition of the Riding and Roadcraft safety manual have now been expanded to include the Snell E2001, so posting of up-to-date information should be upfront under the "Safety" section of the BHS website rather than as an archived news item.

The data used by the BHS regarding accidents and injuries could be collected from county authorities annually. Persistence in the regular surveying of county authorities, where repositories of relevant data reside, would yield information useful for advancing and refining injury prevention initiatives and may also support requests for grants. Regular intervals between surveys would also reinforce an expectation of the exercise to share information for the public good and routinize the survey, which, in turn, may increase response rates. BHS may consider working with the Department of Health since sections 60–62 in the Countryside and Rights of Way Act (2000) direct local highway authorities to provide alternatives to road use in the interest of safety and health promotion among various pedestrian users, cyclists, harnessed horse drivers, and the horse-riding public (Redcar & Cleveland Borough Council, 2005).

A 1993 survey of local authorities in the United Kingdom more recent than the one used by BHS to extrapolate figures for accidents involving horses ridden on roads resulted in a 58% response rate and approximately 348 accidents annually based on figures from the responding authorities (Kerry, 1993). Based on findings from a survey of accidents among "young cyclists," however, the Cumbria County Council discovered that underreporting of accidents could increase their accident statistics by a factor of 6 (Kerry, 1993, p. 5). Horse-related accidents may, therefore, be realistically closer to 2088 in a given year, somewhat less than the figure often cited by BHS (Kerry, 1993). The BHS is well organized and could partner with other equine organizations and university researchers, perhaps through the DfT to address gaps in the research of equestrian safety and evaluation of countermeasures (Finch & Watt, 1996).

The BHS must enhance the Riding and Road Safety Test manual to benefit members by providing education on the recognition of concussion and awareness of the medical risks associated with secondary concussions, however slight, as the consequence of second impact syndrome (severe brain swelling as a result of suffering a second head injury before recovery from the first injury) is permanent brain damage or death (American Riding Instructors Association, 2008). Brain damage can also occur through acceleration-deceleration forces in the absence of impact (Barth, Freeman, Broshek, & Varney, 2001). Pending inclusion in the Riding and Road Safety manual, essential information concerning signs of concussion could be made available as a download on the BHS website. Broshek (2001) (as cited in Northey, 2006) suggested that an optimal strategy would be to have baseline neurocognitive screening of riders and an integral concussion awareness and management program including a neuropsychologist for referrals. While this level of rigor is unlikely to be seen in amateur sport in the near future, it emphasizes the gravity of educating riders about concussion in a sport where head injuries are highly probable.

8.5   Conclusion

The profile of equestrian injury varies depending on the reason for riding; sport, leisure, and work environments place different demographic populations at risk, but there are common mechanisms of injury, such as falls (Newton & Nielsen, 2005; Petridou et al., 2004; Smith, Scherzer, Buckley,

Haley, & Shields, 2004). Falling on the side of the head, which most commonly happens to riders who fall, renders many riding helmets useless as protection against serious or fatal injury (Rumbelow, 2003). A new helmet standard from Snell was recently introduced to provide protection for the side of the head in falls (BHS, 2007). The BHS reports that the new standard is formulated for helmets used in competitive equestrian sport, but no manufacturer yet offers a helmet to these specifications (BHS, 2007). Surrounding the Riding and Road Safety Test are a spectrum of prevention interventions as outlined in Table 8.2.

Commenting on the six levels in the spectrum of prevention, Northey (2006) wrote, "when the initiatives or activities are combined, they are a transformative force for individual, community and societal health" (p. 21). Legislation, as in changes to STATS 19 reporting facilitating statistics for road safety reporting, education, and "environmental modification" form "the holy trinity of injury control" that BHS has implemented (Rivara, 1998). As a safety initiative, the BHS

Table 8.2 The spectrum of prevention

Level	Action
Strengthening individual knowledge and skills	Enhancing an individual's capability of preventing injury or violence
Promoting community education	Reaching groups of people with information and resources to promote health and safety
Educating providers	Training professionals who will transmit skills and knowledge to others
Fostering coalitions and networks	Bringing together groups and individuals for broader goals and greater impact
Changing organizational practices	Adopting regulations and norms to improve health and safety and creating new models
Influencing policy and legislation	Developing strategies to change laws and policies to influence outcomes in health, education, and justice

Note: From Interpreting Human and Horse Interactions: Equestrian Injuries in NZ: A Review Of The Literature, by G. Northey, 2006, New Zealand: Accident Compensation Corporation

Riding and Road Safety Test successfully combines initiatives and actions at all six levels of the spectrum of prevention providing a template for the development of equine safety initiatives elsewhere. The test harmonizes animal welfare and human safety and is much more than the sum of its parts; it is the outcome of the synergistic efforts of many BHS members and the legacy of a safety culture developed with foresight.

Acknowledgments The authors would like to express sincere appreciation to the key informants for this case study: Sheila Hardy, MAIRSO, Senior Executive, Safety of the British Horse Society in Kenilworth, Warwickshire, England and David R. Kerry, FIRSO, MIRSO, MAIRSO, DipASM, Senior Road Safety Officer for Cumbria Highways, Skirsgill, in Penrith, England—whose consultation made this project possible.

BRIO Model: The British Horse Society Riding and Road Safety Test.

Group Served: Recreational and professional horse riders/jumpers/trainers (ages 12–70).

Goal: To educate riders in road safety in order to minimize the risk involved when riding on roads and other common riding environments.

Background	Resources	Implementation	Outcome
Progressive development over 30 years Collaboration with multiple prominent community organizations: Department for Transport, South Essex Insurance Board, V-Bandz Ltd., Thames Valley Mounted Police, Nottinghamshire Mounted Police, Qualifications and Curriculum Authority (QCA) Major goal to reduce and prevent road-related accidents and injuries through education and training	Funding through membership and licensing fees, self-sustaining department Dedicated safety resource team Registered charity status Professional networks (safety and medical fields) In-house accident reporting data collection Accessible online accident reporting system Extensive team of trainers and examiners, required to undergo ongoing standardized training	Multifaceted program involving education and knowledge of theory (written examination), knowledge of practical skills and potential road hazards (simulated road test), and practical exam (road test) Published manuals, leaflets, posters, CD-ROM developed for training and program requirements Awareness campaigns in collaboration with Thames Valley Police Over 50 scheduled examination dates in 2008	Test taken by over 4000 people per year (over 120,000 qualified individuals) Standardization of road safety examination accredited through QCA Program adoption by establishments in other countries (Europe and United States) Three-time recipient of the Prince Michael International Road Safety Award for innovation in safety education Free rider insurance for qualifying BHS members

Life-Space Model: The British Horse Society Riding and Road Safety Test.

Sociocultural: civilization/ community	Interpersonal: primary and secondary relationships	Physical environments: where we live	Internal states: biochemical/genetic and means of coping
Safety is prioritized with oversight from a specialized department of the BHS Connection to the larger community through diverse collaborations Education and testing standardized to maintain quality and integrity and has accreditation through QCA	Comprehensive communications with members through active websites Integrates road regulations and road etiquette with riding lessons and knowledge of horse behavior Relationships with government and local road safety experts used to resolve road use issues and develop the program	Helmet use promoted by recommendation of specific standards used in assessment of helmets Road surfacing issues analyzed by professionals resulting in improved national standards safety	Membership is a source of dedicated volunteer support for teaching and examinations Promotion of high-visibility clothing and accessories to make horses and riders conspicuous to motorists sooner

References

American Medical Equestrian Association News. (2000, September). The University of Texas at Austin.

American Riding Instructors Association. (2008). *Helmets*. Retrieved from http://www.riding-instructor.com/helmets.php

Aronson, H., & Tough, S. C. (1993). Horse-related fatalities in the province of Alberta,1975–1990. *The American Journal of Forensic Medicine and Pathology, 14*(1), 28–30.

Barth, J. T., Freeman, J. R., Broshek, D. K., & Varney, R. N. (2001). Acceleration-deceleration sport-related concussion: The gravity of it all. *Journal of Athletic Training, 36*(3), 253–256.

Be Reflective. (n.d.). *Reflexive leg wrap*. Retrieved from March 4, 2008, from http://www.horses.breflective.com/retroreflective-horse-leg-wrap.php.

British Horse Society. (2003). *Riding and roadcraft* (11th ed.). Addington: Kenilworth Press.

British Horse Society. (2007). Retrieved from http://www.bhs.org.uk

British Horse Society. (2017a). *BHS launches brand new ride safe award*. Retrieved from https://pathways.bhs.org.uk/why-the-bhs/latest-news/bhs-launches-brand-new-ride-safe-award/

British Horse Society. (2017b). *Dead? Or dead slow?* Retrieved from https://www.equestrian-qualifications.org.uk/home/safety-and-accidents/dead-slow

British Horse Society. (2017c). *Horse accidents*. Retrieved from https://www.equestrian-qualifications.org.uk/home/safety-and-accidents/horse-accidents

British Horse Society. (2017d). *Ride safe award*. Retrieved from https://pathways.bhs.org.uk/ride-safe-award/

British Horse Society. (2017e) *Ride safe with the British Horse Society*. Retrieved from http://www.bhs.org.uk/our-charity/press-centre/news/january-to-june-2017/ride-safe-with-the-british-horse-society

Carlton Reckling, W., & Webb, J. K. (1996). Equestrian sports. In R. G. Watkins (Ed.), *The spine in sports* (pp. 527–539). St. Louis, MO: Mosby.

Clarkson, N. (2006) Playing it safe on our roads. Retrieved September 12, 2007, from http://www.horsetalk.co.nz/saferide/roadsafety.shtml.

Department for Transport. (2007). The official highway code. Retrieved September 12, 2007, from https://smartdriving.org/SD_HWC.pdf

Finch, C., & Watt, G. (1996). Locking the stable door: Preventing equestrian injuries. Retrieved September 12, 2007, from https://www.monash.edu/__data/assets/pdf_file/0016/216502/muarc103.pdf.

Firth, J. L. (1985). Equestrian injuries. In R. C. Schneider, J. C. Kennedy, & M. L. Plant (Eds.), *Sports injuries. Mechanisms, prevention and treatment* (pp. 431–449). Baltimore, MD: Williams & Wilkins.

Hardy, S. (2007). *Encouraging education in road safety*. Paper presented at the Road Safety Congress.

Kerry, D. R. (1993). *Equine road safety*. Unpublished manuscript, Manchester College of Arts & Technology.

Moss, P. S., Wan, A., & Whitlock, M. R. (2002). A changing pattern of injuries to horse riders. *Journal of Emergency Medicine, 19*, 412–414.

Newton, A. M., & Nielsen, A. M. (2005). A review of horse-related injuries in a rural Colorado hospital: Implications for outreach education. *Journal of Emergency Nursing, 31*(5), 442–446.

Northey, G. (2006). *Interpreting human and horse interactions: Equestrian Injuries in NZ: A review of the literature*. Wellington: Accident Compensation Corporation.

Petridou, E., Kedikoglou, S., Belechri, M., Ntouvelis, E., Dessypris, N., & Trichopoulos, D. (2004). The mosaic of equestrian-related injuries in Greece. *The Journal of Trauma Injury, Infection, and Critical Care, 56*(3), 643–647.

Pounder, D. J. (1984). The grave yawns for the horseman. Equestrian deaths in South Australia 1973–1983. An Arab proverb. *The Medical Journal of Australia, 141*, 632–635.

Prince Michael International Road Safety Awards. (n.d.). Retrieved 18 March, 2008, from http://www.roadsafetyawards.com.

Qualifications and Curriculum Authority. (2006). *Post-accreditation monitoring report: British Horse Society*. Retrieved from http://dera.ioe.ac.uk/2343/10/qca-07-3075_BHS.pdf.

Redcar, & Cleveland Borough Council. (2005). *Consultation draft equestrian strategy*. Yorkshire: Redcar.

Rivara, F. P. (1998). ISCAIP report: Injury prevention in practice. *Injury Prevention, 4*, S17–S25.

Roadsafe. (2008). A partnership in road safety. Retrieved March 18, 2008, from http://www.roadsafe.com.

Rumbelow, H. (2003, June 7). *Most horseriders' hats 'fail to protect them*. Retrieved 28 October, 2007, from http://global.factiva.comhttp://www.timesonline.co.uk/tol/news/uk/article1139643.ece?

Silver, J. R. (2002). Spinal injuries resulting from horse riding accidents. *Spinal Cord, 40*, 264–271.

Smith, G. A., Scherzer, D. J., Buckley, J. W., Haley, K. J., & Shields, B. J. (2004). Pediatric farm-related injuries: A series of 96 hospitalized patients. *Clinical Pediatrics, 43*, 335–342.

Thames Valley Police. (n.d.). *Darkhorse*. Retrieved March 7, 2008, from http://www.thamesvalley.police.uk/roads/darkhorse/index.htm.

The Pony Club. (n.d.). The pony club. http://www.pcuk.org. Accessed 16 June 2008.

Thomas, K. E., Annest, J. L., Gilchrist, J., & Bixby-Hammett, D. M. (2006). Non-fatal horse related injuries treated in emergency departments in the United States, 2001–2003. *British Journal of Sports Medicine, 40*(7), 619–626.

Volpe, R., Lewko, J., & Batra, A. (2002). *A compendium of effective, evidence-based best practices in the prevention of neurotrauma*. Toronto, ON: University of Toronto Press.

Western Mail and Echo Ltd. (2007, August 28). Retrieved October 28, 2007, from http://global.factiva.com.

Western Morning News. (1998, 3 April). Retrieved October 28, 2007, from http://global.factiva.com.

The 4-H Community ATV Safety Program

Negar Ahmadi and Helen Looker

The purpose of the 4-H Community ATV Safety program is to prevent injuries, such as head and spinal cord, for youth and adult all-terrain vehicle (ATV) riders by providing a wide range of education-based activities to raise awareness for safe riding practices.

9.1 Background

During the early 1980s high numbers of ATV-related deaths and injuries were reported in Alaska, and ATV safety became a concern for the Alaska health and safety officials. As the mortality statistics were released, the Alaska 4-H Youth Development program was beginning to address the issue of ATV safety among local youth (National 4-H Council, 2002). The Alaska 4-H Youth Development program is an essential part of Alaska's public education system and provides youth with access to technological advances in agriculture and life sciences, home economics, human development, and related areas (4-H and Youth Development, 2007). In response to the ATV issue, the Alaska 4-H began collaborating with the local health officials and educators to

create the first training materials and curriculum for an ATV safety program. In order to better expand the ATV safety program across the state of Alaska, the Alaska 4-H asked American Honda Motor Company and local Honda Dealers for support. In fact, as one of the leading ATV manufacturers, Honda contributed significantly to the success of the program in Alaska (National 4-H Council, 2002).

In the meantime, concerns with regard to ATV-related deaths and injuries were raised across the entire nation, as no organization or program was addressing the growing concerns of ATV safety. As a simple solution to the problem in hand, the US Consumer Product Safety Commission (CPSC) was approached by the consumer protection groups and American Academy of Pediatrics to ban ATVs (National 4-H Council, 2002). However, the call to ban ATVs was strongly opposed, not only by the ATV industry and riders across the country but also by the Alaska 4-H. In many rural areas like Alaska, ATVs are the main vehicles of transportation, and a ban on ATVs would pose significant problems for the people in such areas. In 1986, the CPSC was encouraged by the Alaska 4-H, medical associations, and other consumers to host a hearing with regard to the future of ATVs involving all the opposition parties. At the hearing, those opposing the ban strongly expressed their views and even clearly stated their intentions to ignore

N. Ahmadi (✉)
McMaster University, Hamilton, ON, Canada

H. Looker
University of Toronto, Toronto, ON, Canada

an ATV ban if imposed (National 4-H Council, 2002). The CPSC further held a number of other hearings throughout the following years.

At this point, as an alternative solution to reduce ATV-related deaths and injuries, National 4-H Council proposed to expand the Alaska 4-H ATV program nationwide in collaboration with several stakeholders. However, even the initiative to launch a nationwide 4-H ATV program was also not strongly supported by some parties such as state health departments, or the medical associations. Moreover, according to a consent decree signed by the CPSC and the ATV industry in April 1998, the ATV industry was prohibited from supporting any ATV program unless the CPSC was in agreement and supported the design and the implementation of the program. Eventually, National 4-H Council was successful in persuading the CPSC to get involved with the national 4-H safety initiative. In fact, the CPSC shortly established "fit" guidelines based on rider age and ATV engine size that since have been shared through the 4-H Community ATV Safety program. Furthermore, National 4-H Council convinced the CPSC to support Honda's participation in the ATV safety initiative. Ultimately, in August 1989, representatives from various stakeholders gathered at the National 4-H Center for the first 4-H Community ATV Safety program design team meeting. The purpose of the meeting was to allow for all interested parties to discuss the issue at hand and search for an optimal solution. The aim of the design team was to develop the framework for a national program focused at reducing injuries and deaths of youth ATV riders. During the meeting, the CPSC identified the following key ATV risk factors as impact indicators for the program:

1. Not wearing a helmet and other protective gears.
2. Carrying passengers.
3. Riding on pavement.
4. Riding on or alongside of the road (National 4-H Council, 2002).

The first meeting of the design team proved to be a success and laid the groundwork for developing the

4-H Community ATV Safety program. In an effort to develop the 4-H Community ATV Safety program's nationwide team network, in the spring of 1990, teams from 36 states gathered at four regional workshops. The teams prepared state and local action plans to address youth ATV safety. Since then, six other states have also joined the 4-H Community ATV Safety program team network and are training volunteers to become certified hands-on instructors who will train 500 in each state, through the ASI RiderCourses. These teams are establishing new range areas to conduct the RiderCourse and are working with local ATV dealers to secure appropriate-sized ATVs on loan. Over the years, the participating states have successfully modified the program to meet the specific needs of their communities. Although the participating states continue to use the 4-H Community ATV Safety program resources, they have become fairly self-efficient in running their unique ATV safety program. During the regional workshops, the members of the state teams received training in teaching techniques, stages of youth development, and community action strategies. National 4-H Council also provided the state teams with copies of the CPSC "Fit Guidelines" and the Specialty Vehicle Institute of America's (SVIA) "Safety Tips for the ATV Rider" brochure to distribute locally. Nonetheless, the members were encouraged to draft approaches that fit the needs of their communities. The resulting plans included common education-based activities but were unique in design in that they were tailored to the specific needs of each community. Since the program's national launch, it has developed and reached more than six million youth across the Unites States through various means including workshops, 4-H clubs, and ATV rider courses (National 4-H Council, 2002).

The goals of the 4-H Community ATV Safety program are:

1. To educate preteens, teens, and adults riding ATVs about safe operating/riding techniques and practices.
2. To help preteens and teens increase their critical thinking and other life skills as well as enhance their abilities to assess risk and solve problems.

3. To educate parents and other caregivers to protect young operators/riders through supervision and monitoring.
4. To help communities address issues related to safe use of ATVs (4-H ATV Safety Program, 2008a).

9.2 Resources

9.2.1 Stakeholders

The stakeholders who participated in the first 4-H Community ATV Safety program included:

- National 4-H Council: the national nonprofit, private sector of the 4-H and the Cooperative Extension System. National 4-H Council focuses mainly on fundraising, brand management, communications, legal and fiduciary support to national and state 4-H programs, and operation of the full-service National 4-H Youth Conference Center in Chevy Chase, Md., and the National 4-H Supply Service, the authorized agent for items bearing the 4-H Name and Emblem (National 4-H Council, 2008).
- Cooperative Extension System: A nationwide, noncredit educational network that has a state office in every land-grant university and a network of local or regional offices at each US state. These offices provide useful, practical, and research-based information to agricultural producers, small business owners, youth, consumers, and others in rural areas and communities of all sizes (Cooperative Extension System, 2008).
- American Honda Motor Co., Inc., serves as one of the leading ATV manufacturers in the world. The American Honda Motor Company was the main funding body of the 4-H Community ATV Safety program since its initiation until 2004. Since 2004, the support for the program was broadened to include the ATV Safety Institute (ASI) and Specialty Vehicle Institute of America (SVIA).
- State health departments.

- Special interest groups such as American Farm Bureau Federation, health associations, medical professionals' groups, and ATV recreation organizations.
- Federal public land managers.
- US Consumer Product Safety Commission.
- Youth and adult volunteers.

According to Halbert, the former senior vice president of National 4-H Council, one of the important things in initiating a community-based safety effort is recognizing the collective of the various stakeholders and organizations. When developing the National 4-H Community ATV Safety program, each of the stakeholders acknowledged that alone they would be inadequate in addressing the issue of ATV safety. In order for a national program to be successful, they needed the research and ongoing intelligence of the state health departments, outreach to different audiences that the credibility of "special interest groups" brought, the unique outlook and reach of the federal public land managers and the CPSC partner to the general public, and the enthusiasm, commitment, and flexibility of youth and adult volunteers. Halbert further said: "Generally a community/state can be effective by giving adequate resources to a collaborative group that includes representation from the following: ATV industry reps, relevant public agency officials, health professionals—both practitioners and researchers, ATV enthusiasts, non-formal youth groups led by volunteers as well as staff, schools, interest groups with high use of ATVs (e.g., Farm Bureau), and safety education organizations" (S. Halbert, personal communication, July 25, 2008).

However, the stakeholders at the time of the first design meeting had different agendas and opinions. In the initial stages of the program (and still as states and local communities begin this work), organizations come to the table with their views, expertise, and needs as foremost because that's what they "know." As they begin to hear from others, they realize that by themselves they cannot effectively address the confronting problem or issue. For example, the health professionals and agencies can document the problem and provide the evidence that it is growing, but they generally do not have the experience and resources to move out into the community to do something about it. Indeed, according to Halbert: "there was a lot of tension in the early stages among some participants because there is/was not a history that led to trust and viewing each other as partners. In fact, in some cases they had been outright adversaries." One of the important factors that further facilitated the collaboration among the stakeholders was the contribution of Halbert herself to this process. As a skillful facilitator, she brought the entire team members together and worked very hard to allow the team members to go on "side trips" to past experiences as adversarial agencies and organizations. Despite the initial skepticism of the team members, the first meeting resulted in successful collaboration. The fact that the facilitation was done by National 4-H Council and no other powerful organizations (such as Honda or the CPSC), it not only brought all the stakeholders together but also played an important part in reconciling the differences. In fact, the current organizational/interest group partners include categorical representatives of all the same groups as the original design teams, both in the national planning and at the state and community levels. The individuals may change over time, but most successful collaborative efforts still emphasize and include the representation of all the stakeholders (S. Halbert, personal communication, July 25, 2008).

9.2.2 Critical Elements of a Youth ATV Safety Program

Kress has proposed four essential elements that can yield to positive youth development programs (Kress, 2004). The 4-H Community ATV Safety program has taken these elements into account and is designed on the basis of the following four essential elements proposed by Kress (4-H ATV Safety Program, 2008b):

1. Belonging.
   - A positive relationship with a caring adult: In youth programs, an adult can be an

instructor, mentors or other volunteers. Such relationships provide warmth, closeness, caring, support, and good communication.
   - An emotionally and physically safe environment: The program should protect participants from physical or emotional harm. Such environments have clear and consistent rules, structure, continuity, and predictability.

2. Mastery.
   - Opportunities for mastery: Youth participating in the program should feel good about his or her abilities and skills. Mastery can help youth build social, emotional, physical, and intellectual skills and then have opportunities to demonstrate this proficiency. Mastery can be developed over time with repetition.

3. Independence.
   - Opportunities to see oneself as an active participant in the future: Participants should be able to envision a future and see their role within it. A positive youth program should help youth develop a sense of hope and clear vision about the future.
   - Opportunities for self-determination: Youth in the program should become autonomous and empowered and develop a sense of self-worth. Young people need to develop a personal sense of influence over their own lives and exercise their potential to become self-directing adults.
   - Opportunities to experience engagement in learning: The program can help youth understand the subject area and develop understanding. An engaged learner has a higher degree of self-motivation and a large capacity to create.
   - An inclusive environment: The program should be marked by a sense of belonging for all who attend, encouraging and supporting members with positive and specific feedback. Healthy groups celebrate the success of all members and take pride in the collective effort.

4. Generosity.
   - Opportunities to value and practice service to others: The program should help youth provide service to others, which helps them

gain exposure to the larger community. Service to others helps young people develop positive ethics and values.

The 4-H ATV curriculum also focuses on many of the life skills that other 4-H programs also address. These skills include decision making, critical thinking, communication, healthy lifestyle choices, personal safety, problem solving, teamwork, cooperation, social skills, and self-responsibility. The overall goal of the 4-H Community ATV Safety program is to raise awareness about the major risk factors associated with ATVs among youth, parents, and others. The program also helps youth develop critical thinking and decision-making skills to make the right choice and the safe choice when riding ATVs (4-H ATV Safety Program, 2008c). In fact, an implicit goal connected to the objectives of the 4-H Community ATV Safety program is raising awareness of general safety on the roads. As many of the youth ATV riders might later become drivers of automobiles or motorcycles, a training course on ATV safety has the potential to change their behaviors while driving other vehicles on the roads (S. Halbert, personal communication, June 5, 2008).

The American Honda Motor Company provided the initial funding of the program; however, the ATV industry played an important role in funding the 4-H Community ATV Safety program. Since 2004, the support for the program was broadened to include the ASI and SVIA. The funding is allocated to cover the grants, resource materials, training for grantees, and staffing at the national level. The training is provided by the 4-H Community ATV Safety program staff to the 4-H teams. An important contribution to the success of the 4-H Community ATV Safety program has been the involvement of youth and adult volunteers in running the local programs. Enthusiastic youth and adult volunteers come together to form 4-H ATV safety teams, attend training sessions, and initiate local 4-H Community ATV Safety programs to enhance ATV safety among their communities.

The 4-H community ATV safety program involves a wide range of education-based activities to raise awareness about ATV safety among youth. Implementation of the 4-H Community ATV Safety program has been possible mainly due to the grant program offered by National 4-H Council. The grants are awarded to ATV safety teams who then attend the 4-H ATV safety workshops. Grants to local communities and states have been offered and served as an underpinning of program efforts since 1990 through the 4-H Community ATV Safety program. The initial grants were $3500 each and have varied depending on the level of funding and other needs related to building, evaluating, and sustaining the program. In 2005, 4-H Council further began providing grants up to $7500 to the teams determined to implement the 4-H Community ATV Safety program in their communities. The grants can be used towards any of the following activities: workshops, 4-H clubs, staffed exhibits, ATV rider courses, school classrooms, camping programs, and through mass media efforts. The educational programs are run by youth and adult partner ATV safety teams, and optimally the participants would receive 6–8 h of training. The focus in each of the activities mentioned here is ATV safety and teaching strategies to prevent injuries resulting from riding ATVs. The educational sessions include both risk-factor education and hands-on training to the youth and the adults who supervise them (National 4-H Council, 2008).

The 4-H local ATV safety teams are supplemented with various educational materials and implementation strategies to educate youth on ATV safety. The leaders of the ATV safety teams are provided with a *Leader's Guide* book which includes chapters on activities to design and concepts to cover. The *Leader's Guide* encourages the team leaders to follow the experiential learning cycle developed by Pfeiffer and Jones (1983). Figure 9.1 includes a sample taken from the *Leader's Guide*, explaining to the team leaders the process of the experiential learning cycle. The *Leader's Guide* also provides the leaders with the developmental characteristics and implications for safe ATV riding of different age groups. In addition, the 4-H ATV safety teams are provided with copies of the "Fit Guidelines" during training which helps youth in selecting the appropriate size of ATV. A copy of the "Fit Guidelines" is provided in Box 9.1.

Box 9.1 Fit Guidelines Provided to the Local ATV Safety Teams by 4-H Community ATV Safety Program (4-H ATV Safety Program, 2008b)

Follow these guidelines for ATV safety:

Age	Engine
6 and older	To 70 ccs
12 and older	To 90 ccs
16 and older	90 ccs and up

Clearance between the ATV seat and inseam while standing up on footpegs. You must have the right clearance between the seat and your inseam to stand up and properly absorb shocks through the legs while riding your ATV on rough terrain. Proper clearance also keeps the seat from hitting you during a ride, which could throw you over the handlebars. You'll need 3–6 in. clearance between the seat and inseam when you are standing up on your ATV's footpegs. The maximum is controlled by the size of your ATV. The ATV Safety Institute recommends:

Upper legs. The upper portion of your leg—from about the top of your knee to your hip—should be about horizontal to help you control your ATV. A little above or below horizontal shouldn't be a problem, but huge differences—knees significantly below or above the hips—should be checked by an adult. If your knees are quite a bit above the hips, turn the handlebars in both directions and check for contact with knees or legs.

Foot length. Check to see if you can brake correctly. Lock the heel of your right shoe against the footpeg or in the proper position on the running board. Your toe should be able to depress the footbrake with a simple downward rotation of your foot. Check if you have any contact with engine or exhaust protrusions. You should be able to use the brakes consistently without hesitation. The same rule applies to the ATV's left side where the gearshift is located.

Grip reach. To steer and balance correctly, sit normally on your ATV with your hands on the handlebars. Your elbows should have a distinct angle between your upper arm and forearm. If your elbows are straight out, you won't be able to turn the handlebars. Make sure you aren't reaching forward to compensate for a short reach. If your elbows are at less than right angles, you are too large for the ATV and steering and maintaining balance will be difficult.

Throttle reach. Check your throttle reach to control your speed and handling. With your right hand in the normal operating position, check to see if your thumb can easily operate the throttle. Turn the handlebars to the extreme left and right positions. Check again for any interference with easy operation.

Brake reach. Make sure you have good stopping control. Place your hands in the normal operating position with fingers straight out. Check to see if the first joint (from the tip) of your middle finger extends beyond the brake lever. If not, your hand is too small to effectively grasp the lever in an emergency. Make sure your thumb also reaches the engine stop switch. Squeeze the brake lever a few times to be sure you can comfortably use the controls.

National 4-H Council has also launched a website dedicated to 4-H Community ATV Safety program (http://www.atv-youth.org) which provides a variety of resources for both the public and the local 4-H ATV safety teams. The website also features a number of video clips about ATV safety and a number of education materials that can be helpful to the 4-H ATV safety teams. Moreover, the 4-H Community ATV Safety program provides a Safe Riding Tips brochure that is

THE EXPERIENTIAL LEARNING CYCLE

All of the activities in this guide use the experiential learning cycle as a basis for instruction. Experiential learning helps participants process and apply information. The end result is the learner has more knowledge and better skills. See *Reference Guide to Handbooks and Annuals* by J.W. Pfeiffer and J.E. Jones published by John Wiley and Sons, Inc. in 1983.

Most 4-H curricula showcase the model found on this page. Reprinted with permission of John Wiley and Sons, Inc. For an excellent overview that includes teaching and training ideas, see 4-H Afterschool's Teens as Volunteer Trainers, available online at **www.4hafterschool.org/resourceguides.aspx.**

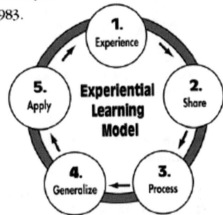

Pfeiffer, J.W., & Jones, J.E., "Reference Guide to Handbooks and Annuals"
© 1983 John Wiley & Sons, Inc.
Reprinted with permission of John Wiley & Sons, Inc.

STEPS OF EXPERIENTIAL LEARNING

Experience: Describe the activity you'll have participants do. Encourage them to think about what they might see or what might happen. Then, let participants experience the activity, perform, or do it.

Share: Ask questions about the activity and the experience after they've completed it. Participants describe the results and their reactions.

Process: Ask questions about something that was important about the experience. Participants analyze the experience and reflect upon the results.

Generalize: Apply the results to real world examples. Ask questions to help participants connect the subject matter to life skills and the bigger world.

Apply: Help participants apply what they learned to their own lives, to give them opportunities to practice these new skills or use the new information.

Fig. 9.1 A sample taken from the *Leader's Guide* on how to design 4-H ATV safety educational activities provided to team leaders (4-H ATV Safety Program, 2008a)

distributed locally. Furthermore, the staff members at the 4-H Community ATV Safety program are constantly trying to develop new and useful resources. One such development is a Resource Guide: How to Develop a Community-Based 4-H ATV Safety Youth-Adult Collaboration. This document provides practical guidelines for those in the process of developing their community

ATV safety programs and can be downloaded from the website.Despite the collaborative and successful efforts of all those involved in the program, there is always a need for more resources. According to Halbert: "It takes money or in-kind donations to expand grants at the local level and support the program with resources like staff and the recently completed guide at the national level. It takes money to get people together for training in how to build collaborative efforts, how to conduct rider training, etc." (S. Halbert, personal communication, July 25, 2008).

9.2.3 Inputs to the Prevention Model

The National 4-H Community ATV Safety program grew out of the Alaska 4-H ATV program, and in some ways, the Alaska 4-H ATV Safety program acted as a pilot project for the national program. As mentioned previously, the 4-H Community ATV Safety program is mainly education based. In fact, from the beginning, the program has been based on learning experiences and public awareness programs focused on early CPSC research when ATV injuries and fatalities were approaching "epidemic proportions" in 1981–1983. The research then indicated risk factors, such as not wearing a helmet or other protective gears, carrying passengers on ATVs meant for one person, riding on or alongside of a road, riding on pavement, riding an ATV that is not the correct size (fit) for the operator, and lack of training in proper/safe techniques. The changes and modifications that have occurred since the initiation of the program have mainly been focused on how to deliver and reinforce the messages and experiences that will change risky/unsafe behaviors. In fact, there have been many creative approaches developed since the initiation of the program. Furthermore, part of the responsibilities of National 4-H Council includes "quality control" which results in providing high-quality resources from the national level. Locally, people cannot often afford to create their own and they use those provided by the council; therefore, the messages delivered will be consistent

(S. Halbert, personal communication, July 29, 2008). The education-based nature of the program as well as the idea of grants to states and local communities has been an ongoing practice by National 4-H Council and has been proven to be effective.

9.3 Implementation

The success of the program lies in its nationwide expansion; in fact, 4-H is a nationwide system of 50+ independent states whose communities usually also act independently. Such a system can allow for an easy dissemination of opportunities, resources, and ideas and includes broad representation. It also allows for decisions to be made at the state and local level. However, collaboration and ongoing, top-notch communication and facilitation are essential every step of the way (S. Halbert, personal communication, July 25, 2008). Although the ATV safety teams are provided with various materials by National 4-H Council, the teams are encouraged to tailor the program to the specific needs of their communities. Since the initiation of the program, such flexibility has led to the development of a number of unique and effective local implementation strategies. The following are examples illustrated in the Evaluation Summary Report of the 4-H Community ATV Safety program (4-H ATV Safety Program, 2003):

- The 4-H Community ATV Safety program in Allen County, Kentucky, has successfully engaged thousands of elementary, middle, and high school students in educational activities focused on ATV safety. Not only do leaders emphasize the importance of wearing the proper gear, they actually help provide helmets to youth who normally would not be able to afford them. The coordinator explained: "Say, for example, that a family can only afford to pay $15. Well, we make up the difference between what we can get the helmets for at wholesale prices through grants like the one we got from National 4-H Council." Young riders also view graphic photographs of riders from accidents who weren't wearing helmets. These strategies are clearly paying off: the percentage of participants in Allen County who "always" wear a helmet increased from 43.5% to 90.9% after the course in 2002 according to Halley Research Study (2004).

- The Bering Strait Community Partnership implemented 4-H Community ATV Safety programs in various remote villages. According to the site coordinator, the major goal was to "show [youth] what happens when you don't follow safety precautions." Youth leaders played an instrumental role in developing the program and designed exercises that would interest their peers. The feedback from the communities has been extremely positive. In fact, the coordinator reported, "Most of the villages want additional classes, and villages that did not get classes want them." The increased demand is not surprising: the number of participants in the Bering Strait communities who "always" wear protective clothing increased from 26.1% to 44%, according to the Halley Research Study (2004).

- The youth and adults who developed the 4-H Community ATV Safety program in Southeast Nebraska organized safety contests, held forums for youth, created a safety booth at the county fair, and, most importantly, offered training camps. The coordinator reported that participants now think differently about the dangers involved in operating ATVs. The research bears out her point: the program increased the percentage of participants in Southeast Nebraska who "never" carry a passenger from 26.3% to 52.6%, according to the Halley Research Study (2004).

- The 4-H Community ATV Safety program in Noble County, Indiana, featured an in-depth, two-day camp that provided training instruction to entire families. Every participant had the opportunity to learn via hands-on experience, effectively putting his or her new safety skills to work right away. "It's been very successful, very rewarding," said the coordinator. "I've had lots of feedback from parents and some of the kids about how useful the training

was." The research supports this claim: the number of youth participants in Noble County who "never" operate ATVs on pavement increased by 25% as a direct result of the program, according to the Halley Research Study (2004).

- The 4-H Community ATV Safety program in Washington County, Kentucky, consisted of a safety course for riders and their parents and Safety Day—a special event held in conjunction with the region's 4-H Camp Week. To reinforce the importance of riding safely, part of the training focused on two recent high-profile ATV accidents in Washington County. As a result, the coordinator stated that "parents have reported they have seen positive changes in their children's ATV-riding behavior." The program has indeed changed behaviors for the better, increasing the number of participants who "never" operate ATVs on or alongside roads from 41.3% to 66.7%, according to the Halley Research Study (2004).

In order for the national program to be successful, systems need to be in place to monitor the ongoing process since all the actions and contributions build the whole. The National 4-H Community ATV Safety program has been successful in engaging organization representatives and recognizing the importance of their contribution. Furthermore, the program allowed for engaging and enthusiastic participation, and it ensured that the various participating organizations felt that their work with National 4-H Council was very important to the overall success of the program. To ensure successful implementation of the program, periodic checks are built into the system whereby grantees submit reports with photos, articles, and links to news articles and websites. Moreover, feedback given to management and frontline workers is structured mainly through reports and presentations. In fact, at the initial stages of the implementation of the program, creative and thorough presentations and reports were prepared for a panel of executives at American Honda Motor Co., Inc., which provided major funding until 2004 (S. Halbert, personal communication, July 25, 2008). Overall, careful program planning, consistent administration, proper management, and continuing evaluation and assessment of effectiveness have led to the successful nationwide implementation of the 4-H Community ATV Safety program. In fact, the evaluations, reports, and interviews proved to be very effective in implementation of the program.

9.4 Outcome

National 4-H Council has evaluated the attainments of the prevention strategies by developing instruments to measure youth behavior and attitude change with expert input from the CPSC staff and university evaluation specialists. The evaluations are done through phone interviews and mail surveys before and after participation in the program. The initial evaluation showed that after just 3 years, 70.6% of youth participants said participating in the 4-H program resulted in changes in their behavior. The most common examples of change in behavior were:

- Taking more care and driving more slowly.
- Wearing more protective gear.
- Wearing a helmet more often (National 4-H Council, 2002).

A thorough evaluation of the 4-H Community ATV Safety program was completed in 2003. The evaluation was performed by Halley Research and assessed change in the behavior and attitudes of youth as the result of participation in the program.

9.4.1 Wearing Helmets and Eye Protection

Helmets are shown to be effective in reducing head injuries in ATV-related accidents. In fact, a CPSC study, looking at helmet safety, found helmets to be effective in reducing 25% of head injuries resulting from ATV accidents. The results of the Halley Research Study found that the number of participants who "always" wear helmets

when operating ATVs increased from 18.8% to 32.1%, and the number of participants who "never" wear helmets decreased by 23.4%. Furthermore, the number of youth who "never" wear eye protection was reduced from 62.4% to 46.9% (4-H ATV Safety Program, 2003). According to one participant: "I didn't think that helmets were such a big deal until I learned that you could die from a head injury, so I wear my helmet now" (4-H ATV Safety Program, 2003).

9.4.2 Wearing Protective Clothing

Knowing what to wear and how to wear it can significantly reduce chances of getting injured during falls from ATVs or ATV accidents. The results of the evaluation showed that the percentage of youth participating in local training program who "always" wear protective clothing when operating ATVs increased from 15.5% to 25.3%. The evaluation also reported that the number of participants who "never" wear protective clothing decreased from 46.1% to 24.5% (4-H ATV Safety Program, 2003).

9.4.3 Carrying Passengers

The evaluation found that the 4-H Community ATV Safety program increased the number of youth who "never" carry passengers from 30.1% to 40% in 2001 (4-H ATV Safety Program, 2003).

9.4.4 Riding on Pavement

ATVs are strictly designed for trail use; therefore riding on pavement is considered extremely dangerous. In fact, 10% of ATV-related injuries and over 25% of ATV-related deaths occur on paved surfaces. The Halley Research Study found that the 4-H Community ATV Safety program increased the number of youth who "never" operated ATVs on pavement from 46.6% to 60% after participating in the program (4-H ATV Safety Program, 2003).

9.4.5   Riding on or Along Roads

Many ATV-related injuries occur as a result of collisions with other vehicles. Therefore, the 4-H Community ATV Safety program educates youth about not riding their ATVs on or alongside public roads. The Halley Research Study found that the percentage of participants who only "sometimes" or "never" operate ATVs on or alongside the road increased from 77% to 84% (4-H ATV Safety Program, 2003).

Overall, the results of the survey showed that the youth who participated in the 4-H Community ATV Safety program were:

1. More likely to wear helmets and eye protection.
2. More likely to wear protective clothing.
3. Less likely to carry passengers.
4. Less likely to ride on paved surfaces
5. Less likely to operate ATVs on or alongside roads (4-H ATV Safety Program, 2003).

Moreover, the Halley Research created a list of exemplary practice for local safety programs:

- Actively involve youth in all phases of the program, including fund development, curricula design, implementation, and follow-up.
- Develop youth/adult partnership teams to foster a greater sense of community interconnectedness.
- Utilize all forms of communication, including radio, TV, billboards, websites, newspapers, newsletters, flyers, bulletin boards, town councils, etc., to recruit new audiences and build community support.
- Find creative ways to provide helmets to youth who cannot afford them.
- Encourage parents and families to fully participate in the training.
- Host panels to discuss differences between unskilled and skilled riders.
- Provide hands-on learning opportunities (e.g., trying on safety gear and practicing safety maneuvers).
- Forge community partnerships to establish trails and safe places to ride. Youth/adult part-

nership teams, 4-H clubs, and trained ATV riders could help local landowners turn unused fields into visitor attractions (4-H ATV Safety Program, 2003).

9.4.6   ATV Injury Rates

Injury reports released by the CPSC show a significant decline in the ATV-related injury rates since concerns about ATV safety were first raised (SVIA, 2005). The following statements are part of the report released in 2003 by the CPSC:

- 31% decline in the ATV injury rate from 1988 to 2002 (SVIA, 2005)
- 5% decline in the ATV injury rate from 2001 to 2002 (SVIA, 2005)
- 14% decline in the fatality rate for the period of 1999 to 2001 (SVIA, 2005)
- 15% decline since 1997 in the proportion of total ATV-related injuries that involve children under 16 (SVIA, 2005)
- 36% decline in emergency department-treated ATV injuries for all ages from 2007 to 2015 (CPSC, 2017)
- 33% decline in emergency department-treated ATV injuries for children younger than 16 years of age from 2007 to 2015 (CPSC, 2017)

The report released by CPSC further shows that ATV use has increased since the initiation of the 4-H Community ATV Safety program, but injury rates have been declining (SVIA, 2005). Furthermore, the stats show a significant decline in the ATV-related injuries involving children under 16. Therefore, it appears that the 4-H Community ATV Safety program has been effective in reducing ATV-related injuries and fatalities particularly among children under 16 years of age.

Moreover, in a study conducted by Bansal et al. (2008) comparing two time periods for ATV-related injuries at the University of California San Diego Medical Center, results indicated a significant reduction of closed-head and spinal cord injuries between 2000–2005 and 1985–1999, but a significant increase in long-bone fractures. Bansal et al. (2008) suggested that an evolving club culture for ATV riders where formal training is available and personal protective clothing and helmets are encouraged accounts for the decline in these types of injuries but made reference to the fact that helmets do not protect against spinal injury. However, one needs to realize that studying rates of injuries is relatively difficult as many factors, including the increase in ATV use, might influence the evaluation. However, it appears that the 4-H Community ATV Safety program has been successful in changing youth behavior and attitude and educating them about the risk factors associated with ATVs.

9.4.7 ATV Safety Social Norms Study

Since the 4-H Community ATV Safety program mainly targets youth, one needs to realize the importance of social norms in delivering the safety message. In fact, social norms can play an important role in shaping behaviors and attitudes in youth. In an effort to recognize the role of social norms in youth's attitudes towards ATV safety, National 4-H Council initiated a study of attitudes of youth towards ATV safety by conducting the ATV Safety Social Norms What Do You Think? survey in 2004. National 4-H Council hoped to use the results of the study to further develop a series of media messages promoting safe behaviors when driving ATVs. The study involved an online survey targeting youth and aimed to study the ways in which social norms influence youth attitudes towards riding ATVs (Halley Research, 2004). The study was conducted at three different sites: Louisiana, Utah, and West Virginia. The survey included questions about wearing helmets, protective clothing, eye protection, carrying passengers, riding on pavement, and riding on or alongside the road. Below are some examples of the questions asked:

What do you think is the most common attitude among other kids your age about wearing helmets?

- Wearing a helmet is always an important thing to do.
- Wearing a helmet is okay, if that's what the person wants to do.
- Wearing a helmet is dumb (not cool).
- I think other kids think wearing helmets when riding ATVs is (enter below):

What do you think is the most common attitude among other kids your age about wearing helmets with some type of eye protection (face shield or eye goggles)?

- Wearing a helmet with eye protection is always an important thing to do when riding ATVs.
- Wearing a helmet with eye protection when riding ATVs is okay, if that's what the person wants to do.
- Wearing a helmet with eye protection when riding ATVs is dumb (not cool).
- I think other kids think wearing helmets with some kind of eye protection when riding ATVs is (enter below):

The results of the 2004 ATV Safety Social Norms Study are summarized below:

- Most youth say wearing a helmet is always an important thing to do.
- Most youth say wearing a helmet with some type of eye protection is always an important thing to do.
- Most youth think that wearing protective clothing when riding ATVs is okay!
- Most youth think it's okay to carry passengers when riding ATVs once in a while, but not all the time.
- Most youth think it's okay to ride ATVs on or alongside the road once in a while but not all the time.

Moreover, the results of the 2004 ATV Safety Social Norms Study also showed that the most effective way to notify youth about the upcoming events or trainings in their community was through TV. The following table (Table 9.1) summarizes the findings with regard to the media

Table 9.1 Percentage of youth reporting each media strategy as a "very good way"

Media strategy	Percent reporting, %
TV	54.7
Newspaper	47.7
Tell my parents	45.1
Radio	33.9
Tell my friends	31.2
Tell my teachers	27.9
Announcement at school	26.0
Flyer handed out at school	18.9
Billboards	18.0
Email	17.2

Note: Halley Research (2004)

strategy and the percent of youth reported the strategy as a "very good way."

The result of this social norm study has helped the 4-H Community ATV Safety program in creating effective messages that target youth and enhance ATV safety within communities and that can also be used with local media outlets.

9.5 Conclusion

A combination of countermeasures must be deployed to reduce the burgeoning burden of injury from ATV-related accidents. ATVs are of growing concern in many places around the world. There is consensus that voluntary standards and self-regulation by industry stakeholders do not work to reduce ATV-related injury and death (Bansal et al., 2008; Helmkamp, Furbee, Coben, & Tadros, 2008). The Canadian Off-Highway Vehicle Distributors Council supports the notion that government overseeing is needed, and legislated safety measures would be effective at reducing ATV-related fatalities in all Canadian provinces, particularly for youth (COHV). In the United Kingdom, HSE occasionally sends inspectors to farms to ensure that quad bikes are well maintained and that riders have training and helmets to use. The HSE

inspectors also canvass ATV dealerships to evaluate the quality of safety information imparted to customers (Newcastle Chronicle & Journal, 2003).

The most common ATV injuries parallel those seen in cycling and motorcycling, but the crash dynamics differ, so injury prevention efforts must be tailored accordingly (Helmkamp et al., 2008). A study commissioned by Governor Joe Manchin in West Virginia broached several ATV-related issues not often cited: that ATVs should not be allowed on public roads, that drivers with suspended licenses be prohibited from utilizing an ATV as alternative personal transport, and that alcohol use must be addressed (Vitello, 2008). Children under 16 years of age remain the most vulnerable ATV riders as they comprise 14% of all riders in the United States, but they suffer disproportionately sustaining almost 47% of total injuries and deaths (Brandenburg, Brown, Archer, & Brandt, 2007). The National 4-H Community ATV Safety program, which was initiated in Alaska and then expanded across the United States, has been shown to be effective in changing youth behavior and reducing risky behaviors among ATV riders.

Program evaluations and injury reports show that the 4-H Community ATV Safety program has changed youth behavior and has contributed to the decrease in injury rates and fatalities. However, it is important to realize that a training program on its own will not solve all the problems. The success of the 4-H Community ATV Safety program lies heavily in the effective collaboration of the various stakeholders involved. In fact, the key to any successful prevention program is in the support and the collaboration of the different parties.

Acknowledgments The authors would like to express sincere appreciation to the key informant for this case study: Shella Chaconas and Susan Halbert of the National 4-H Council in Chevy Chase, MD, USA—whose consultation made this project possible.

BRIO Model: 4-H Community All-Terrain Vehicle (ATV) Safety Program

Group Served: Youth and adult ATV users.

Goal: To prevent head, spinal cord, and any other serious injuries.

Background	Resources	Implementation	Outcome
Children less than 16 years of age account for almost one-third of ATV injury-related emergency department visits and 30% or more of ATV injury hospitalizations Responding to the high number of ATV fatalities in Alaska recorded in 1982, the Alaska 4-H initiated an ATV safety program in collaboration with health officials, educators, and Honda Motor Company In 1986, National 4-H Council offered to expand the program to other US states In 1989, various stakeholders gathered at the National 4-H Center for the first 4-H Community ATV Safety program meeting	Close cooperation of the various stakeholders led to the development of a framework for a nationwide program aimed at reducing key ATV risk factors The CPSC was involved to establish "fit" guidelines based on rider's age and ATV engine size A consent decree between the ATV industry and the CPSC ensured that the ATV industry followed the established safety guidelines A greater involvement of the young people in the design teams reflected the emphasis on youth equal representation Grants ranging from $500 to $7500 have been provided in order to implement local ATV safety programs	Since the program's national launch, 42 states/ localities have implemented the program at various levels The implementation strategies have included workshops, 4-H clubs, staffed exhibits, ATV rider courses, school classrooms, camping programs, and mass media Risk-factor education and hands-on training to young riders and the adults who supervise them are provided options such as workshops and other activities Education and curriculum material and brochures and display boards are provided to the 4-H ATV safety sites Training workshops are offered throughout the year	Statistics from the 2004 4-H research evaluation show that since the initiation of the program, ATV-related injuries have declined by 31% and ATV-related injuries among children under 16 have declined by 15% 2004 evaluations of the program have demonstrated that after just 3 years, 70.6% of youth participants said they made changes in ATV use as a result of the 4-H program Further evaluation of the 4-H ATV program shows that the program increased helmet use and wearing protective clothing, while it reduced the number of youths carrying passengers

Life-Space Model: 4-H Community All-Terrain Vehicle (ATV) Safety Program

Sociocultural: civilization/ community	Interpersonal: primary and secondary relationships	Physical environments: where we live	Internal states: biochemical/ genetic and means of coping
Awareness raising through educational program, video clips, brochures, and guidelines Offering grants to implement the program within local communities Educating communities through 4-H clubs, staffed exhibits, ATV rider courses, school classrooms, camping program, and mass media Adapting the program to the local needs of the communities	Providing training opportunities for local 4-H teams Involving youth and adult volunteers and community members as 4-H ATV safety teams Building relationship between youth in the community and 4-H local ATV safety teams through workshops and education sessions Building a relationship between the program and the ATV industry, CPSC, ASI, and SVIA	Educating youth about the dangers of riding ATVs on pavements and on/along public roads Teaching youth about the importance of wearing helmets and protective gear while riding ATVs Warning children about the dangers of carrying passengers while riding ATVs	Improving youth behavior through promoting safe behaviors and eliminating risky behavior while riding ATVs Identifying the effective means of communicating with youth and using them to deliver safety messages to youth in the community Helping youth develop critical thinking and decision-making skills to make the right choice and the safe choice when riding ATVs

References

4-H and Youth Development. (2007). *What is 4-H?* Retrieved June 20, 2008, from http://www.alaska.edu/uaf/ces/4h/.

4-H ATV Safety Program. (2003). *Evaluation summary report 1990–2003.* 4-H Community ATV Safety Program.

4-H ATV Safety Program. (2008a). *ATV safety leader's guide sample.* Retrieved June 20, 2008, from http://www.atv-youth.org/WorkArea/showcontent.aspx?id=64.

4-H ATV Safety Program. (2008b). Fit Guidelines.. http://www.atv-youth.org/fitguidelines.aspx. Accessed 3 June 2008.

4-H ATV Safety Program. (2008c). Safety Riding Tips Brochure. http://www.atv-youth.org/WorkArea/showcontent.aspx?id=68. Accessed 29 May 2008.

Bansal, V., Fortlage, D., Lee, J., Kuncir, E., Potenza, B., & Coimbra, R. (2008). A 21-year history of all-terrain vehicle injuries: has anything changed? *The American Journal of Surgery, 195,* 789–792.

Brandenburg, M. A., Brown, S. J., Archer, P., & Brandt, E. N. (2007). All-terrain vehicle crash factors and associated injuries in patients presenting to a Regional Trauma Center. *Trauma, 63*(5), 994–999.

Cooperative Extension System. (2008). *About us.* Retrieved June 15, 2008, from http://www.csrees.usda.gov/Extension/.

Halley Research. (2004). ATV *safety social norms what do you think.*

Halley Research Study. (2004). *Consumer product Safety Commission.* https://www.cpsc.gov/PageFiles/84803/atv2006_3.pdf.

Helmkamp, J. C., Furbee, P. M., Coben, J. H., & Tadros, A. (2008). All-terrain vehicle-related hospitalizations in the United States, 2000–2004. *American Journal of Preventive Medicine, 34*(1), 39–45.

Kress, C. (2004). *Essential elements of 4-H youth development.* CSREES, USDA, National 4-H Headquarters.

National 4-H Council. (2002). *ATV safety program summary.*

National 4-H Council. (2008). *National 4-H council.* Retrieved June 20, 2008, from http://www.fourhcouncil.edu/about.aspx.

Newcastle Chronicle & Journal Ltd. (2003). HSE set to launch safety blitz on farm quad bikes. Retrieved July 21, 2008, from http://www.factiva.com.

Pfeiffer, J. W., & Jones, J. E. (1983). *Guide to handbooks and annuals.* Hoboken, NJ: John Wiley and Sons, Inc.

Specialty Vehicle Institute of America. (2005). *New consumer product safety commission report shows decline in ATV injury rate for second consecutive year.* Retrieved July 29, 2008, from http://www.atvsafety.org/SVIAPressReleases/CPSC012605.pdf.

U.S. Consumer Product Safety Commission. (2017). *2015 Annual report of ATV-related deaths and injuries.* Retrieved November 5, 2017, from https://www.cpsc.gov/content/2015-annual-report-of-atv-related-deaths-and-injuries.

Vitello, A. (2008). *Further ATV limits advised. Many deaths occur on paved roads, data show.* Charleston Gazette, Feb. 12. Retrieved July 20, 2008, from http://www.factiva.com.

Bike Safety and Awareness Program

10

Tanya Morton

The Bicycle Safety Awareness Program (BSAP), presently called the bicycle safety program (BSP), is an injury prevention program that teaches youth bicycling safety and rules through comprehensive curriculum and training (The Street Trust, 2017).

10.1 Background

The BSAP is operated under the auspices of the Bicycle Transportation Alliance (BTA), presently referred to as The Street Trust, a nonprofit organization that strives to promote bicycle use and improve bicycling conditions throughout Oregon State. The BTA's activities include programming, education, advocacy, and lobbying for community where people can comfortably meet their daily transportation needs by bicycle (Bicycle Transportation Alliance [BTA], 2008a). The BTA recognizes that strategies to improve the safety of a physical activity are generally outside the realm of what an individual can do alone and therefore strives collectively to "remove obstacles to cycling and to make it safer and higher profile. This also means "adding bike lanes, improving bridge access, and making sure new streets are designed to accommodate bicycles. It means

increasing public awareness of the fact cyclists use the streets and need to be treated safely and respectfully" (BTA, 2000a, 2000b).

Active since 1990, the BTA has grown from a small grassroots organization in the Portland area to a statewide organization with over 4,500 members, hundreds of community volunteers, and a complement of head office administrators, local coordinators, and bicycle safety education instructors (BTA, 2008a). In 1998, the BTA began its Bicycle Safety and Awareness Program (BSAP). The BSAP began with seed money provided by the Oregon Department of Transportation (ODOT), Transportation Safety Division. Although the BTA runs several bicycle programs, the BSAP is the longest running and regarded by the Executive Director Scott Bricker as the "bread and butter" of BTA's overall activities (S. Bricker, personal communication, May 3, 2008). The BSAP has been used to teach over 40,000 students throughout Oregon to cycle more safely (BTA, 2008b). The BSAP's two main goals are to (a) increase safety and awareness around youth bicycling and (b) increase youth bicycle ridership in order to improve safety, community health, and the natural environment.

The theoretical and practical development of the BSAP program began years before its actual implementation. Scott Bricker is a prime developer of the BSAP. He turned his urban planning education and training from graduate school into a more formalized program that became the

T. Morton (✉)
Catholic Children's Aid Society of Toronto,
Toronto, ON, Canada

© Springer Nature Switzerland AG 2020
R. Volpe (ed.), *Casebook of Traumatic Injury Prevention*,
https://doi.org/10.1007/978-3-030-27419-1_10

BSAP curriculum (S. Bricker, personal communication, April 18, 2008). He had a graduate assistantship in the mid-1990s to work on youth transportation issues. While he was working in a community agency on the Urban Ecosystems Project, a grant-funded program for underserved youth, he developed a bicycle club. In addition, he worked as a teacher's aide, providing educational services and making connections between classroom learning and field experience (Bricker, 1998). He began to develop the BSAP curriculum as he biked and worked with children and observed their behavior (S. Bricker, personal communication, April 18, 2008).

In total, Bricker spent two and a half years developing curriculum, with input and oversight from community partners and curriculum committee members including a school principal, teachers, health officials, nonprofit service providers, avid cyclists, and children themselves (BTA, 1999; S. Bricker, personal communication, April 18, 2008). The research and development process of the BSAP began with a national search of evidence-informed bicycle safety programs. Subsequently, the BSAP curriculum incorporated the most effective features of lauded programs in Florida, Montana, Minnesota, and Montana and by national cycling organizations such as the League of American Bicyclists (LAB; BTA, 2003b). Research from the Harborview Injury Prevention and Research Center (HIPRC) that was released at the time of program development suggested that a continuum of traffic safety education is important, with comprehensive rather than brief skills training being most effective (Macarthur, Parkin, Sidky, & Wallace, 1998). The research from the HIPRC helped Bricker determine the scope of the project and the program length (S. Bricker, personal communication, May 8, 2008).

10.1.1 Theoretical Base

A study by Macarthur et al. (1998) from the HIPRC suggested hands-on experiential skills training promotes safe cycling. Hence, Bricker designed a curriculum drawing on action-oriented learning and community-based education theory. Action-oriented learning suggests that children will learn more effectively if participating in hands-on activities. Community-based education theory suggests that children will learn more effectively if participating in activities that allow them to interact with their community (Bricker, 1998).

The program was also based on theories of cognitive development of children. Many researchers have applied Jean Piaget's theories of cognitive development to the study of road safety (Hoffrage, Weber, Hertwig, & Chase, 2003). According to Piaget and Inhelder (1969), children's knowledge is regarded as a function of environmental experience and general cognitive capacity. For example, Piaget demonstrated that when children are in the "concrete operations" stage of development at about age 7–12 years, they show an improved ability to integrate two or more variables (e.g., an object's distance and speed) into a single judgement (e.g., time to arrive). Preoperational children, i.e., under age 7, have difficulties integrating such variables (Cross, 1988; Piaget, 1970; Siegler & Richards, 1979). Parents typically grant their children a greater degree of freedom to travel from home between the ages of 10 and 12. Parents are reasonable to allow children of this age more freedom than before, because children's mental and perceptual abilities and physical coordination are rapidly improving during this period (BTA, 2003b).

For example, children develop the motor skills around the age of 10 that enable them to operate safely on the road. As they progress through Piaget's concrete operations stage, children broaden their range of travel and increase their accuracy of perception and knowledge of the city (Bricker, 1998; Lerner, 2002). The ability to synchronize the motion of self with the motion of objects appears to undertake developmental change up until at least 12 years of age (Hoffmann, Payne, & Prescott, 1980; Savelsbergh & Van der Kamp, 2000). Children also improve their capability to regulate their behavior during the school age years and respond to opportunities to be more capable in decision-making. In spite of these increased capabilities, epidemiological data show children in the fourth to seventh grade exhibit both high bicycle riding activity and high collision rates (BTA, 2003b). Clearly, the cognitive development literature demonstrates that children from fourth to seventh grade are the appropriate target age for bicycle safety programming.

10.1.2 Needs Assessment

As part of his research for his master's degree and bicycle safety program curriculum development, Bricker (1998) underwent an observational needs assessment by riding bicycles with children, observing their on-bike behavior, and noting the bicycle riding activities that they had the most difficulty with, such as left-hand turns or lane positioning. The salient findings to emerge from this needs assessment were that:

- Environmental variables influence middle-school-aged children's decision-making on bicycles. These variables either pertain to addressing the physical infrastructure (i.e., traffic routes) or through providing children with education (bicycle training).
- Age, level of development, parental guidance, physical barriers, and existing travel paths are important determinants of travel patterns.
- Cognition and perception of the urban environment affects travel decisions and behaviors.

The findings of Bricker's needs assessment are corroborated with quantitative research that demonstrates age-related and individual differences in risk perception and motor coordination (e.g., Mathieson, 2007). The implications are that children age 10 and over have acquired the necessary cognitive, perceptual, and coordination skills to begin bicycling in a stimulating and busy environment; however, they require education. Hence this age group is often a target for bicycle training (see Rivera & Metrik, 1998; United States Department of Transportation [USDOT], 2002).

10.1.3 Use of Local Knowledge

The BSAP utilizes local knowledge to shape its program. Illuminating the most prominent safety hazards in a community and any differences between local data and national patterns may provide suggestions about potential preventative interventions and other information likely to reduce injury in a community (Christoffel & Gallagher, 2006). As part of the needs assessment which contributed to Bricker's master's research and curriculum development, he performed one other activity pertinent to the BSAP before the program was implemented: he and his colleagues met with Portland fifth and sixth grade children to discuss their perceptions of bicycling, including potential routes, hazards, and barriers to cycling. Children also hand drew "cognitive maps" of a typical bicycle ride from home to school or other common destinations. The mapping exercise was intended to explore the thinking processes behind children's bicycle travel behavior and desires. The mapping exercise produced findings demonstrating basic trends in children's perceptions of local traffic volumes and speeds, roadway surface conditions, and geography. The results of the exercise were useful to accommodating the needs and desires of children in regard to local transportation policy and planning (Bricker, n.d.). Children's limited understanding of and exposure to the environment are manifested in these cognitive representations and laid the groundwork for programming that promotes safe routes for children, including low-traffic bicycle boulevards and bicycle and pedestrian cut-through paths in neighborhoods for safe and efficient access to schools and parks (Bricker, n.d.). Figure 10.1 shows a cognitive map which demonstrates how children's lesser experience and interaction with the scope of the city vis-à-vis adults are reflected in their perception of the environment.

10.1.4 Program Activities

In addition to receiving initial funding from the ODOT, successful grant writing occurred early in the life of the program for funding from local,

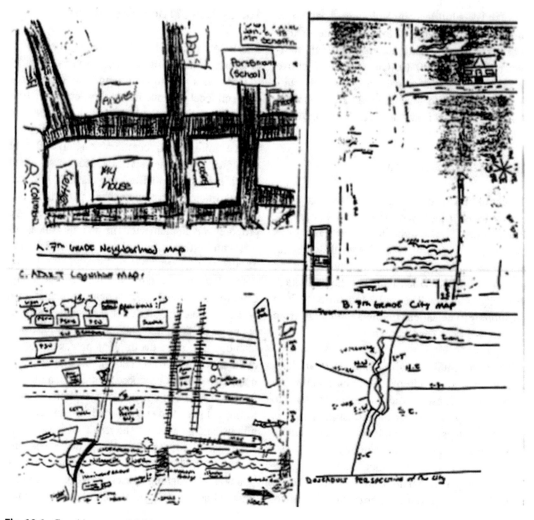

Fig. 10.1 Cognitive map of children's and adults' perceptions of their city

regional, and national organizations and corporations (USDOT, 2002). The BTA gathered statistics and research that demonstrated the need for a comprehensive bicycle safety program in Oregon (BTA, 1999). The BTA adopted the BSAP in 1998 and piloted it in four Oregon communities in 1999. Bricker drove around the state with a truck containing bicycles and delivered the program. An estimated 480 children in total were exposed to the pilot program. The pilot provided an opportunity to see what program components resonated with the children and had the greatest probability of success. After the pilot, the first version of the curriculum was produced. School administrators and teachers that were willing to endorse the program

were recruited by BTA employees (S. Bricker, personal communication, April 26, 2008). Information on the program spread informally through word of mouth (USDOT, 2002). The USDOT (2002) wrote in their good practices review that the BSAP's "widespread popularity has been a measure of its success" (p. 20).

A decision was made to deliver the BSAP during school time rather than as an after-school program in order to maximize program reach. The BTA staff who instruct the program are avid cyclists trained to deliver the program with fidelity (i.e., in the manner it was developed and validated with all the prescribed components and processes). They are also taught child man-

Table 10.1 A timeline for the historical development of BSAP from 1990 to 2001

Year	Development of BSAP
1990	BTA formed as a small grassroots organization in Portland
1996–1998	Scott Bricker conducted research and practiced with students and teachers in three Portland inner city middle schools in the role of a teacher's aide and an employee of the Urban Ecosystems Project (UEP). His goal was to understand students' travel behaviors, concerns, and transportation needs Scott Bricker completed research for his master's degree in urban and regional planning at Portland State University Scott Bricker begins working as a program director at BTA Funding awarded for BSAP from the Oregon Department of Transportation (ODOT), corporations, and local, regional, and national organizations
1999	First test pilot of the BSAP BSAP operated in four Oregon middle schools and reached approximately 235 students
2000	Curriculum revised and reformatted after first year implementation. Evaluation redesigned to put helmet fitting questions on the written test Program expands to three other communities in Oregon
2001	Program adds seven new communities 3,766 students reached in 140 classrooms in about 30 schools Based on feedback from teachers and BTA staff, the curriculum was rearranged to stress on-bike training earlier in the program

Note: This table was created using information from *Project Evaluation Report. Bicycle Safety Education Project* by the Bicycle Transportation Alliance, 1999, 2000a, 2001, Portland, OR: Author, and the *Annual Report*, by the Bicycle Transportation Alliance, 2003a, Portland, OR: Author

agement techniques in order to minimize time wastage due to child behavior problems. Training an instructor is an expensive process, taking two full weeks in addition to shadowing, co-teaching, and liaison. Instructor performance is observed and evaluated by teachers and the BTA (S. Bricker, personal communication, April 26, 2008). School teachers were not selected to deliver the program, largely because the BTA as an organization could have more control over program evaluation if it employed its own instructors. Moreover, schools often want an outside organization to come in to teach the educational component of bicycle safety (A. Koch, personal communication, May 8, 2008). The timeline in Table 10.1 summarizes the measures undertaken to field the BSAP in its early years.

10.2 Resources

10.2.1 Resource Allocation and Strategies

The annual expenses of the BSAP were about $100,000 (BTA, 2006). The BTA's other expenses include outreach and promotion, administration, advocacy, and running its other programs (BTA, 2006). There is always effort required to continue to grow and maintain support. For example, in 2005, Bricker advocated for increasing traffic fines in Oregon while he was working in the capacity of policy director. These increased funds financed traffic safety education. In addition, the revenue for the BTA comes from a variety of other sources, including government, contract work, individual and corporate support, fee for service, and foundations (BTA, 2006). One of the BTA's strengths is the existence of several sources of funding. If the level of support is reduced by one funding source, another is likely to be available to redress the balance (Jones & Offord, 1991).

The BTA's mandate to improve cycling conditions can be broken into three categories: advocacy, programs, and events. The BSAP falls into the program category, but there is overlap among categories. Table 10.2 shows the various strategies of the BTA and examples of how they work together to promote safe cycling.

10.2.2 Expertise

The BTA's Executive Director Scott Bricker has worked at the organization since 1998, starting

Table 10.2 The strategies of the BTA to improve cycling conditions

Strategy		Example
Advocacy	Entails working at the "local, state and national level to make bicycling a safe, convenient option and a part of the community's everyday transportation system" (BTA, 2008a)	Due to BTA legislative campaigns in 2005, two bills were successfully passed: one that gives cyclists more rights on the road and one that launches a statewide Safe Routes to School (SR2S) Program. The Bicycle Boulevards Campaign aims to create a comprehensive network of low-traffic bicycle streets—"bicycle boulevards"—which are safe and welcoming to children, families, and cycling beginners
Programs	An integral part of the BTA's activities is their structured programs that encourage safe walking and biking	The BTA is the program project manager for the city of Portland's Safe Routes to School (SR2S) Program, a coalition-led umbrella program promoting traffic safety. SR2S promotes children walking and biking to school using elements from "4 Es" of injury prevention: encouragement, education, engineering, and enforcement. The BSAP teaches middle school students to cycle properly and safely, by covering topics such as hazard avoidance, proper helmet fitting, and rules of the road (BTA, 2003b)
Events	Offer the cycling community an opportunity to network, socialize, contribute to the cause, and have fun.	Fundraising, organized bicycle rides, and awards ceremonies (BTA, 2008a)

as the original developer and program director for the BSAP. Next, he worked in the capacity of policy director from 2003 to 2007 before becoming Executive Director (S. Bricker, personal communication, May 8, 2008; BTA, 2003b). He and other staff report to a volunteer board that establishes and monitors major policy direction, oversees finances, and helps secure resources (BTA, 2008c).

In order to deliver the BSAP, the BTA brings expertise such as instructors and community volunteers into middle schools. While instructors deliver the program, volunteers help facilitate the community rides with children. On-the-job training is provided for instructors and volunteers. As of 2008, the BSAP had 18 full-time administrative staff at its head office in Portland and four local bike safety education coordinators that work in smaller Oregon communities (BTA, 2008d). The 28 BSAP instructors worked on a full-time year-round, full-time, or part-time seasonal basis. Winter is the slow period for teaching the BSAP and hence some staff may not work, but summer programs such as outdoor camps keep staff busy in summer. The BTA's goal is to keep staff employed as much as possible (S. Bricker, personal communication, May 8, 2008). All BSAP

instructors and coordinators receive opportunities to meet and network for training and debriefing purposes (A. Koch, personal communication, May 8, 2008).

The BTA runs the BSAP with fidelity to the original model in which it was developed and validated (i.e., ten comprehensive classes of 55–60 min each) in spite of pressure to downsize or cut back (S. Bricker, personal communication, May 8, 2008). Bureaucratic pressure to downsize and cut costs is a common occurrence in prevention programs; however, such measures often result in the loss of crucial programmatic components (Jones & Offord, 1991). Bricker is clear that the only way the program will be provided is with adherence to the original model. As there is no other program in the community filling the same niche, the BSAP has some leverage to keep the program faithful to its original design.

Because the head office administrators are not present to oversee the rural statewide Oregon programs with the same vigilance as they can the Portland programs, there is the ability for the statewide Oregon instructors to play the role of coordinators with school representatives. The statewide employees perform a wider variety of tasks than the Portland employees and largely manage their own programs. Hence, they can be responsive to local needs (A. Koch, personal communication, May 8, 2008). However, the administration of the BSAP remains centralized and under the control of the BTA. According to Bourgeois, Noce, Smeh, and Morton (2007), centralization is beneficial; decentralization (i.e., the fragmentation of responsibilities to different agencies) tends to restrict human and fiscal resources. Therefore, if financial support is decreased, resources would be inflexible and not within the implementing agency's control.

10.2.3   Material Resources

Prior to BSAP implementation in a school, a written contract is signed, largely to confirm who provides what items (e.g., permission slips, helmets; S. Bricker, personal communication, April 18, 2008). The BSAP's bicycles are brought into the schools via donated transport because not all children own bicycles or their parents do not allow them to cycle to school. Each community that delivers the program receives a fleet of 25–30 bicycles, the BTA'sFirst Gear instructional DVD, brochures, traffic cones, bicycle maintenance tools, safety vests, a 122-page manual, and other small items (BTA, 2001). Bicycle storage space and assembly are donated. Schools contribute to the BSAP by printing permission slips (S. Bricker, personal communication, May 8, 2008). The BSAP also receives other subsidies, such as below-cost bike helmets (S. Bricker, personal communication, May 8, 2008), or the services of bicycle shop staff that sell bicycles to the program at wholesale cost or perform free bicycle maintenance on the fleet (BTA, 2001). Insurance for bicycles and other equipment is purchased by the BTA. Companies contribute money and resources (S. Bricker, personal communication, May 8, 2008). Due to the material resources amassed by the BSAP, an opportunity is provided to the schools that they would not otherwise have (BTA, 2001).

Although the BSAP is offered in Portland and in several small communities such as Talent, Corvallis, and Gresham, the BTA does not have the resources or mandate to deliver the BSAP to every child in Oregon. Small rural communities find it particularly hard to muster the critical mass of schedule and class demands to set up the program. The BTA lacks the ability to make the BSAP and related programs truly statewide. Ideally, Bricker would like to see the BSAP as part of a statewide continuum of traffic safety education, including pedestrian safety for younger children and driver's safety education for adolescents (S. Bricker, personal communication, April 26, 2008).

10.3   Implementation

10.3.1   Multifaceted Implementation

As previously mentioned in this paper, Bricker incorporated his early research and practice experiences into the BSAP curriculum. These experiences indicated that children make choices and show typical patterns about where and how they cycle, which in turn influences safety. For example, preadolescent children seldom choose to ride in bicycle lanes on busy streets, even though bicycle lanes are often endorsed by urban planners (Bricker, n.d.; S. Bricker, personal communication, April 18, 2008). Children and many adults prefer to cycle on low-traffic routes (Bricker, n.d.; S. Bricker, personal communication, April 18, 2008). If popular children's destinations (e.g., school) could be made accessible to them from multiple low-traffic directions, the numbers of children walking and biking to school would increase and the trend toward chauffeuring to school would be moderated. In the late 1960s the rate of children walking or biking to school in the USA was 65%, and 90% of children living within 1 mile walked or biked. More recently, only 13% of children, and 33% living within 1 mile, walk or bike to school (Center for Disease Control and Prevention, 2000). Chauffeuring children to school increases risk to the children who do walk or bike to school. They are at risk when cars amass in school streets, school parking lots, and local streets (Hunt, 1998; O'Brien, 2004). This awareness of the impact of a car culture and other environmental characteristics on safety was embedded into the BSAP program implementation. As per Bricker's original curriculum development, the program's design acknowledges that altering the social and physical environment can influence bicycle behavior in youth.

The BSAP teaches students to consider environmental influences in terms of hazard avoidance and safe route planning. However, the main focus of the BSAP curriculum is on education, namely, bike handling, helmet and bike fitting, rules of the road, and safety skills. The BTA will also assist with the implementation of environmentally oriented injury prevention strategies when the BSAP is delivered in a school, including an assessment of bicycle parking facilities and working with school staff and administration to support a culture of cycling (BTA, 2003b). The BTA also offers promotional campaigns such as low-cost helmet sales and "bike to school" days (BTA, 2001). BTA attests that citizens' knowledge and awareness of bicycle safety will increase when more children cycle to school. Given that the BTA offers a range of services including advocacy, events, and programs that aim to improve bicycling conditions, it can offer a concomitant range of injury prevention solutions in children's bicycle safety programming.

For example, the BTA is program project manager for SR2S and thus develops, coordinates, and promotes SR2S program elements. SR2S is an umbrella program that was launched in Oregon in 2005 as a 5-year pilot (BTA, 2008e). The BSAP has been made a subsidiary of SR2S, along with sister programs such as the pedestrian safety program that is geared toward children in grades two and three (BTA, 2008e). According to SR2S Director Angela Koch, school administrators often consent to having the BSAP implemented in their school because they would like to obtain the free city-funded engineering components of the SR2S program (which consists of improvements to the school area such as crosswalks, parking controls, curb extensions, and curb cuts). They agree to receive the BSAP in order to obtain the engineering components, but then they realize that the BSAP and other strategies to prevent injury are effective (A. Koch, personal communication, May 8, 2008). As stated by Angela Koch, "just the engineering won't work, just the education won't work. It's holistic" (personal communication, May 8, 2008).

Another resource that is offered as part of the SR2S package is the Pedal Power Squadron. Separate from, yet complementary to, the BSAP, it is an after-school program providing students with skills and the hands-on training to improve their level of safety while cycling and encouraging biking as a means of transportation and recreation. Like the BSAP, the program is delivered on school grounds and on local streets. Some of the children who participate in Pedal Power Squadron have completed the BSAP. Pedal Power Squadron gives these children the opportunity to continue cycling after the BSAP and assumes a mentoring role to the children who have not taken the BSAP (BTA, 2008f). To encourage continued ridership, students from low-income families are eligible to earn a bike and helmet based on completion of the pedal power program.

The range of interventions that the BSAP undertakes correspond to Sleet's categorization of intervention strategies and methods for sports injury prevention. This categorization investigates the determinants of injury using the classic epidemiological model of host, agent, and environment. The injured person is the host, the agent refers to the source of injury, and the environment consists of the social or physical factors surrounding the injury. Whether or not a person becomes injured depends on the interplay of these three factors (Christoffel & Gallagher, 2006; Robertson, 1998).

Using the classic host-agent-environment model, the BTA's targeted use of school-based strategies designed to prevent bicycle injuries among children is categorized according to the framework by Sleet (1994) and expanded upon in Fig. 10.2.

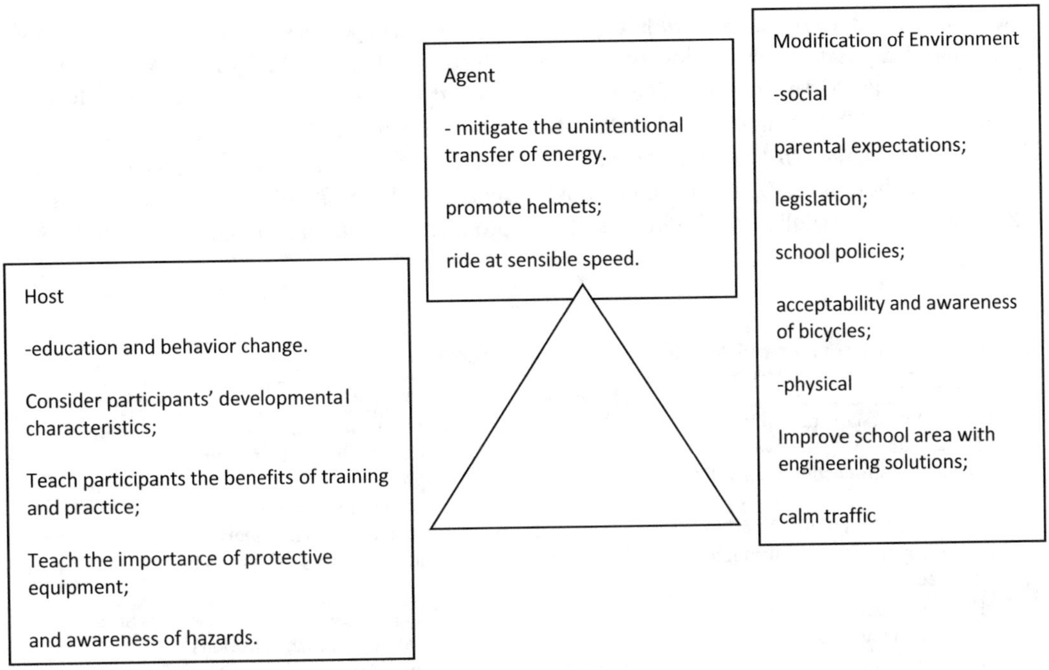

Fig. 10.2 Intervention strategies for preventing bicycle injury according to host-agent-environment model. (Based on *Injury Prevention* by D. A. Sleet, 1994, in The Comprehensive School Health Challenge: Promoting Health Through Education, edited by P. Cortese & K. Middleton, pp. 443–389, Santa Cruz, CA: ETR Associates)

10.3.2 Curriculum

Teaching children cycling skills, such as rules of the road, what to do when approaching intersections, and maneuvering techniques, facilitates safe and predictable biking. Teaching children to understand and interact with their environment through exposure to various access roads teaches youth to map favorable routes to their destinations, including low-traffic streets. In addition, advocating for low-volume, low-speed routes and safe and easy access to children's destinations is important policy implications of the work.

A strength of the BSAP curriculum is that it uses the effective elements of already established curricula. However, the BSAP stresses on-road training, which few curricula do. The BSAP curriculum was developed with an on-bike and hands-on focus, proposing that preadolescents will learn to cycle in traffic properly only while riding bikes with supervision and feedback (BTA, 2003b). Cycling skills are taught incrementally, progressing from the school playground to the street.

In keeping with the evidence that wearing a bicycle helmet is one of the most effective safety measures that a child can take to prevent injury (Rivara, Thompson, Patterson, & Thompson, 1998), the ODOT helmet brochure is consistently used for teaching helmet fit (BTA, 2001). The students undertake a helmet fitting demonstration and exercise early in the program and are taught about the protective effects of wearing a helmet in the event of a crash (BTA, 2003b). However, the program also focuses on the pre-event phase of injury prevention—taking steps to avoid a crash at all is the goal (S. Bricker, personal communication, May 8, 2008).

Plans for evaluation were set forth at the beginning of the program. Establishing the fundamental program tasks and objectives at the beginning of the program has provided the groundwork for a strong evaluation design that is conducive to measuring the implementation and impact of the program. Since initial implementation, the components of the program have remained consistent overall (S. Bricker, personal communication, May 8, 2008), with approximately ten 1-h sessions, consisting of 4 h of classroom learning and 6 h on-bike. The program culminates in a street community ride (USDOT, 2002). During classroom teaching, the ratio of adults to children is 1:10; during community rides the ratio of adults to children is 1:6. Volunteer chaperones add to the level of supervision during the community rides. Volunteers also teach cycling skills on a one-on-one basis to the few children encountered who do not know how to ride a bike at all (S. Bricker, personal communication, May 8, 2008). A summary of the BSAP program curriculum is provided in Table 10.3.

Table 10.3 Overview of the ten class cycling program (60-min classes)

Day	Coverage	Location	Day	Coverage	Location
1	Bicycle ridership and safety Introduction: program overview Optional: introduction to investigation Pre-test Why do we have traffic laws? Riding on the road and through intersections	In class	6	Riding with traffic Predictability: riding on the right Exiting driveways Introduction to intersections Moving through intersections	Street
2	Helmets, gear, and bike parts Optional: melon drop Fitting helmets Signs Bike parts and components Bike gear Optional: video Optional: bike investigation	In class	7	Intersections Introduction to intersections Moving through intersections Three left turns Intersections: putting it all together Optional: intersection practice	Street

3	Laws, hazards, and repair
	Rules of the road (revisited)
	Common reasons for collisions
	Hazards identification
	Fixing flat tires
	Optional: video
	Optional: bicycle investigation
		In class	8	Hazards and emergency avoidance
				Hazards (revisited)
				Emergency avoidance techniques:
				    Railroad tracks
				    Emergency stop
				    Rock dodge
				    Quick turn
				Optional: neighborhood ride
					Playground/street

4	Traffic simulation, fitting bikes Right of way How to drive a car/bike Proper fit of bicycles Basic bicycle maintenance check Optional: secure bicycle locking Optional: bicycle investigation	In class	9	Neighborhood bike ride/bike rodeo Discussion: physically fit lifestyle Neighborhood ride Bicycle rodeo	Street
5	Controlling, stopping, and signaling Bike/helmet check (revisited) Stopping Slalom Learning to look back: riding with one hand Scanning and signaling Gearing Optional: snail race Optional: follow the leader	Playground	10	Neighborhood ride and written test Post-test/evaluation Neighborhood ride	Playground/street

Note: Reprinted from *Safe Routes for Kids Bicycle Safety Program Curriculum Third Edition* (p. xii), by the Bicycle Transportation Alliance, 2003b, Portland, OR: Author. Copyright 2003 by the Bicycle Transportation Alliance

The curriculum has undergone minor iterations due to liaison and discussion among program instructors about how to prioritize and keep the students engaged (e.g., safety messages are taking precedence over teaching how to change a flat tire; there are efforts to get the students on the bikes earlier in the program than previously). Instructor "tips and tricks" that suggest and inform curriculum improvements are documented and shared (S. Bricker, personal communication, May 8, 2008). Angela Koch, Safe Routes to School director and overseer of the BTA's classroom education programs, notes the tension between the instructors following the curriculum with fidelity to the original model and being flexible to adapt to individual situations as they arise. She states that "flexibility is very important. You can't say to someone who will teach the program 'here's our curriculum, here's how you teach it,' and teach them what to say exactly. There's never a level playing field. That's the biggest lesson learned. You need to know the material inside and out and think really fast and figure out what's going to work best in your situation. But, use the curriculum as your guide. There's certain basics you have to get through" (A. Koch, personal communication, May 8, 2008).

10.3.3 Adjustments to the Program

Challenges to program delivery include (a) getting parents involved, (b) the decreasing rate of physical activity among children, and (c) prohibitive levels of traffic and distance between children and their schools. According to S. Bricker (personal communication, May 8, 2008), engaging parents in the program has always been a challenge; however, demands on parents' time have escalated. Moreover, few parents cycle, especially with their children in tow. In order to try to address this challenge, the BTA worked with the city on a strategic outreach to parents (S. Bricker, personal communication, May 8, 2008).

Statistics Canada (2005) demonstrates that decreases in physical activity among children have been associated with increased obesity. Some overweight and obese children have difficulty in participating in the program (e.g., activities such as the 40-min community bicycle ride). The strategy is to encourage overweight children to participate in the program as much as they can and work through the "I can't" mentality that these children may display (S. Bricker, personal communication, April 26, 2008). The same strategy is used for the few children encountered who cannot ride a bike at all (A. Koch, personal communication, May 8, 2008).

As several communities served by BSAP display trends such as increased car traffic and increased distances to school (Bricker, n.d.), the BTA has chosen to address this challenge through their advocacy stream. In addition, to address systemic challenges they have sought out new partners, such as local governments and departments of transport, the national SR2S movement, elected officials, the bicycle industry, and the federal transportation department (BTA, 2008g; S. Bricker, personal communication, May 8, 2008). Combined with implementation strategies such as low-cost helmet sales and community outreach, the BSAP has been able to draw upon a multitude of community resources harnessed and coordinated by the BTA (BTA, 2001).

10.4 Outcome

There are several ways to evaluate bicycle safety program outcomes. Methodological difficulties in the collection of injury and death data related to cycling challenge community-based programs. The collection of such data requires a vast population to garner accurate results. According to Towner and Dowswell (2002), "death as an outcome is too rare an event to provide information on what to target or to be used to evaluate local campaigns" (p. 281). Moreover, it is difficult and expensive for community-based programs to establish injury surveillance systems (Towner &

Dowswell, 2002). Therefore, it is often unrealistic for reduced injury or mortality rates to be the sole outcome measure of a community-based program, even though this is an ultimate goal. However, program effectiveness can be measured by participants' changes in scores on pre- and post-tests, or observations of skills and behaviors. Other ways of assessing program effectiveness are to track the number or types of cyclist crashes that occur, or to track the number of cyclists wearing helmets or the number of cyclists in an area over time (Rivara & Aitken, 1998). For a useful evaluation to occur, there must be "meaningful and consistent" outcome measures used (Towner & Dowswell, 2002, p. 281). The outcome measures used by the BSAP are discussed below.

10.4.1 Crash Statistics in Portland

The BSAP is grounded in the Portland Office of Transportation's (2007) local research that demonstrated that high levels of bicycle ridership are associated with high levels of safety for cyclists. An increase in cycling activity in and of itself improves cyclist safety, largely due to increased awareness and caution on the part of motorists and increased opportunities for motorists and cyclists to learn to function around each other and share the road (Portland Office of Transportation, 2007; Ross, 2008). Hence, the BSAP is part of the BTA's agenda to get more families on bicycles to improve cycling safety for all. In Portland, where the number of cyclists has been regularly tracked, cycling rates have nearly quadrupled since 1990. Between 2005 and 2006, bicycling went up 18% (BTA, 2006; Portland Office of Transportation, 2007). These statistics are corroborated with studies in Portland that track an increase in cycling in non-bridge locations (Portland Office of Transportation, 2007) and studies in other communities that also show that as the number cyclists increases, the roads become safer for them (BTA, 2006). Statistics gathered by the Portland Office of Transportation (2007) showed a decrease in the reported bicycle crash rate, associated with the increase in cycling over Portland bicycle bridges.

10.4.2 Evaluation

To assess the effectiveness of the BSAP, data have been gathered throughout the life cycle of the program. The BSAP has been subject to a higher level of evaluation than most other community-based cycling safety programs. Funding from the Oregon Department of Transportation (ODOT) demanded rigorous evaluation. An estimated ¼ of a full-time equivalency (FTE) per year was spent on evaluation in the BSAP's first 3 years. In year 3 the money spent reached 1/4–1/3 FTE, including tasks such as correcting tests, compiling data, and collating. Not included in these FTE figures is the time required to administer the test in classes (another 1 h per pre-/post-test pair per classroom and evaluation design; S. Dricker, personal communication, July 16, 2008). Although funding bodies gave the program some leeway on evaluation after displaying years of consistent results, the evaluation questions are still asked, and the evaluation results are still compared year to year.

10.4.2.1 Curriculum

One evaluation question asked school teachers if they think the curriculum is effective. Teachers were questioned about the students' response to the curriculum, the instruction techniques, areas of success, and improvements in students' abilities. The results of this evaluation component are used to discuss the effectiveness of the program and any changes that need to occur. Results from the first 3 years of the program indicate that the most frequently mentioned strengths of the program were on-road bicycling, the timing of the classroom instruction, and the resources the BTA brings. The weaknesses mentioned include the weather sensitivity of the program which decreases options if the children cannot go outside, the need for more volunteers, and the administrative time required for evaluation. Overall, the teachers who completed this portion of the evaluation showed strong support for the curriculum. In 2001, the average rating of the program on a 7-point scale was 6.4, with 6.3 for content value. All teachers who participated in the evaluation requested the program again (BTA, 2001).

10.4.2.2 Rules-of-the-Road

The rules-of-the-road evaluation component uses pre- and post-tests to assess children's increases in knowledge and comprehension in such areas as helmet fit, right of way, and traffic signs (BTA, 2003b). The evaluations triangulate different methods of testing in order to tap into different children's learning styles and minimize bias (A. Koch, personal communication, May 8, 2008). The evaluations are comprehensive, consisting of about three pages each. They primarily feature visual tests that require reading, writing, drawing, or multiple-choice responses (BTA, 2006). A sample of participants rather than all participants underwent the pre- and post-testing. Out of the 30 schools in Portland and the 20 other schools across the state that deliver the BSAP, about five classes are selected in Portland and five statewide for pre- and post-testing. Therefore, about ten classes of children underwent pre- and post-testing, with 25–30 children in each class (A Koch, personal communication, May 8, 2008). BTA staff and contractors are taught how to consistently grade the tests, in order to increase reliability of results across communities (BTA, 2001). A 40% increase in children's knowledge has been the consistent evaluation result (S. Bricker, personal communication, May 8, 2008; BTA, 2000a, 2000b, 2001). Although the tests show an improvement from pre- to post-test, The tests have proven challenging for students: data analysis has also revealed that while only 2%–7% of children pass the pre-test, at least 40% pass the post-test (BTA, 2000a, 2000b, 2001). Figure 10.3 gives an example of the rules-of-the-road test.

10.4.2.3 Actively Promote Cycling to School

Activities organized by the SR2S program, such as the BSAP, surveys, walkabouts, mapping, and Walk and Bike to School Day, analyze conditions around the schools and promote the involvement of parents, students, and community groups to help improve the walk or bike ride to school and get more children independently mobile (BTA, 2008e). The BSAP has succeeded in having a higher percentage of children cycle to school than before program implementation. During the 2000–2001 school year, only 4.4% of students in the participating Portland schools cycled to school before the BSAP, while over 11% cycled by the BSAP's final days (Center for Health Training, n.d.). In the smaller communities served by the BSAP, the percentage of students cycling to school increased from 5.9% to 12% from the first and last day of the program. These percentages are in comparison to 1% of children nationally and 2% of children in Portland cycling to school (BTA, 2001). Schools in neighborhoods characterized by busy roads or highways, a perceived long distance to school, many hills, or insecure bicycle parking were found to have more barriers to bicycle ridership than schools without these qualities (BTA, 2001).

10.4.3 Attainments of the Program

The BSAP has garnered external praise in the form of two national awards. The most recent award was from the surgeon general, who presented the BSAP with the 2008 Healthy Youth for a Healthy Future award (BTA, 2008b). In 2003, the BSAP curriculum was recognized for its contribution to bicycling with the Bicycle Education Leadership Award by the League of American Bicyclists (LAB; BTA, 2003a). The BSAP was also profiled in the USDOT's Good Practices Guide for bicycle safety education.

10.5 Conclusion

Via a needs assessment that found that children's perception and cognition of the urban environment affects their travel decisions and behaviors, the curriculum of the BSAP was shaped as an approach to children's bicycle safety that considered environmental factors, the imperatives of child development, and educational goals. The BTA's support has maximized the resources available to the BSAP and given it access to a variety of injury prevention strategies that work together to promote cycling as a safe and enjoyable means of transport.

This test will help us know how well you understand the rules of the road as they apply to bicycles. Read all questions carefully. Questions will ask you to either label pictures, choose the best answer to a question, or list answers. You will receive extra credit where you are able to list more than the requested number of answers.

1. You and the car across from you reach this four-way stop intersection at the same time. You are turning left and the car is going straight. Mark the **one** answer that best explains what you will do.

   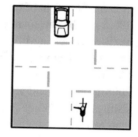

   ○ **A.** Stop, signal left, wait for the car to go first and then turn left

   ○ **B.** Stop, turn through the intersection and then let the car go straight

   ○ **C.** Make eye contact with the driver and make your turn

2. You are riding at night in a properly lighted neighborhood. Mark the **one** answer that best explains what the law requires for night riding.

   ○ **A.** Bright clothes and reflectors

   ○ **B.** Flash light and reflectors

   ○ **C.** Front head light and rear tail light

   ○ **D.** Reflective clothing and front head light

3. Write a brief description of what the following signs mean and label all parts of the traffic signal.

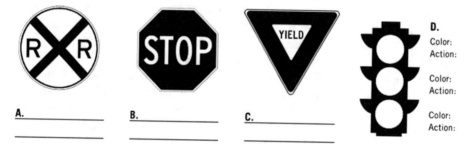

D.
Color:
Action:

Color:
Action:

Color:
Action:

A._____   B._____   C._____

Fig. 10.3 Rules-of-the-road test example. (Reprinted from *Safe Routes for Kids Bicycle Safety Program Curriculum Third Edition* (p. 101), by the Bicycle Transportation Alliance, 2003b, Portland, OR: Author. Copyright 2003 by the Bicycle Transportation Alliance)

Portland remains a city where cycling receives a high profile as a desirable activity (Center for Health Training, n.d.; Ross, 2008). The BSAP's broad program goals, consistent with the positive view of cycling, are to (a) increase safety and awareness around youth bicycling and (b) increase youth bicycle ridership in order to improve safety, community health, and the natural environment. In spite of the methodological difficulties inherent in evaluating community-based cycling programs, the evaluations that do exist for the BSAP indicate that the program is a success. The comprehensive pre- and post-tests triangulate different methods of testing, in order to tap into different children's learning styles and minimize bias. Combined with counts of bicycle ridership, teacher evaluations, and reported crash statistics, the final picture indicates the BSAP is well positioned to continue to offer its curriculum with fidelity to its original model. As cycling continues to be a popular activity for children, the BSAP offers a worthwhile contribution to the injury prevention field.

Acknowledgments The author would like to express sincere appreciation to the key informants for this case study: Scott Bricker and Angela Koch of the Bicycle Transportation Alliance in Portland, OR, USA—whose consultation made this project possible.

BRIO Model: Bike Safety Awareness Program (BSAP)

Group Served: Children from fourth to seventh grade.

Goal: Teaching youth bicycle safety for the prevention of injuries.

Background	Resources	Implementation	Outcome
Children approximately 10–15 years old at greatest risk for bicycle-related injury Bicycle Transportation Alliance (BTA) starts as a small grassroots organization in 1990 to promote cycling BSAP curriculum developed from observational needs assessment and with input from community partners BSAP adopted by the BTA in 1998 and piloted in 1999 Successful grant writing occurred early in the life of the program Curriculum revised and reformatted in 2000 after first year implementation	The annual expenses of the BSAP are about $100,000 Program run by a complement of head office administrators, local coordinators, and bike safety education instructors Substantial investment put into instructor training BSAP has access to the BTA's wider pool of programs, resources, and injury prevention strategies A fleet of bicycles, helmets, and other program materials are received by each community that delivers the program Volunteers, companies, and schools donate time or in-kind goods to the BSAP	A multidimensional approach to injury prevention, including consideration of host, agent, and environment BSAP delivered using effective elements of already established bicycle safety curricula On-bike skills training implemented in accordance with theory and research findings	In 2001, 12% of BSAP-involved children in Portland cycled to school, in comparison to 1% of children nationally and 2% of children in Portland A 40% increase in knowledge of rules-of-the-road from pre- to post-test has been a consistent result In 2001, the average teacher rating of the effectiveness of the program on a 7-point scale was 6.4, with 6.3 for content value. All teachers who participated in the evaluation requested the program again

Life Space Model: Bicycle Safety and Awareness Program (BSAP)

Sociocultural: civilization/community	Interpersonal: primary and secondary relationships	Physical environments: where we live	Internal states: biochemical/ genetic and means of coping
Grounded in local data showing trends in cycling crashes and cycling rates Embedded within the school system's already existing student population and organizational infrastructure Works to improve the acceptability and awareness of bicycles and the numbers of cyclists Rural communities adapt program to fit their local needs	Engages volunteers and community members including teachers, avid cyclists, and city officials Strategic outreach to parents Children's peer relationships enhanced through group riding techniques All BSAP instructors and coordinators receive opportunities to meet and network for training and debriefing	Advocates with the BTA for safer environmental policies and road infrastructure including low-traffic bicycle boulevards and traffic calming Teaches children awareness of surface, collision, and visual hazards while cycling Supports school personnel to work internally to ensure there is secure bicycle parking and safe route planning for students	Normal stages of childhood growth and development provide a guide regarding when and how to deliver the program Develops positive attitude toward and consistent use of helmets Teaches children self-management and social behavior including the application of rules, procedures, and etiquette that promote safe and efficient travel

References

Bicycle Transportation Alliance. (1999). Project evaluation report. In *Bicycle safety education project.* Portland, OR: Author.

Bicycle Transportation Alliance. (2000a). Project evaluation report. In *Bicycle safety education project.* Portland, OR: Author.

Bicycle Transportation Alliance. (2000b). *We're the BTA. Join us [Brochure].* Portland, OR: Author.

Bicycle Transportation Alliance. (2001). *Project evaluation report. Bicycle safety education project.* Portland, OR: Author.

Bicycle Transportation Alliance. (2003a). *Annual report 2003.* Portland, OR: Author.

Bicycle Transportation Alliance. (2003b). *Safe routes for kids bicycle safety program curriculum* (3rd ed.). Portland, OR: Author.

Bicycle Transportation Alliance. (2006). *2006 Annual report.* Portland, OR: Author.

Bicycle Transportation Alliance. (2008a). *About the Bicycle Transportation Alliance.* Retrieved April 20, 2008, from http://www.bta4bikes.org/at_work/index.php.

Bicycle Transportation Alliance. (2008b). *Acting US surgeon general awards BSE program.* Retrieved May 25, 2008, from http://www.bta4bikes.org/btablog/2008/04/10/acting-us-surgeon-general-awards-bse-program/.

Bicycle Transportation Alliance. (2008c). *The BTA's incredible board of directors.* Retrieved May 30, 2008, from http://www.bta4bikes.org/at_work/board.php.

Bicycle Transportation Alliance. (2008d). *The BTA's wonderful staff.* Retrieved May 30, 2008, from www.bta4bikes.org/at_work/staff.php.

Bicycle Transportation Alliance. (2008e). *Safe routes to school.* Retrieved July 15, 2008, from http://www.bta4bikes.org/at_work/saferoutes.php.

Bicycle Transportation Alliance. (2008f). Pedal power squads. Retrieved June 29, 2008, from http://www.bta4bikes.org/at_work/pedalpowersquads.php.

Bicycle Transportation Alliance. (2008g). *Improving Oregon's laws: The BTA and three legislative sessions.* Retrieved 2 July, 2008, from http://www.bta4bikes.org/at_work/legisreview.php.

Bourgeois, R., Noce, M. Smeh, D., & Morton, T. (2007). *Sustainability of community-based health interventions: A literature review.* Unpublished manuscript, University of Toronto, Toronto, ON.

Bricker, S. (1998). *Methods for increasing early-adolescents bicycle ridership.* Unpublished master's thesis, Portland State University, Oregon.

Bricker, S. (n.d.). *Safe routes to school report.* Unpublished manuscript.

Center for Disease Control and Prevention. (2000). *Kidswalk-to-School.* https://stacks.cdc.gov/view/cdc/11316. Accessed 16 Mar 2018.

Center for Health Training. (n.d.). Safe routes to school: Promise and Practice. Retrieved July 18, 2008, from http://www.nhtsa.dot.gov/people/injury/pedbimot/bike/Safe-Routes2004/pages/section-4_portland.htm.

Christoffel, T., & Gallagher, S. S. (2006). *Injury prevention and public health: Practical knowledge, skills, and strategies* (2nd ed.). Sudbury, MA: Jones and Bartlett.

Cross, R. (1988). Application of children's concepts of speed at the kerbside: Accident vulnerability and implications for the teaching of science to young children. In T. Rothengatter & R. de Bruin (Eds.), *International conference on road safety, Aug 1987, Groningen, Netherlands* (pp. 473–481). Assen: Van Gorcum & Co.

Hoffmann, E. R., Payne, A., & Prescott, S. (1980). Children's estimates of vehicle approach times. *Human Factors, 22*(2), 235–240.

Hoffrage, U., Weber, A., Hertwig, R., & Chase, V. M. (2003). How to keep children safe in traffic: Find the daredevils early. *Journal of Experimental Psychology: Applied, 9*(1), 249–260.

Hunt, C. (1998). *Active/safe routes to school.* Ottawa, ON: Canadian Institute of Child Health.

Jones, M. B., & Offord, D. R. (1991). *After the demonstration project.* Paper presented at the 1991 annual meeting of the Advancement of Science, Washington, DC.

Lerner, R. M. (2002). *Concepts and theories of human development* (3rd ed.). Mahwah, NJ: L. Erlbaum Associates.

Macarthur, C., Parkin, P. C., Sidky, M., & Wallace, W. (1998). Evaluation of a bicycle skills training program for young children: A randomized controlled trial. *Injury Prevention, 4*(2), 116–121.

Mathieson, R. (2007). *Personal factors in simulated bicycle accidents.* Unpublished doctoral dissertation, University of Toronto, Toronto, ON.

O'Brien, C. (2004). *Child-friendly transport planning.* Mississauga, ON: The Centre for Sustainable Transportation.

Piaget, J. (1970). *The child's conception of movement and speed.* New York, NY: Basic Books.

Piaget, J., & Inhelder, B. (1969). *The psychology of the child.* New York, NY: Basic Books.

Portland Office of Transportation. (2007). *Improving bicycle safety in Portland.* Portland, OR: Author.

Rivara, F. P., & Aitken, M. (1998). Prevention of injuries to children and adolescents. *Advances in Pediatrics, 45,* 37–72.

Rivara, F. P., Thompson, D. C., Patterson, M. Q., & Thompson, R. S. (1998). Prevention of bicycle related injuries: Helmets, legislation, and education. *Annual Review of Public Health, 19,* 293–318.

Rivera, F. P., & Metrik, B. S. (1998). *Training programs for bicycle safety.* Seattle, WA: Harborview Injury Prevention Research Center.

Robertson, L. S. (1998). *Injury epidemiology: Research and control strategies* (2nd ed.). New York, NY: Oxford University Press.

Ross, W. (2008, July 28). Pedal vs. metal. *Newsweek.*

Savelsbergh, G. J. P., & Van der Kamp, J. (2000). Information in learning to co-ordinate and control movements: Is there a need for specificity of practice? *International Journal of Sport Psychology, 31*(4), 467–484.

Siegler, R. S., & Richards, D. D. (1979). Development of time, speed, and distance concepts. *Developmental Psychology, 15*(3), 288–298.

Sleet, D. A. (1994). Injury prevention. In P. Cortese & K. Middleton (Eds.), *The comprehensive school health challenge: Promoting health through education* (pp. 443–489). Santa Cruz, CA: ETR Associates.

Statistics Canada. (2005). *Canadian community health survey: Obesity among children and adults*. Retrieved June 5, 2008, from http://www.statcan.ca/Daily/English/050706/d050706a.htm

The Street Trust. (2017). *Bicycle safety*. Retrieved September 29, 2017, from https://www.thestreettrust.org/bicycle-safety/.

Towner, E., & Dowswell, T. (2002). Community-based childhood injury prevention interventions: What works? *Health Promotion International, 17*(3), 273–284.

United States Department of Transportation. (2002). *Good practices guide for bicycle safety education*. Washington, DC: Author.

The National Program for Playground Safety

Daniella Semotok

The commitment of the National Program for Playground Safety is to provide parents/caregivers, teachers, and recreation/park coordinators the steps and resources to ensure that playgrounds are developed to be safe and minimize the risk of injuries for children.

11.1 Background

The National Program for Playground Safety (NPPS) was formed in October 1995 to assist communities across the United States in examining the important issues regarding playground safety. The National Action Plan for the Prevention of Playground Injuries is a positive step toward helping to prevent many needless injuries that occur on playgrounds across the world; the purpose of the National Action Plan is to provide a blueprint of action steps to be taken to develop safe playgrounds (Thompson & Hudson, 2002). It is designed in a user-friendly fashion and is intended to be used by parents, teachers, recreation and park personnel, caregivers of children, and other concerned adults. NPPS served as a national resource for the latest educational and research information on playground safety (National Program for Playground Safety, 2005).

D. Semotok (✉)
Toronto District School Board, Oakville, ON, Canada
e-mail: daniella.semotok@tdsb.on.ca

11.1.1 History and Development

In 1995, the University of Northern Iowa established NPPS with funding from the Centers for Diseases Control and Prevention in Atlanta, Georgia (D. Thompson, personal communication, 2005). In the nine years of NPPS's existence, it has become the premier nonprofit organization in the United States to deal with playground safety (NPPS, 2005). In 1996, Dr. Donna Thompson, Dr. Susan Hudson, and Dr. Mick Mack of NPPS, with assistance from the Advisory Board, developed the National Action Plan for the Prevention of Playground Injuries. NPPS felt that the development of this blueprint would assist the public in creating safe playgrounds and prevent countless injuries from occurring (NPPS, 2004a).

11.1.2 Goals of the National Action Plan

The National Action Plan for the Prevention of Playground Injuries provides a unique proposal for tackling the complex issue of playground safety. The National Action Plan is based on four goals, which provide the foundation for playground safety. These goals are to:

- Provide proper Supervision on playgrounds.
- Design age-Appropriate playgrounds.

© Springer Nature Switzerland AG 2020
R. Volpe (ed.), *Casebook of Traumatic Injury Prevention*,
https://doi.org/10.1007/978-3-030-27419-1_11

- Provide proper Fall surfacing under and around the playground equipment.
- Properly maintain Equipment and surfacing.

Although the goals are presented separately, they are intended to interact with one another toward creating a SAFE play space. Each section features one major goal and outlines actions to be taken to achieve that goal. This is a dynamic model, and action in one area affects the other areas.

11.1.2.1 Goal: Provide Proper Supervision On Playgrounds

- Action 1: Appraise current supervision plans.
- Action 2: Specify the supervision methods to be used.
- Action 3: Enhance supervision practices.

According to NPPS, more than 40% of playground injuries are a result of inadequate supervision (Thompson & Hudson, 2002). Both adults and children play an important role in creating a supervised playground. Adults need to be responsible for surveying the playground environment for potential hazards and should be on alert for dangerous behavior. Also, children need the guidance of adults to help them make appropriate choices about safe play equipment, behavior, and activity. NPPS indicates that an important focus on safe playground practices should be emphasized at the beginning of the school year. As indicated by Thompson and Hudson (2002), local agencies reduce injuries by providing "safe playgrounds days" programs at school playgrounds during the first few weeks of a new school year or at public playgrounds during the beginning of summer when most injuries occur.

11.1.2.2 Goal: Design Age-Appropriate Playgrounds

- Action 1: Assess the age-appropriate design of playgrounds.
- Action 2: Choose age-appropriate equipment.
- Action 3: Advocate that all playgrounds being designed are age appropriate.

Designing an age-appropriate play environment means that play equipment is suitable for the children's size, strength, and decision-making abilities (Thompson & Hudson, 2002). Developing children have these needs: physical (i.e., strength, grip, height, and weight), emotional (i.e., risk taking and exploration), social (i.e., cooperation, sharing, and accepting), intellectual (i.e., decision making, inquisitiveness, and creativity) and accessibility (i.e., mobility) (Thompson & Hudson, 2002).

NPPS recommends that equipment for preschool children be separate from equipment for school-aged children (NPPS, 2004b; Thompson & Hudson, 2002). When there are not separate areas for young children, they are able to access equipment that is not developmentally appropriate for them, and thus the risk of injury increases. When designing play environments, it is important to keep in mind that playgrounds should provide challenging opportunities for children, but there must be consideration for whether or not the equipment is developmentally appropriate for the children using the play area.

11.1.2.3 Goal: Provide Proper Fall Surfacing Under and Around Playground Equipment

- Action 1: Evaluate current surfacing situations.
- Action 2: Select proper surfacing under and around equipment.
- Action 3: Improve surfacing for the future.

Falls to the surfaces of playgrounds are a major contributor to playground injuries (Thompson & Hudson, 2002, 2004). According to NPPS, "the lack of proper surfacing under and around playground equipment is cited as a contributing factor in over 70% of the reported incidents by the United States Consumer Product Safety Commission" (Thompson & Hudson, 2002). Although falls on playgrounds cannot be entirely prevented, good surfacing can assist in preventing the severity of an injury. Research indicates that there are poor surfaces under and around playground equipment. These include asphalt, concrete, dirt, and grass (Thompson & Hudson, 2002, 2004). Playgrounds with these surfaces need to be replaced by impact-attenuating surfacing and must be considered in terms of environmental conditions, management requirements, characteristics of the users, maintenance requirements, and characteristics of the play equipment (Thompson & Hudson, 2002).

11.1.2.4 Goal: Properly Maintain Equipment and Surfacing on Playgrounds

- Action 1: Review maintenance policies and procedures.
- Action 2: Improve maintenance practices.

The proper maintenance of playground equipment can assist in protecting children from injuries. According to NPPS, "it is estimated that poor maintenance is a contributing factor in at least 30% of playground injuries" (Thompson & Hudson, 2002). It is essential to establish regular preventative care and maintenance of all equipment and surfaces. Playground equipment must be checked for rust, splinters, protruding bolts, missing or broken parts, and gaps (which could entrap the head of a child). Older equipment made from wood and metal (as opposed to plastic) appear to have the most maintenance problems. Once a playground is built, there needs to be proper maintenance of the playground environment, which includes scheduled programs of inspection and maintenance of equipment and surfaces. It is recommended that this be done by a trained inspector with the necessary resources (Thompson & Hudson, 2002).

11.2 Resources

11.2.1 Collaborators

The National Action Plan for the Prevention of Playground Injuries was co-authored by members of the faculty of the School of Health, Physical Education, and Leisure Services at the University of Northern Iowa, Cedar Falls, Iowa. The key collaborators of the National Action Plan were Donna Thompson, Ph.D., Director; Susan Hudson, Ph.D., Education Director; and Mick Mack, Ph.D., Project Coordinator. The key col-

laborators at NPPS are Donna Thompson, Ph.D., Executive Director; Susan Hudson, Ph.D., Education Director; and Heather Olsen, M.A. Project Associate (D. Thompson, personal communication, 2005).

11.2.2 Stakeholders

There are a number of stakeholders involved with NPPS. The stakeholders include child care personnel, elementary school personnel, park personnel, board members, parents, grandparents, children aged 2–12, and legislators interested in playground safety. The associated stakeholders presently perceive the program with high regard and value the success of NPPS (D. Thompson, personal communication, 2005).

11.2.3 Resources to Implement Prevention Strategies

At the time of the initial development of NPPS, The Centers for Disease Control and Prevention was involved and provided funding. Others who have supported NPPS include Senator Tom Harkin, Senator Chuck Grassley, and Congressman Jim Nussle (D. Thompson, personal communication, 2005). Also, a great amount of support was provided by the University of Northern Iowa (D. Thompson, personal communication, 2005).

Continuing support has been provided by The Centers for Disease Control and Prevention between the years of 1998 and 2001. Another cycle of support from CDC was from 2001 to 2004. In May 2004, NPPS was notified that the funding from CDC would be ending in September 2004 due to other priorities of CDC (NPPS, 2004b). CDC agreed to provide funding for 2005–2006.

In terms of advocacy, NPPS has been established to bring about attention to the need for playground safety through the United States. In order to gather support across the United States, NPPS staff contacted governors in each state to sign a proclamation, resulting in an average of 40 states per year participating in the program (NPPS, 2004b).

11.2.4 Support from NPPS Products and Services

Major support for NPPS comes from the sales of their products and services (D. Thompson, personal communication, 2005). The products that NPPS provides are age-appropriate playground signs, lapel pins, apparel such as a slogan hat and slogan T-shirt, magnets, safety packs, videos, CD-ROMS, Safe Playground Supervision kits, brochures, and books and monographs (NPPS, 2005).

There are also a number of services that NPPS offers. Safety School is a service that NPPS provides where participants review playground safety issues, learn to plan and design areas for safe play, and discover ways to affect change in their communities (NPPS, 2005). NPPS also provides a supervision training workshop where participants learn the essential aspects of playground supervision. The workshops are conducted by a certified instructor, and participants receive a workbook of playground supervision information (NPPS, 2005). In addition, NPPS offers consultations regarding playground design and development (NPPS, 2005). The sales from videos and proceeds from workshops have provided a major source of support for NPPS, and these resources have assisted in their study of the safety of America's playgrounds (NPPS, 2004b).

11.3 Implementation

11.3.1 Actors in the Decision Making and Planning

The current actors involved in the decision making and planning include Dr. Thompson, Executive Director; Dr. Hudson, Education Director; and Ms. Hudson, Operations Director. In addition, a board of directors is also consulted from time to time, and some individuals related to various projects are also consulted (D. Thompson, personal communication, 2005).

11.3.2 Effective Practices

Focus on local, state, and national levels—the four goals outlined in the S.A.F.E. Model from the National Action Plan are aimed at the three areas of government. NPPS emphasizes that successful playground safety programs require a partnership between these three levels (Thompson & Hudson, 2002). This plan is developed on the understanding that different groups of individuals participate in all three levels. Table 11.1 outlines how the National Action Plan targets the different areas of government.

Table 11.1 National action plan at three levels of government

Local level	State level	National level
At the local level, the National Action Plan refers to community agencies and organizations. These include schools, park and recreation departments, child care centers, parent and teacher associations, and community groups such as Kiwanis, Lions Clubs and other nonprofit organizations	At the state level, the plan asks professional organizations to assist in providing information and education about playground safety. These state organizations may be associated with preschool children, schools, parks and recreation departments, teacher education, medical professionals, etc. Also, state governmental departments in education, natural resources and parks, health, and human services are asked to become involved in playground safety	At the national level, the plan outlines actions to be taken by professional organizations such as the American Alliance of Health, Physical Education, Recreation and Dance (AAHPERD); Association for Childhood Education International (ACEI); National Association for Education of Young Children (NAEYC); National Recreation and Park Association (NRPA); National Safety Council (NSC); National Safe Kids Campaign (NSKC); and others to ensure that the nations' playgrounds are safe

Note: The table was created using information from the National Program for Playground Safety website, by the National Program for Playground Safety (2005)

11.3.3 Ongoing Evaluation of Prevention Strategy

NPPS practices both pre- and postevaluations on a regular basis. For example, in 2000, NPPS issued its first national report card on the safety of America's playgrounds. The report card was based on data collected from a comprehensive survey of child care facilities, schools, and park playgrounds conducted between 1999 and 2000 (Thompson & Hudson, 2004). The results of this data indicated the conditions of the nation's playgrounds during this time period and the areas for improvement. Since this time, another evaluation was conducted in 2003, and the results of this survey indicate an improvement of America's playgrounds (NPPS, 2004b; Thompson & Hudson, 2004). However, since playground safety is an ongoing effort, NPPS hopes to see an even greater improvement in future years (Thompson & Hudson, 2004).

11.3.4 Increased Awareness

The increase in awareness of playground safety by NPPS has been tremendous. The importance of playground safety has not only expanded within the United States, but it has also extended to other areas within the world. In June 1999, NPPS was invited by the U.S. Air Force to conduct a playground safety school in Hawaii for those who are involved in child care and school-age playgrounds. The results from this showed that there needed to be serious alterations to the existing playgrounds, and NPPS worked with the community to improve the conditions (NPPS, 2004b). As a result of the work with the Air Force in Hawaii, NPPS provided a Safety School at Wright-Patterson Air Force Based in Ohio and another at Ramstein Air Force Base in Germany (NPPS, 2004b).

11.3.5 Additional Program Services

NPPS serves both playground professionals and the public by allowing them to have direct access to an ongoing assortment of program services. Several of these services include (NPPS, 2005)

- An interlibrary loan service of publications and documents from the University of Northern Iowa's Rod Library.
- A national information hotline (800-554-PLAY) about playground injury prevention.
- Pamphlets, brochures, and other resource materials for use by service clubs, organizations, and agencies.
- In-depth educational opportunities through the National Playground Safety School and workshops.
- A network of professionals to contact to provide specific information to local communities around the country.

11.4 Outcome

11.4.1 Evaluation

America's playground safety report card: Year 2000—in 1998, NPPS conducted its first of two nationwide evaluations of child care facilities, parks, and school playgrounds (Thompson & Hudson, 2004). The purpose of the evaluation was to determine the safety of America's playgrounds and to outline possible areas of improvement. NPPS has been the only organization to conduct a scientific study of children's centers, schools, and parks in the United States (NPPS, 2004b). The survey has been based on the S.A.F.E. Model (Supervision, Age-Appropriate Design, Fall Surfacing, and Equipment Maintenance), as outlined in the National Action Plan for the Prevention of Playground Injuries (NPPS, 2004a; Thompson & Hudson, 2004). During the survey in 1998, there were 3052 child care, park, and school playground sites that were visited for evaluation. These playgrounds were located in all 50 states across the United States.

In the year 2000, the results from this survey were released in the form of a report card. At this time, the nation received a grade of C (Thompson & Hudson, 2004). Given that all 50 states were surveyed, NPPS also developed regional and state differences.

The 2000 report outlined a number of issues regarding playground safety in America (Thompson & Hudson, 2004):

- Ninety percent of playgrounds did not have rules or information posted concerning the importance of playground supervision.
- Fifty-nine percent of playgrounds did not have separate equipment for children aged 2–5 and 5–12.
- Fifty-three percent of playgrounds did not have adequate loose-fill surfacing materials at a sufficient depth needed to cushion falls.
- Thirty-five percent of playgrounds did not have surfacing materials in the proper stationary equipment use zones.
- Twenty-five percent of playgrounds had equipment pieces with gaps that pose entanglement problems.
- Twenty-two percent of playgrounds had inadequate fall surfacing materials under and around the equipment.
- Twenty-one percent of playground equipment had potential head entrapments.

The results from this study drew immediate attention from news outlets such as NBC, CBS, FOX, and CNN (NPPS, 2004b). NPPS was pleased with the increase in awareness regarding playground safety that their report generated but also realized that playground safety is a definite "work in progress" (NPPS, 2004b).

America's playground safety report card: Year 2004—a second evaluation was conducted in the spring of 2003, and NPPS replicated its first survey by revisiting the same playground sites (due to construction repairs, only 2993 of the original 3052 sites were revisited). Staff and consultants of NPPS dedicated themselves to flying over 35,000 miles and spent over 3600 h visiting playground sites (NPPS, 2004b).

When visiting playgrounds for this study, NPPS found that there had been an increase in new playground structures since the previous study in 1998. The installation of new playground equipment indicates that there are improvements

toward safety because playground manufacturers must adopt the Consumer Product Safety Commission's guideline and use the American Society for Testing Materials standards when developing equipment. This specifies that new playground installations are meeting the minimum safety standards (Thompson & Hudson, 2004). However, this does not necessarily mean that the playgrounds meet the S.A.F.E. Model.

11.4.2 Summary of S.A.F.E. from 2004 Report Card

Supervision—this is one area where NPPS found a decrease from the 2000 report (Thompson & Hudson, 2004). The reason for the decrease is that with the installation of new play structures, there seems to be an increase in crawl spaces and areas on the equipment where children cannot be easily viewed (Thompson & Hudson, 2004). NPPS recommends that when playground manufacturers are designing equipment, they need to keep in mind that children must be observed from all areas of the equipment. The second recommendation of NPPS is that playground owners and operators should provide signage reminding the public of the importance of adult supervision (NPPS, 2004b; Thompson & Hudson, 2004).

Age-appropriate design—NPPS indicates that the rise in composite structures since the 2000 report card has thus increased the likelihood of mixed-age usage of playground equipment (Thompson & Hudson, 2004). When there are mixed-age playground areas, there is an increased chance that younger children will access areas that are not safe for them to use. NPPS recommends that all new playground areas designed for ages 2–12 should have two distinct play areas: one for younger children of ages 2–5 and another section for older children of 5–12 years (Thompson & Hudson, 2004). Another recommendation of NPPS is that there should be signage for adults regarding the appropriateness of equipment (Thompson & Hudson, 2004).

Falls to surface—NPPS indicates that proper surfacing under and around playground equipment is determined by four factors: (1) suitable surfacing materials, (2) height of the equipment, (3) depth of loose fill surface materials, and (4) placement of suitable materials at the adequate depth of playground use zones (Thompson & Hudson, 2004). In the 2004 evaluation, only 18% of playgrounds had unsuitable surfacing materials. This indicates that there has been an increase in awareness of the importance of suitable surfacing material (Thompson & Hudson, 2004). Another notable improvement is that the height of playground equipment has remained under eight feet tall in accordance to the CPSC guidelines (Thompson & Hudson, 2004). However, one clear area of concern is in relation to the surfacing material as cushioning agent. According to NPPS, "In order to be effective, the depth of loose fill materials must be sufficient to absorb a fall proportionate with the height of the equipment" (Thompson & Hudson, 2004). Less than 20% of the playgrounds surveyed had the sufficient depth of loose fill materials (Thompson & Hudson, 2004). NPPS did note progress with surfacing materials in the proper use zone; 71% of playgrounds had proper use zones for playground equipment (Thompson & Hudson, 2004).

NPPS has made several recommendations based on the surfacing portion of the report card. First, owners and operators must provide suitable surfacing materials under and around all playground equipment. In addition, owners and operators must increase their efforts to maintain loose-fill surfacing materials in order to ensure that it is at the appropriate depth. The last recommendation is that children should not be allowed to play in areas where the depth of the surfacing is less than 9 in. (Thompson & Hudson, 2004). It is clear that these recommendations are geared toward the owners and operators of the play equipment. However, parents and other concerned adults can be aware of these recommendations and can make inquiries at their local playgrounds.

Equipment and surfacing maintenance— NPPS has found that the maintenance of playground equipment made of metal or wood is difficult in comparison to equipment made of plastic (NPPS, 2004b). There has been an increase in equipment made of plastic in cases where playground sites are renovated. NPPS found that head entrapments continue to be a concern for 21% of the playgrounds visited (NPPS, 2004b). NPPS made several recommendations in relation to equipment and surface maintenance. The first is that there should be consideration to replace all equipment installed prior to 1991. Another suggestion by NPPS is that playground owners and operators should follow a schedule for routine maintenance, repair, and replacement of equipment. In addition, owners and operators should ensure that playground equipment is inspected to meet CPSC guidelines before allowing children to use the area (NPPS, 2004b).

11.4.3   Results from 2004 Report Card

The overall findings from the study indicated that there has been an increase in playground safety across the country since the first study conducted in 1998 (NPPS, 2004b). The United States received an overall grade of C+ for the 2004 report card, and this is an improvement from the grade of C received from the 2000 report. According to NPPS, "over half the states in the study improved their safety scores significantly" (NPPS, 2004b). While NPPS acknowledges that the movement toward a grade of C to C+ does not sound like much, it is a step in the right direction. In terms of regional differences in the United States, three of the regions have increased their scores (Midwest, Northeast, and Southeast) since the 2000 report card. One region (Southwest) remained the same from the 2000 report, and one region (Northwest) decreased (Thompson & Hudson, 2004). For a more specific look at the improvements made from the 2000 report, Florida's score went from a D− in 2000 to a B+ in 2004 and Michigan increased its score from D+ to B (NPPS, 2004b; Thompson & Hudson, 2004). Both of these states, as well as many others, have been working with NPPS to improve the safety of the playgrounds in their areas.

11.4.4 Long-Term Outcomes of NPPS

NPPS has undertaken to prevent playground injuries by focusing on three areas: education, research, and advocacy. Since the origination of the program in 1995, NPPS has had great success in these three areas. The following is a summary of accomplishments from October 1995 to September 2004: (NPPS, 2004a).

11.4.4.1 Education
- Distributed over 100,000 National Action Plans for the Prevention of Playground Injuries.
- Created 25 informational brochures and pamphlets.
- Developed a clearinghouse containing over 5000 citations (1984–present).
- Conducted 26 sessions of the National Playground Safety Schools, including schools held in Germany, Hawaii, Ohio, and Kentucky.
- Published.
  - Nineteen books/monographs
  - Twenty-one book chapters
  - One hundred and three professional articles
  - Eighteen technical reports
- Produced.
  - Thirteen public service announcements
  - Eight videos
  - Two CD-ROMs
- Provided 265 presentations across the country at professional conferences and/or before professional groups.
- Developed a Playground Supervision Kit.
- Created the Kidchecker program and assessment tool.

11.4.4.2 Research
- Received funding for 23 grants/contracts for research and assessment projects.
- Conducted four studies on surfacing:
  - Loose-Fill surfacing (led to changes in the ASTM F-1292 protocol).
  - Impact Attenuation of common surfaces found in the inside of play environment.
  - Iowa SAFE Surfacing Initiative (2003–2004).

- Iowa SAFE Surfacing Initiative (2004–2005).
- Conducted two comprehensive studies regarding the risk factors found on playgrounds:
  - First Study (1998–2000).
  - Second Study (2003–2004).
- Assessed 64 child-care and school-age sites for the U.S. Air Force.
- Developed three theoretical models.
  - S.A.F.E. Model.
  - Risk/Challenge Model.
  - S.A.F.E. Surfacing Design Model.
- Participated with the University of Northern Colorado in a study of playground safety on Indian school sites in Wyoming.
- Assessed Airport Playgrounds for the Iowa Air Space Consortium.
- Conducted a study concerning supervision practices found in elementary schools in Iowa.
- Conducts a National Playground Study, which involves visiting randomly selected playgrounds around the country to look at a variety of playground surfaces and collect data on the types of playground equipment, as well as observes the conditions of the surface materials. The study will utilize equipment called the Triax Tripod System, which helps give information on the condition of the playground surface. It calculates speed, time, and impact (NPPS, 2017).

11.4.4.3 Advocacy
- Received over 1.5 website visits, fielded over 30,000 phone calls on 800 hotline.
- Generated over 30 million dollars of P.R. value.
- Made seven major television appearances on ABC, CBS, CNN, FOX, and NBC.
- Created National Playground Safety Week.
- Involved in the following American Society for Testing and Materials standard committees:
  - Development of standards for children under the age of two.
  - Committee on public use playground equipment.
  - Committee on surfacing under and around playground equipment.

- Provided information for the revision of CPSC Handbook for Public Use Playgrounds, 1997.
- Involved in the revision of the CPSC Handbook for Public Playgrounds, 2005.

11.4.5 Recommendations

Suggestions for improving the safety of playgrounds—NPPS recommends that all public child care facilities, school, and park playgrounds adopt the Consumer Product Safety Commission Public Use guidelines when developing children's playgrounds (Thompson & Hudson, 2004). The results from the latest survey of the nation's playgrounds indicate that there are areas for improvement within the S.A.F.E. Model:

11.4.5.1 Supervision
1. Children need to be supervised while on playground equipment.
2. Adequate sight lines need to be present to allow the observation of children on equipment, especially on tube slides and crawl spaces.

11.4.5.2 Age-Appropriate Design
1. Playgrounds should be designed so that there is a distinct separation between areas for children aged 2–5 and 5–12.
2. Signage/labels should be present to direct children and adults to equipment that is appropriate for developmental levels of the children.

11.4.5.3 Fall Surfacing
1. Appropriate surface materials are used (as outlined in the CPSC handbook) under and around the playground equipment.
2. Proper depth of appropriate loose-fill materials is in place.

11.4.5.4 Equipment Maintenance
1. Playground equipment is routinely inspected and repaired.
2. All equipment is free from gaps or spaces for head entrapments.

11.5 Conclusion

The National Program for Playground Safety is an organization dedicated to preventing injuries among children; this is clearly displayed through their education, research, and advocacy. The National Action Plan for the Prevention of Playground Injuries has been shown to meet exemplary practice criteria, providing effective opportunities for avoiding unnecessary that which occur every day on playgrounds across the United States, in Canada, and worldwide. The application of exemplary practice criteria to this multilevel initiative is tabled at the end of this chapter.

Adaptive change in the incidence of playground injury is seen as more than a function of the independent properties of the person and the environment. According to NPPS, "There are still public playgrounds around the country that are putting children at significant risk for injury through improper supervision, inappropriate design, lack of adequate surfacing, and non-existent maintenance" (Thompson & Hudson, 2004). NPPS views playground safety as a "work in progress," so there are still many actions to be taken to improve the conditions of children's playgrounds. As an exemplary practice, NPPS is necessarily an opportunity rather than a template, one that encourages adaptation and improvement. NPPS is optimistic that in the years ahead, there will be even greater improvements in the conditions of playgrounds.

11.5.1 Life Space Model: Playgrounds

Among children and youth, unintentional falls often result in serious injury and are actually the number one cause of hospitalization. Falls at home decline as children get older, while falls occurring in educational, sports, and recreational environments increase. Most commonly, almost half of children younger than five years treated for playground injuries at the emergency room have injuries to the head or face. Older children's injuries typically result in fractures.

Boys more often experience falls that lead to injury than girls, possibly due to the difference in risk-taking behavior. In childcare settings, younger children are at higher risk for injury than older children, especially boys. Previous exposure to injury also plays a part in parents' perception of risk-taking behavior, which is thought to be a contributor to subsequent injury.

Injury on the playground is complex since safety is influenced by many factors, such as the playground environment, supervision, and behavior of the child. Most injuries occur on school and public playgrounds. Falls represent the majority of playground injures and typically occur during summer months on school days. More childhood deaths occur on home playgrounds. Swings are responsible for the majority of these injures.

One important way to secure a safe home playground is to ensure that there are shock-absorbing surfaces under and around play areas. The height of playground equipment and the severity of injury are also positively related. Proper maintenance and inspection of equipment is therefore an important aspect of playground safety. Injury risk increases when children use equipment that is not appropriate for their strength and size. Inadequate visual and auditory supervision increases this risk, as does a lack of parental physical proximity. Unfortunately, compliance to standards that ensure safe design and installation is currently only voluntary, except in areas mandated by legislation.

Childhood injury on the playground can be prevented by addressing the elements that contribute to playground safety. The National Program for Playground Injuries targets surface, height, maintenance, supervision, and age-appropriate concerns regarding child safety in the playground.

NPPS was formed in 1995 to assist U.S. communities in making playgrounds safer for chil-dren. With the assistance of its advisory board, the National Action Plan for the Prevention of Playground Injuries was born. Through education, research, and advocacy, the program provides a blueprint on the steps needed to be taken to develop safer playgrounds. The plan is intended to be used by parents, teachers, recreation and park personnel, child caregivers, and other concerned adults.

The overall goals of the program are intended for the creation of a SAFE play space. Supervision, Age-appropriate playgrounds, Fall surfacing, and Equipment maintenance form a dynamic model and represent the main features to be addressed by the program.

Funding for the program came from the Centers for Disease Control and Prevention; services, such as supervision training workshops and products such as lapel pins, are a source of support as well. NPPS is currently seeking larger financial support to extend the program.

The goals of the SAFE model from the National Plan of action are aimed at local, state, and national levels of government. Currently, the program is advocated by governors across the United States.

NPPS continues to identify the transformative processes and conditions that contribute to injury; elements within relevant systems entailed in playground safety inevitably interact and change over time (see Life Space Table). It has been successful in raising awareness and encouraging safe practice within the complex adaptive system of the playground in the United States and internationally. With this initial success, greater improvements in the prevention of childhood playground injury are anticipated in the future.

Acknowledgments The author would like to express sincere appreciation to the key informant for this case study: Dr. Donna Thompson of the National Program for Playground Safety, School of Health, Physical Education and Leisure Services, at the University of Northern Iowa in Cedar Falls, IA, USA—whose consultation made this project possible.

BRIO Model: National Program for Playground Safety

Group Served: Children ages 2–12 years.

Goal: Improve playground safety for children and prevent injuries.

Background	Resources	Implementation	Outcome
Most childhood injuries occur on the playground Falls represent the majority of playground injuries and are a number one cause of hospitalization among children Injury on the playground is a complex problem involving consideration of the environment, supervision, and child behavior Areas of improvement involve attending to concerns regarding Supervision, Appropriately aged playgrounds, Fall surfacing, and Equipment maintenance	Program designed to assist communities in making playgrounds safer for children Funded by Centers for Disease Control and Prevention	Goals of the program are aimed at local, state, and national levels of the government The program is advocated by governors across the US Program practices are evaluated on pre- and postlevels. Areas of improvement are suggested, and success is surveyed	Nation Plan for Playground Safety has increased national awareness and encouraged safe play Increases in playground safety have been observed since initiative inception

Life Space Model: National Program for Playground Safety

Sociocultural: civilization/ community	Interpersonal: Primary and secondary relationships	Physical environments: where we live	Internal states: biochemical/ genetic and means of coping
Younger children are at higher risk for fall-related injuries than older children Falls at home decline as children get older, but falls incurred through recreational activities increase Boys experience falls more often than girls There is a need for a model that can summarize and direct action regarding the complex issues contributing to playground injury	SAFE model summarizes safety issues that need to be addressed by governments, parents, city staff, children, teachers, and the community Education and advocacy efforts dictate that networking prevents playground injuries	Program targets playground injury; most childhood injuries occur on the playground Proper maintenance, inspection, height of equipment, parental or caregiver supervision, lack of compliance to safety standards are examined	Disseminating materials and advocating the program through various venues ensures that others will feel empowered to increase safe play Empirically assessed materials promote community knowledge and competence in effecting change

References

National Program for Playground Safety. (2004a). *National action plan for the prevention of playground injuries*. Retrieved from http://www.uni.edu/playground/plan.html.

National Program for Playground Safety. (2004b). *Nine years of excellence 1995–2004*. Cedar Falls, IA: Author.

National program for Playground Safety. (2005). *National program for playground safety*. Retrieved from http://www.uni.edu/playground/home.htm.

National Program for Playground Safety. (2017) *National playground study*. Retrieved from http://playground-safety.org/node/696.

Thompson, D., & Hudson, S. (2002). *National action plan for the prevention of playground injuries* (3rd ed.). Cedar Falls, IA: National Program for Playground Safety.

Thompson, D., & Hudson, S. (2004). *How safe are America's playgrounds? A national profile of child-care, school, and park playgrounds*. Cedar Falls, IA: National Program for Playground Safety.

Part II

Fall-Related Traumatic Injury Prevention: Falls Across the Life-Span

Overview of Fall-Related Traumatic Injury Prevention: Falls Across the Lifespan

Rachel Monahan

Falls pose a significant, and yet preventable, threat to the lives and well-being of individuals worldwide (see Fig. 12.1 for an illustration of fall-related fatality rates mapped geographically across the United States) across their lifespan. A fall can have a "devastating physical and psychological effect on a person resulting in disability, chronic pain, loss of independence, reduced quality of life, and even death" (Volpe, 2014, p. 26). Additionally, the financial, time, and psychological burden of a fall-related injury often extends beyond the individual to include their family members, friends, and coworkers (Volpe, 2014).

Definition—the Centers for Disease Control and Prevention (CDC, 2017a) note that a fall-related injury is one that is "received when a person descends abruptly due to the force of gravity and strikes a surface at the same or lower level" (¶ 8). Within injury databases, fall injuries "exclude those due to assault and intentional self-harm," as well as "falls from animals, burning buildings and transport vehicles, and falls into fire, water, and machinery" (WHO, n.d., ¶ 1). Therefore, for the purpose of this section, the use of the term fall-related injury may be understood as borrowing from this definition and refers only to unintentional injury.

Moreover, since an injury is a result of a complex system of interrelated factors, clarification about what constitutes a fall injury is necessary. According to the Centers for Disease Control and Prevention (CDC, 2017a), "the cause, or mechanism, of injury is the way in which the person sustained the injury; how the person was injured; or the process by which the injury occurred" (¶ 3). Also, the CDC (2017a) discerns between direct and underlying causes of injury:

> The underlying cause is what starts the chain of events that leads to an injury. The direct cause is what produces the actual physical harm. The underlying and direct causes can be the same or different. For example, if a person cuts his or her finger with a knife, the cut is both the underlying and direct cause. However, if a child falls and hits his head on a coffee table, the fall is the underlying cause (the action that starts the injury event), and the contact with the table is the direct cause (the action that causes the actual physical harm). (¶ 3)

Further, the CDC (2017a, ¶ 4) explains that underlying causes are significant to injury prevention because "without the underlying cause, there would be no direct cause" (CDC, 2017a, ¶ 4). While the cause of the injury is often quite complex due to the compounding nature of risk, it is clear that if we can prevent the fall—the underlying cause—then we prevent the injury. However, if we were to instead just move the coffee table (the direct cause in our sample scenario above) the child will still hit something else (likely the ground) which could easily

R. Monahan (✉)
Applied Psychology and Human Development, Ontario Institute for Studies in Education, University of Toronto, Toronto, ON, Canada
e-mail: rachel.monahan@mail.utoronto.ca

© Springer Nature Switzerland AG 2020
R. Volpe (ed.), *Casebook of Traumatic Injury Prevention*,
https://doi.org/10.1007/978-3-030-27419-1_12

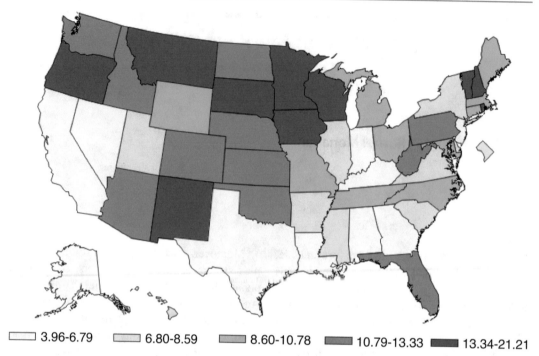

Fig. 12.1 2008–2014 Unintentional, fall-related death rates (per 100,000 population) by state. The overall (i.e., the entire country as a whole) annualized rate of unintentional deaths due to a fall (per 100,000) between 2008 and 2014 was 8.86. (From "Fatal Injury Mapping," by the Centers for Disease Control and Prevention, 2015)

Legend: 3.96-6.79 | 6.80-8.59 | 8.60-10.78 | 10.79-13.33 | 13.34-21.21

become the new direct cause of a similar injury. As such, the fall offers a more effective place to focus prevention efforts.

Incidence—falls account for half of all injury-related hospitalizations and 3.6 times the hospitalizations of any other injury (CDC, 2017e). Falls commonly result in fractures, broken bones, sprains, strains, head injuries, cuts, and abrasions, as well as fear, guilt, and depression (CDC, 2017b). They are the most common cause of traumatic brain injury (CDC, 2016b) and, according to data from Canada, are the leading cause of permanent and temporary disability (Volpe, 2014). In the year of 2015 alone, 33,381 Americans died; 1,203,694 Americans were hospitalized; and 9,368,778 Americans visited an emergency department due to a fall (CDC, 2017c, d, e).

Fatal falls typically involve trauma to the head or multiple body parts (National Safety Council, 2015). Worldwide, falls remain the second leading cause of accidental injury deaths resulting in an estimated 646,000 fatal falls per year (WHO, 2018). In the United States, falls are the third leading cause of unintentional-injury-related mortality and the leading cause of nonfatal unintentional injury. See Table 12.1 for data from Canada that illustrate the frequency of falls according to type and severity. While injury statistics show overwhelming odds, falls and/or injuries resulting from falls are not inevitable. Many of these falls and related injuries/fatalities are both predictable and preventable.

There is no question that falls are the cause of significant fatal and nonfatal injury across the lifespan with a debilitating individual and societal impact. However, falls particularly impact young children and older adults (National Safety Council, 2015; Volpe, 2014). For Americans age 65 and older, falls are the leading cause of both unintentional-injury-related death and nonfatal injury (CDC, 2016a).

Moreover, falls cause some of the most expensive injuries resulting in significant economic impact on individuals (see Table 12.2), their communities, and private sector businesses (National

Table 12.1 Canadian incidence, type, and severity of falls in 2010

Types of falls	Severity				
				Disability	
	Deaths	Hospitalization	ER visits	Partial	Complete
Total falls	4071	128,389	1,036,079	23,236	1969
On the same level	327	37,660	330,199	7235	532
On stairs	393	12,404	130,747	2968	287
From furniture	280	7794	61,863	1107	93
From ladders and scaffolding	15	4189	64,597	1384	106

Note: The data in this table is from Canada in the year 2010. Created using data from *The Cost of Injury in Canada*, by Parachute (2015), Toronto, Canada: Author. Copyrighted by Parachute

Table 12.2 Cost and extent of unintentional falls injury in 2010

Severity	Total		Cost		
			Medical	Work lost	Combined
Death	26,009	Average	$23,925	$255,975	$279,900
		Total	$622 million	$6.6 billion	$7.3 billion
Hospitalization	992,452	Average	$38,925	$56,690	$95,615
		Total	$38.6 billion	$56.3 billion	$94.9 billion
ER[a] treatment and release	8,043,684	Average	$2552	$3764	$6316
		Total	$20.5 billion	$30.3 billion	$50.8 billion

Note: Adapted from the "Cost of Injury Report," by the Centers for Disease Control and Prevention, 2014
[a]ER stands for emergency room or emergency department

Safety Council, 2015; Volpe, 2014). In the United States, direct medical costs alone for Americans age 65 and older due to falls account for an estimated $31 billion dollars annually (CDC, 2017b), and the average cost of hospitalization to an individual age 65 or older is over $30,000 (CDC, 2016b). Additionally, falls are a leading cause of missed work days (National Safety Council, 2015). In 2011, falls accounted to about one quarter of the direct workers compensation cost burden—$13.5 billion (National Safety Council, 2015).

12.1 Lifespan Approach to Fall Prevention

Fall injuries are the result of interrelated factors that accumulate throughout the lifespan (Volpe, 2012). Some factors stay constant across the lifespan (e.g., physical and social environment), while others change with age (e.g., balance; Grey Bruce Health Unit, 2017). Figure 12.2 illustrates American fatality and hospitalization rates due to unintentional falls across the lifespan. Taken together, the developmental and transactional nature of fall injury signifies the necessity to consider prevention holistically from a developmental approach. "The life[span] approach views health as a product of risk factors, protective factors, and environmental agents that we encounter throughout our lives, and that have cumulative impacts on health outcomes" (Grey Bruce Health Unit, 2017, p. 10). This approach treats fall-related injury prevention as a lifelong effort, specifically aiming prevention in, across, and between developmental stages (Grey Bruce Health Unit, 2017). Additionally, higher quality prevention will "actively address broader social and ecological determinants of falls injuries" (Volpe, 2014, p. 52), such as health inequities or safety culture.

Many falls that occur in both public and private spaces can be prevented by making changes to those environments. Environmental changes are an important component of the multifactorial prevention programs presented in this section. This is an example of an area where policy changes (e.g., building codes) have the potential to significantly influence fall prevention (Grey

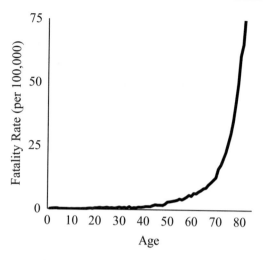
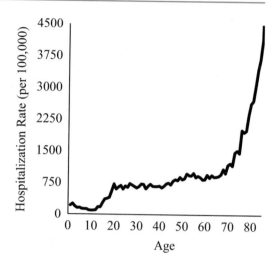

Fig. 12.2 These two graphs show the rate of unintentional injury due to falls resulting in fatalities (graph one) or hospitalization (graph 2) plotted across the lifespan. These rates represent data from the United States in the year 2015. The data represented in graph 1 is from "Fatal Injury Reports," by the Centers for Disease Control and Prevention (2017d). The data represented in graph 2 are from "Nonfatal Injury Reports," by the Centers for Disease Control and Prevention (2017e)

Bruce Health Unit, 2017). A successful implementation of the Stay On Your Feet fall prevention program (Chap. 15) in Burnaby Western Australia is an excellent example of how policy has been incorporated to further improve an exemplary prevention program. Overall, the success of the programs presented in this section are much in part due to the implementation of both behavioral and environmental prevention.

Likewise, to increase success, fall-related injury prevention programs should also consider the complex relationship between the social determinants of health and injury so that they might effectively meet the needs of the population. For example, consider that socioeconomic status may affect the ability to afford safe housing. Other examples of the influence that social factors have on fall injury risk include gender—i.e., adult women fall more often than men, young boys fall more often than young girls—and employment. Several of the cases (e.g., Kids Can't Fly and the Fall Safe program) in this section engage with social determinants of health.

Certain stages of life pose a specific risk to falls for reasons associated with age and development. This is evidenced graphically in Fig. 12.2. Ideally a combination of separate prevention programs that focus on falls across the lifespan and programs that focus on specific developmental stages would most effectively prevent overall unintentional fall injury and death. The prevention programs in this section focus mostly on specific developmental periods. As such, the case studies are ordered by the developmental period that they address. In the following paragraphs, the cases are introduced alongside a brief explanation of the pertinent fall-risk factors relevant to their associated developmental period.

12.2 Section Chapters

12.2.1 Early Childhood

Alongside rapid physical and cognitive development, young children under five are learning those gross motor skills that adults take for granted, including sitting, standing, crawling, walking, running, jumping, and climbing. As they attempt these things for the first time while gaining basic balance and stability, it is not surprising that children at this age fall down frequently. Most of these falls are an insignificant part of the learning process; nevertheless, traumatic injury can happen (see Table 12.3 for early childhood fall injury incidence). As such, fall prevention for children under the age of five must account for this learning curve.

Additionally, an understanding of risk factors must account for the complexities of the social determinants of health. For example, the severity of injury due to a fall during childhood has been shown to be related to the socioeconomic status of parents (Grey Bruce Public Health Unit, 2017). In addition, inadequate supervision is a commonly cited cause of childhood fall injury (WHO, 2018). However, the relationships between these factors and fall risk are complex. A prevention program that does not take this complexity into consideration chances missing the mark completely. To illustrate, the Gray Bruce Health Unit (2017, p. 14) provides the example of "a child [falling] down the stairs because his parent was not providing adequate supervision. Using [this example], the parent may not have the

Table 12.3 Incidence and severity of unintentional injury due to a fall in early childhood (ages 1–4)

Severity of injury	Amount	Rate per 100,000	Percent of young children's total injuries[a], %
Fatalities	30	0.19	2.4
Emergency department visits	770,250	4835.45	43.7
Hospitalization	10,940	68.68	37.5

Note: These results reflect data from the year 2015 in the United States. Created using data from "Fatal Injury Reports," by the Centers for Disease Control and Prevention (2017d); the "Non-Fatal Injury Reports," by the Centers for Disease Control and Prevention (2017e); the "Leading Causes of Fatal Injury Reports," by the Centers for Disease Control and Prevention (2017d); and the "Leading Causes of Non-Fatal Injury Reports," by the Centers for Disease Control and Prevention (2017e)

[a]This is the percent of the total overall unintentional injuries of the specified severity of injury for children aged 1–4 that was caused by an unintentional fall (i.e., 43.7% of the total number of emergency department visits, for an unintentional nonfatal injury, by children aged 1–4, were caused by an unintentional fall)

financial means to live in safer housing, or to purchase a proper safety gate for the stairs, or the social connectedness to have support for home improvements." The early childhood case study in this section, Kids Can't Fly, is a model prevention program that accounts for the social determinants of health by considering the complexity of the person–environment relationship in context.

Kids Can't Fly (Chap. 13) is a prevention program from Boston aimed at preventing the phenomena of very young children falling out of windows. Kids Can't Fly targeted the needs of the highest risk population—i.e., those who are of low socioeconomic status. In so doing, Kids Can't Fly addresses the complex relationship between adequate supervision and socioeconomic status by combining environmental interventions, a safety device for the window, with effective modes of disseminating both information and the safety device itself. Kids Can't Fly worked with community stakeholders and experts to choose, provide, and install a device in windows that would physically stop children from falling out. Also, Kids Can't Fly worked with local agencies to communicate to parents about the real prevalence of this problem. This prevention program achieved remarkable results.

A note on risk taking—risk is a primary developmental aspect of all child and youth fall risk. "Paradoxically, risk-avoidance can put children at greater risk long-term because they may miss out on important developmental benefits" (Grey Bruce Health Unit, 2017, p. 22). Through risky play, children develop the ability to manage risk and avoid injury by learning skills that sustain risk management. When participating in risk taking, children learn to recognize their own limits and recognize risk; they also gain resilience, persistence, and decision-making skills. Risky play has important developmental and learning benefits as well (Grey Bruce Health Unit, 2017). Nevertheless, any consideration of risk and its benefits must not outshadow the reality of the economic disparity prevalent in determining what "risk" is. This trend of seeking out risk in play does seem to be a markedly privileged one—when risk is a part of a person's daily lived experience, they are less likely to actively seek out more. Therefore, it is important that fall prevention programs balance risk appropriately, respecting the entire complexity of an individual's life.

12.2.2 Mid Adulthood

Fall injury prevention has often overlooked young and mid-life adults choosing to focus instead on the young and the elderly (Volpe, 2014). This is a result of the increased risk of fatality to these age groups; however, this is a grave oversight. In the U.S., for adults, falls are the leading cause of hospitalization and nonfatal injury (CDC, 2017d). They are also the third leading cause of accidental injury fatalities for this age group (CDC, 2017e). See Table 12.4 for fall injury incidence in mid-life.

Of further note, "those in the mid-life age range comprise a group whose fall injuries, though they are less likely to be fatal, have a considerable cost to the social and economic climate of the wider community" (Volpe, 2014,

Table 12.4 Rates of fatal and nonfatal unintentional injuries due to a fall in mid-life (ages 19–24)

Severity of injury	Amount	Rate per 100,000	Percent of mid-life adult's total injuries[a], %
Fatalities	4793	2.45	5.4
Emergency department visits	3,977,702	2031.57	22.5
Hospitalization	309,966	158.31	25.8

Note: These results reflect data from the year 2015 in the United States. Created using data from "Fatal Injury Reports," by the Centers for Disease Control and Prevention (2017d); the "Non-Fatal Injury Reports," by the Centers for Disease Control and Prevention (2017e); the "Leading Causes of Fatal Injury Reports," by the Centers for Disease Control and Prevention (2017d); and the "Leading Causes of Non-Fatal Injury Reports," by the Centers for Disease Control and Prevention (2017e)
[a]This is the percent of the total overall unintentional injuries of the specified type for the specified age group that was caused by an unintentional fall (i.e., 35.5% of the total number of hospitalizations, for an unintentional nonfatal injury, by adults aged 40–64, were caused by an unintentional fall)

p. 39). This age group represents most of the workforce and is responsible for the most significant contributions to the economy. As a result, while fall injuries are statistically less severe for adults (ages 20–65), they have the most substantial economic impact (Volpe, 2014).

The Grey Bruce Health Unit (2017) identifies "four key risk factors for falls in this age group during everyday activities: (1) individual differences in risk taking behavior, (2) alcohol and drug use, (3) unsafe work conditions, and (4) environmental factors such as snow, ice, uneven sidewalks and unsafe stairs" (p. 20). There are clear workplace hazard trends that demonstrate how certain occupations offer an increased risk of falls (see Fig. 12.3). Occupation is among the major fall-risk factors for mid-life adults, and the mid-life fall prevention program case study offered in this section addresses this area.

Within the construction industry, which has some of the most dangerous occupations in the United States, falls are consistently cited as the leading cause of death and injury (Occupational Safety and Health Administration, n.d.). Nevertheless, effective safety and preventive measures to protect against falls are not being implemented in the workplace (Occupational Safety and Health Administration, n.d.). The Fall Safe Intervention for Construction Workers (Chap. 14) is an exemplary fall injury prevention program aimed at increasing the use of established fall prevention practices and technology in the construction industry. This program targeted contractors through a certification program that incentivized safety practices by supporting the contractor's reputation. This program involved policy, education/training for workers and supervisors, a multilevel accountability system, and a hazard-management auditing tool that is currently being replicated and repurposed in other industries. Hazard management puts the ownership for safety in the hands of individuals within the company while simultaneously implementing passive environmental changes, which resulted in a significant increase in contractors' use of safety measures. The purpose

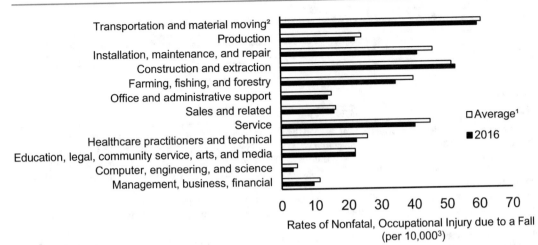

Fig. 12.3 Rates of nonfatal, occupational injury due to a fall by industry across the United States. The data represented in the graph are from "Occupational Injuries and Illnesses and Fatal Injuries Profiles," by the Bureau of Labor Statistics, U.S. Department of Labor (n.d.). This is public data. (1) Average rate calculated across 2011–2016. (2) Transportation fall injury data were unavailable for 2014–2015. "Incidence rates represent the number of injuries and illnesses per 10,000 full-time workers and were calculated as: $(N/EH) \times 20{,}000{,}000$ where, N = number of injuries and illnesses, EH = total hours worked by all employees during the calendar year, $20{,}000{,}000$ = base for 10,000 full-time equivalent workers (working 40 h per week, 50 weeks per year)" (Bureau of Labor Statistics, n.d.)

of this program was to work with construction companies to create a safety culture by supporting them to take ownership over their relationship to the environment.

Fall Safe focused on increasing safety culture in the construction industry by reaching out to workers and personalizing education to reach the audience. A need for a more positive safety culture was evident as, within the construction industry, effective prevention methods already existed but were not being implemented. Other exemplary occupational fall prevention programs with industries that demonstrate similar circumstances (e.g., The Kentucky ROPS program, see Cole & Westneat, 2001) have likewise focused on increasing safety culture. However, each program has used a different model to achieve this goal: Fall Safe can be seen establishing ownership over the person–environment relationship, whereas the Kentucky ROPS applied more of an overall community-based participatory prevention model. Together they establish a foundation for other prevention programs concerned with safety culture.

12.2.3 Older Adults

Scotti (2016) indicates that "on average, an older adult dies every 20 minutes or obtains treatment in an emergency room every 13 seconds as a result of unintentional falls" (¶ 1). Adults over the age of 65 are especially vulnerable to injury and death related to falls. Table 12.5 shows the falls severity incidence for individuals over the age of 65. This increased vulnerability is related to a combination of potential factors related to a normal aging process, including ability to recover, age-related changes to the body (i.e., muscular changes, vision changes, and balance loss), and taking multiple medications (Grey Bruce Health Unit, 2017). Ultimately, it is the accumulation of multiple risk factors combined that is problematic (Ontario Injury Prevention Resource Centre, 2008). Nevertheless, falling is not simply an inevitable part of the aging process. Falls within this population are preventable. The most effective fall prevention programs for older adults are those that use a multifactorial, community-based approach (Ontario Injury Prevention Resource

Table 12.5 Rates of fatal and nonfatal unintentional injuries due to a fall in older adulthood (age 65+)

Severity of injury	Amount	Rate per 100,000	Percent of older adult's total injuries[a], %	Percent of USA's total fall-related injury represented by this older adults[b], %
Fatalities	28,486	59.64	55.4	85.3
Emergency department visits	3,037,550	6359.92	64.4	32.4
Hospitalization	851,715	1783.29	79.2	70.8

Note: These results reflect data from the year 2015 in the United States. Created using data from "Fatal Injury Reports," by the Centers for Disease Control and Prevention (2017d); the "Non-Fatal Injury Reports," by the Centers for Disease Control and Prevention (2017e); the "Leading Causes of Fatal Injury Reports," by the Centers for Disease Control and Prevention (2017d); and the "Leading Causes of Non-Fatal Injury Reports," by the Centers for Disease Control and Prevention (2017e)

[a]This is the percent of the total overall unintentional injuries of the specified type for adults age 65+ that was caused by an unintentional fall (i.e., 55.4% of the total number of unintentional fatal injury, by adults age 65+, were caused by an unintentional fall)

[b]Percent of the overall population total of fall-related injuries (of the specified type) that was by a person 65+ (i.e., 85.3% of the population's total fall-related, unintentional fatalities were people age 65+)

Centre, 2008). The older adult case studies, Stay On Your Feet and the Melbourne Extended Care and Rehabilitation Services (MECRS) patient fall prevention program, are examples of effective multilevel/−factorial approaches to fall injury prevention.

The Stay On Your Feet (SOYF) Seniors Falls Prevention Program (Chap. 15) targets older adults (65+). It has gained international influence and popularity over the years due to its proven effectiveness, sustainability, and wide reach. SOYF employs a multifaceted approach, involving a wide array of health professionals and community members and includes the active involvement of seniors in both implementation and planning. Its implementation strategies include "awareness raising, community education, policy development, home hazard reduction, media campaigns, and working with health professionals—all aimed at using local knowledge, leadership and expertise, fostering community ownership and input into solutions, and sustainability" (Volpe, n.d., Stay On Your Feet section, ¶ 1). SOYF's positive health message aims to educate seniors about the fact that falls are preventable, not just an inevitable part of aging. SOYF is of particular significance because this program manages to address all four quadrants of the life-space model (sociocultural, interpersonal, physical environment, and internal states;

see Chap. 1 for more information on this model and its significance).

Moreover, this senior-fall prevention program is unique for its international presence. Fall injuries remain a leading worldwide health concern that particularly impact adults over the age of 65 (WHO, 2018). This case study is presented in a slightly different, more extensive, format than others in this book so that it can address some of its exemplary implementations from various locations around the world. These subcases are a unique opportunity to gain insight into how effectively a program can be implemented in a new community with unique needs. The transferability of this program brings forth both sustained and discontinued implementations that might be considered when duplicating or adapting a program within a new environment.

The Melbourne Extended Care and Rehabilitation Services Patient Falls Prevention Program (Chap. 16) was initiated due to a high rate of falls in hospital settings and limited knowledge about risks or prevention measures. This comprehensive prevention program framework looked at the interactions between many different and wide-ranging potential factors to assess risk. The thorough risk assessment tool developed during the program has expanded its reach internationally and has also been adapted for use outside of the hospital to address falls in the community. Resulting prevention measures were equally exhaustive and addressed fall hospital prevention holistically. The MECRS prevention program is a model of the strength that a process-evaluative framework brings to an injury prevention program. Because of this process-evaluation framework and commitment to learning, the MECRS hospital prevention program contributed to fall-prevention knowledge.

The Otago Exercise Program (Chap. 17) was designed by the Falls Prevention Research Group at the University of Otago Medical School. Two physical functioning assessments are used to assess lower limb muscle strength and balance. If a person is unable to complete either task, it indicates deficits in their strength and balance. The participant is instructed to carry out the set of exercises three times a week and to walk twice a week for 30 min. The exercise instructor conducts four home visits over a period of 2 months with the exercise instructor allowing up to 1 h for each visit. Overall, the data indicated that the Otago Exercise Program was effective in reducing the number of falls and fall-related injuries by 35%. In terms of injurious falls prevented, the program was more effective for participants aged 80 years and older than for those 65–79. Participants with and without a history of a previous fall benefited equally from the exercise program. Combining the results from the four trials demonstrated the fact that the program prevented the most falls and injuries in those aged 80 years who had fallen in the previous year.

12.3   For What Follows

Falls have a significant cost to individuals, families, communities, and nations. Falls are the leading cause of nonfatal, unintentional injury and third leading cause of unintentional fatality in the USA. Fall injuries can have a significant impact on quality of life. The factors associated with falls are multifaceted and, thus, best understood from a lifespan perspective that goes beyond the immediate visible risks and considers social determinants and ecology. Volpe (2012) states that "development is conceived of as a conse-

quence of both the person and the environment, a result of the joint functioning of individuals and their context" (p. 16). The nature of the person–environment interaction is, therefore, central to an effective fall prevention program and is highlighted throughout the following cases. The recognition of development in context allows us to appreciate injury as "associated with a number of interrelated components, including personal, cultural, and environmental factors that accumulate throughout the lifespan" (Volpe, 2014, p. 53). Fall prevention programs that extend across the lifespan to target primary prevention before risks accumulate with age may have the most significant benefit. Therefore, when reviewing the cases in the following section, keep in mind the complexity of fall risk and protective factors from a developmental perspective.

References

Bureau of Labor Statistics U.S. Department of Labor. (n.d.). *Occupational injuries and illnesses and fatal injuries profiles.* Retrieved February 25, 2018, from https://data.bls.gov/gqt/InitialPage.

Centers for Disease Control and Prevention. (2016a). *CDC Newsroom: Falls are the leading cause of injury and death in older Americans.* Retrieved January 15, 2018, from https://www.cdc.gov/media/releases/2016/p0922-older-adult-falls.html.

Centers for Disease Control and Prevention. (2016b). *Home and recreation safety: Costs of falls among older adults.* Retrieved January 25, 2018, from https://www.cdc.gov/homeandrecreationalsafety/falls/fallcost.html.

Centers for Disease Control and Prevention. (2017a). *Definitions of nonfatal injuries.* Retrieved February 3, 2018, from https://www.cdc.gov/injury/wisqars/nonfatal_help/definitions_nonfatal.html.

Centers for Disease Control and Prevention. (2017b). *Home recreation and safety: Important facts about falls.* Retrieved January 25, 2018, from https://www.cdc.gov/homeandrecreationalsafety/falls/adultfalls.html.

Centers for Disease Control and Prevention. (2017c). *National center for health statistics: Accidents or unintentional injuries.* Retrieved January 25, 2018, from https://www.cdc.gov/nchs/fastats/accidental-injury.htm.

Centers for Disease Control and Prevention. (2017d). *WISQARS: Fatal injury data.* Retrieved January 25, 2018, from https://www.cdc.gov/injury/wisqars/fatal.html.

Centers for Disease Control and Prevention. (2017e). *WISQARS: Nonfatal injury data.* Retrieved January

25, 2018, from https://www.cdc.gov/injury/wisqars/nonfatal.html.

Cole, H. P., & Westneat, S. (2001). *The Kentucky ROPS Project. Final technical report for partners in prevention: Promoting ROPS and seat belts on family farm tractors.* Lexington, KY: University of Kentucky, Southeast Center for Agricultural Health and Injury Prevention.

Grey Bruce Public Health Unit. (2017). Working collaboratively to prevent falls across the lifespan. Grey Bruce, ON: Author.

National Safety Council. (2015). *Injury facts.* Retrieved January 20, 2018, from http://www.nsc.org/Membership%20Site%20Document%20Library/2015%20Injury%20Facts/NSC_InjuryFacts2015Ed.pdf.

Occupational Safety and Health Administration. (n.d.). Fall protection. Retrieved October 5, 2017 from https://www.osha.gov/SLTC/fallprotection/index.html

Ontario Injury Prevention Resource Centre (2008). *Falls across the lifespan: Evidence based practice synthesis document.* Ottawa, ON: Queen's Printer for Ontario.

Parachute. (2015). *The cost of injury in Canada.* Toronto, ON: Author.

Scotti, S. (2016). Preventing elderly falls. *National Conference of State Legislatures Legisbrief Briefing Papers on the Important Issues for the Day, 24*(17). Retrieved February 10, 2018, from http://www.ncsl.org/documents/health/lb_2417.pdf.

Volpe, R. (2012). *The conceptualization of injury prevention as change in complex systems.* Toronto, ON: Smartrisk.

Volpe, R. (2014). *Best practices in the prevention of midlife falls in everyday activities.* Retrieved January 25, 2018, from http://onf.org/system/attachments/294/original/MLF_COMBO_RS_Fin_Dec_14.pdf.

Volpe, R. (n.d.). *Implementation and evaluation projects.* Retrieved February 18, 2018, from https://wordpress.oise.utoronto.ca/richardvolpe/research/implementation-and-evaluation-projects/#SOYF.

World Health Organization. (2018). *Falls.* Retrieved January 15, 2018, from http://www.who.int/mediacentre/factsheets/fs344/en/.

World Health Organization. (n.d.). *Falls.* Retrieved January 15, 2018, from http://www.who.int/violence_injury_prevention/other_injury/falls/en/.

Kids Can't Fly: A Childhood Injury Prevention Program

13

Daria Smeh and Tanya Morton

Kids Can't Fly is an injury prevention program designed to help prevent young children from falling out of windows through the use of safety guards.

13.1 Background

In 1993, the Boston Globe announced that a spate of window falls was afflicting young children, with 18 children falling from unprotected windows in the Boston area between June and December. These alarming statistics published by the Boston Globe prompted the mayor to initiate the creation of the window fall prevention program, Kids Can't Fly, targeted to protect all children in Boston aged 0–6 years old (US Department of Health and Human Services, 1998). However, the program did target minorities and low-income neighborhoods because these groups have an increased risk and incidence of falls (E. Christiansen, personal communication, April 23, 2007). Three months of planning

and organization was required to create the foundation for the program. The timeline in Box 13.1 outlines the measures undertaken to mount the Boston prevention program.

> **Box 13.1 A Timeline for the Historical Development of Kids Can't Fly**
>
> June–July 1993
>
> The Mayor of Boston marshalled a Roundtable Conference to conduct an assessment of the window fall problem.
>
> A series of meetings was held by the Office of Public Safety (Commonwealth of Massachusetts).
>
> The consequent plan identified window guards as the solution to the problem and determined that existing state building codes enabled the installation of window guards.
>
> The Office of Public Safety delegated the responsibility of window fall prevention to the Boston Public Health Commission's Childhood Injury Prevention Program (CIPP).
>
> The CIPP established Window Falls Prevention Task Force, which undertook the following steps:

(continued)

D. Smeh (✉)
LoyalTeam Environmental, Toronto, ON, Canada

T. Morton
Catholic Children's Aid Society of Toronto, Toronto, ON, Canada

© Springer Nature Switzerland AG 2020
R. Volpe (ed.), *Casebook of Traumatic Injury Prevention*,
https://doi.org/10.1007/978-3-030-27419-1_13

(continued)

- Examined the New York City program "Children Can't Fly"[1] and
- Addressed the issues specific to Boston's environment: determined whether to make window guards mandatory and selected the type of guard that met the fire department's approval

August 1993:

The Mayor announced the formal initiation of a city-wide Window Falls Prevention Program entitled Kids Can't Fly.

A rationale for the program was established using the injury statistics gathered from June to December 1993, which provided the following:

- The justification for targeting low-income communities, including subsidized housing developments
- The need for heightened vigilance during the summer months
- An understanding of the potential severity of injuries, and
- Consideration of the role of building height

US Department of Health and Human Services (1998)

According to the Kids Can't Fly Strategy Transfer Guide from the Models That Work campaign (US Department of Health and Human Services, 1998), eight goals were outlined during the development of the program. The goals are as follows:

1. Increase awareness of the danger posed by open windows by conducting city-wide education and outreach efforts
2. Expand outreach and make available information and technical assistance to the public on the devices that might mitigate this serious problem
3. Provide a forum for discussion with industry representatives on the design and manufacture of an operable window guard and improved designs thereafter
4. Expand interagency cooperation and involvement
5. Encourage property owners to voluntarily install window safety guards on windows and dwellings occupied by children aged 6 years and under
6. Identify and track voluntary installation of window guards
7. Improve coordination among local hospitals for accurate tracking of incidents
8. Participate in industry discussion on product specifications and standards

The goals were created based on consideration of the initial barriers encountered by program developers. These include a lack of awareness about the danger of open windows, difficulty in identifying and reaching out to high-risk groups, a diversity of languages and cultures, and the lack of a product acceptable to Boston building standards and the fire department (Boston Public Health Commission [BPHC], n.d.-a).

During the development of the program, only a fixed window guard was available, which did not enable emergency egress. Therefore, the Window Falls Prevention Task Force was reluctant to endorse this product. Eventually, a guard was selected that met the approval of all stakeholders and was affordable for residents and property managers. From the process of selecting a guard, a national industry and government subcommittee was struck to develop standards for window guards and continue the process of improving their designs, which was active until the late 1990s (US Department of Health and Human Services, 1998).

---

[1]In 1971, the initiative "Children Can't Fly" was created by the New York City Health Department to address the alarming incidence of child mortality and morbidity due to window falls. The program is an example of a holistic falls prevention program that includes a comprehensive reporting system for hospital emergency rooms, the enforcement of law obligating landlords to install window guards in apartments with children, and an education and media campaign.

After the selection of a window guard, staff from the CIPP conducted research on existing legislation across the country. As much of the draft of the ordinance was based on existing New York City legislation, the process of deriving legislation for Boston took only 1 year. Following the creation of that draft legislation, the Window Falls Prevention Task Force members, fire service personnel, and real estate representatives were consulted for feedback regarding the feasibility of the ordinance. The result of active involvement by stakeholders was an ordinance that promoted voluntary compliance to window guard installation, with an emphasis on community education (Box 13.2).

Box 13.2 City of Boston Ordinance for Establishing a Window Falls Prevention Programs in the Department of Health and Hospitals

CITY OF BOSTON

AN ORDIANCE

Be it ordained by the City Council of Boston, as follows:

City of Boston Code, Ordinances, Chapter IX is amended by inserting after section 9-9.10, the following new section 9-9.11

Section 1. Definitions

For the purposes of this ordinance, the following terms shall have the following meaning:

Child: a person age 6 years and under.
Board: The Board of Health and Hospitals.
Department: The Department of Health and Hospitals.
Installation: the proper equipping of windows with window safety guards in accordance with regulations issued by the department of health and hospitals.
Owner: person, who alone or severally has legal titles, or has charge or control of

any capacity including but not limited to agent, executor, administrator, trustee or guardian, or any officer or trustee of a real estate trust or association of unit owners.
Tenant: a lessee, or other regular occupant of a dwelling unit with or without a lease.
Window safety guard: a device designed to restrict passage or access through a window of a child 6 or under.

Section 2. There shall be a Window Falls prevention program established within the Department of Health and Hospitals. The purpose of said program shall be as follows: educating the public about the danger to children, age 6 years and under, of falling from windows, and encouraging the voluntary installation by owners of window safety guards on windows in dwellings occupied by children age 6 years and under.

Section 3. The program shall conduct city-wide education and outreach efforts promoting awareness about the dangers to children, age 6 years and under, from falling from open or otherwise unprotected windows. Information and technical assistance shall be made available to the public on the steps and devices that may mitigate this serious problem. The Program shall work with any and all existing agencies and departments involved with children in its outreach efforts. The Window Falls Prevention Program will also encourage owners to voluntarily install window safety guards on windows in the dwellings occupied by children age 6 years and under.

Section 4. The Board is empowered to oversee the Program and may meet to develop regulations regarding window safety guards. In so doing, the Board will work with all appropriate agencies to ensure compliance with existing state building codes and fire department codes.

Based on the ordinance, a plan for window guard distribution and installation was developed. Retailers, property owners and managers, health centers, and community organizations provided free guards to families or subsidies and discounts to purchase guards. In 1994 and 1995, the retailer Home Depot donated 1000 guards to the program and also sold guards at cost for the entire summer. Home Depot even produced a 15-min educational video from which a 30-s PSA was developed (US Department of Health and Human Services, 1998). Property managers and homeowners were invited to participate in instructional workshops on installation at home improvement stores. The Boston Housing Authority (BHA) played a central role since the beginning of the program because they set an internal policy to make window guard installation mandatory in the housing they manage (BPHC, n.d.-a; US Department of Health and Human Services, 1998).

In 1997, the Children's Hospital in Boston created the yearly Adopt-a-Building campaign to assist low- and moderate-income families. The campaign required hospital personnel to select an apartment building from a pool of applicants; the selected building was outfitted with window guards at the hospital's expense (US Department of Health and Human Services, 1998). The Adopt-a-Building program stopped providing financial resources to install window guards in 1999, but it still distributes educational materials (E. Christiansen, personal communication, April 4, 2007). Currently, the guard is subsidized to residents through the Matching Buy Program by the CIPP and the Area Planning Action Council (APAC), a community antipoverty and health promotion agency (E. Christianson, personal communication, July 9, 2007).

After addressing the legalities and technicalities of the program, further key barriers were identified and addressed by the CIPP so as to promote the social and environmental changes that are necessary to ensure that children are protected from window falls (Table 13.1).

To address the problems listed in Table 13.1, two dedicated program champions spearheaded an initiative. City of Boston Mayor Menino, who launched the initiative over a decade ago, and the CIPP. Mayor Menino provided stable funding and constant political support for the CIPP. Subsequently, the cooperation of various agencies and individuals was marshalled during program

Table 13.1 Problems faced during the development of Kids Can't Fly and the responses to the problems

Problem	Response
Windows were still not recognized as a potential hazard by many parents and caregivers.	A comprehensive education and outreach campaign was repeatedly delivered to remind parents and caregivers about the importance of window safety.
The number of people reached through the free window guard giveaway over a 2-year period was relatively small; furthermore, a very small percentage of recipients actually installed the guards due to lack of tools, knowledge, or motivation.	The Matching Buy Program was created to target property managers of mid-sized, low- and moderate-income complexes. This program resulted in more families receiving guards and ensured proper installation. Consequently, the responsibility to distribute the guards was delegated to property management companies.
Local availability of guards was limited; for example, stores discontinued selling window guards after the initial promotion of the program because of lack of sale volume or lack of interest from retailers.	Regular monitoring of retailers who offer window guards as monitoring is necessary to provide information on availability.
Standard reporting and referral system was required so that the total number of incidents is known to hospitals and agencies.	Accurate reporting of injury statistics can be challenging because Boston possesses a number of hospitals. Therefore, a standardized reporting and referral system remains a future task for the next generation of injury prevention professionals.

Note. From *Kids Can't Fly: Strategy Transfer Guide. Models that Work* by the U.S. Department of Health and Human Services, 1998. Bethesda, MD: Department of Health and Human Services Bureau of Primary Health Care

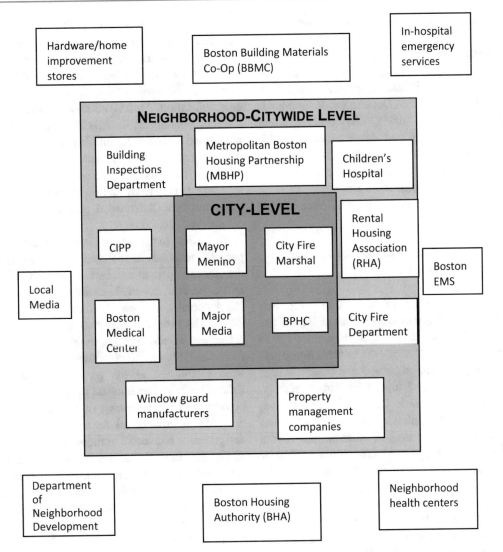

Fig. 13.1 Organizational chart of Boston stakeholders involved in Kids Can't Fly. The size of the boxes, which encase each stakeholder group, is not indicative of their degree of importance and involvement in the program. Also included are the public and private sector stakeholders that partnered with the city to with the objective to reduce window falls

development and initial implementation (Vish, Powell, Wiltsek, & Sheehan, 2005). Given that the BPHC and Mayor Menino were the primary players in the program, they are featured at the center of the organizational chart in Fig. 13.1.

Prior to the program's development in 1993, a need assessment of Kids Can't Fly was undertaken by the CIPP in order to promote the program's sustainability in the long term. In so doing, the CIPP ensured that information resources addressed real community needs (e.g., accommodating language preferences, easy level of comprehension of key safety messages). During deployment, the CIPP ensured that all systems were suited to the capabilities of the users and to the constraints of the community. For example, following an assessment by the BPHC of the window guard give-away initiative, it was discovered that the distribution of free window guards to caregivers of children did not transfer into installation because caregivers did not always have the time or expertise to install the guards. However, when property managers and owners were engaged, adherence to the program increased (E. Christiansen, personal communication, April 2007; U.S. Department of Health and Human Services, 1998). The involvement of property managers and owners was a notable departure from New York's Children Can't Fly program. The involvement of these additional stakeholders complimented the voluntary compliance promoted under the ordinance created in Boston.

13.2   Resources

The annual budget of Kids Can't Fly was $60,000 in 1998 (US Department of Health and Human Services, 1998). Currently, the CIPP is granted a budget of $250,000 for three injury prevention programs—a car seat and bicycle helmet program share the budget with Kids Can't Fly. The budget for Kids Can't Fly encompasses staffing, office supplies, marketing and education materials, and the cost of window guards (the Matching Buy Program). The office of Mayor Menino issued funding on behalf of the City of Boston. The $250,000 budget has remained consistent due to an agreement between the city council and the BPHC with respect to the fiscal needs of the program (E. Christiansen, personal communication, April 23, 2007).

External funding has never been sought for Kids Can't Fly because shared responsibility is expected between property owners/managers and the BPHC/the city (E. Christiansen, personal communication, April 23, 2007). Yet the financial resources of the program enable the CIPP to equally share the cost of window guards with property managers or owners through the Matching Buy program. The subsidy denotes that the cost of the window guard is split equally between the CIPP and the property managers and residents. One potential drawback of having a single funding body is that if the level of support is reduced, another is unavailable to redress the balance (Jones & Offord, 1991).

Currently, three full-time staff members and two part-time staff members run the program.[2] The current program director has worked in the CIPP for over 6 years, and 4 of those years she worked as the director (E. Christiansen, personal communication, April 23, 2007). Staffing at the CIPP is generally stable. All CIPP staff members are housed in the BPHC building, which provides office equipment and information systems supplied by the city government. Therefore, no expenditure is made from the program budget on these items (E. Christiansen, personal communication, April 26, 2007).

According to the former program director, the program responds to the changing dynamics of the city and operates successfully on a consistent basis, despite minimal staffing and funding (K. Antonellis, personal communication, May 1, 2007). The program is able to run successfully regardless of resource constraints because the fundamental tasks and objectives of the program were established at the program's inception. Establishing the fundamental program tasks and objectives at the beginning of the program has provided the groundwork for a strong evaluation design that is conducive to measuring the impact of the program. Consequently, a decision has been made to keep the tasks and objectives of the program consistent, regardless of any changes in human resources. The new director simply adds energy to the program (K. Antonellis, personal communication, May 1, 2007).

Stable and favorable external socioeconomic and political factors translate into a consistent

---

[2]Before the Kids Can't Fly program was an official initiative (i.e., in 1991), window safety was the responsibility of a part-time director and a part-time outreach worker in Boston Public Health. At the program's inception in 1993, seven staff members were employed at the CIPP: a part-time director, a full-time assistant director, and five support staff (K. Antonellis, personal communication, April 30, 2007); while, in 1998, BPHC consisted of a director who was responsible for program administration; an Outreach Worker who conducted community workshops; support staff who responded to phone requests and prepared mailings; and a consultant with a technical background who developed educational and media materials, developed a public relations plan, and assisted in guard design review (US Department of Health and Human Services, 1998).

level of funding and reliable capacity of human resources (Bourgeois, Noce, Smeh, & Morton, 2007, p. 17). Since the inception of Kids Can't Fly, the CIPP has maintained financial and political support from the Mayor. Furthermore, the administration of Kids Can't Fly has remained centralized and under the control of the CIPP. According to Bourgeois et al. (2007), decentralization (i.e., the fragmentation of responsibilities to different agencies) tends to restrict human and fiscal resources. When financial support is decreased, resources are inflexible and not within the implementing agency's control.

13.2.1 External Resources

Almost all the current stakeholders have been involved in the Kids Can't Fly program since its inception. Although some stakeholders are less active now than compared to their involvement at the inception of the program, all stakeholders will be consulted if changes are made. By 1998, the stakeholders included politicians (the Mayor, City Council), administrators (Rental Housing Association, property management companies), professionals (window guard manufacturers, the media), the community (Boston residents, East Boston Neighborhood Health Center and other neighborhood health centers, hardware/home improvement stores), consumers (residents), and public service agencies (Boston Building Materials Co-Op; Boston Housing Authority; Boston EMS, Boston Fire Department, Boston Medical Center, Children's Hospital; Inspectional Services Department) (US Department of Health and Human Services, 1998).

Information about Kids Can't Fly is distributed by the BPHC through official brochures and flyers. Some stakeholders provide vouchers for window guards that hardware stores provide, while others keep abreast of window guard technology (US Department of Health and Human Services, 1998). By 2001, the same stakeholders remained involved, but, again, some to a lesser degree; also, by 2001, the Department of Neighborhood Development was added as a partner (Boston Public Health Commission, n.d.-a). Not only have new stakeholders joined the initiative, but all of the existing and past stakeholders remain supportive of the program and play consultative roles to varying degrees (E. Christiansen, personal communication, April 23, 2007).

Due to the strategic position of the BPHC as a health and government agency and the CIPP as a specialized branch of that organization, both the BPHC and the CIPP can make their roles and the roles of the stakeholders multifaceted. For example, building managers install the window guards, but they also act as mediators to provide information about safety to residents (E. Christiansen, personal communication, April 23, 2007). In addition, the director of the CIPP, not only oversees program administration but also acts as a trainer at the local level (i.e., visiting daycares to provide information and training sessions to caregivers on window guard safety).

The CIPP's position as a health organization and a government agency also positions them to reinforce voluntary compliance. Participation in the program is voluntary, as dictated by the ordinance. Although the ordinance translates into no legal consequences if ignored, it is still considered legislation taken seriously by the City of Boston. The program director states that because an ordinance is in place, it is easy for her to encourage landlords (or their legal representatives) who are attempting to avoid installation to comply with the ordinance. Christiansen states that when landlords are not willing to comply, she not only informs them about the ordinance but also educates them about past lawsuits that arose after preventable window falls occurred (E. Christiansen, personal communication, April 4, 2007). As the CIPP is a public health organization and not an enforcement agency, it can only strongly encourage compliance (E. Christiansen, personal communication, April 23, 2007) by building trust with collaborators.

Since initial implementation, the components of the program have remained consistent overall. The ordinance to install window guards has not become mandatory because positive results were achieved without changing the position of the law. The design of the window guard has remained the same since 2000 because this design is satisfactory to all stakeholders, particularly the Fire Department. The tools to provide education have also remained consistent; however, the program adds new languages to its repertoire when new cultural-linguistic groups are identified in Boston. The relationship with the stakeholders is extremely stable, although some contact may occur on an as-needed basis. Regardless of the infrequency of communication, the CIPP still boasts the ability to gather all stakeholders easily as they all possess a willingness to communicate and participate. The CIPP also has continued to accept the main responsibility for program direction, despite low-level funding for the program (E. Christiansen, personal communication, April 4, 2007; K. Antonellis, personal communication, May 1, 2007).

13.3 Implementation

13.3.1 Education, Awareness Raising, and Advocacy

In Kids Can't Fly, public outreach and education are essential tools used to communicate with communities, agencies, and industries in order to raise awareness. A comprehensive education campaign was developed to ensure an understanding by the community that precautions are required to protect children from window falls. Efforts are made to keep program visibility high. Christiansen suggests that adequate planning and resources are required to communicate fall risk to individuals who hail from diverse geographic and cultural backgrounds (personal communication, 23 April 2007). For example, Christiansen states that CIPP staff members attend outdoor fairs that are hosted by different cultural groups in spring and summer. At these fairs, CIPP staff members set up a table with multilingual information brochures and have a translator in attendance (E. Christiansen, personal communication, April 26, 2007). Another strategy to bring attention to Kids Can't Fly is the media release published by the office of Mayor Menino. The Mayor's office disseminates the release to the BPHC and local media outlets. The content includes safety information, outlines future work of the program,

and highlights the historical success of Kids Can't Fly in Boston. The last media release was issued in spring 2004. Subway advertisements also contribute to program visibility. Christiansen states that inquiries about the program were made specifically to her as a result of subway advertisements (E. Christiansen, personal communication, April 26, 2007). Table 13.2 displays a breakdown of the comprehensive education and outreach strategies that are targeted to various segments of the population.

The wording of the brochure used by Kids Can't Fly has remained the same since the inception of the program. However, as a way to revitalize the message of window safety, the CIPP created a new logo in 2005 (M. Nicastro, personal communication, April 30, 2007). A rationale for redesigning the brochure and launching the new logo was to revitalize the safety message by replacing the old logo of two children standing behind a window guard with a "happier" flower logo (E. Christiansen, personal communication, April 4, 2007). The brochure currently used by Kids Can't Fly is provided below in Fig. 13.2.

13.3.2 Window Guard Technology

Windows that are open just 4 in. pose a danger to children 10 and under; even a closed window can be dangerous—falling through glass can cause serious and often fatal injuries. Window safety guards are made of aluminum or steel bars with 4-in. spacing from the guard to the bottom half of the window. Guards are designed to withstand 150 lb of pressure (The Metropolitan Boston Housing Partnership, 2005). As such, a properly installed window guard is recommended as an established method to prevent window falls (New York City Department of Health and Mental Hygiene, 2007). Although designed for double-hung windows, the window guard chosen for Kids Can't Fly (Fig 13.3) can be cascade mounted one on top of the other for sliding and casement windows. The guard is for use with double-hung windows of openings from 23″ to 35″ wide, the height is 21 3/8″, and bar spacing is 3 7/8″ (See ChildSafetyGates.com, 2007 for a picture of the

Table 13.2 Overview of educational and outreach strategies and target population, Kids Can't Fly

Strategy	Description	Target population
Posters, newsletters, and brochures 1993–present	Multilingual: includes English, Spanish, Chinese Haitian Creole, and French New logo launched in 2005 Provides information about the window fall problem and basic safety, demonstrates window guard installation, provides information about Kids Can't Fly and contact information for the CIPP	General population Immigrant populations Illiterate populations
Public service announcements Radio: 1993–2005 TV: 1993–present Newspapers: 1993–present	Radio—60-s message Airplay increased free of charge because message is a public service Television Multilingual: English, Spanish Airs June–August, several times per day	Immigrant populations Illiterate populations Radio listeners and television viewers Commuters in cars
Press conferences 1993–1999	Unilingual: English Involves the print and digital media Held by the mayor at spring/summer season to commence program Highlights Mayor's safety message Provides information about the window fall problem Media used to provide widespread coverage and generate mass awareness	Television viewers
Billboards 2004–present	Unilingual: English Six erected in residential neighborhoods Provides information about basic safety messages and Kids Can't Fly	Commuters using cars Residential neighborhoods with buildings
Subway advertisements 2000–present	Unilingual: English Posted during summer months Provides information about the basic safety messages and information about Kids Can't Fly Summer 2005: new design launched over four weeks with 120 posters	Subway commuters Low-income people
Vendor Information Sheets 2000–present	Unilingual: English Provides information on Matching Buy program and window guard installation	Retailers and property managers

vertical and horizonal "Guardian Angel Window Guards–Model 2335" manufactured by Automatic Specialties, Inc., 2007).

As of 2007, the last meeting with the window guard manufacturing industry to improve window guard design and specification was before 2000. The CIPP has continued to promote the same window guard for years because no malfunction in design has been discovered. Any change in technology would be the decision of the director, who does independent research on the varying costs of the different products offered by Home Depot and other retailers (E. Christiansen, personal communication, April 4, 2007).

Housing managers in higher income properties have expressed concerns about the aesthetic look of window guards. In response, the director of the CIPP researched security screens as an alternative to the guards. Manufacturers constructed heavy-duty metal screens and claim that the product can prevent falls. However, the fire department does not recommend window screens because the screen can act as a barrier during an emergency. The CIPP also does not support the use of these screens as they are costly, which would restrict accessibility in low-income neighborhoods (E. Christiansen, personal communication, April 23, 2007). Thus, the CIPP has researched and justified its decisions in response to the concerns of the community.

A strong partnership with the East Boston Neighborhood Health Center (EBNHC) began in 1996 in order to disseminate educational

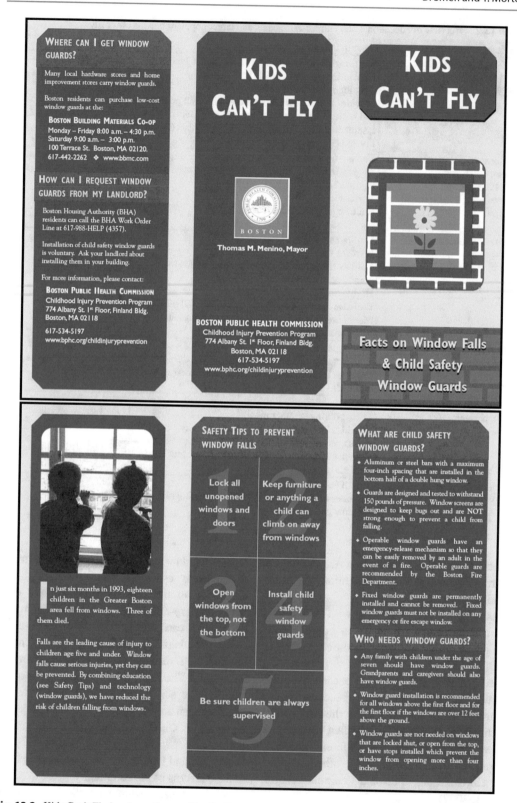

Fig. 13.2 Kids Can't Fly brochure, front and back. (From "Kids Can't fly. Facts on window falls and child safety window guards" by the Boston Public Health Commission, 2007)

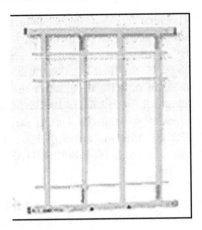 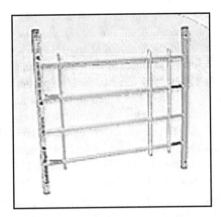

Fig. 13.3 The guardian angel window guard, manufactured by Automatic Specialties, Inc. The first image shows the vertical guard, and the second shows the horizontal guard. (From "Guardian Angel Window Guard—Model 2335" manufactured by Automatic Specialties, Inc., 2007. Retrieved May 2007 from www.child-safety-gates.com)

information on installation. Currently, the Health Center targets low-income families with toddlers (M. Nicastro, personal communication, April 4, 2007). Mr. Michael Nicastro describes his task as Director of Community Safety Programs of the EBNHC in Box 13.3. According to M. Nicastro, a translator accompanies him to the mini-workshops in the pediatric department of the Health Center. Since the program began at the EBNHC in 1996 to 2007, the Health Centre has distributed over 1200 window guards in the East Boston community (personal communication, April 12, 2007).

> **Box 13.3 Window Falls Safety and Kids Can't Fly Instruction, Mr. M. Nicastro, EBNHC, April 12, 2007**
>
> I conduct mini workshops providing parents with safety tips to help prevent their children from falling from windows. In addition to the safety tip workshops, I give window guard installation demonstrations as well as free window guards to those who attend the workshops and installation demonstrations. The workshops can take place in our Pediatric department waiting area or at some of the child day care sites in East Boston and our surrounding communities.

> Typically, when I set up shop in our Pediatric waiting area, I'll identify parents with toddler-age children and ask if they are interested in window guards for their home. If they accept, I'll spend some time going over the safety tips and then give them a window guard installation demonstration using a model window frame and the actual guards we give away. Once the demonstration is complete, I will give the parent a voucher indicating they have attended the installation demonstration. The parent takes this voucher to our local Area Planning Action Council (APAC), which has the parent sign a waiver form and then distributes two window guards per family.

The BHA was particularly praised for its involvement at the inception of the program. According to BPHC (n.d.-a), the BHA was a "major force in the success of voluntary installations and serves as a national model for other housing associations" (p. 3) because it set an internal policy prioritizing the installation of window guards. In recent years, the BHA has become decentralized because each BHA housing complex has become increasingly governed by individual management (E. Christiansen, personal communication, April 26, 2007). In spite of the increased decentralization of the BHA, the CIPP maintains occasional contact with the BHA and its clients. For the past 2–3 years, the director of the program has received occasional calls from residents living in public housing managed by the BHA. These residents voiced concern that their window guard had not been installed. The director followed up with the BHA in order to ensure that the guards were installed (E. Christiansen, personal communication, April 4, 2007). Importantly, the calls from concerned public housing residents suggest that they believe that the program has value and are willing to exercise their roles as agents.

According to Christiansen, the most effective strategy of the program is collaborating with various agencies and families across the city (personal communication, April 26, 2007). Collaboration and community-based interests inform the policies of the CIPP. Resources are distributed among stakeholders top to bottom and bottom to top in an iterative process. In other words, the involvement of both experts and community laypeople are integral to the success of this program (E. Christiansen, personal communication, April 26, 2007). Although experts have developed program content and evaluation designs, the influence of the intended beneficiaries inform program content and evaluation.

13.4 Outcome

Local epidemiological data gathered from outcome evaluations enable evaluators to make judgements about the effects of a program (Tard, Ouellet, & Beaudoin, 1998). The CIPP has evaluated its own program by collecting outcome data on the incidence of window falls and the degree of educational outreach through media campaigns. In other words, outcomes may be measured in terms of the change in window fall incidence from year to year or by the reach of educational campaigns, such as the number of brochures distributed or the number of PSA's shown.

Outcome data show that the trend of falls from windows among Boston's children has consistently remained at less than four per year from 1998 to 2005 (BPHC, 2006). "Kids Can't Fly" resulted in an 83% decrease in the number of window falls from 1993 to 1995, a 50% decrease between 1993 and 1997 (US Department of Health and Human Services, 1998), and a 95% decrease between 1993 and 2000 (BPHC, n.d.-a; Fig. 13.4).

To assess the effectiveness and sustainability of Kids Can't Fly, data have been gathered throughout the lifecycle of the program. A thorough foundation in empirical research helps the implementation process by identifying the etiology of injuries, where they are occurring, and who are most affected (Durlak, 1997). In fact, Kids Can't Fly has garnered positive reviews from both internal and external evaluators. The internal evaluations consist of reviews done within BPHC, including the Window Guard Giveaway Program Assessment, the Health Centre Survey (US Department of Health and Human Services, 1998), and the actual tracking of child window falls (BPHC, n.d.-b). External praise has come from reviews in academic journals (e.g., American Academy of Pediatrics; Vish et al., 2005) and the federal government (e.g., Models That Work). Federal review lauded the ability of Kids Can't Fly to adapt to local needs and conditions. Therefore, Kids Can't Fly was deemed a Models That Work Competition special honoree in 1998 for its "creative, community-driven solution to significant health challenges, developed by building partnerships and maximizing existing capacities within the community" (US Department of Health and Human Services, 1998, p. 2).

In the year 2017, the Boston Public Health Commission (n.d.-b) continued to provide education on window fall injury prevention on their website.

13.4.1 Program Sustainability

Kids Can't Fly has adhered to principles that previous research has shown to be associated with program sustainability (e.g., Johnson, Hays,

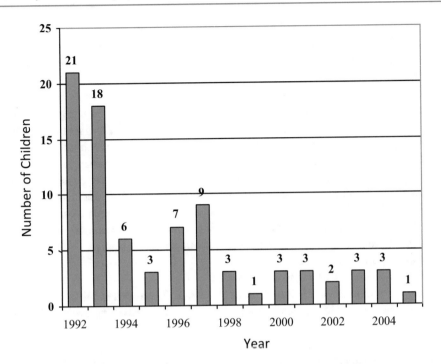

Fig. 13.4 Boston Experience 1992–2005, Number of children fallen from windows. (From *Boston Experience 1992–2005: Number of Children Fallen from Windows* by the Boston Public Health Commission, 2006)

Table 13.3 Principles and examples of sustainability, Kids Can't Fly

Principle of sustainability	Example
The coalescing of private–public partnerships that facilitate public investment	Partners included the Mayor, Fire Marshal, property management companies, the media, and hardware/home improvement stores (US Department of Health and Human Services, 1998).
Response to the needs of the community	Cultural and language-specific outreach efforts, local professionals performing community education, awareness campaigns, and outreach programs are tailored to the demographic characteristics of their communities (US Department of Health and Human Services, 1998).
Designing programs with consideration of local capability	When local families had difficulties installing the guards, distribution of guards and responsibility for installation shifted to property managers (US Department of Health and Human Services, 1998).
Ongoing internal evaluation of outcomes by the BPHC and the CIPP	The availability and affordability of guards is monitored; actual injuries are tracked in spite of challenges with standardized reporting and referral systems (US Department of Health and Human Services, 1998).
Ongoing external evaluation of outcomes by academics and outside agencies	The Models That Work program, supported by the U.S. Department of Health and Human Services, evaluated and lauded the program. Academics such as Vish et al. (2005) reference "Kids Can't Fly" as a model program.

Center, & Daley, 2004). Several strategies used by Kids Can't Fly that adhere to the principles of sustainability are presented in Table 13.3. Key examples of sustainability will be further discussed in this section.

The CIPP ensures that as much as possible can be learned about the effects of the intervention in a real-world environment where randomized studies are usually impossible (Bourgeois et al., 2007). An organization "must be willing to monitor, assess, and evaluate its objectives and strategies and modify these in the best interest of those involved" (Bourgeois et al., 2007, p. 17). For example, in Kids Can't Fly, the initial strategy was to distribute window guards through a giveaway program. In 1996, the giveaway program was reassessed after installation rates were found to be low among residents. This reassessment prompted a new strategy that engaged and obligated property managers to install the guards and therefore led to an increase in the number of installations. Evaluation suggests that Kids Can't Fly has had considerable reach (US Department of Health and Human Services, 1998): by 1997, approximately 11,400 window guards were installed in the Boston area (Matching Buy program: 2600; Health Centers: 2300; Adopt-a-Building: 1500; and Boston Housing Authority: 5000).

The CIPP recognizes that positive outcomes are realized through strategically planning the timing and reach of the education and outreach campaign. For example, the campaign increases in intensity in the spring and summer due to the increased risk for window falls during that time (E. Christiansen, personal communication, April 26, 2007). By 1998, the media campaign reached an estimated 381,000 people through major and local newspapers. There have been 7,520,000 public service radio announcements in English, Spanish, and Haitian Creole (US Department of Health and Human Services, 1998). By 2007, multiple forms of media have been utilized, but the key to a sustained reduction in window falls has resulted from continuous safety reminders delivered during high-risk seasons.

Kids Can't Fly has moved beyond initial project interventions by continuously engaging individuals (e.g., Boston residents, property managers), communities (e.g., neighborhood health centers), and local organizations (e.g., BHA, BMRC). As previously discussed in this paper, the director of the CIPP provides safety consultations at cultural fairs with translators,

the staff members of the BPHC conduct group training on installation in day cares, and the CIPP director accepts phone calls from concerned residents if their window guards have not been installed and follows up with the Boston Housing Authority. Future goals of Kids Can't Fly are to engage families not yet recruited by the program (e.g., new immigrants and isolated parents that are not connected with a child care group or health care center). Therefore, the CIPP allocates time and financial resources to maintain the program's sustainability by building capacity with residents and community and public service agencies.

13.4.2 Transportability to Other Community and Cultural Contexts

Kids Can't Fly is a successful replication of New York City's Children Can't Fly program. Kids Can't Fly has mirrored the overwhelming response that Children Can't Fly received for resident participation and lower incidence of window falls. The principal safety messages of Kids Can't Fly were then transported to several U.S. states, including, for example, Connecticut, Iowa, Florida, Illinois, Virginia, and Oregon (Connecticut Safe Kids, 2006; Iowa Department of Public Health, 2002; Screen Manufacturers Association, 2007; Fairfax County Fire and Rescue Department, 2006; Inova Regional Trauma Center, 2002; Oregon Health Services Unit, n.d.; Vish et al., 2005). Likewise, in 2005, the French Institute for Public Health Surveillance conducted a study on the etiology of window falls in Paris. The study found that prevention campaigns are needed to raise adult awareness of the risk of children falling from windows. Both Children Can't Fly and Kids Can't Fly were deemed pioneering programs that had prevention principles transferable to the French context.

13.4.3 Conceptual Guidelines

The "Kids Can't Fly" program combines the efforts of various community members and professionals (e.g., parents, local merchants, property managers, politicians, policymakers, and medical personnel) in order to accomplish the goals of the program (E. Christiansen, personal communication, April 23, 2007; U.S. Department of Health and Human Services, 1998). The support and consultation of local citizens by community organizations can result in programs that are responsive to local needs (Boyle & Willms, 2002). However, research indicates that expert knowledge enhances community programs through the imposition of a structure, including scientifically based recommendations for program content, dosage, intensity, and maintenance (Boyle & Willms, 2002; Howell, Devaney, McCormick, & Raykovich, 1998). The involvement of experts enhances program development and implementation because they can facilitate adherence to certain recommendations that incorporate the core tenets of many successful prevention programs. These core tenets include frequent and intensive exposure to the program; broad, multifaceted approaches to meeting identified needs; and maintenance of the program to support sustained results (Ramsey & Ramsey, 1998). Strong leadership encourages adherence to these tenets (Howell et al., 1998); furthermore, leadership complemented by clear communication between professionals and non-professionals alike facilitates good long-term relationships that promote program sustainability (Bourgeois et al., 2007).

13.5 Conclusion

As children develop and respond to changes in their environment, keeping them safe in the home is an ongoing, dynamic, and changing process. Likewise, program sustainability requires ongoing effort. Although the goals of Kids Can't Fly have remained constant, program planners have endeavored to stay current by constantly monitoring and evaluating the various components of the program and responding to changes in the outside world. Overall clear leadership and coordination, the effective uses of existing community and agency skills, and stakeholder buy-in have all informed the positive outcomes and sustainability of Kids Can't Fly. The evidence suggests that the physical injury and death of many children by window falls has been prevented by Boston's well-planned holistic program.

Acknowledgments The authors would like to express sincere appreciation to the key informants for this case study: Erin Christiansen of the Boston Public Health Commission in Boston MA, USA; Mike Nicastro of East Boston Neighborhood Health Centre in Boston MA, USA; and Kim Antonellis of the Boston Public Health Commission in Boston, MA, USA—whose consultation made this project possible.

BRIO Model: Kids Can't Fly

Group Served: Children aged 0–6.

Goal: Prevent young children from falling out of windows through the use of safety guards.

Background	Resources	Implementation	Outcome
1971: New York residents express concern about the epidemic of window falls among children; Children Can't Fly program is created and sustained 1993: Boston residents express concern about a similar epidemic. New York Program provides a model for the inception of Kid's Can't Fly 1994: Ordinance developed in Boston to promote voluntary compliance 1996: Kids Can't Fly program assign primary responsibility for guard installation to property owners and managers rather than residents 1998: The annual budget was $60,000US. Funded consistently by the office of Mayor Menino	Currently the CIPP is granted a budget of $250,000US for three injury prevention programs Childhood Injury Prevention Program (CIPP) equally share the cost of window guards with property managers or owners Program run by three full-time staff members and two part-time staff members CIPP continues to accept the main responsibility for program direction Variety of stakeholders provide significant human capital Program has a range of media at its disposal for educational purposes (e.g., brochures, advertisements, mini-workshops)	Range of educational and outreach strategies employed to reach target populations A variety of cultural and linguistic groups are targeted A suitable window guard was selected and recommended by Boston Public Health A range of stakeholders participate in various components of the program's implementation Community residents and property managers played an active role Data has been gathered on stakeholder involvement, rates of guard installation, sales levels, and injury rates Voluntary Adopt-a-Building campaign further facilitated guard installation	By 1997, 11,400 guards were installed in the Boston area By 1998, the media campaign reached an estimated 381,000 people through major and local newspapers There have been 7,520,000 PSA radio announcements in English, Spanish, and Haitian Creole Kids Can't Fly resulted in an 83% decrease in the number of window falls from 1993 to 1995; and a 50% decrease between 1993 and 1997 (US Department of Health and Human Services, 1998) In 2000, there was a 95% reduction in window falls since the inception of the program and a total of three falls in 2000 In 2005, there was only one reported fall from a window

Life Space Model: Kids Can't Fly

Sociocultural: civilization/community	Interpersonal: primary and secondary relationships	Physical environments: where we live	Internal states: biochemical/genetic and means of coping
Awareness raising that window falls do occur and are preventable Use of public health agencies to deliver and promote prevention messages Policy development and legislative support for a falls prevention program Multi-faceted approach that includes community health practitioners, residents, property managers and owners, local merchants, housing agencies, and local and city-level governments	Relationship among caregivers and community health and housing agencies to increase knowledge and education of window fall risk and prevention Relationship between property managers/owners and the CIPP to share responsibility for window guard installation	Hard surfaces in the urban landscape Laws of gravity Evaluation of the characteristics of the built environment to adopt appropriate preventative measures Adoption of appropriate window guard technology	Empowerment of caregivers and property managers and owners by offering training on installations Ownership of safety initiatives by property managers/owners through a "buy-in" program of window guards

References

Boston Public Health Commission. (2006). *Boston experience 1992–2005: Number of children fallen from windows*. Boston, MA: Author.

Boston Public Health Commission. (2007). *Kids can't fly. Facts on window falls and child safety window guards* [Brochure]. Boston, MA: Author

Boston Public Health Commission. (n.d.-a). *Childhood injury prevention: Kids can't fly*. Boston, MA: Author.

Boston Public Health Commission. (n.d.-b). Windows falls prevention. Retrieved from http://www.bphc.org/whatwedo/childrens-health/injury-prevention/safe-at-home/Pages/Window-Falls-Prevention.aspx#

Bourgeois, R., Noce, M., Smeh, D., & Morton, T. (2007). *Sustainability of community-based health interventions: A literature review*. Unpublished manuscript, University of Toronto, Toronto, ON.

Boyle, M., & Willms, J. D. (2002). Impact evaluation of a national, community-based program for at-risk children in Canada. *Canadian Public Policy, 28*(3), 461–481.

ChildSafetyGates.com. (2007). *Guardian angel window guard-model 2335*. Retrieved May 10, 2007 from www.child-safety-gates.com

Connecticut SafeKids. (2006). *For Parents, Kids can't fly* [Brochure]. Connecticut: Author.

Durlak, J. A. (1997). *Successful prevention programs for children and adolescents*. New York, NY: Plenum Press.

Fairfax County Fire and Rescue Department. (2006). *Kids can't fly: Make your windows no-falls zones!* [Brochure]. Fairfax, VA: Author.

Howell, E. M., Devaney, B., McCormick, M., & Raykovich, K. T. (1998). Back to the future: Community involvement in the Healthy Start Program. *Journal of Health Politics, Policy and Law, 23*(2), 291–317.

Inova Regional Trauma Center. (2002). *Annual report. Inova-Fairfax Hospital for Children*. Falls Church, VA: Author.

Iowa Department of Public Health. (2002). *Iowa health focus. Keep kids safe: Watch those windows* [Brochure]. Des Moines, IA: Author.

Johnson, K., Hays, C., Center, H., & Daley, C. (2004). Building capacity and sustainable prevention innovations: A sustainability planning model. *Evaluation and Program Planning, 27*(2), 135–149.

Jones, M. B., & Offord, D. R. (1991). *After the demonstration project*. Paper presented at the 1991 annual meeting of the Advancement of Science, Washington, DC.

Metropolitan Boston Housing Partnership. (2005). *Mbhp@home: Kids can't fly* [Brochure]. Boston, MA: Author.

New York City Department of Health and Mental Hygiene. (2007). *Window falls prevention program: Frequently asked questions*. Retrieved April 23, 2007 from http://www.nyc.gov/html/doh/html/win/winfaq.shtml

Oregon Health Services Unit. (n.d.). *Kids can't fly: Protect your child from window falls*. Retrieved April 4, 2007, from www.ohsu.edu/trauma/injuryprevention.html

Ramsey, C. T., & Ramsey, S. L. (1998). Early intervention and early experience. *American Psychologist, 53*(2), 109–120.

Screen Manufacturers Association. (2007). *SMA safety programs*. Retrieved March 29, 2007, from www.sma-central.org/safety/html

Tard, C., Ouellet, H., & Beaudoin, A. (1998). *Program evaluation for organizations under the Community Action Program for Children (CAPC). Introductory manual*. Quebec, QC: Université Laval Centre de recherché sure les services communautaires.

U.S. Department of Health and Human Services. (1998). *Kids can't fly: Strategy transfer guide. Models that work*. Bethesda, MD: Department of Health and Human Services Bureau of Primary Health Care.

Vish, N. L., Powell, E. C., Wiltsek, D., & Sheehan, K. M. (2005). Pediatric window falls: Not just a problem for children in high rises. *Injury Prevention, 11*, 300–303.

Fall Safe Project: West Virginia

Kim Ceurstemont

The Fall-Safe intervention program aims to reduce workplace falls in the construction industry. The program educates contractors through a certification program and implements accountability measures to increase and improve the use of established fall prevention practices and technologies.

14.1 Background

14.1.1 Becker and Fullen's Fall-Safe Intervention

It is known that most injuries in construction are caused by falls; many of these result in severe neurotrauma and spinal cord injury. Still, workers are passively observing safety practices, and existing prevention initiatives are not being consistently implemented in the workplace (Musick, 2016). In fact, in the 2016 fiscal year, the Occupational Safety, and Health Association (OSHA) ranked fall protection as the number one violation for the sixth straight year (Musick, 2016). As a result, the OSHA consistently cites falls as the leading cause of death in the construction industry (Occupational Safety and Health Administration [OSHA], n.d.).

The Fall-Safe intervention established by Becker, Fullen, Akladios, and Hobbs (2001) represents an exemplary practice in occupational fall prevention. It is presented here as a multilevel case study and should be viewed from the perspective of an opportunity for improvement in practice and research on falls in the construction industry. The nature of the Fall-Safe intervention, which entails an ecological setting, is such that it does not lend itself very easily to the control required by experimental research. Nonetheless, the authors used a quasi-experimental method employing both control and experimental groups, which is a rare occurrence in this field of study. The Fall-Safe intervention therefore stands apart from other fall-prevention strategies mentioned in the literature, which do not have data to support their efficacy.

The Fall-Safe intervention was initiated in 1998 in response to an evident gap in fall prevention literature (Becker et al., 2001). It is an initiative developed by the Safety and Health Extension at West Virginia University (WVU), an organizational intervention. Fall-Safe targets construction contractors and, through education, aims to increase the use of established fall prevention practices and technologies.

The Fall-Safe program uses a contractor certification program to improve the use of existing fall prevention practices. The program involves developing or rewriting a company fall protection policy, worker and supervisor training, and

K. Ceurstemont (✉)
Toronto, ON, Canada

R. Volpe (ed.), *Casebook of Traumatic Injury Prevention*,
https://doi.org/10.1007/978-3-030-27419-1_14

implementation of the Fall-Safe fall hazard management system. Fall-Safe involves two kinds of accountability systems: supervision by competent workers within the contracting companies and supervision by an independent third party (WVU staff).

The Fall-Safe training program and hazard control audits are based on the fall protection standards of the OSHA. The main OSHA requirements applicable to construction contractors are as follows:

1. Where protection is required, select fall protection systems appropriate for given situations
2. Use proper construction and installation of safety systems
3. Supervise employees properly
4. Use safe work procedures
5. Train workers in the proper selection, use, and maintenance of all protection systems (U.S. Department of Labor, 1996)

These standards identify areas where fall protection is needed (e.g., at an elevation of 6 ft or where there is a danger of falling into dangerous equipment).

Various fall protection measures are acceptable, such as guardrail systems, safety net systems, personal fall arrest systems (see Fig. 14.1), positioning device systems, and warning line systems. Employers must select a fall protection measure that is compatible with the type of work being performed.

14.1.2 Project Aims

The intervention focused on the reduction of falls in the construction industry. As discussed above, fall-related accidents are the leading cause of fatalities and injuries in this occupational setting (OSHA, n.d.). These fatalities are preventable (OSHA, n.d.).

Effective fall-prevention procedures are available; the safety literature advocates countless fall-prevention practices, such as placing railings around roofs (National Institute for Occupational Safety and Health [NIOSH], 1989) and the use of

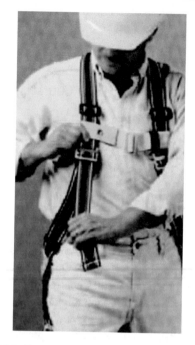

Fig. 14.1 Strategy to reduce fall-related injuries: *Personal protective equipment. Falls. Construction Safety*, by the Construction Safety Association of Ontario, 2003

personal protective equipment (International Safety Equipment Foundation [ISEA], n.d.; Musick, 2016).

However, the use of such safety practices and technologies are not widely and consistently implemented among construction contractors (ISEA, n.d.). There remains an evident need for an intervention like Fall-Safe, which aims to improve contractors' adherence to fall-prevention procedures.

The comprehensive objectives of the Fall-Safe intervention are as follows:

- Decrease incidence of construction falls in West Virginia
- Improve the ability of contractors to manage and control construction fall hazards
- Determine if the pilot model for Fall-Safe developed in West Virginia can be successfully marketed and implemented in other parts of the nation
- Determine if the Fall-Safe Partnership offers sufficient benefits to contractors to become economically self-sufficient

- Determine if implementation of the Fall-Safe Partnership leads to an increase in the quality of site-specific fall prevention plans
- Determine if implementation of the Fall-Safe Partnership leads to an improvement in fall prevention audit scores at construction sites belonging to Fall-Safe contractors
- Determine if implementation of the Fall-Safe Partnership leads to fewer construction fall injuries as measured by claims made to Workers' Compensation (West Virginia University [WVU], 2002)

14.2 Resources

14.2.1 Financial Resources

The Fall-Safe intervention was funded by the National Institute for Occupational Safety and Health (NIOSH) and the Center to Protect Workers' Rights (CPWR) in Washington, D.C. At the onset of the program, NIOSH provided a $2.41 million grant, and CPWR provided over $1.1 million in grants. The Construction Safety Council (CSC) and St. Paul Fire and Marine Insurance Company (St. Paul FMIC) have served as sponsors for the extension of the Fall-Safe program in the Midwest. The program was fully funded by grants, and there were no fees to the contractors for participation.

Overall, the Co-Principle Investigator of Fall-Safe estimated that, in the early 2000s, the approximate cost to run the program was $12,000 per contractor, per year. For a construction company to engage in such an intervention independently, it was estimated at the time of publication (Becker et al., 2001) that the cost could be $10,000. This amount includes the costs to the company, as well as the fees to a third-party partner.

14.2.2 Human Resources

Key informant—Mark Fullen, one of Fall-Safe's two principle researchers, is well respected in the field of public health. He has worked for over 10 years in the domain of occupational safety and health. Among his experiences in the field, Fullen has worked as a safety director and safety engineer for construction companies. Additionally, Fullen has worked at West Virginia University (WVU) as a construction safety and health specialist and clinical instructor. He has developed and taught many safety and health classes to a wide range of students, including business owners and managers. As of the updates made to this case in 2017, he is now an associate professor at WVU and simultaneously holds the position of WVU's Extension Director of Safety and Health.

Many groups of people from various vocational backgrounds were involved in the operation of Fall-Safe. The Principle Investigator (PI) of the intervention was Paul Becker and the Co-PI was Mark Fullen. Both were professors at WVU. The PI developed the intervention model and conceived the audit tool architecture. He also conducted statistical analyses and was the first author of the publication on Fall-Safe. The Co-PI was the field person or change agent. He worked directly with the contractors conducting training sessions, field audits, annual meetings, and administering the partnerships with the CSC and St. Paul FMIC.

Over the time the program was run, there were on average 2.25 other WVU staff members assisting with the project. One faculty member was employed to conduct audits, one employed as support staff, and 0.25 of a person employed to help with marketing. Assistant professor Brandon Takacs assisted the PI in the final analyses of the program, including the measurement of injury reduction.

The WVU Health and Safety Extension acts as a certifying organization for construction contractors in West Virginia. During the time of this program, WVU staff also assumed the role of a third-party mediator or a team of overseers external to the company. They assisted contractors in developing a site-specific handbook of fall prevention and spent 8 h training company supervisors and 2 h training other company workers. Furthermore, the WVU team monitored compliance with all aspects of the program by conducting quarterly surprise audits, which included a thorough inspection of the construction site.

Another major component of the intervention involved incentives for the construction companies. In addition to training and consultation on fall prevention, WVU staff provided the contractors with marketing and public relations assistance, which helped to increase their revenue.

The contractors themselves played a major role in the intervention. Many different supervisors were designated within each construction company: site-specific supervisors who monitored the construction site for fall hazards on a daily basis, company supervisors who conducted weekly audits, and a Fall-Safe committee that conducted monthly inspections (see Fig. 14.2). Furthermore, the intervention involved regular meetings. Supervisors were able to consult with the WVU team as needed.

Fall-Safe was piloted by the Health and Safety Extension of WVU. The initial success of the pilot intervention drew the attention of the CSC and St. Paul FMIC. These organizations became franchise partners for the expansion of the intervention. Hence, Fall-Safe was a partnership between WVU, CSC, and St. Paul FMIC.

14.3 Implementation

14.3.1 The Contractors

The program involves a partnership between WVU and West Virginia construction contractors. Sixteen contractors agreed to participate under the conditions specified by the WVU Fall-Safe coordinators. The duration of the first implementation phase was 1.5 years.

The first implementation of Fall-Safe began in 1998 and consisted of ten experimental contractor companies and six control companies. They were selected based on willingness to participate in the program. The stipulations of the program were outlined in a handbook (participant's handbook) made available to contractors. The type of construction work carried out by the selected contractors ranged from general contract work to roofing and highway contractors. The yearly employment of the contractors was estimated to range between 50 and 250 employees.

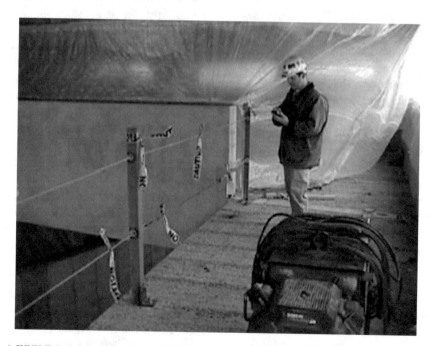

Fig. 14.2 A WVU Fall-Safe coordinator audits a guard rail at a Fall-Safe contractor's site. Reprinted from *NIOSH Construction Compendium: Intervention*, by the National Institute for Occupational Safety and Health, 2002

14.3.2 Awareness Raising

Substantial project resources were devoted to marketing the intervention to contractors. The coordinators of Fall-Safe ensured that there were adequate incentives for contractors such that their earnings would increase as a result of their participation. Intensive marketing and public relation strategies were implemented regarding the contractors' efforts to reduce fall-related morbidity and mortality. WVU obtained the endorsement of the Appalachian Construction Users Council (ACUC), the regional organization of industrial plants who regularly use construction services. The ACUC sent letters to all potential construction companies in support of the Fall-Safe program.

A Fall-Safe logo was designed (see Fig. 14.3). Paraphernalia imprinted with the Fall-Safe logo was manufactured (e.g., cups, clipboards, pencils, participation cards, etc.). WVU Fall-Safe signs were made for participating contractors to place on construction sites. An inauguration ceremony was held, and press releases were issued to contractors' local media in order to publicize the beginning of the Fall-Safe program.

Fall-Safe coordinators at WVU also established a website and published a series of Fall-Safe Newsletters. The newsletters published the names of participating contractors and informed participating parties of updates, particular accomplishments, and other news.

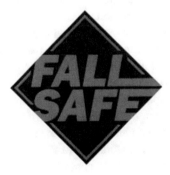

Fig. 14.3 The Fall-Safe logo. Reprinted from *NIOSH Construction Compendium: Intervention*, by the National Institute for Occupational Safety and Health, 2002

14.3.3 Procedures

In addition to providing valuable incentives and marketing to the contractors, the developers of Fall-Safe had postulated that two other elements were crucial to the success of the program. First, the intervention should be fairly intense in order to produce a measurable outcome. Second, the intervention should involve well-established accountability systems to ensure the ongoing adherence to safety practices.

At the onset of the intervention, participating contractors were asked to sign a contractual agreement (see Box 14.1) whereby they agree to implement the fall hazard management system developed by WVU. They were given the public status of Fall-Safe contractor. To retain this status, they had to maintain an acceptable level of compliance with the program.

Box 14.1 The Fall-Safe Contract
Contractual agreement

In order to decrease falls in the construction industry, WVU Safety and Health Extension and [name of contractor] enter into the following agreement.

Contractor's Name

Agrees to carry out the Fall-Safe program as described in the participant's handbook.

Agrees to allow and facilitate examination and audit of the contractor's Fall-Safe performance as described in the participant's handbook.

May terminate this agreement with 2 weeks' written notice.

West Virginia University Safety and Health Extension

Agrees to provide consultation to participating contractor as described in the participant's handbook.

Agrees to provide training and materials to participating contractor as described in the participant's handbook.

Agrees to audit and report results to participating contractor as described in the participant's handbook.

(continued)

(continued)

Authorizes participating contractor to use the designation West Virginia University (WVU) Fall-Safe participant.

May terminate authorization above with a 2-week written notice if participating contractor is found by WVU Safety and Health Extension staff to be in significant non-compliance with this agreement.

The duration of this agreement is 1 year.
From..
To..
Paul Becker for WVU [signature]
Date..
Contractor's Representative [signature]
Date..

Reprinted from "Prevention of Construction Falls by Organizational Intervention," by P. Becker, M. Fullen, M. Akladios, G. Hobbs, 2001, Injury Prevention, 7.

hazards. Company-wide competent persons performed inspections every week, and the Fall-Safe committee performed inspections every month.

The second accountability system involved WVU staff, who acted as third-party overseers. To ensure safety, the WVU staff audited adherence to hazard control in terms of training, inspections, and meetings. Six surprise audits were carried out by the WVU staff over the 1½ years of the program (i.e., one audit approximately every 3 months). Each time the company was evaluated based on the OSHA requirements. Each potential hazard was evaluated for effective control, and a score was given for each hazard location and jobsite. If the company did not meet a criterion score of 70% on two successive audits, they were no longer eligible to participate in the program. The WVU coordinators also ensured that the required training, inspections, and meetings had taken place. Feedback was provided to the contractor.

Knowledge dissemination was another important element of the Fall-Safe intervention. WVU staff provided 8 h of fall prevention training for all supervisors and 2 h for all workers. The program content complies with OSHA's fall regulations for the construction industry, and the WVU team provided consultation as needed regarding fall prevention.

The WVU staff and contractors worked together to develop a company fall protection policy and to write a site-specific fall prevention program. Several members of the company staff took an active role in the program. In addition to having site supervisors, each company designated company-wide and site-specific competent persons and established a labor management Fall-Safe committee. Regular hazard-control meetings were held.

Fall-Safe involved two kinds of accountability systems. The first accountability system was within the contracting company. Competent persons within each company engaged in safety planning prior to construction and monitored hazards as each job was carried out. Site supervisors performed daily jobsite inspections of fall

14.3.4 Program Tracking

The dependent variable (i.e., fall safety practices) was tracked via the use of a handheld auditing computer. The device was equipped with special software designed to catalogue all possible fall hazard conditions on a construction site. The auditing device was used daily by the contract companies and by the WVU staff when they performed quarterly inspections of the job site.

Information entered into the auditing tool was used to evaluate contractors' fall prevention practices and their compliance with OSHA standards related to construction falls. The data entered into the auditing tool was compiled and could be used to analyze changes in scores over time. The scores were also used to compare Fall-Safe contractors to contractors in the control condition.

The impact of the pilot intervention was also measured via the administration of opinion and activity questionnaires to the company owners, supervisors, and workers. For the ten experimental groups and the six control groups, questionnaires were filled out at the preintervention stage, as well as at the postintervention stage (after

1.5 years). Fall-Safe extended its project to compare the actual rate of fall-related injuries between intervention and control groups. Workers' Compensation claims for falls were examined.

14.4   Outcome

14.4.1   Data Analyses

Becker et al. (2001) examined the data to determine the presence of differences between the experimental and control contractors. Audit data were aggregated for experimental and control groups and examined using a one-way analysis of variance (Becker et al., 2001).

Figure 14.4 depicts the hazard control audit scores of the contractors. Becker et al.'s (2001) analysis of hazard control scores revealed no statistically significant difference between the experimental and control groups at baseline. By the last inspection, there was a greater improvement in hazard control by the experimental group (11 percentage points) versus the control group (5 percentage points); however, the difference was slightly below the level required for significance ($p = 0.06$; Becker et al., 2001).

Figure 14.5 depicts the program audit scores of the contractors, which measure practices such as training, inspection, and meetings (Becker et al., 2001). By the last inspection, there was a greater improvement in program implementation

by the experimental group (21 percentage points) versus the control group (8 percentage points); the difference was statistically significant ($p = 0.02$; Becker et al., 2001). Furthermore, there was a significant relationship between "practice" scores and hazard control scores (Becker et al., 2001). Thus, there is statistical evidence that the Fall-Safe intervention is effective in improving the fall prevention practices of construction contractors (Becker et al., 2001).

14.4.2   Feedback

Fall-Safe was well received by the participating companies. The contractors felt that Fall-Safe would reduce their Workers' Compensation premiums and result in increased market share value for their companies (Becker et al., 2001). The positive public relations generated by Fall-Safe in the local communities were also desirable to the contractors. A high percentage of companies reported that they would be willing to pay for the program internally. Fuller started but did not publish a qualitative study of the intervention, and the comments from contractors were overwhelmingly positive. They especially liked the third-party auditing of worksites and the subsequent feedback for improvement. Hence, the program was successfully marketed to the contractors, and they held that it benefited them.

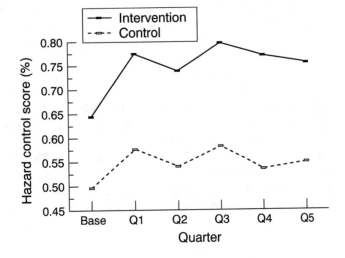

Fig. 14.4 Mean contractor hazard control audit scores by quarter. Reprinted from "Prevention of Construction Falls by Organizational Intervention," by P. Becker, M. Fullen, M. Akladios, G. Hobbs, 2001, Injury Prevention, 7, i66

Fig. 14.5 Mean contractor program audit scores by quarter. Reprinted from "Prevention of Construction Falls by Organizational Intervention," by P. Becker, M. Fullen, M. Akladios, G. Hobbs, 2001, Injury Prevention, 7, i66

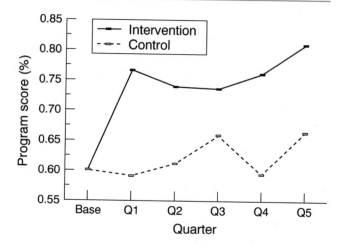

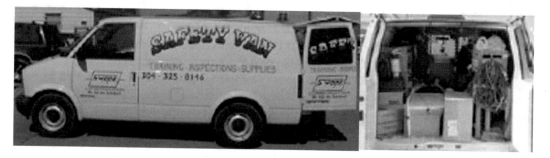

Fig. 14.6 The swope safety van. Reprinted from the Fall-Safe Newsletter, 2002

The positive reception of the program by the contractors can be demonstrated by the development of a special Swope Safety Van by Swope Construction, one of the participating companies (see Fig. 14.6). The company workers proudly drove it to the Fall-Safe training center at WVU to show the staff this vehicle, which is fully stocked with safety equipment. This undertaking was reported in the Fall-Safe newsletter.

Although Fall-Safe did not track the incidence of fall-related injuries over the course of the intervention, an event occurred that qualitatively demonstrated the efficacy of the intervention. In 2001, a construction worker fell off a roof, and another worker fell 24 ft from a bridge. Fortunately, both workers were saved from serious injury because appropriate fall protection was in place. They both worked for construction companies using the Fall-Safe program.

14.4.3 Expansion

WVU received additional grants in 1999 permitting the Fall-Safe coordinators to extend the intervention to more contractors. The university had the opportunity to work with 16 additional contractors. Overall, WVU worked with contractors in the following states: West Virginia, Virginia, Pennsylvania, Maryland, Washington DC, and Ohio. Fall-Safe was expanded in follow-up studies to Chicago, St. Paul FMIC (St. Paul, MN), and a larger group in the West Virginia area. These data were never published (M. Fuller, personal communication, 2017).

The report by Becker et al. (2001) mentioned that a follow-up study was in progress, in which additional audit data were being collected such that the long-term efficacy of the program could be evaluated. Although these results are not yet available, the authors report that the outcomes are very similar to those published in 2001. The author also noted that they were unable to measure actual changes in fall incidents or injuries at the time. Future reports will include multiple analyses of Workers' Compensation claims for falls in both intervention and control groups. Intervention groups will also be compared to other similar contractors in the Workers' Compensation database who have not received the intervention. Preliminary investigations of worker compensation claims indicated that Fall-Safe contractors reduced claims with respect to falls. This, in turn, resulted in lower insurance premiums. The success of Fall-Safe also led to the further development of computer-based audit equipment. New audit systems permit construction companies to monitor their own jobsites.

Further, the audit system developed in the Fall-Safe program led to further research (M. Fullen, personal communication, October 18, 2017). Some of the further research included an electrical standard study. This program used a different audit philosophy than the Fall-Safe program. In the electrical standard study, the audit was in the hands of a competent worker and a foreman would sign off on this. The Fall-Safe program, comparably, was a management-driven system with feedback from workers. There were also some other research groups that used the Fall-Safe audit system. For example, one group used the audit system as an instrument to collect data for a resident home builders project.

M. Fullen (personal communication, October 18, 2017) also mentioned that his research group received funding in 2016 for a new project in the logging industry, Timber Safe, which will again build off of the audit system from Fall-Safe. For this project, they have fine-tuned the audit system further and developed it into a mobile application (M. Fullen, personal communication, October 18, 2017). The development of this application has been published in a technical journal. It would allow for jobsite audits to focus on relevant aspects in detail. The goal for this application is that researchers could collect data across a range of disciplines (M. Fullen, personal communication, October 18, 2017).

14.5   Conclusion

Fall-related injuries in the construction industry account for a large proportion of occupational morbidity and mortality; however, there is a scarcity of appraised programs aimed at reducing the incidence of falls in the construction industry. The coordinators of Fall-Safe must therefore be commended for their contribution to the field. Although there was no direct measure of injuries due to falls during the study by Becker et al. (2001), the abovementioned results implied that the program had potential to reduce the incidence of fall-related injuries and effectively promoted adaptive change within the systems involved in injury. The research component of Fall-Safe demonstrated that its methodology was able to improve the fall prevention practices in construction companies.

The Fall-Safe program included three main effective strategies: training, inspections, and incentives. Training all workers within the companies ensured that all employees were aware of the OSHA standards and fall-protection equipment. A notable element of the Fall-Safe program was its two-part accountability system: internal accountability within the contracting companies and external accountability by an independent third party (WVU staff). Moreover, as evidenced by the contractors' comments, the incentives were necessary to ensure that the companies would obtain tangible benefits from the work invested.

The Fall-Safe strategies have been found to be important in the occupational safety literature. Inadequate training has been implicated in workplace falls (Hsiao & Simeonov, 2001), and fall hazard inspections have been found to decrease the claim rate for fall-related injuries (Nelson, Kaufman, Kalat, & Silverstein, 1997). The inclusion of incentives was an insightful addition to the Fall-Safe program, and the combination of three strategies was indubitably important in achieving the observed change in practices and hazard controls.

As a field research project, Fall-Safe's practicality should be emphasized. The positive outcomes of the intervention demonstrate its applicability to real-life conditions. Moreover,

Becker et al. (2001) used a research model that is not often employed in testing methods in construction. This study is an inspiration for more researchers in this area to employ experimental methodologies.

While the use of quasi-experimental methodology by Becker et al. (2001) is laudable, there are some limitations inherent in this methodology. First, random assignment is unattainable, and recruiting contractors as controls is difficult. Second, there can be contamination of the control group if a Fall-Safe trained employee moves to a control side. Also, the inspection of the Fall-Safe auditor may have an impact on the control group.

The success of the Fall-Safe intervention resulted in support by funding organizations and expansion across the U.S. While the original Fall-Safe is no longer used, it did inspire other prevention programs, and various parts of it are still used (M. Fullen, personal communication, October 18, 2017). Given the high rate of fall accidents, it is evident that Fall-Safe is a cost-effective prevention program when the cost of accidents is compared with the cost of the intervention. In 2001, a single fall-related accident could cost hundreds of thousands of dollars, whereas Fall-Safe was estimated, at the time, to cost $10,000 per company per year.

Acknowledgments The author would like to express sincere appreciation to Mark Fullen and Brandon Takacs of the West Virginia University Safety & Health Extension in Morgantown, WV, USA, who consulted as the key informants on this case study.

BRIO Model: Fall Safe

Group Served: Construction Workers.

Goal: To prevent avoidable injury from falls on construction sites.

Background	Resources	Implementation	Outcome
Most deaths in the construction injury are caused by falls which have been shown to result in head trauma and death Non-fatal falls also have serious repercussions: permanent disability, lost time and wages, long treatments, and rehabilitation Most falls are preventable Existing fall prevention programs are not being used and fall prevention techniques are not being implemented Programs are needed to increase the use of existing fall prevention practices and techniques Strategies include training, inspections, and incentives Training component is based on the fall prevention standards of the OSHA	Funded by the National Institute for Occupational Safety and Health, also the Center to Protect Workers' Rights Operated under West Virginia University Crucial to the success of the program: intervention needed to involve a combination of strategies, it needed to be intense to provide measurable outcomes, and include well-established accountability systems to ensure adherence to safety practices	Adherence to and evaluation of OHSA standards were tracked with an auditing computer (pilot) Impact of pilot was also measured through opinion and activity questionnaires distributed to company owners, workers, supervisors	Program effective in significantly improving use of prevention practices Incidence reductions are assumed through increased use of safe practices and observations of prevented injury at individual construction sites Program was deemed practical and applicable and was well received by participating companies West Virginia has extended the intervention to more construction contractors and further development of computer-based audit equipment

Life Space Model: Fall Safe

Sociocultural: Civilization/community	Interpersonal: Primary and secondary relationships	Physical environments: Where we live	Internal states: Biochemical/genetic and means of coping
Raised awareness of fall risk factors and preventative practices among workers, companies, and governing bodies Program impacts the way in which falls are viewed by the entire construction industry Program components decreased company and societal costs associated with fall-related injury	Multilevel program involvement has the potential to create positive relations and networks The way in which all tiers of the construction industry relate to one another will incorporate program knowledge	The identification of multi-factorial antecedents to falls contribute to safety Empirical assessment of risk for falling protects safety Use of auditing computer organizes the environment and facilitates safety	Program can increase the quality of life, security and self-efficacy among workers, companies, contractors, governing bodies Reception of incentives in combination with work involved reinforces safe behavior and increases self-confidence and ability

References

Becker, P., Fullen, M., Akladios, M., & Hobbs, G. (2001). Prevention of construction falls by organizational intervention. *Injury Prevention, 7*(Suppl I), i64–i67.

Construction Safety Association of Ontario. (2003). Falls. Construction safety, Special Issue (B039), 1–8.

Fall-Safe Newsletter. (2002, Spring). Retrieved January 28, 2005 from www.wvu.edu/~exten/depts/she/vol31.pdf

Hsiao, H., & Simeonov, P. (2001). Preventing falls from roofs: A critical review. *Ergonomics, 44*(5), 537–561.

International Safety Equipment Foundation. (n.d.). *Personal protective equipment use in heavy construction trends upward.* Retrieved January 28, 2005, from http://www.safetyequipment.org/workzone/survey.htm

Musick, T. (2016, November). OSHA's top 10 most cited violations for 2016. Safety and Health Magazine, 194(6), pp. 44–52. Retrieved October 2, 2017, from www.safetyandhealthmagazine.com

National Institute for Occupational Safety and Health. (1989). *Preventing worker deaths and injuries from falls through skylights and roof openings* [DHHS 90-100]. Washington, DC: U.S. Government Printing Office.

National Institute for Occupational Safety and Health. (2002). *NIOSH construction compendium: Interventions.* Retrieved January 28, 2005, from http://www.cdc.gov/elcosh/docs/d0100/d000107/interventions.html

Nelson, N., Kaufman, J., Kalat, J., & Silverstein, B. (1997). Falls in construction: Injury rates for OSHA-inspected employers before and after citation for violating the Washington state fall protection standard. *American Journal of Industrial Medicine, 31*, 296–302.

Occupational Health and Safety Administration. (n.d.). *Welcome to OSHA's fall prevention campaign.* Retrieved October 2, 2017, from www.osha.gov

U.S. Department of Labor. (1996). *Construction Safety and Health Outreach Program: Fall protection.* Retrieved January 28, 2005, from http://www.osha.gov/doc/outreachtraining/htmlfiles/subpartm.html

West Virginia University – Extension Service. (2002). *Annual report of accomplishments and results, fiscal year 2001: October 1, 2000–September 30, 2001.* Morgantown, WV: Author.

The Stay On Your Feet (SOYF) New South Wales Program

15

Gilla K. Shapiro

Stay on Your Feet (SOYF) is a multifactorial prevention program aimed at reducing the incidence of falls experienced by people over 60 years old.

15.1 Background

The rapid acceleration of aging has important implications for public health, health systems, and health expenditure (World Health Organization [WHO], 2015). The frequency of falls and serious associated consequences increases with age and frailty (WHO, 2007). The Stay on Your Feet (SOYF) program was developed in New South Wales, Australia, in 1992 in response to the need for an evaluated fall prevention program based on published epidemiological evidence (Kempton et al., 1998). The aim of this program was to decrease the number and severity of falls experienced by individuals over 60 years of age through a multistrategic, population-based prevention approach where success could be measured (Garner, Kempton, & van Beurden, 1996). SOYF was designed to be a community-level intervention operating through community mobilization to reduce injury. This program targeted individuals who were living in the community, in other words living in accommodation that they control (not in institutional settings; Kempton et al., 1998). A community intervention was thought to be more effective than targeting high-risk subgroups because the incidence of falls and related injury is substantial among otherwise healthy older individuals, and most fall-related risk factors are relatively common (McClure et al., 2010). The principles underpinning the SOYF program stem from the Ottawa Charter for Health Promotion (WHO, 1986) and the Jakarta Declaration for Health promotion (WHO, 1997), which declares that health promotion efforts should develop personal skills, create supportive environments conducive to health, strengthen community action for health, reorient health services toward health promotion and disease prevention, and build public policy directed toward achieving these aims (Powell, Wilkins, Leiper, & Gillam, 2000).

The initial SOYF program was implemented from 1992 to 1996 on the North Coast of New South Wales (NSW), Australia. This area was strategically chosen because the proportion and growth rate of the older population exceeded the Australian national average. The population of older adults on the North Coast included 90,000 (or 21% of the entire population) individuals who were noninstitutionalized and aged 60 years and over (Garner et al., 1996; Hahn, van Beurden, Kempton, Sladden, & Garner, 1996; Sladden, 1993). The rate of falling among older North

G. K. Shapiro (✉)
Department of Supportive Care, Princess Margaret Cancer Centre, University Health Network, Toronto, ON, Canada
e-mail: gilla.shapiro@uhnresearch.ca

© Springer Nature Switzerland AG 2020
R. Volpe (ed.), *Casebook of Traumatic Injury Prevention*,
https://doi.org/10.1007/978-3-030-27419-1_15

Coast's residents was high, and approximately 2 in 9 individuals experienced a fall each year (approximately 20,000 individuals; Garner et al., 1996). The initial evaluation of 2,000 older adults from the intervention region was compared to 1,600 older adults living on the Sunshine Coast, Queensland, where there were no existing fall prevention activities (van Beurden, Kempton, Sladden, & Garner, 1998). The regions were otherwise similar from a demographic and geographic standpoint. The evaluation of SOYF demonstrated a significant 20% reduction rate of fall-related hospital admissions (van Beurden et al., 1998). The reported success of SOYF has resulted in wide replication and adaptation of the SOFY program in other states of Australia and internationally (Beard et al., 2006).

15.1.1 Program Objectives

The aim of the SOFY program was to reduce falls and subsequent injury among older persons (60 years and over) in the general, noninstitutionalized, community (Hahn et al., 1996; Kempton et al., 1998). SOYF planned to develop a multistrategic prevention approach that addressed the lifestyle and medical causes of elderly falls and evaluate the cost-effectiveness, sustainability, and outcome of the program. This process involved many stages, including (Kempton et al., 1998; van Beurden et al., 1998):

- A literature review and community consultation to ascertain the extent of knowledge on fall prevention and strategies (in 1992).
- Analysis of health data regarding North Coast fall demographics and determining a baseline of the levels of fall risk factors on the North Coast.
- An assessment of community needs through focus group discussions.
- An overview of current fall prevention policy and practice in North Coast local government.
- Inclusion of specific principles in relation to health promotion with older people as identi-

fied in the Ottawa Charter for Health Promotion.
- Determining delivery methods for interventions that are sustainable.
- Developing an exemplary model for community-based fall interventions that is cost-effective and sustainable.
- Undertaking an evaluation of exemplary strategies by using a pre/post intervention repeated measure design with comparison to national, state, and local fall-related data.
- Refining the model based on research outcomes.
- Disseminating findings.

15.2 Resources

The total cost of the 4-year SOFY program (in Australian dollars) was $600,000, including evaluation (Kempton, van Beurden, Sladden, Garner, & Beard, 2000). According to the Interbank rate, the cost of SOYF in Australian dollars equaled $406,800 American dollars on January 1, 1994 (Ganz & Wu, 2007). Using the inflation calculator at the Bureau of Labor Statistics website (www.bls.gov), this equals $594,792.66 in 2010 US dollars.

This calculation of total cost does not reflect all the costs associated with the program, including the contributory costs incurred by community networks such as government agencies, health promotion agencies, medical organizations, and nongovernment organizations focused on seniors. For example, the Community Health Education Groups (CHEGS), a nonprofit, incorporated organization, received ongoing support and training from health promotion workers (Kempton et al., 1998). CHEGS took a community development approach by recruiting and training local seniors to run classes on fall prevention, recovering costs of class leaders by charging participants a fee. Further, the reported cost of SOYF does not include the time of clinicians (GPs), community health staff, and volunteers (Beard et al., 2006). According to Beard et al. (2006), "it was not possible to estimate a number of costs borne by the community arising from the program. Neither the cost of travel to classes nor the costs of home modification were recorded" (p. 744). This implies that the cost of running SOYF is greater than what was reported.

On the other hand, innovative schemes proposed in the original implementation of SOYF created savings that (likely) would not be present in future program replications. For example, awareness-raising partnerships were made with commercial networks to decrease distribution costs (Kempton et al., 1998). In one endeavor, SOYF proposed putting fall prevention messages on 316,000 milk cartons. This not only was an effective marketing mechanism but also resulted in the dairy company absorbing the distribution cost. Replications of SOYF may have to subsidize distribution and other costs that were avoided in the initial implementation.

Funding for SOYF was obtained from the NSW Health Department, and funding for the evaluation of SOYF was obtained from the National Health and Medical Research Council. Table 15.1 shows the monetary input of running SOYF. From the outset, evaluating SOYF was an integral aim of the program. The evaluation cost $145,000, and $137,000 of which was received from external funding (Table 15.1).

15.3   Implementation

15.3.1 Overview

SOYF planned to reduce elderly falls by addressing eight recognized lifestyle and medical causes for falling. These factors are insufficient physical activity, inadequate management of medications (especially when multiple drugs are used), poor and deteriorating vision, unsafe footwear, an underlying physical condition, muscle weakness, poor balance and gait, and home and public environmental hazards (Kempton et al., 1998; Tinetti, 2003; van Beurden et al., 1998).

Mindful of the salient risk factors, SOYF used an umbrella model that was designed to allow for a wide range of strategies. Five co-occurring strategies were integrated to ameliorate the risk of falling using different mechanisms. The program aimed to (1) raise awareness about the problem of falls and disseminate information on fall prevention, (2) increase community education, (3) reduce home hazards, (4) develop partnerships with health professionals, and (5) develop fall prevention policies (Hahn et al., 1996; Kempton et al., 1998). These major strategies were phased in during the implementation of the program, each encompassing numerous activities (as described below).

15.3.2 Individual Strategies to Implement SOYF

15.3.2.1   Public Awareness

Many older adults believe that falls are an unpreventable aspect of the aging process. Raising awareness among the target population was therefore undertaken in the earliest phase of the program to counter this view. The awareness campaign, which was also important in creating a SOYF brand identity, had two key messages: (1) falls are a significant health issue, and (2) falls are preventable (Kempton et al., 1998). This information was distributed through media outlets including television, radio, newspapers, milk

Table 15.1 Cost of the Stay on Your Feet Program (1992–1997)

	1992/1993	1993/1994	1994/1995	1995/1996	1996/1997
Salaries/wages	$79,076	$38,229	$62,222	$44,000	$18,625
Goods/services	$87,801	$53,500	$55,500	$86,000	$8750
Evaluation external grants		$50,000	$8000	$32,000	$55,000
Total	$166,877	$141,729	$125,722	$162,000	$82,375

Note: Data for this table are from *Stay on Your Feet Final Report: 1992–1996* by Kempton et al., 1998, Lismore, South Wales, Australia: Northern Rivers Health Service Institute of Health and Research. The data from 1996 to 1997 are from E. van Beurden, personal communication, n.d.

cartons, calendars, and fridge magnets (Kempton et al., 1998).

Media advertisement and the distribution of resources were the main methods for raising awareness. For example, on television, a series of 15 s community service messages that "life is better without a fall" were telecasted throughout 1993. In addition, a set of six community-service radio dialogues about fall prevention measures were developed and broadcasted on community radio networks (Kempton et al., 1998). Media strategies also informed the public about fall prevention activities through print outlets. The local radio stations also conducted interviews whereby community educators discussed fall prevention and the SOYF programs. Local newspapers also publicized SOYF activities. Another interesting venture was the organization of fall prevention expositions in several major towns and smaller communities.

Specialty products carrying fall prevention messages were distributed broadly to raise awareness. For example, a calendar was produced for each of the first 3 years of the program and distributed free of charge through pharmacies, general practitioners, and community health and education networks. A total of 47,000 calendars were distributed with positive images of older people, SOYF cartoons, and fall prevention messages (Kempton et al., 1998). A further 316,000 milk cartons carried fall prevention messages for 3 months in 1993 (Kempton et al., 1998).

Once the target group had been made aware that falls were preventable, the program began to provide clear, concise information about measures to prevent falls. Information dissemination activities involved the community in many ways. One initiative was providing a 3-year action plan to health workers and service providers within five health districts, as well as to government and nongovernment agencies. In 1993, SOYF also distributed 24,000 books on falling prevention to older people throughout the North Coast. Another book, published in 1994, distributed 30,000 copies by 1996.

SOYF also trained advisors in diverse areas who were responsible for disseminating information to the target group. Fall prevention advisors were aged 50 and older (mostly aged 60 and older). Advisors gave interviews about their work and assisted with SOYF efforts (e.g., by staffing expos and stalls). The fall prevention advisers could reach approximately 3,000 older people through talks and expositions at clubs and other venues (Kempton et al., 1998). Another initiative was the training and employment of nine Medication Workshop Leaders who, facilitated discussion groups on safe medication use on a part-time basis. Approximately 500 older adults attended these workshop sessions. Furthermore, 15 home safety advisors were trained to give presentations on fall prevention strategies and home safety products.

15.3.2.2 Community Education

As well as the face-to-face instruction given by fall prevention advisers, medication workshop leaders, and home safety advisors, the North Coast Community Health Education Groups (CHEGS) took several measures to orchestrate education at the community level (Kempton et al., 1998). SOYF used both health professionals and trained older individuals as community educators (Kempton et al., 1998). Fall prevention days were scheduled to educate the community about unsafe footwear, gentle exercise, and other fall prevention techniques. A "pill spill" campaign was a popular initiative that encouraged older people to dispose of outdated medication.

Workshops that focused on various aspects of fall prevention were also popular. For example, 950 older adults attended a 9-week gentle exercise workshop where they improved their balance and leg strength throughout the workshop. An interesting and well-received venture was the "Walking on Air" workshop. This program focused upon the care of feet by incorporating a massage, foot/ankle exercises, and a discussion about safe and unsafe footwear. Other community education efforts included belly dancing classes and walking stick decoration classes.

15.3.2.3 Home Safety Measures

A home safety checklist that provided a list of home modifications and safety products was developed. A 1993 seed grant enabled a community nurse and two students to trial a home safety checklist (Kempton ct al., 1998). Another initiative, the Home Safety Month, saw high participation from community businesses, with 90% of the 48 hardware stores and 100% of the 19 tile stores situated in the area participating in this project (Kempton et al., 1998). Furthermore, three quarters of the stores believed that the intervention was beneficial to their customers and staff, and half of the stores were later found to be stocking fall safety products (Kempton et al., 1998).

15.3.2.4 Health Professional Involvement

Both general practitioners (GPs) and community health nurses (CHNs) are key to a fall prevention strategy (Barnett et al., 2003; Kempton et al., 1998). This is partly because GPs and CHNs are an important source of health information (Barnett et al., 2003). As part of a SOYF initiative, a North Coast GP developed educational tools and outreach education to other GPs throughout the intervention region. This package included educational materials that addressed medications, patient fall-risk assessment, physical inactivity, foot problems, vision, and home hazards. In addition, information evenings were organized in conjunction with their Divisions of General Practice and the Certified Medical Education program (Kempton et al., 1998). One hundred GPs attended these information evenings, each receiving Certified Medical Education points.

Another venture was the development of a referral pad by which community health nurses could refer at-risk older clients to a range of additional services important to fall prevention, such as occupational therapists, podiatrists, optometrists, gentle exercise classes, and general practitioners. This referral pad provided a well-researched response with great potential to reduce falls and related injuries.

15.3.2.5 Policy Development

Policy development involved working collaboratively with government and nongovernment organizations, including the Department of Housing and local councils (Kempton et al., 1998). Policy initiatives included encouraging local council to adopt a fall prevention policy for public places, hospitals to implement fall prevention procedures for patient management and ward environments, and the Department of Housing to implement fall-safe building codes. Notably, SOYF developed a set of guidelines entitled *Preventing Falls in Public Places: Challenges and Opportunity for Local Government*, which was distributed to all councils on the North Coast (Kempton et al., 1998). This document sought to assist local governments in understanding the issue of senior's falls and initiatives that could prevent falls in the future.

In addition, in 1993, four North Coast local councils received seed grants from the Public Health Unit. Each council (i.e., Bellingen Shire Council, Hastings Shire Council, Kempsey Shire Council, and Nambucca Shire Council) could undertake their own fall prevention activities to identify and rectify fall hazards within local town centers. For example, the Nambucca Shire Council began conducting safety audits of businesses and provided proprietors with a copy of the safety assessment, as well as documents demonstrating how fall safety and access could be improved.

In the Final Report of SOYF, Kempton et al. (1998) note that SOYF would have benefited from an earlier introduction of policy development strategies. Though, as mentioned above, a few local councils were early partners with SOYF, most partnerships with local councils only occurred in the last year of the intervention.

15.3.3 Key Considerations for the Implementation of SOYF

Throughout the implementation of SOYF, there was an emphasis on the involvement and empowerment of older adults (Garner et al., 1996). SOYF employed an older woman as the falls prevention coordinator, which Kempton et al. (1998) believed added to SOYF's "credibility and acceptance" (p. 62). Seniors were involved in planning risk reduction, educating other seniors, and evaluating the results. In 2009, Peel and Warburton reflected on the innovativeness and effectiveness of this approach. Although the results of SOYF cannot solely be attributed to this single component, Peel and Warburton (2009) argued that peer education provides effective communication, positive role models, and a cost-effective, sustainable approach for fall prevention (Peel & Warburton, 2009).

SOYF also worked with existing community networks and structures and considered the community's own perception of their needs. Specific aims of this approach included utilizing local knowledge, leadership, and expertise; fostering community ownership of the problem and input into solutions; allowing for a mix of strategies; and planning for future sustainability.

Garner et al. (1996) report that the key to the success of SOYF's implementation was the inclusion of the following:

- Widespread involvement of older people in program delivery
- Development of effective partnerships and networks
- Well-researched and appropriate resources
- Carefully targeted media messages
- Employment and training of peer-group community educators
- Use of seeding grants as local government incentives
- Harnessing of established links between older people, their general practitioners, and other health workers
- Strategies based on formative research and regular monitoring and improvement of those strategies

These components can be usefully incorporated in replications of SOYF.

A further point of consideration is that part of the initial success of an intervention is its novelty and the eagerness of staff. Replications should be mindful of recapturing these components. Another final note made by the Final Report on SOYF recommends that future adaptations target a specific age group, rather than attempting to create programs that target all people over 60 (Kempton et al., 1998). In this pursuit, it is important to be mindful that different age groups would likely benefit from different strategies.

15.4 Outcome

Evaluation strategies of SOYF were wide-ranging to examine diverse outcomes. The SOYF 5-year evaluation budget was $1,480,000 (see van Beurden et al., 1998) and involved a large-scale demonstration program with the availability of evaluation expertise. Strategies to evaluate SOYF included surveys of annual reach, local government policy and practice, and the knowledge and attitudes of the target group toward falls. A comparison of hospital admissions in the intervention area with the rest of NSW and with the Queensland control area was also obtained and analyzed (Kempton et al., 1998; van Beurden et al., 1998).

The methodology used in the evaluation of SOYF was comprehensive. The control area (Sunshine Coast, Queensland) was carefully selected to match NSW's intervention area in terms of geography (coastal, rural region with urban centers), demography (high proportion of retirees), and climatic factors while at the same time being remote enough not to be influenced by the interventions (Kempton et al., 2000). The control area did not have any systematic fall prevention interventions in place at the outset of SOYF, and the health service providers in the control area agreed to stay intervention free for the duration of the program (Kempton et al., 2000). The control area was used to compare fall-related hospital morbidity data from the two regions. In addition, a longitudinal telephone risk-factor survey was conducted among 2.5% of North Coast (intervention area, $n = 2000$) and Queensland (control area, $n = 1600$) residents. Phone calls lasted a maximum of 20 minutes and were used to obtain information regarding the knowledge, attitudes, fall incidence, and fall outcomes (van Beurden et al., 1998). Focus-group discussions were also conducted with nine groups of 8–10 older people to gauge opinions, beliefs, and perception about falls (van Beurden et al., 1998).

After the 1992–1996 SOYF fall prevention program ended, the cost-effectiveness and sustainability of the program were examined (Beard et al., 2006). These later analyses provided information regarding the long-term outcome of the SOYF program.

15.4.1 Specific Outcomes of Interest

Hospitalizations—the evaluation of SOYF revealed measurable gains in health outcomes (Kempton et al., 2000). At the final year of follow-up for hospitalizations (1994/1995), age-standardized fall-related admissions for North Coast residents aged 60 years and over was 20% lower than admissions for the Sunshine Coast (control group) residents (rate ratio − 0.80, 95% CI 0.76–0.84, $p < 0.01$; Kempton et al., 2000). A similar result was observed when comparing North Coast residents with the rest of the state of NSW. See Table 15.2 for the rates of falls per 100,000 for the years between 1991/1992 and 1994/1995.

The reduction in falls was similar for males (23%) and females (19%). As expected from an aging cohort, the mean fall incidence (baseline versus follow-up) rose in both intervention (0.297–0.365 falls/person/year) and control

group (0.280–0.413 falls/person/year; Kempton et al., 2000). This may be due to an increase in age, as well as an increase in medication use, which may cause unsteadiness (Hahn et al., 1996).

The statistically significant 20% reduction in falls was found in both a comparison to the control community and the state of NSW (Kempton et al., 1998, 2000, Table 15.2). This figure is arguably a conservative estimate of effect, given that the data for the final year of the intervention (1995/1996) were not available (Kempton et al., 1998) and was therefore not included in this calculation (Barnett et al., 2003, 2004; Kempton et al., 2000; McClure et al., 2010).

Self-reported falls—at follow-up, there was a lower rate of self-reported falls in the intervention cohort compared with the control cohort (Kempton et al., 2000). A multivariate analysis, which controlled age and gender differences, showed that the impact of the intervention was a 22% reduction in self-reported falls; however, this analysis was not significant (Kempton et al., 2000). The lower rate of self-reported falls, although nonsignificant, has been thought to support the statistically significant 20% reduction in hospitalization (Kempton et al., 2000).

Attitudinal and behavioral changes—SOYF was found to have a significant influence on attitudes toward falls (Hahn et al., 1996; Kempton et al., 2000). Using telephone interviews, Hahn

Table 15.2 Direct Age Standardized Falls-Related Hospital Separation rates per 100,000 persons in New South Wales North Coast (NC), Queensland Sunshine Coast (SSC), and NSW total residents aged 60 years and over (1991/1992 to 1994/1995)

Year	NC rate/100,000 (±95% CLs)	SSC rate/100,000 (±95% CLs)	Total NSW rate/100,000 (±95% CLs)	NC vs. SSC rate ratio (±95% CLs)	NC vs. Total NSW rate ratio (±95% CLs)
1991/1992	1653.5 (1640.3, 1667.3)	1666.0 (1651.8, 1680.9)	1808.8 (1801.6, 1816.1)	0.99 (0.94, 1.05)	0.91 (0.86, 0.96)*
1992/1993	1732.4 (1719.2, 1746.2)	1649.4 (1635.4, 1664.0)	1919.1 (1911.8, 1926.4)	1.05 (0.99, 1.11)	0.90 (0.85, 0.95)**
1993/1994	1712.2 (1699.2, 1725.8)	1822.6 (1808.5, 1837.4)	2017.7 (2010.4, 2025.1)	0.94 (0.89, 0.99)*	0.85 (0.80, 0.89)**
1994/1995	1641.8 (1629.1, 1655.0)	2051.2 (2036.8, 2066.2)	2016.5 (2009.2, 2023.8)	0.80 (0.76, 0.84)**	0.81 (0.77, 0.86)**

Note: North Coast rate ratio 1991/1992 (baseline) versus 1994/1995 (follow-up): females = 0.96, males = 1.12, persons = 0.99. Data for this table are from *Stay on Your Feet Final Report: 1992–1997* by Kempton et al., 1998, Lismore, South Wales, Australia: Northern Rivers Health Service Institute of Health and Research
$*p < 0.05$, $**p < 0.01$

et al. (1996) found that after only 18 months of SOYF intervention, there was a 6% reported increase in the belief that falls are preventable (Hahn et al., 1996). The full effect of 4 years of SOYF produced a statistically significant 34% increase in awareness that falls are preventable and a 31% increase in elderly respondents, considering that they were at moderate or high risk of having a fall (Kempton et al., 2000). These attitudinal changes are reflected in many behavioral changes, and there was a significant increase in intervention subjects wearing safer footwear (35%) and nonsignificant improvements in other aspects of behavior, including more frequent vision checks, increased physical activity, and fall-safe changes to the home (Kempton et al., 2000). At the outset of SOYF, Kempton et al. (1998) thereby concluded in SOYF's final report that "the program has raised the awareness of older people regarding the risk of falling, improved their perceptions in relation to the preventability of falls and increased their knowledge of risk factors" (p. 1).

Reach: the program had demonstrable success in terms of its reach. Program reach was tracked annually from 1994 to 1996 in cross-sectional, random sample telephone surveys in the intervention area only (Kempton et al., 2000). These surveys aimed to identify what fall prevention strategies were most effective in increasing awareness in older adults (see Table 15.3; Kempton et al., 2000). The gender ratio was 2:1 (for females to males), and the age distribution was 71% for ages 60–74, 24% for ages 75–84, and 5% for ages over 85 years (Kempton et al., 2000).

The final survey results for reach of the SOYF program, from a random (0.8%) sample of 744 North Coast residents aged 60 and over, are available in Table 15.3 (Kempton et al., 1998). In comparing 1996 with the previous two annual reach surveys, dramatic and significant increases in the awareness of, and participation in, the various components of SOYF were evident (Kempton et al., 1998). Over half of the respondents in 1996 had heard of the SOYF program, which is a statistically significant increase from 1994 whereby only 27% of respondents had heard of the SOYF

Table 15.3 Cross-sectional surveys of SOYF program reach, indicating target population exposure to different SOYF components

SOYF component	1994 $n = 494$ No. (%)	1995 $n = 709$ No. (%)	1996 $n = 744$ No. (%)
Seen, read, or heard about falls prevention	212 (43.0)	399 (56.4)	504 (67.7)**
Heard of SOYF	117 (23.7)	310 (43.7)	378 (50.8)**
Seen a falls TV ad	119 (24.1)	238 (33.5)	248 (33.3)**
Seen a falls newspaper item	100 (20.2)	168 (23.7)	294 (39.5)**
Received a SOYF book	60 (12.1)	155 (21.8)	233 (31.3)**
Received a SOYF calendar	37 (7.5)	NA	64 (9.0)*
Heard a SOYF radio ad	NA	NA	98 (13.2)
Used a "pill bag"	NA	36 (5.1)	69 (9.3)*
Attended a SOYF talk about falls	28 (5.7)	39 (5.5)	46 (6.2)*
Attended a gentle exercise class	26 (5.3)	37 (5.2)	59 (7.9)*
Had a SOYF home safety check	11 (2.2)	30 (4.2)	81 (10.9)*
Attended a Medication Workshop	7 (1.4)	4 (0.6)	18 (2.4)**
Attended a SOYF falls Expo	1 (0.2)	2 (0.2)	NA
Involved with any SOYF component	255 (51.6)	480 (67.7)	572 (76.9)**

Note: Data from "Older People Can Stay on Their Feet: Final Results of a Community-Based Falls Prevention Programme," by Kempton et al., 2000, *Health Promotion International*, *15*(1)
NA: not available (interventions not conducted in these years)
*$p < 0.05$, **$p < 0.001$ (x^2 test comparing first and last instances: $df = 1$)

program. About one third of older people had received a copy of the SOYF book (31%), which increased significantly from 1994 ($p < 0.001$).

The effectiveness of media releases and promotions was reflected in the steady increase to almost 40% of respondents reporting reading a newspaper item about falls and one third reporting viewing a TV advertisement about falls, by 1996. Radio advertisements were less effective, and only 13% of respondents reported hearing a SOYF radio advertisement, by 1996. The reach surveys indicate that awareness-raising strategies had significant reach among older North Coast residents, reaching approximately a third to half of older residents (Kempton et al., 2000). Kempton et al. (2000) reported that significant reach influenced outcomes: "there were greater improvements in falls rate, wise medication use, physical activity and balance among subjects whose attitudes or knowledge had improved" (p. 32).

Reach in the SOYF intervention area was also compared to the control area. Over half of participants in the intervention area (52.4%) had seen, read, or heard about fall or fall prevention, which is greater than the control area (17.7%; Kempton et al., 1998).

Local government policy and practice change—this survey indicated that though the content of hazard-related complaints remained consistent from 1992 to 1996, the number of complaints rose dramatically throughout the intervention. Kempton et al. (1998) believe that this is the result of greater fall prevention awareness and prioritization among the target population, as well as an increased awareness of the local government's responsibilities. The most common complaint was about providing and improving footpaths, improving lighting, improving surface finish, providing ramps, and improving access to facilities. During the program, there was also a rise in specific protocols for dealing with reported falls (i.e., for insurance and hazard rectification). In this regard, the guideline that SOYF published was cited by 6 (of 13) local councils as a useful tool in developing fall prevention strategies (Kempton et al., 1998).

Cost-effectiveness—in 2005, Kannus and colleagues explained that a major difficulty with multifactorial fall prevention strategies is that they can be labor intensive and thereby may not yield a cost-effective strategy to prevent fall and related injuries. Contrary to this view, it has also been argued that for the cost of one hip replacement (approximately $40,000), you can run SOYF for a year (Corlett & Warren, 2006; Kempton et al., 2000).

To accurately determine the economic utility of SOYF, Beard et al. (2006) conducted a thorough cost-benefit analysis that was published in *Public Health*. This analysis (1) compared the estimates of savings from avoided hospital admissions in the intervention region to the control group and (2) compared the hospital utilization in the intervention region with the state of NSW. In this assessment, Beard et al. (2006) considered direct costs (i.e., inpatient costs, medical services, pharmaceutical benefits, nursing homes expenses, and allied health services), as well as indirect costs (i.e., time lost due to illness, pain, and suffering). Both methods in Beard et al.'s investigation showed a net savings of 5.4 million AUD (direct costs alone) to $16.9 million AUD (direct and indirect costs). As a result, this research group concluded that SOYF was a highly cost-effective fall prevention program.

Though Beard et al. (2006) argue that "well designed interventions for falls prevention among older people can be highly cost effective and a wise investment for all levels of government" (p. 750), this does not necessarily denote that the cost benefit of SOYF cannot be improved upon further. For example, Kannus, Sievanen, Palvanen, Jarvinen, and Parkkari (2005) points out that one limitation of a multidisciplinary fall prevention intervention (like SOYF) is the inability to locate which part of an intervention is most effective. Accordingly, it is possible that one or two of the components of SOYF is largely responsible for the significant reduction in elderly falls. If this is the case, the surplus spent on additional components may be superfluous from a cost-benefit perspective, though deemed important as part of SOYF's multistrategic plan. Independent calculations of the cost-effect for different components of the program would be recommended in the future (Beard et al., 2006). Nevertheless, given the substantial cost of falls and related injuries, it is promising that a prevention program like SOYF can yield dramatic savings.

Sustainability—sustainability is an important aspect of the quality of health promotion programs, which provides enhanced health benefit and enables a program to sustain itself after funding has elapsed (Hanson, Salmoni, & Volpe, 2009). The systematic study of program sustainability has been proposed as "in its infancy" (Barnett et al., 2004) whereby even the definition of sustainability is dependent on the view of stakeholders (Hanson et al., 2009). Those who have evaluated the sustainability of SOYF have defined sustainability as incorporating program sustainability, agency sustainability, and sustainability of program effects (Crisp & Swerissen, 2002). Several years after the original SOYF intervention was completed, Barnett et al. (2004) assessed the sustainability of SOYF among multiple community stakeholder groups, including general practitioners, pharmacists, community health staff, local councils, and the original target group (older adult participants).

Barnett et al. (2004) found that 74% of GPs who had heard of SOYF believed that the program had influenced their practice. The most common activity of GPs was checking for medication that may contribute to an increased risk of falling in older patients (Barnett et al., 2003, 2004). Barnett et al. (2003) found that more than half of GPs did not give advice to their patients about fall prevention, and more than one quarter never used gentle exercise or walking groups in their referrals (both of which are beneficial for preventing falls). Pharmacists had less recall than GPs (45%), but many of those who had remembered SOYF reported being somewhat influenced by the program (79%; Barnett et al., 2003). Like physicians, pharmacists' main activity was checking patient medication and urging clients to dispose of out-of-date medication.

Community health staff demonstrated the highest degree of sustainable activities. Medication checks and gentle exercise classes were sustained at greater than 50%. Barnett et al. (2004) explain that this is especially encouraging, given that a 60% rate of sustained activities has been considered a reasonable achievement (Bracht et al., 1994). It is also encouraging that more than half of older adults described behavioral changes they made due to SOYF. The intervention strategies were designed to be self-sustaining (Garner et al., 1996), and it is heartening that daily walking, improving home safety, footwear changes, eye checkups, and other behavioral changes were continued past the life of the original program.

The least sustainable of SOYF activities was among local government (shire councils and their access committees). Though regular checks on footpaths and other safety policies were sustainable, Barnett et al. (2004) believe that this was "most likely directly related to fear of litigation" rather than a result of SOYF (p. 286). In support of this view, it was found that only one of the ten councils reported still using SOYF's manual, *Preventing Falls in Public Places*, as a guideline. To increase sustainable changes in local government, future adaptations are recommended to concentrate on key policy changes, as opposed to manuals that may or may not be adhered to (Barnett et al., 2004).

Of course the sustainability of a program will be influenced by the prioritization and reach of a program. In the later regard, Kempton et al. (2000) showed that the reach for SOYF was extensive. In addition, other internal factors within organizations, personal interest, and influence from other sectors will be influential (Barnett et al., 2004). However, though the sustainability of SOYF had varying degrees of success depending on the stakeholders, Barnett et al. (2004) conclude that SOYF has demonstrated immediate outcomes, as well as long-term sustainability. This is especially true when considering the approach of health practitioners and the behavioral changes in the original target group. In future studies, it would be important to determine whether program sustainability translates into a continual reduction in fall-related hospital admissions (Barnett et al., 2004).

It has been noted that SOYF NSW's period of evaluation finished in 1997; however, the NSW SOYF program has led to a statewide fall prevention program with adaptations and replications worldwide. National policies, in Australia and New Zealand, have also increased the benefit and sustainability of SOYF. Furthermore, SOYF has extended beyond Australia and New Zealand and is being implemented in various communities in countries throughout the world, including the United States and Canada. In 2017, platforms such as YouTube make SOYF exercise videos and informative videos easier and cheaper to disseminate.

15.4.2 Methodological Advantages and Limitations of Evaluating SOYF

There are some notable methodological limitations of evaluating SOYF. For example, the estimations of hospital rates may be subject to annual fluctuations (Kempton et al., 2000). Also, similar to other community-based fall prevention approaches, SOYF was not a randomized study (Kempton et al., 2000; McClure et al., 2005). It would be difficult to ensure compatibility of different randomized communities and to standardize SOYF in each locality. A randomized intervention design was also deemed to be unsuitable, given that awareness raising through media outlets would affect neighboring control areas (van Beurden et al., 1998). Instead, SOYF utilized a prospective, longitudinal evaluation design whereby cohort subjects were randomly selected from the intervention and control areas that were comparable for key demographic attributes, and multivariate methods were used to adjust for potential confounders (Kempton et al., 2000). However, importantly, the problem of a cohort design is that repeat measurements might influence the responses of cohort participants.

Another limitation of a cohort design is attrition, which is an obvious concern, considering that reasons for attrition in SOYF may be associated with study outcomes (e.g., fall incidence; van Beurden et al., 1998). Problems of attrition are expected in cohort studies, particularly in elderly cohorts (persons over 60) whereby morbidity, mortality, and relocation (or move to nursing homes) provide a further difficulty in participant follow-up. To counter this problem, SOYF evaluations attempted to locate persons who moved prior to the follow-up. Adjustments were also made for baseline differences through a covariate analysis (van Beurden et al., 1998). A further methodological limitation of SOYF's evaluation is the difference, albeit small, in the age distribution between the control and intervention groups. The control group had 5% more individuals who were 60–64 years old and 5% less of 80–84 years old ($p < 0.001$ and $p < 0.02$; Kempton et al., 2000).

Notwithstanding these limitations, Kempton et al. (1998) and other research groups have since credited SOYF as a well-executed and comprehensively evaluated community intervention program, which demonstrated measurable gains. For example, a Cochrane meta-analysis examined the effectiveness of community-wide, multistrategy initiatives aimed at reducing falls in older adults (McClure et al., 2005). McClure et al. (2005) were only able to identify 5 studies (out of 23 identified studies) that met the criteria for inclusion in their analysis. The only Australian fall prevention program effective to date (with a rigorous evaluation) was SOYF, which had the largest study among those reviewed and one of the highest-reported success rates in reducing falls (McClure et al., 2005).

15.4.3 Summary of SOYF Outcomes

The extensive evaluations and clear presentation of the SOYF program has distinguished SOYF in the field of fall prevention. According to Kempton et al. (1998), "Stay on Your Feet has demonstrated that a well-planned, well executed, and comprehensively monitored and evaluated community intervention to reduce falls can achieve measurable gains in both intermediate and health outcomes" (Kempton et al., 1998, p. 1).

It is encouraging that health outcomes in SOYF are corroborated from different sources and all indicators are linked in an integrated framework that reinforce each other. For example, the 20% reduction in hospitalization because of falls is corroborated by a (nonsignificant) 22% reduction in self-reported falls (see above). SOYF conducted an evaluation on multiple levels (e.g., process, formative, and outcome) using quantitative and qualitative methods (e.g., telephone and written surveys, hospitalization data) and diverse approaches (e.g., cost-benefit and sustainability analyses) to fully understand the impact of the SOYF program (van Beurden et al., 1998). The broad and in-depth approach taken in the evaluation of SOYF adds credibility to the program, as does the many publications of SOYF's findings in academic journals (Ganz & Wu, 2007).

The result of SOYF's evaluation—of reach, cost, sustainability, fall reduction, and changes in attitudes and knowledge surrounding falls—illustrates measurable gains in intermediate and lasting health outcomes from a community fall prevention program (Kempton et al., 2000). The reported success of this program has helped SOYF gain intersectoral support by obtaining grants for extended implementation and evaluation and has made SOYF a model for fall prevention programs (van Beurden et al., 1998).

15.5 Adaptations of SOYF

Though the funding for the initial SOYF program ceased in 1997, the program continued to be replicated and adapted and be a major influence in the field of elderly fall prevention. There are multiple factors that vary among newer SOYF programs, expertise; however, the breadth and diversity of these programs attest to SOYF's worldwide impact on the field.

15.5.1 Australia

New South Wales—as detailed above, the SOYF program began on the North Coast in NSW. NSW continued its fall prevention efforts. In 2006, 3 years of funding was received from the NSW Health Department to adapt the most successful aspects of SOYF to Gosford and Ryde/Hunters Hill. This program retained a multistrategic approach to raise awareness and education among local partners and within the community. In NSW, SOYF awareness campaigns target adults over 65, while physical exercise campaigns are offered to those aged 50 and over (H. Kale, personal communication, n.d.). The aim of SOYF NSW is to promote active and positive aging. Implementation of SOYF NSW involved increasing physical activity, conducting home safety checks, and improving vision in older adults.

The awareness campaign in SOYF NSW took on an inventive strategy whereby a single risk factor was focused on for 3 months at a time before progressing to another risk factor. This approach was conducted to retain interest in the SOYF message by continually providing new and useful materials, as well as allowing the organizers to effectively network with partner organizations specific to each risk factor. Awareness campaigns also involved educational talks to seniors concerning falls, prevention of falls, and the fear of falling. Furthermore, resource kits were developed and included a shopping bag with the SOYF logo, practical resources (e.g., pill cutters), fact sheets, and other fall awareness materials (H. Kale, personal communication, n.d.). In addition, newspaper, banners, advertisements on buses, community radio interviews, and other media outlets were utilized. The brand identity of SOYF saw an increase in recognition, and the organizers reported witnessing a change in seniors' behavior (H. Kale, personal communication, n.d.).

Working with local partners was emphasized throughout the program and was manifest in the SOYF NSW implementation (S. Miten-Lewis, personal communication, n.d.; H. Kale, personal communication, n.d.). For example, Gosford involved ambulances and libraries in disseminating information regarding falls and fall prevention. Local optometrists were enlisted to promote regular eye checkups. Furthermore, incentives reinforced the SOYF message. For example, between March and April 2008, older community members who had an eye examination or obtained new glasses from participating optometrists received a free fall prevention information pack. The SOYF NSW program encouraged GPs, Community Nurses, densitometry technicians, and other healthcare workers to refer patients. Patients also received free passes to Tai Chi classes, which was believed to be an important incentive (H. Kale, personal communication, n.d.). Another initiative, regarding home safety, was encouraging local hardware stores to promote and display home safety products and give away fall prevention information packs to their customers. A similar initiative occurred in the summer of 2008 whereby pharmacies gave out kits and promoted the "manage your medicines" message to their customers.

In terms of physical activity and exercise promotion, SOYF NSW has developed Staying Active Directories that contain a local list of physical activity opportunities in the community. After 400 people responded to a Tai Chi ad in the Gosford local paper, 27 Tai Chi classes in 18 locations were established. These classes were particularly popular (approximately 200 individuals attended classes weekly; H. Kale, personal communication, n.d.). The success of this program may be due to the initial receipt of (one to three) free classes, the low cost of classes, and the enlistment of health professionals to refer patients to the program.

In Ryde/Hunters Hill, SOYF NSW worked directly with public housing residents to increase physical activity and initiate exercise classes. Furthermore, multiple Staying Active expos were held where people could try out various types of exercise and gather information from guest speakers and stalls. Events like the Walking Challenge, where participants tested and increased physical activity over a 4-week period with the help of pedometers, were extremely popular.

The SOYF NSW program has been highly regarded; however, one significant challenge was the large percentage of non-English speakers in Ryde/Hunters Hill. This challenge was addressed by translating resources (e.g., the home safety fact sheets) into six different languages and by distributing these resources to libraries, service clubs, and community organizations. Furthermore, presentations in Ryde/Hunters Hill were given to non-English-speaking local community groups. For example, in September 2008 SOYF, NSW organized a Tai Chi "taste test" for an Italian-speaking women's group. Another challenge was providing physical activity to those who are financially disadvantaged. In response, SOYF NSW developed partnerships and allowed participants to "come and try" events. Further, SOYF funded exercise programs at each site, which led to increased access.

Western Australia—Stay On Your Feet Western Australia (SOYFWA) is a statewide fall prevention program that began in 1996 in the South West region following the successful NSW implementation of SOYF. In 1998, the Department of Health Injury Prevention Branch officially adopted the Stay on Your Feet WA® model and registered the trademark. SOYFWA was funded by the Department of Health Western Australia (K. Moore, personal communication, n.d.). The Department of Health Western Australia funded personnel costs (approximately $100,000/annum), printing and distributing of SOYF® Resources (approximately $30,000/annum), and other advocacy and promotional activities (approximately $700,000/annum).[1]

SOYFWA was driven by various collaborative groups working in partnerships within government and nongovernment organizations, across multiple sectors, and with key stakeholder with broad representation. Volunteers were an active and vital component of SOYFWA's success. SOYFWA maintained its collaborative approach when it was consolidated with the formation of the Falls Prevention WA Health Network in 2006. This network developed a model of care, giving advice regarding the location and general mechanism of fall prevention measures in WA, with SOYFWA taking a leading role in this effort.

SOYFWA focused on three primary services: (1) awareness raising, (2) volunteer management, and (3) orchestrating a SOYFWA Week on an annual basis. Awareness raising efforts included expos (in areas populated by the target group), community presentations, viewings of SOYFWA's video, as well as publishing and disseminating the quarterly SOYFWA newsletter and e-newsletter. SOYFWA also provided information on fall prevention to governmental, health, and community organizations. SOYFWA utilized volunteers to spread messages of fall prevention. Through a peer role modeling and education program, volunteers participated in industry committees, networks, and meetings where appropriate. Furthermore, SOYFWA had a multifaceted communication strategy to disseminate its message. In so doing, television, radio, print, and other resources were utilized. Volunteers were also involved in other educational promotional activities through the

---

[1] The funds presented in this paragraph are all measured in United States Dollars.

principles of positive aging. Culturally and Linguistically Diverse (CALD) materials were developed and disseminated as part of awareness-raising efforts. SOYFWA ran an April No Falls Day, and its SOYFWA Week included participation from the local government, local health services, and regional communities. In SOYFWA Week, healthcare workers, volunteers, and staff disseminated fall prevention materials and merchandise and discussed fall prevention with community members.

One venture that is particularly attention worthy occurred in Burnbury, WA. In Burnbury, a group of participating seniors, called the Safety Walks Group, would meet to go for walks and survey the safety of different locations. A report of the group's experience would then be later given to the local government or businesses for rectification. This venture, which evolved from SOYF, was supported by the local government, where, partially due to a prevention awareness policy, the group was allocated $20,000 from the local government budget for hazard identification and rectification (Powell et al., 2000). The Safety Walks Groups targets behavioral and environmental changes across the five strategies set out by SOYF. For example, aside from the walking group being a forum for exercise, it strived to work with local authorities to remove public hazards in pedestrian areas, businesses, houses, and accommodations. Seniors were trained in four 2-h sessions about the risks of falls and fall prevention strategies. Over 18 months the group identified and rectified 86 hazards (Powell et al., 2000). Powell et al. (2000) believe that the success of this group was due to the funding and commitment of the local government, community empowerment, and the partnerships between agencies, people, and communities.

Evaluation of SOYFWA was process driven with broader outcome evaluation undertaken by the fall prevention health network. Accordingly, feedback was collected on SOYFWA's resources, presentations, and events. Furthermore, the number of presentations, resources disseminated, and other activities were tracked.

The SOYFWA® program became recognized nationally and worldwide with requests received from both government and nongovernment agencies to use the program to help develop area-specific literature and programs.

Queensland—Queensland Health and Injury Prevention Control Australia Ltd. conducted a 5-year fall prevention trial project from 2001 to 2006 called "Stay Active, Stay Independent, Stay on Your Feet" in the Wide Bay/Burnett region. This program targeted individuals aged 60 years and over who were living independently in the Wide Bay/Burnett community. The Wide Bay/Burnett region was chosen for this trial because it has Queensland's highest proportion of individuals aged 60 years and over. This program was a direct cooperation and collaboration effort with the Northern Rivers NSW SOYF program. SOYF Wide Bay/Burnett spanned 21 local government authority areas and involved a range of communities.

In implementing this program, a few focal principles guided SOYF Wide Bay/Burnett practice (Queensland Health, 2008), including the following:

- Encouraging local involvement and ownership
- Being inclusive, accessible, simple, and practical
- Starting from what is already in place and aiming to enhance and extend the reach
- Being guided by research

In practice, SOYF Wide Bay/Burnett program efforts translated into an awareness campaign, a volunteer program, community fall prevention education and training, and an emphasis on physical activity. Other SOYF Wide Bay/Burnett strategies included the message of safe footwear, home modification, medication review, and public safety (McClure et al., 2010). The awareness campaign that aimed at raising the profile of SOYF among local older people and stakeholders was involved with updating, creating, and distributing fall prevention fact sheets, brochures, One Step Ahead booklets, display boards, calendars, as well as publishing a bimonthly community newsletter. In addition, a 30-s television advertisement on three regional television networks ran from June to November 2005 and January to April 2006. This was developed jointly with the Northern Rivers Area Health Service. In addition, SOYF Wide Bay/Burnett implemented an Ambassadors Program whereby older community members were trained to volunteer to promote independence and activity by sharing fall prevention information and supporting older adults in an informal, friendly, and nonthreatening manner (McClure et al., 2010). SOYF Wide Bay/Burnett also provided local education and training for workers who provide in-home services.

Physical activity was an emphasis in the SOYF Wide Bay/Burnett program. Physical opportunities were promoted widely, and numerous "come and try" days were held in many locations across 33 communities and 21 Local Government Authority areas. Furthermore, new physical activity events were developed by training local leaders (77 local leaders were trained in 20 communities). Inventive physical activities to get older adults involved included Nordic Pole Walking, Life Ball, Tai Chi for Arthritis, and Gentle Exercise classes. Another useful adaptation to improve access and reach was a library loan system for physical activity equipment and resources on physical education.

The outcome of this 5-year trial project (2001–2006) resulted in an increased proportion of older people who agreed that falls are preventable, which was also accompanied with behavioral changes in older adults (e.g., increased calcium intake and reported changes to home environments). Furthermore, due to SOYF's efforts, more local activities were organized, particularly those relating to physical activity. An evaluation of the program revealed that there was no significant improvement in the incidence of self-reported falls or fall- related injury based on self-reports, hospital admissions, or mortality data. However, as Queensland Health (2008) point out, "benefits may require several years to accrue." SOYF Wide Bay/Burnett has made some very useful recommendations on improving its program. These recommendations can be viewed at http://www.health.qld.gov.au/stayonyourfeet/documents/soyf_exec_summary.pdf.

South Australia—SOYF Whyalla was a fall prevention demonstration project that was also funded from 2002 to 2005 under the National Falls Prevention for Older People Initiative of the Australian Government Department of Health & Ageing. This project was one of five similar funded initiatives (including Adelaide West) in Australia between 2002 and 2005 (Dollard & Fuller, 2005). The funding for $270,000 (Australian dollars) was distributed over two stages between March 2002 and March 2005.

Whyalla is a regional city in South Australia, 4 h from the closest capital city. Accordingly, the aim of SOYF Whyalla was to adapt the SOYF program to a community-based regional setting. The project aimed to establish an improved fall prevention system, to make that system sustainable, and to disseminate the lessons learned (Dollard & Fuller, 2005). A gap analysis was conducted prior to the commencement of the project. This analysis revealed the need for a way to systematically detect individuals at risk of falling and the need for developing a wider range of physical activity opportunities. SOYF Whyalla therefore developed and implemented a range of strategies: (1) screening and referral, (2) workforce development, (3) community promotion, and (4) physical activity development and promotion (Dollard & Fuller, 2005).

To improve screening and referral, a self-completed Falls Risk Checklist (FRC) was adapted and widely disseminated among GPs and other healthcare workers (Dollard & Fuller, 2005). Along with other tools provided to healthcare providers, the FRC was used to more systematically screen and assess clients. Many educational activities were also designed to engage the community and local health professionals in fall prevention, including providing discipline-specific resources. Furthermore, community promotion was sought by developing and disseminating fall prevention materials for community use (e.g., posters, brochures, newspaper, radio copy, talks to community groups, and volunteer peer educators). This awareness campaign was perceived to be very effective (especially the use of newspaper and brochures) and influenced the target group's value of exercise and other beliefs about falls. SOYF Whyalla also encouraged supervised physical activity options for older people (e.g., Tai Chi for Arthritis groups; Dollard & Fuller, 2005).

As SOYF Whyalla planned to demonstrate system improvement rather than a reduction in falls, a process-focused (rather than outcome) initiative was undertaken (Dollard & Fuller, 2005). This approach allowed for frequent assessments and recommendations to improve the program, make the program more sustainable, and disseminate the lessons learned.

15.5.2 New Zealand

Wellington—from April 2004 to December 2006, Sport Wellington set up a contract for Stay on Your Feet Greater Wellington in New Zealand with the aim of reducing the incidence and consequence of falls in older people in the Greater Wellington/Hutt region. The program was jointly funded by Capital and Coast and Hutt Valley District Health Boards and the Accident Compensation Corporation. Due to funding differences, the deliverable outputs from the program differed by region. The annual cost of the program was $43,975.50 (New Zealand Dollars).

The SOYF Greater Wellington program was an authentic replication of SOYF in its aim to provide a holistic and comprehensive fall prevention program. The program was involved in health promotion through awareness raising; exercise to improve strength, gait, and balance; and improving fall-related policy. SOYF Wellington was organized by a qualified coordinator (e.g., physiotherapist), while support and guidance were provided through a steering committee.

In general, the age range targeted by this program was 60–75 years. However, the organizer's observation that Maori "age earlier" than European New Zealanders was taken into account, and the fall prevention services were made available to Maori people younger than age 60 when it was appropriate. Referrals to the service were made by medical practitioners, nurses, or community organizations or through self-

referral. The program also initiated a program where individuals were "prescribed" an exercise routine by their GPs.

Individual assessment allowed the prevention programs to match and best serve their unique needs and circumstances. For example, if an individual has many risk factors for a fall, an individualized exercise program and home management assessment was seen to be the most beneficial intervention. For others, attending a group-based exercise session, e.g., a modified Tai Chi class, twice a week was the best management option. At times, a medication review would be suggested to its GP for implementation. It was also recognized that there are some people who are at a particularly high risk of falling due to a combination of factors such as reduced strength, multiple medications, and environmental hazards. When there is an especially increased risk, it was more appropriate for the individual to be referred to a geriatrician.

Based on referrals and risk assessments, individuals were recommended an appropriate intervention to increase strength, balance, and gait. These include a group exercise class (for low-risk individuals), individualized classes by an appropriately skilled peer trainer (for medium-risk individuals), and individualized classes by a fall coordinator or other health professionals (for high-risk individuals). To deliver multiple classes, physiotherapists trained volunteers, peer trainers (friends, family, or neighbors), and residential care exercise facilitators in proven fall prevention exercises to be conducted individually or in groups. Most of the classes offered were Tai Chi or a modification of the Otago Exercise Program, and both have been proven to be effective. In addition to providing classes, the coordinator also referred individuals to other services for appropriate interventions, such as vision checks, use of hip protectors, home hazard identification and modification, and a medication review.

SOYF Wellington ceased when it was incorporated into a national fall prevention strategy, which is reflected in New Zealand Injury Prevention Strategy (NZIPS; B. Hislop, personal communication, n.d.). Wellington has lost the

SOYF branding in this more widespread implementation of fall prevention; however, Wellington retained the SOYF umbrella model of fall prevention in its implementation.

15.5.3 Canada

Ontario: original implementation—in 2004, SOYF was launched in three diverse Ontario communities: (1) Kingston, Frontenac, Lennox, and Addington (KFL&A); (2) Grey Bruce; and (3) Elliot Lake (Corlett & Warren, 2006). These three communities were selected after assessing their planning and proposed programs (Volpe, 2004). As SOYF was already considered to have proven success in Australia, the Ontario implementation focused on assessing whether and how SOYF could be adapted to three diverse communities in Ontario (Corlett & Warren, 2006). Because of the diversity of the chosen areas, each center adopted a different model for their implementation. For example, KFL&A is an urban center that is supported by a Public Health Unit and therefore adopted an urban model. In contrast, Grey Bruce developed a rural model because of its rural composition of many decentralized towns and small villages with some support from a Public Health Unit. A business model was utilized by Elliott Lake because this isolated northern community had no support from a Public Health Unit but gained most of its support from a major corporation that attracts seniors and retirees to the community (i.e., Elliot Lake Retirement Living; Corlett & Warren, 2006).

The Ontario Neurotrauma Foundation (ONF) provided a seed grant for up to $100,000 for each of the three selected communities, $50,000 to be spent per year, for 2 years. The goals of the grant were (1) to enable sustainability of SOYF beyond the 2-year project,[2] (2) to work in coordination with other interested stakeholders, and (3) to create an agenda for policy advocacy and long-term

funding with the Government of Ontario and other stakeholders for the implementation of SOYF in communities across the province (Corlett & Warren, 2006). In additional to ONF funding, in-kind or cash contributions from SOYF partners were received. The amount of these funds depended on each site, with Elliot Lake receiving over three times the value of the grant, Grey Bruce receiving almost four times the value of the grant, and KFL&A receiving an estimated ten times the value of the ONF grant (Corlett & Warren, 2006). Though in-kind funding was very generous, program leaders found the SOYF initial grant was critical to the generation of additional in-kind contributions. ONF also added an additional, one-time grant of $10,000 for program evaluation.

One commonality between the three sites was the ONF provision that all initiatives consider SOYF's umbrella model, containing each of the five thematic areas of implementation into their effort. Each site developed plans, initiated activities under the five SOYF strategies, and provided updates on their progress and achievements. In this respect, the program was in keeping with the initial Australian implementation. The implementation process in Ontario began in September 2003. Eric van Beurden, a research and evaluation coordinator for the original SOYF program, assisted in ONF's aim of exemplary practice transfer (Volpe, 2004).

During the implementation process, the communities described unique barriers in implementing SOYF. Elliot Lake had difficulty distributing its information to French-speaking seniors and relocated seniors. Grey Bruce reported challenges in distributing its materials among its population that has a low-literacy rate and is culturally diverse (including Aboriginals and Amish individuals). Lastly, Kingston reported the challenge of serving a population that is very isolated (i.e., where 30–50% of seniors live alone) and therefore is at elevated risk of falls and other serious health outcomes (Culmer & O'Grady, 2005). The difficulty of reaching rural and isolated low-income seniors was an important obstacle. The two rural groups, Elliot Lake and Grey Bruce, not

---

[2] In so doing, the role of public health units in organizing and maintaining the program beyond its original funding was essential (Corlett & Warren, 2006; H. Gagné, personal communication, n.d.).

surprisingly also had difficulty due to geographical distance, lack of adequate transportation systems, and poor weather. Initiatives in Ontario since this time have benefited from the implementation of the three originally funded ONF sites (Corlett & Warren, 2006). Though an umbrella approach was the goal, due to capacity issues, more selected strategies were implemented (e.g., home safety, exercise) with the hope that other strategies would be included at a later stage (H. Gagné, personal communication, n.d.).

The concerns that Corlett and Warren (2006) expressed regarding the sustainability of SOYF in Elliot Lake once the seed grant finished were partially realized. On the other hand, both Grey Bruce and KFL&A were able to continue fall prevention efforts and move into a phase of revitalization (M. Thomas, personal communication, n.d.). In so doing, liaisons with healthcare workers and other fall prevention programs in these regions have been an asset (M. Thomas, personal communication, n.d.). In addition to the initial ONF-funded communities, SOYF projects were extended into other Ontario regions such as Parry Sound, North Bay, and Sudbury. Ongoing efforts in these sites included supporting fall prevention theater troupes (which experienced success in other sites), arranging fall prevention commercials, and printing SOYF calendars, brochures, and books.

North Eastern Ontario: further implementation—the North Eastern Ontario SOYF regional fall prevention strategy operates across five communities spanning a large, and often secluded, geographical area (North East Local Health Integration Network [NE LHIN], 2017b). This area is over 154,000 square miles but only contains 4% of Ontario's population (NE LHIN, 2017b). Of this population, over 20% are 65 years or older (NE LHIN, 2017b). The health needs of these communities are served locally at the policy level by individual Public Health Units (PHU), as well as one Local Health Integrated Network (LHIN) (NE LHIN, 2017a). The LHIN and these PHUs must respond to the challenge of serving such a large and often inaccessible geographical area (some areas are accessible only by plane) with a small and culturally diverse population (NE LHIN, 2017a).

Based on research and the previous experience of implementing SOYF in Ontario, the five PHUs and the LHIN together committed to collaboratively implement SOYF in 2014 (NE LHIN, 2017b). In 2015, these five PHUs and the LHIN entered into a 3-year common memorandum of understanding that outlined an agreement for their working partnership (NE LHIN, 2017a). They agreed to coordinate locally and to work together to identify and act upon regional needs—thereby reducing the duplication of work (NE LHIN, 2017a).

The LHIN invests $540,000 annually to fall prevention through SOYF (NE LHIN, 2017b). Of this money, $100,000 goes locally to the individual PHUs, and the remaining $40,000 is used to support operating funds and the region as a whole (NE LHIN, 2017b). Locally, the PHUs divide funding toward purchasing resources and employing a full-time position to SOYF (NE LHIN, 2017b). Also, they match the contribution with PHU resources and staff (NE LHIN, 2017b).

Likewise, according to the memorandum, key responsibilities are divided on a local and regional level. The LHIN operates regionally. The committee that oversees the SOYF strategy is multifactorial and dedicated to ensuring community ownership and action (NE LHIN, 2017b). They address priority topics (such as evaluation) through regional workshops (NE LHIN, 2017b). The PHUs are responsible for all local SOYF planning, implementation, and evaluation, as well as for supporting regional initiatives (NE LHIN, 2017b). To accomplish these goals, the PHUs work with local multifactorial coalitions made up of local stakeholders (e.g., agencies, volunteers, and older adults; NE LHIN, 2017b). At this level, the groups identify local priorities and make regional recommendations.

A multilevel evaluation framework was determined at the initiation of the memorandum. The goal of evaluation was to ensure that SOYF was implemented as intended; to allow for continuous feedback, communication, and thus quality improvements; and to assess how the LHIN will continue to implement fall prevention at the end of the 3-year agreement (NE LHIN, 2017b). Evaluations from the fall of 2017 indicate an overall downward trend in hospitalizations in the region. However, this evaluation has also discovered several factors that should be incorporated into future SOYF implementations.

One aspect of the North Eastern Ontario implementation of SOYF that makes it especially interesting is the way it coincided with a key partnership (the LHIN and PHUs under the memorandum) and that this partnership was evaluated. Evaluation of the memorandum partnership showed that the advantage of the collaboration is that it allowed for the leveraging of each partners' specific strengths (NE LHIN, 2017b). Collaboration and sharing of workloads allowed for greater reach and ability to move forward with initiatives, resulted in innovation, and allowed linking to nontraditional partners (NE LHIN, 2017b). Moving forward, evaluation led to an understanding that future partnerships needed to better reflect and respect the diversity of the different regions and that decision-making processes need explicit a priori clarification (NE LHIN, 2017b).

Some of the most valuable lessons attained from this initial 3-year agreement pertain to the reach and usefulness of information and classes. The resources and information designed were of high quality; however, their usefulness was limited because of various cultural factors (NE LHIN, 2017b). To expand the reach and dissemination of this information, these resources need to be designed in a way that accounts for the unique needs of the cultural groups living in a region (NE LHIN, 2017b). Likewise, educational and exercise classes are only useful if community members are attending them. While the classes were free and advertised locally and regionally, attendance remained low (NE LHIN, 2017b). Methods of encouraging participation in this type of complex geographical and cultural environment need further exploration. So far, the NE LHIN (2017b) has reported a few specific barriers to participation, such as the following: having the class in a retirement home may be unappealing, posters may not entice enough motivation, and providers may not have enough time to encourage participation (NE LHIN, 2017b).

In addition to exercise classes, the NE LHIN offers a skill-based class called Stand Up! that teaches gross motor skills that prevent falls. Stand Up! is another exemplary practice program that this partnership integrated into its SOYF fall prevention strategy (NE LHIN, 2017b). Unlike the exercise classes offered, the Stand Up! classes are well attended (NE LHIN, 2017b). The NE LHIN (2017b) found that a follow-up class is needed for older adults to maintain gains. In response, a Still Standing postclass is currently being pilot tested, and it is exploring more culturally sensitive ways to offer this program to the indigenous communities it serves (NE LHIN, 2017b). The exercise program (Stand Up!) that the communities implemented as a part of SOYF demonstrated a range of improvements (NE LHIN, 2017b).

15.5.4 United Kingdom

Mid Hampshire—from 2002 to 2006, a multiagency alliance, led by Mid Hampshire Primary Care Trust (MHPCT), implemented a Stay on Your Feet program to prevent elderly falls using a multiinterventional strategy (Owen, 2003). Accordingly, SOYF Mid Hampshire considered fall prevention with attention to the greater context of local health and community priorities. Throughout its programming, SOYF Mid Hampshire encouraged older adults' participation, as demonstrated by frequent informal discussions and focus groups on fall awareness, as well as lunches for older adults whereby participants completed questionnaires on falls and fall prevention. Furthermore, feedback was sought from health professionals (e.g., senior occupational therapists, practice nurses, district nurses), care homes (e.g., nursing care team, nursing home managers), and voluntary sector and community groups that offer health and social care locally (e.g., alliance members). This feedback was beneficially incorporated into SOYF Mid Hampshire's activities.

SOYF Mid Hampshire raised awareness through distributing bookmarks, SOYF packs, and leaflets for health professionals. These resources contained information on falls and fall prevention. As of May 2004, adapted versions of SOYF Falls Prevention Packs were carried by Hampshire's ambulance vehicles so that fallers who were not in need of hospitalization received information to prevent repeated falls (Owen, 2006). Another productive awareness initiative in Mid Hampshire was the linking of SOYF with other health campaigns across Winchester. For example, fall prevention leaflets were provided to district nurses to distribute to older people receiving flu immunizations. Furthermore, information about Stay on Your Feet workshops and other project activities ran in newspapers, in local newsletters, and on the radio. In addition, the Stay on Your Feet Times, a popular newsletter to update alliance members on SOYF activities and fall prevention, was developed and produced quarterly (Owen, 2004).

SOYF Mid Hampshire also focused on training older adults through seminars in the local community and home visits. On average, SOYF Mid Hampshire delivered two Falls Awareness events/seminars a month to people over 65 years attending community clubs (Owen, 2004). These sessions focused on fall prevention measures, risk assessment, and guidance about how to get up following a noninjurious fall. SOYF Mid Hampshire also carried out home safety and security checks, arranged minor safety repairs, and provided guidance on grant aid assistance and home energy savings. In addition to events with the public, awareness raising, training, and consultation events were organized for partners, voluntary agencies, and caregivers. For example, an accredited workshop for health professionals and general practitioners was held in November 2002. The aim of this event was to examine local provisions to prevent elderly falls and to consider the issues relevant to the development of fall prevention guidelines.

The Stay on Your Feet Alliance, which included members from a broad spectrum of organizations and community groups, met every 2 months and provided an important forum for sharing information, expertise, and resources. In collaboration with GPs, the Stay on Your Feet Alliance usefully developed easy-to-use screening tools and Risk Assessment Guidelines. These tools were an all-encompassing assessment of older people's needs, so procedures were not needlessly duplicated by different agencies. Especially notable in this effort (as well as other efforts) of SOYF Mid Hampshire is cross-agency collaboration (e.g., clinicians, public agencies, and patients), which was usefully incorporated throughout the program (S. Owen, personal communication, n.d.).

A key challenge that was identified by SOYF Mid Hampshire, but is not restricted to this prevention program, was the difficulty in finding accurate measures to evaluate success in fall prevention and isolating these measures from confounding variables that also contribute to fall and related injury (S. Owen, personal communication, n.d.). Internal evaluations through annual reports were submitted to key stakeholders and funding bodies (S. Owen, personal communication, n.d.). Feedback on training programs, screening, and assessment tools were also collected and incorporated.

The annual cost of SOYF was approximately £32,000. SOYF Mid Hampshire recommended that future SOYF programs increase fall prevention activity in primary care, ambulance, and pharmacy services; increase osteoporosis awareness in primary care services; maintain links with older people's forums and groups to assess the impact of fall services; collaborate, train, and support practitioners, volunteers, informal caregivers and older people; and identify and utilize hotspots to disseminate information and resources to older adults who are housebound (i.e., mobile library services; Owen, 2004). Diverging from the original SOYF target group, SOYF Mid Hampshire also recommended that future SOYF programming target older adults who live in residential care (Owen, 2004). As the in-kind contribution was believed to be a particular strength of the project, future collaborations are also encouraged (S. Owen, personal communication, n.d.).

Though SOYF Mid Hampshire was a successful program, SOYF programming ceased in October 2006 because Mid Hampshire Primary Care Trust was merged into the larger Hampshire Primary Care Trust (S. Owen, personal communication, n.d.).

Warrington, Cheshire—in 2007, the Warrington Community Services Unit created a SOYF exercise program that targeted adults over 65. This 8-week gentle exercise class had an educational and exercise components. The purpose of the class was to deliver a physical activity program that would prevent falls and improve independence in older individuals living in the community. In 2007–2008, the program was allocated £75,000, which allowed SOYF Warrington to provide the course and transport free of charge (H. Anderson, personal communication, n.d.).

Each week, a health professional attended the group to provide a 30-min discussion on various topics (e.g., foot care, weight management, fall prevention, etc.). Also, there was a 1-h varied exercise class (e.g., Tai chi, using resistance bands, etc.). SOYF Warrington reported strong collaborations within the health care system. This was demonstrated by the program's requirement that individuals be referred to the program by a GP or practice nurse so as to ensure that the individual was fit to attend the class. Individuals were excluded from this program if they were very frail, had an unstable health condition, or did not consent to the referral.

Physical improvement, program completion, sustainability, and patient satisfaction were tracked using surveys (H. Anderson, personal communication, n.d.). After completing this program, individuals had the option to remain in the program for another 8 weeks. After an additional 8 weeks, individuals were invited to participate in other active community programs such as Reach for Health.

Wokingham, Berkshire—another SOYF adaptation occurred in Wokingham, Berkshire. In October 2009, Wokingham incorporated the SOYF branding into its already-existing fall prevention program. The emphasis of SOYF Wokingham was to raise awareness on fall prevention and home safety, though it was also involved in promoting exercise and conducting multifactorial risk assessments (K. Arding, personal communication, n.d.). The target group was individuals over 60 years of age who were referred to Wokingham's fall advisory services by their GPs, district nurses, physiotherapists, senior groups, or family members or were self-referred. SOYF Wokingham incorporated SOYF's message of putting a positive spin on fall prevention (K. Arding, personal communication, n.d.).

The initial major effort of SOYF Wokingham was the adaptation of a SOYF booklet from Western Australia to make this resource relevant to the Wokingham population. This adaptation included making the 56-page self-help booklet's wording more suitable to British individuals, changing the relevant contact details, and adding information about local hazards and home hazard prevention. It cost approximately £3200 to print 5000 booklets (K. Arding, personal communication, n.d.). Funding was received from a Wokingham Borough Council Prevention Grant. Booklets were distributed during talks at seniors' clubs or disseminated through Wokingham's fall advisory services at the time of an assessment. Satisfaction forms were included inside the SOYF booklet, and this feedback was used to improve this resource (K. Arding, personal communication, n.d.).

15.5.5 A Note on SOYF Adaptations

Adaptations of SOYF are an excellent way to transport the original success of the North Coast's fall prevention program. However, as seen above, most of SOYF's adaptations are less intensive than the original program (in scope and implementation period), yet these programs have not conducted an outcome evaluation to establish that their adaptation of the program has the same impact. These less comprehensive programs may be more sustainable and cost-effective, but they also may not have the same anticipated success in reducing falls. McClure et al. (2010) sought to investigate whether these "less ambitious" adaptations of SOYF could deliver comparable outcomes to the original SOYF program. McClure et al. (2010) investigated self-reports, mortality, and hospital separations in two different SOYF program adaptations in Australia: Wide Bay, Queensland, and Northern Rivers, NSW. As mentioned above, both programs used the motto "Stay Active, Stay Independent, Stay on Your Feet," with the project called Stay on Your Feet (or SOYF) in Wide Bay but Stay Active, Stay Independent (or SASI), in Northern Rivers. The goal of both programs was to reduce fall-related injury by incorporating SOYF fall prevention strategies into existing community structure and services. The implementation of these strategies varied, but both programs took place between 2002 and 2006.

McClure et al. (2010) found that neither of the interventions, in Wide Bay or Northern Rivers, decreased the rate of fall-related injuries among older adults, though there was some reduction in women's reports of multiple falls. This research group therefore concluded that an intensive, multistrategic, public health approach is important for SOYF's success (McClure et al., 2010). In support of this view, systematic reviews by Gillespie et al. (2003), Chang et al. (2004), and Gates, Lamb, Fisher, Cooke, and Carter (2008) similarly suggest that the beneficial effects of fall prevention programs are more pronounced in intensive multistrategic interventions. Though many SOYF practitioners take the view that "something is better than nothing," an intensive and multistrategic intervention with an effective implementation should be the aim of a SOYF replication (Fixsen, Naoom, Blase, Friedman, & Wallace, 2005).

In addition to being intensive and multistrategic, SOYF adaptations should also not be "stuck in time." Progressing the SOYF program requires incorporating emerging evidence-informed research and demographic trends that may be useful in improving upon the initial program. For example, until recently, sleep disruptions were an unrecognized cause of falls (Studenski, 2010). Sedatives, daytime sleepiness, and nocturnal sleep conditions (e.g., low levels of light) contribute to balance disorders and fall risk (Ancoli-Israel & Ayalon, 2009; Studenski, 2010). Susceptibility to falls increases because sleep disruptions cause reduced alertness and attention (Studenski, 2010). A SOYF adaptation may usefully work with GPs, healthcare workers, and the target group to increase awareness that sleep problems are not an inevitable part of aging and that by treating sleep disorders it is possible to prevent falls. For example, GPs could ask their patients about their sleep quality, as common poor sleep self-reports are often good indicators of a sleep problem (Studenski, 2010). Research on Vitamin D supplements and medication use could also be usefully incorporated into a SOYF program. New and insightful research regarding the cause of falls or fall prevention practice also has the possibility to enhance the SOYF program.

15.6 Conclusion

The reasoning for fall preventative programs is self-evident when considering the growing population of older adults, the high prevalence of falls in this age group, and the health and fiscal implications of falls (McClure et al., 2010). The Stay on Your Feet program is a multistrategic (i.e., umbrella model) intervention that aims to reduce elderly falls by addressing fall awareness, community education, home hazards, healthcare management, and fall prevention policies. Through the implementation of these diverse strategies, the program is consistent with the Ottawa Charter for health promotion (1986) and the Jakarta Declaration (1997), which seek to strengthen community action. The initial SOYF program (1992–1996) was extensively evaluated and found to be successful at increasing awareness and decreasing fall-related hospitalizations. The program also demonstrated cost-effectiveness and sustainability (especially in community education and behavioral changes among older adults). As an additional marker of its success, the SOYF program received international attention and has become a model for fall prevention strategies worldwide.

Despite the replications and adaptations of SOYF, the effectiveness of most of these alternative programs in preventing falls has yet to be evaluated and published. The immense potential of SOYF to reduce the rate of falls and the substantial associated health costs is potentially watered down by smaller and fragmented adaptations. It is important that modified SOYF programs evaluate and publish their findings in academic journals and disseminate their findings to older adults and caregivers by using media and other appropriate communication outlets. Furthermore, very few of the adaptations of SOYF have specifically aimed to increase access to fall prevention strategies among neglected populations (e.g., Aboriginal or disadvantaged communities), which should be a priority. Nevertheless, research to date has demonstrated that SOYF is a feasible, collaborative, and intensive fall prevention program and an effective direction for fall prevention among older adults. For optimal implementation of SOYF, it is necessary to have an integrated and multistrategic framework on the local, state, and national levels.

Acknowledgments The author would like to express sincere appreciation to the key informants for this case study: Eric van Beurden of the Health Promotion Team, Population Health Planning & Performance Management Division North-Coast Area Health Service in Lismore, NSW, Australia; Suzanne Mitten-Lewis of the Stay on Your Feet Community Falls Prevention, Northern Sydney Health Promotion in NSW, Australia; Helen Kale of Stay on Your Feet Community Falls Prevention, Northern Sydney Central Coast Health in NSW, Australia; Karina Moore of the Health Network Branch in Subiaco, WA, Australia; Joanne Dollard of the University of Adelaide in Adelaide, Australia; Barry Hislop of the Accident Compensation Corporation in Wellington, New Zealand; Marguerite Thomas of the Ontario Neurotrauma Foundation in Brussels, ON, Canada; Hélène Gagné of the Ontario Neurotrauma Foundation in Toronto, ON, Canada; Helen Anderson of Warrington Primary Care Trust in Birchwood, Warrington, England; Karen Arding of Community Care Services in Wokingham, England; and Sara Owen of the National Health Service Hampshire in Scotney, Hampshire, England—whose consultation made this project possible.

BRIO Model: Stay On Your Feet

Group Served: noninstitutionalized, elderly people (60 years and older) in the community.

Goal: to reduce the incidence and injury from falls in elderly people.

Background	Resources	Implementation	Outcome
Falls are a major cause of unintentional injury and death among people aged 65 years and over. Previous studies were inadequate to evaluate community programs for fall prevention. Objectives of this program included utilizing local knowledge, leadership, and expertise; fostering community ownership of the problem and input into solutions; allowing for a mix of strategies; and, providing for future sustainability.	The total cost of the first 5 years of the Stay on Your Feet program was $678,703, which included a $137,000 external funding grant. Additional costs also were incurred by community networks such as government agencies, health promotion agencies, medical organizations, and nongovernment organizations focused on seniors. Second phase of the program was funded by the Australian National Health and Medical Research Council.	Phases of implementation included awareness raising, information dissemination, policy development, home safety measures, and the involvement of health professionals. Evaluations included formative, process, outcome, and sustainability assessments.	Fall-related hospitalizations decreased by 20%. The intervention produced a 34% increase in the odds of respondents considering fall preventable and a 31% increase in respondents considering that they were at a moderate or high risk of experiencing fall. Program had a wide reach, and 52.4% of the respondents had seen, read, or heard about fall prevention.

Life Space Model: Stay On Your Feet

Sociocultural: civilization/community	Interpersonal: primary and secondary relationships	Physical environments: where we live	Internal states: biochemical/genetic and means of coping
Raising awareness that falls are preventable and not a natural part of aging. Use of community health services to deliver prevention messages. Policy development of fall prevention in public places Multifaceted approach that included general practitioners, community health nurses, podiatrists, occupational therapists, exercise trainers, local businesses, and the government.	Healthcare provider/patient relationships through the inclusion of a broad base of community health systems. Peer relationships through the active involvement of older individuals in leadership roles and as volunteers.	Safety audits of home and public areas. Participation of stores to present fall prevention displays and stock preventative devices (such as antislip tile and hand bars).	Empowerment of individuals through the inclusion of seniors in the planning and implementation of the program.

References

Ancoli-Israel, S., & Ayalon, L. (2009). Diagnosis and treatment of sleep disorders in older adults. *American Journal of Geriatric Psychiatry, 7*, 98–105.

Barnett, L. M., van Beurden, E., Eakin, E. G., Beard, J., Dietrich, U., & Newman, B. (2004). Program sustainability of a community-based intervention to prevent falls among older Australians. *Health Promotion International, 19*(3), 281–288.

Barnett, L., van Beurden, E., Eakin, E., Dietrich, U., Beard, J., & Newman, B. (2003). Falls prevention in rural general practice: What stands the test of time and where to from here? *Australian and New Zealand Journal of Public Health, 27*, 481–485.

Beard, J., Rowell, D., Scott, D., van Beurden, E., Barnett, L., Hughes, K., et al. (2006). Economic analysis of a community-based falls prevention program. *Public Health, 120*, 742–751.

Bracht, N., Finnegan, J. R., Rissel, C., Weisbrod, R., Gleason, J., Corbett, J., et al. (1994). Community ownership and program continuation following a health demonstration project. *Health Education Research, 9*, 243–255.

Chang, J. T., Morton, S. C., Rubenstein, L. Z., Mojica, W. A., Maglione, M., Suttorp, M. J., et al. (2004). Interventions for the prevention of falls in older adults: Systematic review and meta-analysis of randomized clinical trials. *British Medical Journal, 328*, 680–683.

Corlett, S., & Warren, R. (2006). Evaluation of Stay on Your Feet (SOYF): A senior falls demonstration project. Prepared for the Ontario Neurotrauma Foundation.

Crisp, B., & Swerissen, H. (2002). Program, agency, and effect sustainability in health promotion. *Health Promotion Journal of Australia, 13*, 40–42.

Culmer, L., & O'Grady, D. (2005). *Stay on Your Feet executive summary (KFL&A)*. Retrieved from http://www.stepsafe.com/pdf/05soyfyearend.pdf

Dollard, J., & Fuller, J. (2005). *Whyalla falls prevention project 'Stay on Your Feet Whyalla': Final report*. Prepared for the National Falls Prevention for Older People Initiative, the Community Demonstration Projects, and the Commonwealth Department of Health and Aged Care.

Fixsen, D. L., Naoom, S. F., Blase, K. A., Friedman, R. M., & Wallace, F. (2005). *Implementation research: A synthesis of the literature*. Tampa, FL: University of South Florida, Louis de la Parte Florida Mental Health Institute, The National Implementation Research Network.

Ganz, D. A., & Wu, S. (2007). *Reducing the risk of falls and fall-related injuries among older people*. Paper presented at the Workshop on the Social Detriments of Adult Health and Mortality, Washington, DC.

Garner, E., Kempton, A., & van Beurden, E. (1996). Strategies to prevent falls: The Stay on Your Feet program. *Health Promotion Journal of Australia, 6*, 36–43.

Gates, S., Lamb, S. E., Fisher, J. D., Cooke, M. W., & Carter, Y. H. (2008). Multifactorial assessment and targeted intervention for preventing falls and injuries among older people in community and emergency care settings: Systematic review and meta-analysis. *British Medical Journal, 336*, 130–133.

Gillespie, L. D., Gillespie, W. J., Robertson, M. C., Lamb, S. E., Cumming, R. G., & Rowe, B. H. (2003). Interventions for preventing falls in elderly people. *Cochrane Database Systematic Reviews*, (4), CD000340.

Hahn, A., van Beurden, E., Kempton, A., Sladden, T., & Garner, E. (1996). Achievements of a community-based falls prevention programme in 18 months. *Health Promotion International, 11*, 203–211.

Hanson, H. M., Salmoni, A. W., & Volpe, R. (2009). Defining program sustainability: Differing views of stakeholders. *Canadian Journal of Public Health, 100*(3), 304–309.

Kannus, P., Sievanen, H., Palvanen, M., Jarvinen, T., & Parkkari, J. (2005). Prevention of falls and consequent injuries in elderly people. *The Lancet, 366*, 1885–1893.

Kempton, A., Garner, E., van Beurden, E., Williams, A., Sladden, T., McPhee, L., et al. (1998). *Stay on Your Feet final report: 1992–1996*. Lismore, South Wales: Northern Rivers Health Service Institute of Health and Research.

Kempton, A., van Beurden, E., Sladden, T., Garner, E., & Beard, J. (2000). Older people can stay on their feet: Final results of a community-based falls prevention programme. *Health Promotion International, 15*(1), 27–33.

McClure, R. J., Hughes, K., Ren, C., McKenzie, K., Dietrich, U., Vardon, P., et al. (2010). The population approach to falls injury prevention in older people: Finding of a two community trial. *BioMed Central Public Health, 10*(79), 1–9.

McClure, R., Turner, C., Peel, N., Spinks, A., Eakin, E., & Hughes, K. (2005). Population-based interventions for the prevention of fall-related injuries in older people. *Cochrane Database Systematic Reviews*, (1), CD004441.

North East Local Health Integration Network. (2017a). *Stay on your feet evaluation report – October 2017 draft*.

North East Local Health Integration Network. (2017b). *Stay on your feet evaluation report – November 2017 draft*.

Owen, S. (2003). *Stay on Your Feet alliance annual report 2002/2003*. Health improvement and social inclusion report.

Owen, S. (2004). *Stay on Your Feet alliance annual report 2003–2004*. Health improvement and social inclusion report.

Owen, S. (2006). *Stay on Your Feet alliance annual report 2005–2006*. Health improvement and social inclusion report.

Peel, N. M., & Warburton, J. (2009). Using senior volunteers as peer educators: What is the evidence of effectiveness in falls prevention? *Australasian Journal on Ageing, 28*(1), 7–11.

Powell, J., Wilkins, D., Leiper, J., & Gillam, C. (2000). Stay on Your Feet Safety Walks Group. *Accident Analysis and Prevention, 32*, 389–390.

Queensland Health. (2008). *Executive summary, Wide Bay/Burnett Stay on Your Feet trial project*. Retrieved from http://www.health.qld.gov.au/stayonyourfeet/documents/soyf_exec_summary.pdf

Sladden, T. (1993). *A picture of health and disease on the North Coast*. Lismore, South Wales: North Coast Public Health Unit.

Studenski, S. A. (2010). Sleep and falls in the elderly. In S. R. Pandi-Perumal, J. M. Monti, & A. A. Monjan (Eds.), *Principles and practice of geriatric sleep medicine* (pp. 299–306). Cambridge, UK: Cambridge University Press.

Tinetti, M. E. (2003). Preventing falls in elderly persons. *New England Journal of Medicine, 348*, 653–654.

van Beurden, E., Kempton, A., Sladden, T., & Garner, E. (1998). Designing an evaluation for a multiple-strategy community intervention: The North Coast Stay on Your Feet program. *Australian and New Zealand Journal of Public Health, 22*, 115–119.

Volpe, R. (2004). *The best practice approach to strategic funding: Stay on Your Feet (SOYF)/Ontario implementation evaluation (year one)*. Toronto, ON: University of Toronto.

World Health Organization. (1986). *The Ottawa charter for health promotion*. Retrieved from http://www.who.int/healthpromotion/conferences/previous/ottawa/en/

World Health Organization. (1997). *Jakarta declaration on leading health promotion into the 21st century*. Retrieved from http://www.who.int/healthpromotion/conferences/previous/jakarta/declaration/en/

World Health Organization. (2007). *WHO Global Report on Falls Prevention in Older Age*. Retrieved from https://www.who.int/ageing/publications/Falls_prevention7March.pdf?ua=1

World Health Organization. (2015). *World report on ageing and health*. Retrieved from https://apps.who.int/iris/bitstream/handle/10665/186463/9789240694811_eng.pdf;jsessionid=CF5F750A791BF013F7B7F7475B3BC878?sequence=1

Melbourne Extended Care and Rehabilitation Service Falls Prevention Project

16

David Gentili

The Melbourne Extended Care and Rehabilitation Service (MECRS) falls prevention program was a multidisciplinary, comprehensive, and holistic program designed to prevent falls in hospitals. The components of this program included education, risk assessment, and environmental interventions.

16.1 Background

16.1.1 History and Development

In response to a growing concern about injuries due to falls in hospitals, the Melbourne Extended Care and Rehabilitation Service (MECRS) center of the Royal Melbourne Hospital (RMH) designed a Falls Prevention Project to fill the research gap. This was built on developmental activities undertaken previously at the MECRS. While MECRS no longer exists in the RMH, the falls prevention program they designed is still an excellent example of a hospital falls prevention program.

The program acknowledged falls prevention as a multifactorial problem that required "a multidisciplinary solution" (National Ageing Research Institute [NARI], 2002, p. 8). Early on, the program adopted the slogan "fall prevention is everybody's responsibility" (NARI, 2002, p. 8). The project team involved collaborations between researchers with expertise in falls prevention, skilled practitioners from the MECRS Falls and Balance Clinic team, and practitioners from the broad range of allied health disciplines with a key role in falls prevention. These included a geriatrician, physiotherapist, occupational therapist, nurse, podiatrist, dietitian, and clinical psychologist. This mix of research and clinical skill included funding, dedicated project time for practitioners, and ensured support and endorsement of project activities by hospital staff as they were implemented.

The project incorporated a number of individual components, including workforce (staff) training (SPLATT Attack), an advanced falls prevention trainee program, action research, patient and career focus groups, validation and implementation of a falls risk assessment tool, an environmental safety audit process review, podiatry audits of patients' feet and footwear problems, a review of nutrition and falls risk of patients, a bed/chair alarm trial, fear of falling review in rehabilitation patients, and an interaction with falls prevention activities within the acute setting at Melbourne Health.

This falls prevention program is based on the available research evidence and expert opinion.

D. Gentili (✉)
Toronto, ON, Canada

© Springer Nature Switzerland AG 2020
R. Volpe (ed.), *Casebook of Traumatic Injury Prevention*,
https://doi.org/10.1007/978-3-030-27419-1_16

16.1.2 Project Aims

The primary aim of the project was to reduce the rate of falls within MECRS. The target initially set was a 30% reduction in all falls rates. To achieve this goal, a number of supporting secondary aims were also established, relating to individual components of the project. These were the following:

- To raise staff, patient, and family/career awareness of falls risk factors and falls prevention strategies that falls are often multifactorial in nature, that falls prevention strategies can be effective, and that falls are preventable.
- To validate and implement a recently developed falls risk assessment tool for hospitalized older people.
- To evaluate the effectiveness of an action research approach in improving staff ownership and participation in falls prevention activity.
- To identify and develop strategies to address barriers to effective falls prevention in the hospital setting.
- To identify and support enablers which facilitate uptake of falls prevention activities within the hospital setting.
- To evaluate the effectiveness of specific falls prevention equipment (such as bed alarms and hi/lo beds) within the subacute setting, to promote their use, and to investigate the provision of hip protectors to those deemed at risk of injurious falls.
- To evaluate existing resources for falls prevention in the hospital setting (including posters and brochures) and, if required, develop additional resources addressing identified areas of need.
- To develop a framework for interaction and preliminary falls prevention activity between the subacute falls prevention program and the falls prevention team at MECRS and staff in medical wards at the RMH (K. Hill, personal communication, 2004; F. Vrantsidis, personal communication, 2004).

Clearly, the MECRS Falls Prevention Project was an ambitious initiative to design, implement, and empirically test a balanced and multipronged program for reducing falls in healthcare settings.

16.2 Resources

16.2.1 Stakeholders and Collaborators

The MECRS provided healthcare services to older people who lived in the northern and western metropolitan regions of Melbourne, Australia. As the hub of the Aged Care and Rehabilitation Program of the city of Melbourne, the MECRS offered programs in rehabilitation, geriatric evaluation and management, specialist community-based programs, mental health services, and residential care services. MECRS also endeavored to cater to diverse cultural and linguistic groups.

The MECRS aimed to be the center of excellence in the provision of aged care and rehabilitation services. There were approximately 150 inpatient beds at MECRS located in six wards, including three geriatric evaluation and management (GEM) wards, a rehabilitation ward (primarily amputee and neurological patients), an aged transitional care unit, and a complex residential care unit (cared for residents with acquired brain injuries). The MECRS acted as the base for Aged Care Assessment Services, a community rehabilitation center, a day activities center, and Community Support Services. Additionally, it had specialist medical outpatient clinics that deal with pain, falls and balance, memory, continence, and wounds[1]. The MECRS was also involved in teaching current and future healthcare professionals from all disciplines.

The National Ageing Research Institute (NARI) has developed a strong record of accomplishment for a range of projects, including

---

[1] While these same services still exist at the RMH, they are no longer housed under the name of MECRS and the organization is different. For more information about current rehabilitation and extended care services at the RMH, please visit their website: www.thermh.org.au

those conducted in the biological, clinical, public health, and education fields. The NARI is associated with researching key health problems related to ageing. In particular, these include falls, memory impairment, pain, and wound healing. At the time of this case, NARI had completed a review of the research evidence in falls and falls injury prevention in the community, residential aged care, and hospital settings. It was also a national appraisal of activity in falls prevention for the Commonwealth Department of Health and Aged Care. NARI has also developed a national database of falls prevention programs in the community setting for the Public Health and Development Division, Victorian Department of Human Services.

The MECRS/NARI Falls and Balance Clinic was the first fully multidisciplinary specialist Falls and Balance Clinic developed in Australia, commencing operation in 1988 (Hill, Smith, & Schwarz, 2001). The staff included those with both clinical and research backgrounds. The clinic published research and presented at many nationally and internationally at conferences. The clinic's assessment process and management procedures were used as the basis for many clinics that developed in Victoria. Finally, the clinic provided training for allied health students and regularly hosted visitors from the Victoria area, interstate, and overseas.

16.2.2 Funding

The MECRS Falls Prevention Project was funded through the Department of Human Services (DHS) Quality Improvement Funding (QIF), built on some developmental activities undertaken in a 4-month project at MECRS in 2000, and funded by the DHS Aged Care Division.

An important component of any hospital-based falls prevention project is staff education. The project was a good opportunity to raise the profile of falls prevention in the hospital and to provide a base on which subsequent initiatives could be implemented.

A range of resources were produced during the implementation; these include the SPLATT Attack general staff training handouts, advanced falls prevention training manual, footwear and clothing information sheet (as part of the action research process), footwear safety checklist, and list of suppliers, falls prevention poster, summaries of recommendations for falls prevention education sessions for patients and families, introduction of patient information bed charts as part of the action research process, and a validated falls risk assessment tool, which was published and is still in use internationally.

The MECRS Falls Prevention Project was really a joint implementation of previously existing initiatives. In this paper, the educational components will be found under implementation, though they could also be considered resources.

16.3 Implementation

A retrospective evaluation of falls-related incident forms for the 6 months prior to the project commencement was undertaken to identify a baseline for comparison during the 12-month project duration. During this baseline period, there was an average of 16.0 falls/1000 bed days. Based on this data, 95% confidence intervals were established, which indicated that the rate of falls would need to be reduced to below 13.9 falls/1000 bed days for a statistically significant reduction in falls (NARI, 2002).

16.3.1 General Staff Training

SPLATT Attack. During this 12-month project, two rounds of general staff training were undertaken at MECRS using the popular interactive and experiential approach developed as part of the falls prevention program at MECRS in 2000. The so-called SPLATT Attack Expo involved staff working through seven workstations in small groups and interactively exploring key falls prevention messages. The first round was held in September 2001, and follow-up sessions, targeting new staff or those who missed the first round, were held in March 2002. The workstations included environment (general and bedside), psychosocial and sensory considerations, medications, feet and footwear, nutrition, transfers, mobility and gait aids, and fear of falling.

One hundred and fifty-four people attended the 2001 Expo, and a further 64 attended the 2002 sessions. Staff feedback was very positive about this approach to falls prevention training, and the Expo attracted visitors from many other hospitals interested in using the approach (NARI, 2002). The SPLATT Attack program has been successfully translated into another falls prevention project in the acute hospital setting at Western Health.

Advanced Falls Prevention Training Program. To support the general staff training, an advanced training program was developed to provide several staff in each ward with a high level of knowledge and skill to support ongoing falls prevention activities on the wards beyond the duration of the project. The training program consisted of ten sessions conducted by specialists in falls prevention, over a 1-h period for 5 weeks. An additional session discussed issues related to organizational culture and practice change management, with the aim of creating facilitators who would foster practice change in their own respective area. Nineteen staff from all wards and representing five professional health groups attended the training. The training program was rated as very good or excellent by most trainees, and a follow-up meeting was held 3 months after the training program to identify actions being undertaken and barriers and facilitators to planned activities (NARI, 2002).

16.3.2 Action Research

Action research provided a means for staff to identify the issues they perceive to be most relevant to an issue (in this case falls prevention) in the context of their unique environment and to develop strategies to address these, observe the outcomes, and reflect and modify actions if required. Many problems were identified, with priorities being to target inappropriate shoes and clothing, improved communication between staff and between staff and family, and environmental hazards on the ward. Several outcomes were achieved through the action research process, including developing a footwear and clothing information sheet and implementation of an information chart for each patient to display key information including mobility and falls risk, set out over the patient's bed.

16.3.3 Patient and Family/Career Focus Groups

Patient and family/career focus groups were planned to explore falls-related issues and to identify perceptions on strategies to effectively promote the falls prevention message. Most participants had firsthand experience with falls and subsequently highlighted the devastating effect a fall could have. Participants considered the link of falls prevention with maintenance of independence to be important. Also, participants reviewed the falls prevention in hospital brochure developed in the 2000 MECRS project and considered its content and layout to be very good (NARI, 2002). Recommendations for falls prevention education sessions were developed based on feedback from participants.

16.3.4 Validation and Implementation of the FRHOP

The Falls Risk for Hospitalized Older People (FRHOP) falls risk assessment tool was developed as part of the 2000 MECRS falls prevention project for use in subacute settings. Prior to implementation on the wards, a research project investigating prediction accuracy of the FRHOP was conducted. Unfortunately, recruitment for the research was slower than anticipated, resulting in a smaller than desired sample size (44 subjects were recruited). The FRHOP identified a range of levels of falls risk on each of the falls risk factors (and for the overall falls risk score). At the time of publication, moderate to high retest and inter-rater reliability were demonstrated for the overall falls risk score on the majority of the items on the FRHOP (NARI, 2002). The small sample size limited prediction accuracy; however, using a cutoff score of 23 or greater, sensitivity of 0.43 and specificity of 0.68 were achieved (NARI, 2002). Using a rating of 3 (high) or 4 or more risk factors resulted in a sensitivity of 0.57 and specificity of 0.68 (NARI, 2002). The FRHOP was introduced to all wards at MECRS in the later stages of the project when the validation project neared completion (NARI, 2002).

16.3.5 Environmental Hazards Process Review

The project occupational therapist provided input to the review of the environmental safety audit tool at Melbourne Health to ensure issues relevant to falls prevention were fully incorporated. In this way, the environmental safety audit could address environmental hazards for both occupationalhHealth and safety issues as well as falls prevention (NARI, 2002).

16.3.6 Bed/Chair Alarm System Trial

Two bed and chair alarm systems were introduced to wards. Previous studies suggest that these systems are not suitable for all patients but for patients at highest risk for falling. In this way, they appear to be a valuable tool in improving monitoring and thereby reducing falls (NARI, 2002).

16.3.7 Nutrition Audits

Most patients participating in the FRHOP validation study also underwent a brief nutritional assessment by the project dietitian (77%). Forty-one percent of the sample were at risk of malnutrition, and a further 24% were identified as malnourished. When results of the nutrition screen were compared with the FRHOP results, a trend was evident that those with increased risk of falling also had increased risk of malnutrition.

These results highlight the need for falls prevention programs in hospitals to consider nutritional needs, particularly as they impact upon patients' bone strength and ability to exercise (NARI, 2002).

16.3.8 Podiatry Audits

Given the importance of feet and footwear in falls prevention, an audit was undertaken to review feet and footwear problems among inpatients on two wards at MECRS. Forty-four patients were included in the review. Eighty-six percent were rated as having inappropriate footwear (NARI, 2002). Almost all patients had one or more foot problems requiring podiatry care. Recommendations were made to patients regarding change in footwear and need for regular podiatric care. A footwear checklist identifying qualities of good footwear and a list of footwear suppliers were distributed to wards and made readily available.

16.3.9 Fear of Falling Survey

An additional area of work that commenced late in the project was a review of the problem of fear of falling among rehabilitation patients at the time of discharge home.

16.3.10 Involvement with Falls Prevention in the Acute Setting at Melbourne Health

A small component of the project concerned the interaction with falls prevention activities at the Royal Melbourne Hospital. Project staff provided a forum for staff on one of the medical wards outlining the project activities and discussing options for translation into the acute setting. Several staff from the Royal Melbourne Hospital also attended the SPLATT training sessions at MECRS to consider ways this may be able to be conducted in the acute setting (NARI, 2002).

16.4 Outcome

The project achieved a great range of positive outcomes within each of the project areas described. Outcomes associated with specific project components have been previously discussed and can be found in sections of the report pertaining to these components. This section focuses on outcomes associated with the overall goal; however, the entire BRIO framework used to profile this case is summarized in table format at the end of this chapter.

The entire project was designed as a pilot and carefully measured from stage to stage. In terms of the primary goal, falls among inpatients at MECRS reduced from an average of 16.0 falls/1000 bed days in the period prior to project commencement to 14.6 falls/1000 bed days during the 12-month project intervention (NARI, 2002). This 9% reduction in falls rates equates to 66 less falls during the 12-month period.

16.4.1 Future Directions

While the MECRS no longer exists, fall prevention remains a priority at the RMH as evidenced by the continued existence of the falls prevention clinic.

The FRHOP is now a well-established risk assessment tool used and validated in hospital setting in many countries across the world. In fact, the Taiwan version was published in August of 2017 (Chang, Chang, Pan, Kao, & Kao, 2017). As well, it has been used as a basis to further research and create other assessment tools. One notable example is the Falls Risk for Older People-Community Setting risk assessment tool, which has also been taken up internationally (Russell et al., 2009).

Acknowledgments The author would like to express sincere appreciation to the key informants for this case study—Keith Hill and Freda Vrantsidis of the National Aging Research Institute in Parkville, Victoria, Australia—whose consultation made this project possible.

BRIO Model: MECRS Hospital Falls Prevention

Group Served: Patients in hospitals, mainly elderly patients.

Goal: Assess causes of falls in hospital settings and subsequently act to prevent them.

Background	Resources	Implementation	Outcome
Risk of neurotrauma from falls is highest among those over 65 years of age Falls in subacute and rehabilitation settings can be associated with complications, psychological effects, and permanent institutionalization and can extend length of stay or necessitate diagnostic procedures Rates of falls in subacute settings is high with limited knowledge available about how to prevent them The program aimed to reduce falls within Melbourne Extended Care and Rehabilitation Service	Program was built on developmental activities already in existence at the institution. The DHS Aged Care Division at Melbourne funded this aspect The program the Department of Human Services Quality Improvement funded it	Retrospective evaluation of falls formed a baseline for the project Program included workforce, training workstations (SPLATT), research, patient and career focus groups, validation and implementation of a falls risk assessment tool, an environmental safety audit process review, audits of patients' foot wear, review of patient nutrition, a bed/chair alarm, a fear of falling review, and an interaction with falls prevention activities	Feedback from the training initiative (SPLATT) was positive Advanced falls prevention training program was rated as very good or excellent by participants The action research component yielded several problems related to falls; strategies to address shoes, clothing, communication, and environmental hazards were developed Recommendations for fall prevention education were obtained via family/career focus groups Linkages between nutrition and falling were made

Life Space Model: MECRS Hospital Falls Prevention

Sociocultural: civilization/community	Interpersonal: primary and secondary relationships	Physical environments: where we live	Internal states: biochemical/genetic and means of coping
Raised awareness of fall risk factors and preventative practice among staff, patients, and families. Program impacts the way in which falls were viewed by all involved in the Melbourne community	Interactive program design has the potential to create positive relations and networks among patients, families, and staff. The way in which family and staff interact with patients will incorporate program knowledge	The identification of multifactorial antecedents to falls contribute to safety. Empirical assessment of risk for falling protects safety. Environmental audit process review makes the environment safer	Program can increase the quality of life, security, and self-efficacy among older patients

References

Chang, Y. W., Chang, Y. H., Pan, Y. L., Kao, T. W., & Kao, S. (2017). Validation and reliability of Falls Risk for Hospitalized Older People (FRHOP): Taiwan version. *Medicine, 96*(31), e7693.

Hill, K., Smith, R., & Schwarz, J. (2001). Falls clinics in Australia: A survey of current practice, and recommendations for future development. *Australian Health Review, 24*(4), 163–174.

National Ageing Research Institute. (2002). Preventing adverse events in sub-acute care: Changing practice to prevent falls. Report to the Metropolitan Health & Aged Care Services Divisions, Department of Human Services.

Russell, M. A., Hill, K. D., Day, L. M., Blackberry, I., Gurrin, L. C., & Dharmage, S. C. (2009). Development of the falls risk for older people in the community (FROP-Com) screening tool. *Age and Ageing, 38*(1), 40–46.

The Otago Exercise Program: A Home-Based, Individually Tailored Strength and Balance Retraining Program

17

Georgios Fthenos

The issue of falls and fall-related injuries among older adults is a serious public health concern. Falls and fall-related injuries among older adults result in longstanding pain, functional impairment, disability, hospital admissions, premature nursing home admissions, and death. Moreover, they represent a significant burden on individuals, families, society, and the health-care system. In recognizing that falls are one of the most costly and complex injury issues facing older adults, it is important for government, health agencies, service providers, and nongovernment and community organizations to support and promote research and programs to prevent senior falls (Report on Seniors Falls in Canada, 2005). In addition, public awareness, health education, and a safe environment can help prevent and reduce the number and severity of falls among older adult populations.

With a strong record of falls prevention research, a research team at the University of Otago Medical School in New Zealand developed the Otago Exercise Program, a program specifically designed to prevent falls in older adults, consisting of leg muscle strengthening and balance retraining exercises.

17.1 Background

17.1.1 Falls: The New Zealand Context

According to the Accident Compensation Corporation (ACC), falls resulting in injury are the leading cause of hospitalization and one of the top three causes of injury-related deaths in New Zealand. In young adulthood, hospital admissions resulting from falls are uncommon, but with advancing age, the incidence of fall-related hospital admissions increases at an exponential rate (Australian and New Zealand Falls Prevention Society). After the age of 40, the admission rate due to falls for men increases by 4.5% per year; for women the rate increases by 7.9% (Australian and New Zealand Falls Prevention Society).

More than 381,000 people were hospitalized for an unintentional injury; of these, 162,900 (43%) were fall related (Accident Compensation Corporation, 2005). It is also important to note that in these years:

- Fourteen thousand children aged 0–4 years were hospitalized for unintentional fall-related injuries; of these 52% of these falls occur in the home.
- Thirty-five thousand children aged 5–14 years were hospitalized for unintentional fall-related injuries.

G. Fthenos (✉)
Toronto, ON, Canada

© Springer Nature Switzerland AG 2020
R. Volpe (ed.), *Casebook of Traumatic Injury Prevention*,
https://doi.org/10.1007/978-3-030-27419-1_17

- Fifty-five percent of all hospitalized unintentional fall-related injuries were accounted for those aged 65–69 years, 65% for those aged 70–74 years, and 82% for people aged 75 and older.
- Fifty-two percent of hospitalizations for unintentional fall-related injuries are accounted for by females.

The issues of falls and fall-related injuries are considered a particularly serious public health issue among the older adult population in New Zealand. In order to contribute to the reduction of these rates, the Otago Medical School Falls Prevention Research Group created the Otago Exercise Program, an intervention strategy which has effectively been proven to reduce the rate of falling among older persons who participate in the program.

17.1.2 The Otago Exercise Program

The Otago Exercise Program has been tested in four controlled trials and shown to reduce fall and fall-related injuries in older people aged 80 years and older. The benefits of this program, in comparison to competing fall prevention programs, are that (a) no other program has been tested in such a comprehensive way and (b) the program has been tested beyond a research setting and proven effective when delivered from registered healthcare professionals (Otago Exercise Manual, 2003). The program's four distinct premises also make it distinct and set it apart from other intervention strategies (see Box 17.1).

> **Box 17.1 The Four Premises of the Otago Exercise Program**
> 1. The program needs to be individually tailored because older people vary considerably in their physical capacity and health and in their response to exercise.
> 2. The program will need to be increased in difficulty, because there will be initial improvement in strength and balance.
> 3. A stable, sustainable program should be established after a series of visits from the exercise instructor and will need checking two to three times a year thereafter.
> 4. A walking program to increase physical capacity should complement the strength and balance program.
>
> Source: Gardner, Buchner, Robertson, and Campbell (2001)

The following section will (a) explore the background of the program (i.e., the history, environment, and events that have shaped the program development), (b) investigate the program design and resource allocation, particularly how the program achieves its objectives, (c) discuss program implementation, specifically how the program design is practiced, and (d) determine the impact of the program, specifically the short-term and long-term outcome measures.

17.2 Resources

The Otago Exercise Program was designed by the Falls Prevention Research Group at the University of Otago Medical School. The following individuals have played an important role in the implementation of the Otago Exercise Program:

- Professor John Campbell, MD, FRACP, Professor of Geriatric Medicine
- M. Clare Robertson, PhD, Senior Research Fellow
- Melinda Gardner, Research Physiotherapist, New Zealand Falls Prevention Research Group
- David M. Buchner, VA Puget Sound Health-Care System

Stakeholders: The following stakeholders were responsible for encouraging and supporting the Otago Exercise Program's initiative to prevent falls and fall-related injuries. The agencies involved include as follows:

- Accident Rehabilitation and Compensation Insurance Corporation (ACC)
- The New Zealand Lottery Grants Board
- The Health Research Council of New Zealand
- Health Funding Authority Northern Division
- The Ministry of Health

Preventing Injury from Falls: The National Strategy 2005–2015: The Otago Exercise Program is part of the Preventing Injury from Falls: The National Strategy 2005–2015. The strategy aims to reduce the incidence and severity of injury from falls and the impact of fall-related injuries.

The Accident Rehabilitation and Compensation Insurance Corporation is the lead agency for the National Falls Prevention Strategy (NFPS). The National Falls Prevention Strategy has two aims: (1) to reduce the incidence and severity of injury from falls and (2) act as a guide for coordinating activities of government, health agencies, service providers, nongovernment, and community organizations (ACC, 2005). By improving knowledge, building effective leadership, and developing effective interventions and resources, such as the Otago Exercise Program, the incidence of falls and fall-related injuries will be reduced.

Prior to the development of the strategy, various individuals and organizations (i.e., researchers, service providers, advocacy groups, government and nongovernment agencies, community groups, professional associations) conducted research in the area of falls prevention. However, there was little coordination and collaboration on the research conducted. In order to remedy this situation, a national strategy was developed. The strategy focuses on (a) identifying a strategic vision, (b) identifying the goals to achieve the vision, (c) detailing the objectives that will help achieve the goals, and (d) proposing actions for managing and delivering the prevention initiatives.

17.2.1 Economic Evaluations

17.2.1.1 Case Study: Dunedin Study A: Costs to Implement Exercise Program

The Otago Exercise Program's cost-effectiveness has been established in two health-care settings. Table 17.1 outlines in detail the cost for implementing the Otago Exercise Program for Dunedin Study A.

In the first year, the exercise program costs $173 per person. In the second year, the program costs $22 per person, for the 71 exercise group participants who remained in the study. The resources used to implement the exercise program included those for recruiting the physiotherapist (health-care professional) who administered the exercise program, program materials (i.e., instruction booklets, ankle cuff weights utilized during leg strengthening exercises), and overhead costs (i.e., University of Otago services).

17.3 Implementation

17.3.1 Requirements to Participate in the Otago Exercise Program

In order to participate in the Otago Exercise Program, a person must be referred to the program by their general practitioner or registered health professional. All participants are required to meet specific referral criteria. These include the following:

- Be aged 80 years and over
- Display at least one fall risk factor
- Had a fall in the past year
- Leg muscle weakness
- Impaired balance
- Fear of falling
- Be able to walk (with or without an aid)
- Live in the community

Table 17.1 Incremental costs of implementing the exercise program

Cost item	Resource use	Unit cost ($)	Total cost ($)
Year 1 (n = 116)			
Recruiting costs	Details available from authors		1895
Prescribing the program			
Exercise instructor time	4 h/person	16.61/h	7707
Exercise instructor transport	2980 km	0.56/km	1669
Materials for the program			
Ankle cuff weights	180 weights	9.85/weight	1773
Instruction booklet	116 folders, paper	3.71/booklet	430
Participant follow-up costs			
Exercise instructor time	10 min telephoning 4 times/person	16.61/h	1285
General practitioner time	Total 1 h	146.36/h	14,905
Overhead costs	University of Otago services	35% of total costs	5217
Total exercise program implementation costs for year 1			20,122
Year 2 (n = 71)			
Exercise instructor time	10-min telephone, 2 monthly/person	16 61/h	1179
Overhead costs	University of Otago services		
Total exercise program implementation costs for year 2			1592
Average cost per person year 1			173
Average cost per person year 2			22

Note. Robertson et al. (2001)

Average exchange rate in 1995 New Zealand $1.00 = UK £0.42, USA $0.66

17.3.1.1 Identification and Assessment of Impaired Strength and Balance

Gardner et al. (2001) identify key fall risk indicators that can be used to determine those people who are at the highest risk of falling. These include:

- Age 80+ years
- Female
- Recent illness
- Impaired strength
- Previous falls
- Recent surgery
- Impaired balance

Two physical functioning assessments are used to assess lower limb muscle strength and balance: the chair stand test and the four-test balance scale. If a person is unable to complete either of these tasks, it indicates deficits in their strength and balance (Boxes 17.2 and 17.3).

Box 17.2 Chair Stand Test
- A straight-backed chair with no armrests should be used.
- Place the chair with a wall behind for safety.
- Instruct the person to stand up and sit down as quickly as possible, five times with the arms folded.
- Using a stopwatch, record in seconds the time taken to stand up and sit down five times.
- Allow a maximum of 2 min to complete the test.

Source: Gardner et al. (2001)

Box 17.3 Four-Test Balance Scale
The four-test balance scale includes four timed static balance tasks of increasing

(continued)

(continued)
difficulty that are completed without assistive devices (the tasks are illustrated in Fig. 17.1).

- No practices are allowed for any of the four tests and they should be carried out in bare feet.
- The person can be helped by the assessor each time to assume the position and the person should then indicate when (s)he is ready to begin the test unaided.
- If the person cannot assume the position, the test is failed at that stage.
- Each position must be held for 10 s before the person progresses to the next level of difficulty.
- Timing is stopped if (1) the person moves their feet from the proper position, (2) the assessor provides contact to prevent a fall, or (3) the person touches the wall with a hand.

Source: Gardner et al. (2001)

17.3.1.2 Exercise Program Schedule

The exercise instructor conducts four home visits over a period of 2 months; in the trials (discussed in Sect. 17.4), home visits were made at weeks 1, 2, 4, and 8, with the exercise instructor allowing up to 1 h for each visit (Gardner et al., 2001). Following the home visits, booster visits were conducted every 6 months. This allowed the exercise instructor to individually prescribe and develop the muscle strengthening and balance retraining exercises, as well as walking plan, for the OEP participant. Between home visits, the exercise instructor telephones the participants to check on progress, maintain motivation, and collect reports of any problems (Gardner et al., 2001). Table 17.2 outlines in detail the OEP schedule.

17.3.1.3 Program Resources

There are few resources required to implement the Otago Exercise Program. Each participant receives

FEET TOGETHER STAND

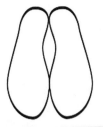

SEMI-TANDEM STAND

- The person chooses which foot is placed in front
- Hold for 10 seconds

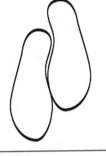

TANDEM STAND

- The person chooses which foot is placed in front
- Hold for 10 seconds

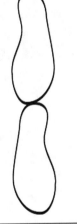

ONE LEG STAND

- The person chooses which foot to stand on
- Timing starts as soon as the person raises one foot off the ground
- We chose to extend the maximum length of time of the one leg stand test from 10 seconds to 30 seconds to lessen the ceiling effects of this test

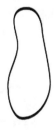

Fig. 17.1 Four-test balance scale (Gardner et al., 2001)

Table 17.2 Otago Exercise Program schedule

Month			1	2	3	4	5	6	<Monthly>	12
Week	1	2	4	8						
Home exercise visits	X	X	X	X				X		X
Telephone follow-up					X	X	X	X		
Monitoring of exercises completed			X	X	X	X	X	X	X	X
Monitoring of any falls			X	X	X	X	X	X	X	X

Note. Otago Exercise Manual (2003)

an exercise booklet and ankle cuff weights (Gardner et al., 2001). The exercise booklet provides instructions and illustrations for each exercise prescribed by instructor (Boxes 17.4, 17.5, and 17.6 and Figs. 17.2, 17.3, and 17.4). The ankle cuff weights provide resistance for the strengthening exercises.

> **Box 17.4 Examples of Instruction and Illustration from the Exercise Booklet: Trunk Movements**
>
> *Trunk Movements* (see Fig. 17.2)
>
> – Stand up tall and place your hands on your hips.
> – Do not move your hips.
> – Turn as far as you can to the right, comfortably.
> – Turn as far as you can to the left, comfortably.
> – Repeat five times to each side.
>
> Source: Otago Exercise Manual (2003)

> **Box 17.5 Examples of Instruction and Illustration from the Exercise Booklet: Side Hip Strengthening Exercise**
>
> *Side Hip Strengthening Exercise* (see Fig. 17.3)
>
> – Strap the weight on to your ankle.
> – Stand up tall beside the bench.
> – Hold onto the bench.
> – Keep the exercising leg straight and the foot straight forward.

> – Lift the leg out to the side and return.
> – Repeat _____ times.
> – Strap the weight on to the other ankle.
> – Turn around.
> – Repeat the exercise _____ times.
>
> Source: Otago Exercise Manual (2003)

> **Box 17.6 Examples of Instruction and Illustration from the Exercise Booklet: Knee Bends-Hold Support**
>
> *Knee Bends-Hold Support* (see Fig. 17.4)
>
> – Stand up tall facing the bench with both hands on the bench.
> – Place your feet should-witch apart.
> – Squat down half way, bending your knees.
> – The knees go over the toes.
> – When you feel your heels start to lift, straighten up.
> – Repeat the exercise times.
>
> Source: Otago Exercise Manual (2003)

17.3.1.4 Main Features of the Otago Exercise Program

The Otago Exercise Program addresses three major areas—strength, balance, and endurance. The strength aspect of the program consists of leg strengthening exercises, with up to four levels of difficulty. The balance aspect consists of balance retraining exercises, with up to four levels of difficulty. The endurance aspect is achieved via a

Fig. 17.2 Trunk movements (Otago Exercise Manual, 2003)

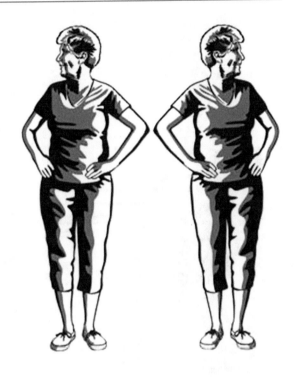

Fig. 17.3 Side hip strengthening exercise (Otago Exercise Manual, 2003)

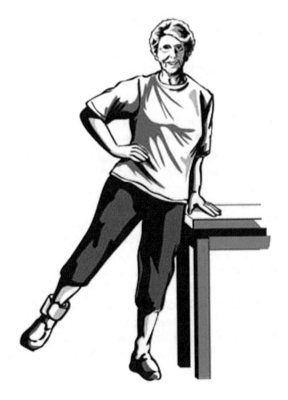

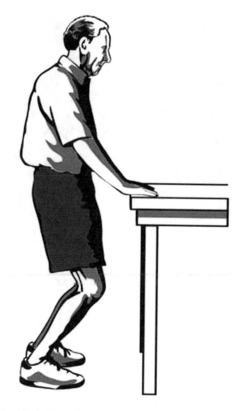

Fig. 17.4 Knee bends-hold support (Otago Exercise Manual, 2003)

walking plan. The main features of the OEP are listed in Table 17.3.

17.3.1.5 Components of the Otago Exercise Program

Prior to beginning the OEP strength and balance exercises, participants perform warm-up exercises. The main purpose of warm-up exercises is to help increase the body's core and muscle temperature; by increasing muscle temperature, it makes the muscles loose and pliable, decreasing the likelihood of injury. An effective warm-up also has the effect of increasing the participant's heart and respiratory rate. This increases blood flow, which in turn increases the delivery of oxygen and nutrients to the working muscles; this helps to prepare the muscles, tendons, and joints for more strenuous activity. The warm-up exercises include:

- Head movements
- Neck movements
- Back extensions
- Trunk movements
- Ankle movements

17.3.1.6 Strength Training Component of the Otago Exercise Program

The OEP provides participants with moderate-intensity strength training by targeting the major muscles of the leg. The focus on strength training is an important component of the OEP, as strengthening the lower body is important for the prevention of falls. The strengthening exercises include (for details see Table 17.4):

- Front knee strengthening exercise
- Back knee strengthening exercise
- Side hip strengthening exercise
- Calf raises—hold support/no support
- Toe raises—hold support/no support

The strengthening exercises focus on the major lower limb muscles (i.e., knee flexors, knee extensors, hip abductors, ankle dorsiflexor muscles, ankle plantar flexor muscles). The hip extensor, knee extensor, hip abductor, and ankle muscles are targeted, as they are important for functional movements (i.e., standing up from a chair and walking) (Gardner et al., 2001). The ankle dorsiflexor and plantar flexor muscles are targeted as they play an important role for recovery of balance. In order to facilitate strength training, the ankle cuff weights are used to provide resistance to the hip abductor, knee flexor, and knee extensor muscles; the ankle dorsiflexor and plantar flexor muscles are strengthened by the participants body weight (Gardner et al., 2001).

The duration and frequency of strength training is recommended 3 days a week. Participants are advised to allow a day of rest between muscle strengthening exercises, as it allows for muscle recuperation and development.

Table 17.3 Main features of the Otago Exercise Program

	Strengthening	Balance retraining	Walking
Activities	5 leg muscle strengthening exercises, with up to 4 levels of difficulty[a]	12 balance retraining exercises with up to 4 levels of difficulty[a]	Advice about walking
Assessment	The amount of weight in ankle cuff should allow 8–10 repetitions before fatigue	Set each exercise at a level that the person can safely perform unsupervised	Discuss present walking activities
Intensity	Moderate	Moderate	Usual pace with usual walking aid
Progressions[a]	Increase to 2 sets of repetitions, increase the weight of the ankle cuff	From supported exercise to unsupported exercise	
Frequency	At least 3 times a week, with a rest day between	At least 3 times a week	At least 2 times a week
Duration	Approximately 30 min to do the flexibility, strength, and balance exercises; exercises can be divided up over the day		30 min; can be broken down to three 10-min walks throughout the day

Note. Otago Exercise Manual (2003)
[a]The exercises at each level of difficulty are shown in Tables 17.4 and 17.5

Table 17.4 Levels and number of repetitions for the strengthening exercises

Strengthening exercises	Levels	
	All 4 Levels	
Knee extensor (front knee strength)	Ankle cuff weights are used to provide resistance to the muscles and 10 repetitions of each exercise are carried out	
Knee flexor (back knee strength)		
Hip abductor (side hip strength)		
	Level C	Level D
Ankle plantar flexors (calf raises)	10 repetitions, hold support, repeat	10 repetitions, no support, repeat
Ankle dorsiflexors (toe raises)	10 repetitions, hold support, repeat	10 repetitions, no support, repeat

Note. Otago Exercise Manual (2003)

17.3.1.7 Balance Retraining Component of the Otago Exercise Program

The OEP provides participants with balance exercises. The balance exercises are dynamic—stretches that use speed of movement, momentum, and active muscular effort to bring about stretch—as opposed to static (Gardner et al., 2001). Balance exercises are important for everyday lifestyle activities and function, for example, moving from a sit to a stand position, walking and turning around, and knee bends. The balance training exercise include (for details see Table 17.5):

- Knee bends—hold support/no support
- Backward walking—hold support/no support
- Walking and turning around
- Sideways walking
- Heel toe standing—hold support/no support
- Heel toe walking—hold support/no support
- One leg stand—hold support/no support
- Heel walking—hold support/no support
- Toe walking—hold support/no support
- Heel toe walking backward
- Sit to stand—two hands/one hands/no hands
- Stair walking

The purpose of the balance exercises is not only to maintain balance but also to recover balance by using legs rather than grasping for supporting structures (i.e., furniture) with arms. Therefore, in addition to helping maintain balance, the balance exercises improve the recovery of balance.

Table 17.5 Levels and number of repetitions for the balance retraining exercises

	Level A	Level B	Level C	Level D
Knee bends	10 repetitions, hold support	(1) 10 repetitions, no support *or* (2) 10 repetitions, hold support, repeat	10 repetitions, no support, repeat	3 × 10 repetitions, no support
Backward walking		10 steps, 4 times, hold support		10 steps, 4 times, no support
Walking and turning around		Walk and turn around (make figure of 8) twice, use walking aid	Walk and turn around (make figure of 8) twice, no support	
Sideways walking		10 steps, 4 times, use walking aid	10 steps, 4 times, no support	
Tandem stance (heel toe stand)	10 s, hold support	10 s, no support		
Tandem walk (heel toe walk)			Walk 10 steps, hold support, repeat	Walk 10 steps, no support, repeat
One leg stand		10 s, hold support	10 s, no hold	30 s, no hold
Heel walking			10 steps, 4 times, hold support	10 steps, 4 times, no support
Toe walk			10 steps, 4 times, hold support	10 steps, 4 times, no support
Heel toe walking backward				Walk 10 steps, no support, repeat
Sit to stand	5 stands, 2 hands for support	(1) 5 stands, one hand or (2) 10 stands, 2 hands for support	(1) 10 stands, no support or (2) 10 stands, 1 hand for support, repeat	10 stands, no support, repeat
Stair walking	As instructed	As instructed	As instructed	As instructed, repeat

Note. Otago Exercise Manual (2003)

The OEP balance exercises progress from holding onto a stable supporting structure (i.e., heavy furniture) to performing the exercises independent of support. The starting level of each exercise is dependent upon the baseline physical functioning and health status of the older person; not all older people will necessarily start at the same level or be prescribed all the balancing exercises (this is where the individually prescribed component is integrated into the OEP; Gardner et al., 2001). The duration and frequency of balance retraining is recommended 3 days a week.

17.3.1.8 Walking Component of the Otago Exercise Program

The OEP encourages participants to include a walking component as part of the exercise program. In implementing this component, participants are encouraged to aim for 30 min of walking, twice per week. If the participant is unable to walk the prescribed duration and frequency, they are encouraged to start with 10-min walks broken up over period of the day; as strength and endurance increases, the participant can progress to the prescribed duration and frequency (Gardner et al., 2001).

17.3.1.9 Study Population of the Four Trials

In order to identify participants for the four trials, general practitioners utilized computer practice registers. The potential participants identified received a letter from their general practitioner inviting them to take part in the strength and balance training intervention (Robertson, Campbell, Gardner, & Devlin, 2002). Following the referral from the general practitioner, the potential participant received a telephone call from the exercise instructor or research staff (Robertson et al., 2002).

The only criteria for exclusion in the intervention trials were inability for the participant to walk around their residence, if they were receiving physiotherapy at the time of recruitment, or if they were unable to understand the trial requirements (Robertson et al., 2002). The study population characteristics differed: age groups differed in each trial; the Dunedin Study A included women only and the Dunedin Study B included only persons currently taking psychotropic medication, as withdrawal of these medications was an intervention in this trial (Robertson et al., 2002).

17.3.1.10   Participant Recruitment

The patient's general practitioner or a registered health professional approves participation in the program. Of the individuals invited to participate, some choose to participate, some declined, and others were not eligible to participate. In order to ensure that each study participant had a fair and equal chance of receiving the intervention, the participants were separated into study groups via randomization (Robertson, Devlin, Gardner, & Campbell, 2001).

17.3.1.11   Health Outcome Measures

Falls were defined as "unintentionally coming to rest on the ground, floor, or other lower level" (Robertson et al., 2002). In order to monitor falls, participants were asked to return preaddressed, prepaid, tear-off monthly postcard calendars for each month (Robertson et al., 2002). If the card was not returned, the research staff telephoned the participant. The monthly post card calendars and follow-up contact with participants was found to be the best method for reporting falls. In the instance a fall was reported, the date and circumstances were recorded by completing a fall event form by telephone (Robertson et al., 2002). Falls were classified as resulting in "serious" injury if the fall resulted in a fracture, admission to the hospital, or stitches were required; a moderate injury if the fall resulted in bruising, sprains, cuts, abrasions, or reduction in physical function for at least 3 days; or a fall resulting in no injury (Robertson et al., 2002).

17.4   Outcome

17.4.1 An Evidence-Based Approach to Falls Prevention

The Otago Exercise Program has been tested in four separate controlled trials (for details see Table 17.6). The main results from each of the four trials (Dunedin Study A, Dunedin Study B, West Auckland Trial, Southern New Zealand Trial) are detailed below.

17.4.1.1   Trial 1: Dunedin Study A

The Otago Exercise Program was first tested in a randomized controlled trial of women aged 80 years and older. The results of the study indicated that after the first year of implementation, the program was effective in reducing the risk of falling by 32% and the risk of a fall-related injury by 39% (Campbell et al., 1997). Due to the excellent results, the trial was extended for a second year; a significant reduction in falls and fall-related injuries continued.

17.4.1.2   Trial 2: Dunedin Study B

The Dunedin Study B investigated two interventions to prevent falls in people aged 65 and older; (1) the gradual withdrawal of psychotropic (sleeping) medication and (2) the Otago Exercise Program. The results of the study indicated there was a 66% reduction in falls for participants who withdrew from their psychotropic medications, in comparison to those who continued on their prescribed medication regimen (Campbell, Robertson, Gardner, Norton, & Buchner, 1999). The permanent withdrawal was difficult to achieve for 46% (8 of 17) of participants; 1 month after the trial's completion, these individuals restarted their medications (Campbell et al., 1999). There was no evidence that the Otago Exercise Program reduced falls and fall-related injuries.

17.4.1.3   Trial 3: West Auckland Trial

In both Trial 1 and Trial 2, the Otago Exercise Program was delivered by a qualified health professional (i.e., physiotherapist) in a controlled research setting. In order to test the exercise program in a "real life" situation, two additional trials were implemented in routine health-care service settings (West Auckland Trial and Southern New Zealand Trial).

The participants in the West Auckland Trial were men and women aged 75 years and older. The purpose of the trial was to investigate the effectiveness of the individually prescribed home exercise program, administered by a trained dis-

Table 17.6 Summary of the four trials

Trial features	Dunedin Study A	Dunedin Study B	West Auckland Trial	Southern New Zealand Trial
Trial sample	Women aged ≥80	Women and men aged ≥65 currently taking psychotropic medication	Women and men aged ≥75	Women and men aged ≥80
Sample size	Year 1: 233 Year 2: 152	93	240	450
Trial design	Randomized controlled trial	Randomized controlled trial 2 × 2 factorial design 4 groups	Randomized controlled trial	3 exercise centers 4 control centers
Interventions	(1) Exercise program (n = 116) vs. (2) Social visits and usual care (n = 117)	(1) Exercise program (2) Gradual withdrawal of psychotropic medication—a double blind intervention	(1) Exercise program (n = 121) vs. (2) Usual care (n = 119)	(1) Exercise program (n = 330) vs. (2) Usual care (n = 120)
Exercise instructor	Physiotherapist	Physiotherapist	Community nurse	General practice nurse
Number of home visits	4	4	5	5
Setting	Research	Research	Community health service	General practices
Fall events monitored	2 years	44 weeks	1 year	1 year
Key results	Exercise program reduced falls by 32% in year 1 For those who kept exercising, benefit continued in year 2	Falls reduced by 66% in those who withdrew from psychotropic medication Exercise program did not reduce risk of falling	Exercise program reduced falls by 46%	Exercise program reduced falls by 30%

Note. Otago Exercise Manual (2003)

trict nurse, in reducing falls and fall-related injuries, as well as provide an estimate of the cost-effectiveness of the program (Robertson, Gardner, Devlin, McGee, & Campbell, 2001).

The results indicated a reduction in falls by 46%, with fewer participants reporting a serious injury, compared with those receiving usual case (Robertson, Devlin, Scuffham, et al., 2001). Furthermore, the findings demonstrated that falls were reduced for participants aged 80 and older, but there were no significant reductions in falls and fall-related injuries for participants aged 75–79 years (Robertson, Devlin, Scuffham, et al., 2001). In other words, the program was cost-effective in participants aged 80 years and older compared with younger participants. In addition, the trial verified that the home exercise program, successfully administered by a physiotherapist in the Dunedin A and B studies, was also effective

in reducing falls when delivered by a trained nurse from with a home health service.

17.4.1.4 Trial 4: Southern New Zealand Trial

In the Southern New Zealand Trial, participants were men and women aged 80 years and older. The purpose of this trial was similar to that of the West Auckland Trial, that is, to investigate the effectiveness of the individually prescribed home exercise program, administered by a trained district nurse, in reducing falls and fall-related injuries, as well as provide an estimate of the cost-effectiveness of the program (Robertson, Gardner, Devlin, et al., 2001).

The results of the study indicated a 30% reduction in falls and a 28% reduction in moderate and serious injuries combined, as compared with usual care (Robertson, Devlin, Scuffham, et al., 2001). Due to the effectiveness and ease of implementation of the program, approximately 70% of participants continued exercising at the end of the trial, with 43% continuing with the individually prescribed exercises (Robertson, Devlin, Scuffham, et al., 2001). In addition, the results of the West Auckland and Southern New Zealand trial demonstrate that trained district nurses, closely supervised by an experienced physiotherapist, were able to deliver the exercise program with beneficial results.

17.4.2 Combining the Results: Meta-Analysis of Individual-Level Data

A meta-analysis combined the data from all four trials. Robertson et al. (2002) conclude:

- Overall, the data indicated that the Otago Exercise Program was effective in reducing the number of falls and fall-related injuries by 35%.
- In terms of injurious falls prevented, the Otago Exercise Program was more effective for participants aged 80 years and older than for those 65–79.
- Participants with and without a history of a previous fall benefited equally from the exercise program.
- Both men and women benefited equally from participating in the exercise program, with an overall 35% reduction in falls.
- Combining the data provided an opportunity to determine which subgroups in the trials benefited most from the exercise program shown in Table 17.7.
- In terms of the number of falls and injurious falls prevented by the exercise program, those aged 80 and older and those with a previous fall benefited most.
- Combining the results from the four trials demonstrated the fact that the program prevented the most falls and injuries in those aged 80 years who had fallen in the previous year.
- Two simple physical assessments, the chair stand test and four-test balance scale, showed

Table 17.7 Combined analysis of the four trials: number of fall events prevented in subgroups

Subgroup	Falls prevented per 100 person years	Injurious falls prevented per 100 person years
Aged ≥80, fall(s) in previous year	54.0	28.8
Fall(s) in previous year	44.3	20.9
Aged ≥80	40.8	20.1
All participants (aged 65–97 years)	33.9	15.8
Aged ≥80, no fall in previous year	25.8	11.6
No fall in previous year	23.6	11.0
Aged 65–79	5.4	−2.3

Note. Robertson et al. (2002)

improved strength and balance in exercise group participants.
- There were very few adverse events in the trials due to the exercise program.

17.5   Conclusion

There is good research evidence that the Otago Exercise Program reduces falls and fall-related injuries in older people. The evidence indicates that the exercise program is effective in reducing the number of falls and fall-related injuries by 35% in older adults. Furthermore, the results from the four trails combined indicate that the exercise program is most effective in preventing falls and injuries in those aged 80 years who have fallen in the previous year. The program's cost-effectiveness has been established in two health-care settings and is most beneficial in high-risk groups (i.e., individuals over 80 years of age with previous falls). Although tested as a stand-alone intervention, the Otago Exercise Program could be delivered as part of a multifactorial falls prevention program. An additional benefit is that manual and program are ready for implementation.

Acknowledgments The author would like to express sincere appreciation to the key informant for this case study—M. Clare Robertson of the Dunedin School of Medicine, University of Otago in Dunedin, New Zealand—whose consultation made this project possible.

BRIO Model: Otago Exercise Program

Group Served: The program serves senior adults who have history of a fall.

Goal: The program aims to prevent reinjury from falls through an exercise program.

Background	Resources	Implementation	Outcome
According to the Accident Compensation Corporation (ACC), falls resulting in injury are the leading cause of hospitalization and one of the top three causes of injury-related deaths in New Zealand A complex interaction of risk factors contributes to falls. The risk factors can be grouped into three categories: (1) biological and medical, (2) behavioral, and (3) environmental The Otago Exercise Program is an individually tailored muscle strengthening and balance retraining exercise program	The Otago Exercise Program was designed by the Falls Prevention Research Group at the University of Otago Medical School The Otago Exercise Program is part of the Preventing Injury from Falls: The National Strategy 2005–2015. The strategy aims to reduce the incidence and severity of injury from falls and the impact of fall-related injuries The Otago Exercise Program's cost-effectiveness has been established in two health-care settings The resources used to implement the exercise program include those for recruiting the physiotherapist who administered the program, program materials, and overhead costs	Two physical functioning assessments are used to assess lower limb muscle strength and balance: the chair stand test and the four-test balance scale. If a person is unable to complete either of these tasks, it indicates deficits in their strength and balance The participant is instructed to carry out the set of exercises three times a week and to walk twice a week for 30 min The exercise instructor conducts four home visits over a period of 2 months; in the trials (discussed in Sect. 17.4), home visits were made at weeks 1, 2, 4, and 8, with the exercise instructor allowing up to 1 h for each visit	Overall, the data indicated that the Otago Exercise Program was effective in reducing the number of falls and fall-related injuries by 35% In terms of injurious falls prevented, the Otago Exercise Program was more effective for participants aged 80 years and older than for those 65–79 Participants with and without a history of a previous fall benefited equally from the exercise program Combining the results from the four trials demonstrated the fact that the program prevented the most falls and injuries in those aged 80 years who had fallen in the previous year

Life Space Model: Otago Exercise Program

Sociocultural civilization/community	Interpersonal primary and secondary relationships	Physical environment where we live	Internal states biochemical/genetic and means of coping
The evidence indicates that implementing this program reduces falls and injuries in older people The Otago Exercise Program is administered in a home-based community setting The effect of the exercise program was a 35% reduction in the number of falls and a 35% reduction in the number of fall-related injuries The program was more effective for those aged 80 and older than for those 65–79 years old, especially in terms of injurious falls prevented	Fosters relationships between general practitioners and patients The program can be combined with group programs (i.e., meeting once a week with other participants to complete the strength and balance retraining exercises) The program involves family members, as they are an important role in the reinjury process	According to the Accident Compensation Corporation (ACC), falls resulting in injury are the leading cause of hospitalization and one of the top three causes of injury-related deaths in New Zealand In young adulthood hospital admissions resulting from falls are uncommon, but with advancing age, the incidence of fall-related hospital admissions increase at an exponential rate After the age of 40, the admission rate due to falls for men increases by 4.5% per year, while for women the rate increases by 7.9%	Individuals who make physical activity and exercise a part of their daily lives experience the benefit throughout their life span Although the Otago Exercise Program is concerned with strength and balance retraining, the exercise program provides participants with both physical and mental benefits In addition to the physical component of reinjury, a fall can result in the loss of independence and confidence, a reluctance to undertake certain activities, reduced quality of life, and a fear of falls happening again

References

Accident Compensation Corporation. (2005). *Preventing injury from falls: The National Strategy 2005–2015.*

Campbell, A. J., Robertson, M. C., Gardner, M. M., Norton, R. N., & Buchner, D. M. (1999). Psychotropic medication withdrawal and a home-based exercise program to prevent falls: A randomized controlled trial. *Journal of the American Geriatrics Society, 47*, 850–853.

Campbell, A. J., Robertson, M. C., Gardner, M. M., Norton, R. N., Tilyard, M. W., & Buchner, D. M. (1997). Randomised controlled trial of a general practice program of home based exercise to prevent falls in elderly women. *British Medical Journal, 315*, 1065–1069.

Gardner, M. M., Buchner, D. M., Robertson, M. C., & Campbell, A. J. (2001). Practical implementation of an exercise-based falls prevention program. *Age and Ageing, 30*, 77–83.

Otago Exercise Manual. (2003). Otago Medical School, University of Otago.

Report on Senior's Falls in Canada. (2005). Division of Aging and Seniors, Public Health Agency of Canada, Minister of Public Works and Government Services Canada.

Robertson, M. C., Campbell, A. J., Gardner, M. M., & Devlin, N. (2002). Preventing injuries in older people by preventing falls: A meta-analysis of individual-level data. *Journal of the American Geriatrics Society, 50*, 905–911.

Robertson, M. C., Devlin, N., Gardner, M. M., & Campbell, A. J. (2001). Effectiveness and economic evaluation of a nurse delivered home exercise program to prevent falls. 1: Randomised controlled trial. *British Medical Journal, 322*, 697–701.

Robertson, M. C., Devlin, N., Scuffham, P., Gardner, M. M., Buchner, D. M., & Campbell, A. J. (2001). Economic evaluation of a community based exercise program to prevent falls. *Journal of Epidemiology and Community Health, 55*, 600–606.

Robertson, M. C., Gardner, M. M., Devlin, N., McGee, R., & Campbell, A. J. (2001). Effectiveness and economic evaluation of a nurse delivered home exercise program to prevent falls. 2. Controlled trial in multiple centres. *British Medical Journal, 322*, 701–704.

Part III

Road Traffic-Related Traumatic Injury Prevention Programs

Overview of Road Traffic-Related Traumatic Injury Prevention Programs

Raganya Ponmanadiyil

Transportation is arguably one of the most predominant and essential aspects of everyday life. Individuals all over the world—regardless of age, class, race, and ability—require transportation in some way, shape, or form for a variety of tasks and situations. Unfortunately, the prevalence of transportation comes with significant potential danger. Whether traveling by foot, bicycle, or motorized vehicle, transportation systems and routes pose threats to not only the quality of life but life itself. Despite originally falling under the responsibility of the transport sector, which is often a collection of traffic safety agencies within a governmental department, road safety has increasingly become part of the public health sector. Thus, road safety has become a collaborative effort of medicine, biomechanics, epidemiology, sociology, behavioral science, criminology, education, economics, and engineering (Volpe, 2004).

Injuries from transportation collisions are, more often than not, unintentional in nature. Transportation is the second leading cause of unintentional injury-related death in the United States (Centers for Disease Control [CDC], 2015). This is significant as unintentional injury

was the third leading cause of death in general (CDC, 2015). Globally, approximately 1.3 million individuals die in road crashes every year (Road Crash Statistics, 2018). Despite the modern transportation advancements and safety measures of today, fatalities continue to transpire at alarming rates.

18.1 Rates of Road Injury

18.1.1 Canada

Canada experienced 2620 deaths and 290,782 emergency room visits in the year 2010 alone as a result of transportation-related incidents (see Table 18.1; Parachute, 2015). In 2015, the number of motor vehicle fatalities decreased from 1858 to 161,902 injuries. This has resulted in a rate of 5.2 deaths per 100,000 (Canadian Motor Vehicle Traffic Collision Statistics: 2015, 2017).

Transportation-related incidents create significant economic burden. Considering both direct and indirect costs, such as hospital visits and unemployment, experts suggest that in 2010, transportation-related injuries cost Canadians a total of $4298 million (Parachute, 2015). Table 18.2 (Parachute, 2015) displays the breakdown of costs as a result of transportation incidents.

R. Ponmanadiyil (✉)
Ontario Institute for Studies in Education, University of Toronto, Toronto, ON, Canada

© Springer Nature Switzerland AG 2020
R. Volpe (ed.), *Casebook of Traumatic Injury Prevention*,
https://doi.org/10.1007/978-3-030-27419-1_18

Table 18.1 Incidences of death, hospital visits, and disability as a result of collisions in 2010

	Deaths	Hospitalization	ER visits	Partial disability	Permanent disability
Transportation incidents (total)	2620	28,350	290,782	7204	699
Motor vehicle	1119	14,437	161,977	3534	360
Bicycle	92	4112	59,815	1240	113
Pedestrian	369	2902	17,725	673	76

Note. These results reflect data from 2010 in Canada. This table was created using data from The Cost of Injury in Canada, by Parachute, 2015, Toronto, Canada: Parachute

Table 18.2 Economic costs[a] (direct and indirect) as a result of transportation incidents

	Total costs ($ millions)	Direct costs ($ millions)	Indirect costs ($ millions)
Transportation incidents (total)	4289	2145	2144
Motor vehicle	1190	987	2177
Bicycle	293	213	506
Pedestrian	234	225	458

Note. These results reflect data from 2010 in Canada. This table was created using data from The Cost of Injury in Canada, by Parachute, 2015, Toronto, Canada: Parachute
[a]Economic costs are divided into direct costs (healthcare costs arising from injuries) and indirect costs (costs related to societal productivity losses—reduced productivity due to hospitalization, disability, and premature death)

Table 18.3 Incident rates of road collisions leading to death and nonfatal injuries in 2013

	Deaths	Nonfatal injuries
Total road incidents	35,500	4,300,000
Car	14,800	3,260,000
Bicycle	1000	120,000
Pedestrian	6100	160,000
Other[a]	13,600	760,000

Note. These results reflect data from 2013 in the United States from road collisions leading to death or nonfatal injury. This table was created using data from Injury Facts, 2015 Edition by the National Safety Council, 2015
[a]"Other" indicates injury from collisions with fixed objects, non-collisions, railroad train, and other minor types

18.1.2 Australia

Australia has relatively low rates of fatalities and injuries as a result of road incidents, with a total of 1352 fatalities in 2010 (Henley & Harrison, 2015). In the same year, they had a total of 42,583 serious incidents that lead to some level of serious injury (Henley & Harrison, 2015; see Table 18.3; Henley & Harrison, 2015).

18.1.3 The United Kingdom

The United Kingdom (UK) had lower numbers of serious road injuries when compared to the incidence rates in Canada or Australia in categories such as automobile, motorcycle, bicycle, and pedestrian. Nonetheless, in 2014, the United Kingdom had a total of 1775 fatalities and 22,807 total serious injuries as a result of transportation-related incidents, an increase of 4% compared to the year before (Department for Transport, 2015).

18.1.4 The United States

While these Canadian, Australian, and British figures are problematically high, they pale in comparison to the United States. Between 2008 and 2014, the averaged death rates per 100,000 individuals ranged between 6.28 and 24.89 across the country (CDC, 2015). In 2016 alone, the United States experienced 38,748 deaths resulting from motor vehicle collisions, costing the country over $288 billion (CDC, 2017; National Safety Council, 2015). Incident rates from 2013 across the United States are displayed in Table 18.3.

Road collisions are the principal cause of neurotrauma injuries. Motor vehicle crashes are responsible for 30–50% of all brain and spinal cord injuries, which can lead to partial or complete disability or death (Ontario Brain Injury Association Review [OBIA], 2002). From 2008 to 2014, transportation-related traumatic brain injury across the United States ranged from 1.80 to 10.46 injuries per 100, 000, with an annualized rate of 4.09 (CDC, 2015).

With road-related incidents being a leading cause of serious injury and death, it is essential to understand some major issues affecting traffic safety today. These risk factors provide areas of focus for prevention and intervention programs to address for the purpose of increasing road safety. Listed below are several major road safety issues as expressed by the National Safety Council (2015):

- Occupant protection.
- Alcohol and drug influences leading to impairment.
- Speeding.
- Distracted driving: This includes using a cell phone or text messaging while driving.
- Large trucks.
- Motorcycles.
- Young drivers: This includes those between the ages of 15 and 20.
- Pedestrians.

Prevention efforts are difficult without fully comprehending the reasons contributing to transportation incidents. Among the variety of factors involved, most commonly, unintentional incidents are rooted in an existing inconsistency between driver behavior, road environments, and/ or vehicle characteristics. Thus, there is inevitable susceptibility to the impact of road-related threats; however, certain factors are preventable—to varying degrees. Driver characteristics and road environments, or more broadly internal and external factors, need to be considered.

Effective prevention appears to require attention to interactions and transactions among and between people and their environments, which unfortunately leads to complexity. The performance level of a driver varies as it is impacted by factors such as fatigue, drowsiness, illness, and lack of concentration. In turn, the road environment varies due to factors such as traffic flow rates, geometric features of the road, and road type. To accommodate for this, the driver must adapt their performance based on demands of the road system. An incident occurs when there is a discrepancy between the driver's performance and their adaptability to the demands of the road environment (Haddon, 1968). The safety margin between the driver's performance level and the demands of the road environment can be increased through engineering improvements in the road design.

The "Haddon Matrix" can be used as a device for sorting out the pieces of the motor vehicle loss problem and preventive measures directed at its reduction (Haddon, 1968). Building on this matrix, road trauma prevention seeks to identify and rectify the major sources of error or design weaknesses that contribute to fatal and severe injury crashes. As well, prevention efforts attempt to mitigate the severity and consequences of injury by reducing exposure or risk, preventing road traffic crashes from occurring, reducing the severity of injury in the event of a crash, and reducing the consequences of injury through improved post-collision care.

Similarly, the life-space approach (Volpe, 2004) aims to determine the sociocultural, interpersonal, physical, and internal factors to determine the effectiveness of a prevention program (Volpe, 2004). Evident here is a dynamic interplay of complex systems, where injury involves complex person-environment interactions. The shortcoming of most discipline-based research is that it does not take into consideration this complexity, usually favoring a reductionist account by separating causes of injury into distinct component parts. Injury prevention should be focused on the holistic nature of human change and the importance of timing in understanding human adaptation as a part of complex contextual system (Volpe, 2004). Fortunately, some programs are in practice today that understand the complexity of road safety.

18.2 Section Chapters

This current section will review nine case studies that demonstrate exemplar practices and programs aimed at preventing motor vehicle and road trauma-related injuries. Across all programs is the understanding of an incorporated systems approach and the life-space approach. This section will attempt to preview the case studies that will follow in this chapter under two main qualities: external and internal factors to the individual.

By understanding these exemplary programs from their conceptions to their current situations, the world can be one step closer to the fantasy of road trauma incidents being a thing of the past.

18.2.1 Factors External to the Individual

Considering the variety of external factors that could affect road trauma incidents is essential. Such external factors include infrastructure of roads, engineering, and technological additions. Since human error can occur at any moment during walking, biking, or driving, it is essential to control as much as possible without the unpredictability of human inaccuracies affecting overall safety.

An example of such a comprehensive approach to road safety lies within the program Vision Zero (Chap. 19) (Vision Zero Canada, n.d.). This exemplar program, first developed in Sweden, has contributed to the country's reputation of having some of the safest roads in the world (European Commission, 2005). Now a multinational initiative, Vision Zero aims to create a world where there are zero road-related traumas and deaths, by understanding that humans make mistakes and the road system should be designed to protect individuals from those mistakes, utilizing a "safe system approach" (City of Toronto, 2017). This is a result of understanding that a safe road system consists of engineering, enforcement, education, and technology initiatives (Business Sweden, n.d.). Vision Zero breaks up the system into road users, roads/roadsides, vehicle, and speed and aims to tackle the factors not susceptible to human error as much as possible while also providing education to combat those issues. Internationally, many of these goals and practices are being implemented to the ultimate goal of zero road-related deaths (Business Sweden, n.d.).

This allows for a certain capacity of give and take in order to be more forgiving of potential human error by controlling factors that can be managed and manipulated. For example, controlling in-car activity is relatively difficult and unpredictable, but having rumble strips or a large shoulder on the side of the highway can help combat serious injury as a result of losing control on the road (Swedish National Road Administration [SNRA], 2006; City of Toronto, 2017). This program is sensational in its comprehensiveness, many initiatives, and exemplar in its ability to incorporate the four quadrants of the life-space model. As effective as Vision Zero has proven to be, it is a vast and highly comprehensive program with a variety of aspects required to be implemented, which may be difficult for some to apply.

Similarly, another effective program that highlights the importance of combating external factors stems from Australia. The Black Spot Program (Chap. 20) understands the holistic approach to road safety and aims to combat it by studying trends in driver and collision behavior. However, in an altered approach, high-risk locations, referred to as hazardous or "black spots," are identified, which are complicated by many factors including the degree and type of risk, road characteristics, traffic exposure, and crash severity. Accordingly, black spot projects are road improvement treatments that focus on reducing the number of casualties at a particular location on a road network through the most cost-effective means (Bureau of Transport Economics, 2001). Typically, black spot programs focus on reduction factors such as fixed roadside objects that infringe on traffic lanes, unsealed shoulders, high traffic volumes and minimal traffic control, poor visibility, and pedestrians (Bureau of Transport Economics, 2001). The program is highly implemented across Australia as it is approvingly funded by the federal government.

In a less intricate fashion, introducing and instigating technology advancements to roads are effective in minimizing road-related trauma risks. Some programs continue to understand the rounded approach to road safety while having more explicit emphases. The United Kingdom (UK) initiated the implementation of External Vehicle Speed Controls (EVSC)/Intelligent Speed Adaptations (ISA; Chap. 21) to control traffic flow and improve road safety. The technology allows for the speed of cars and other motorized vehicles to be presented roadside while driving for the benefit of the driver. Being distracted or zoning out regarding one's speed while driving is common, and therefore having visual reminders of staying within the speed limits have proven to be advantageous.

Comparable to the Black Spot Program, Ontario's COMPASS (Chap. 22) program focuses on critical areas concerning traffic congestion that threaten safety on the road. The COMPASS initiative was designed based on successful programs in Los Angeles and Detroit to manage recurring and non-recurring congestion. COMPASS is utilized to smooth out the flow of traffic to deflect from stop-and-go driving conditions (Korpal, Rayman, & Masters, 1994). Incident detection is utilized and undertaken by COMPASS with automatic and manual methods. COMPASS is an empirically proven method of reducing accidents on freeways cited as primary locations for transportation-related injury, in and around major urban areas, such as Toronto, Canada (Ontario Road Safety Annual Report, 2001).

18.2.2 Factors Internal to the Individual

When it comes to human behavior, it is difficult to control factors that are internal to an individual. Regarding road safety, internal factors include alcohol consumption, distracted driving, as well as age. Some of these factors are relatively easily preventable and a variety of prevention programs exist to either educate or legally reprimand negative outcomes. By dividing internal factors further into those related to age and capability, preventative measures can be more comprehensively tackled.

18.2.2.1 Age Related: School-Aged Children

Traffic fatalities are a leading cause of injury death in Canada for children over the age of 1 year (Canada Safety Council, 2004; Canadian Institute of Child Health [CICH], 2000; Organisation for Economic Co-operation and Development [OECD], 2004). Worldwide, road traffic injuries account for the second leading cause of death of 130,835 children between the ages of 5 and 14 years (World Health Organization

[WHO], 2004). Based on their physical growth and development, children are much more susceptible to severe injury when involved in a collision (Liu & Yang, 2003). Furthermore, a greater head rotational velocity results in more severe traumatic brain injuries resulting in head injuries to a 6-year-old child being more severe than those sustained by a 15-year-old child in the same collision (Liu & Yang, 2003).

In addition to the frequency and severity of child pedestrian injuries, it is also important to distinguish where and how these injuries typically occur. Among 5- to 9-year-old pedestrians, 48% of injuries occurred at mid-block, non-intersection locations and most of these resulted from stepping out from between parked cars (Rivara & Barbar, 1985). Older children tend to have a higher injury rate, which is typically due to their greater mobility when compared to younger children. In the 10–14 age category, 56% of injuries occurred at intersections, and only 10% of victims were accompanied by an adult at the time of injury (Hunt, 1998; Rivara & Barbar, 1985).

Interestingly, and vital for prevention, is to understand the relation of child road-related injuries and school. Based on a Canadian study done in 1991, 6% of child injuries happened to children on their way to school compared to 30% that occurred on their way home (Joly, Foggin, & Pless, 1991).

It is necessary to have a vision of prevention that is able to meet the needs of all members in a community as "injury prevention is about culture and society, communities and neighborhoods, families and friends, lifestyles, and ways of thinking" (Volpe, 2004). One such exemplar program targeting the issues pertaining to child pedestrian road safety is Ontario's Active and Safe Routes to School (ASRTS; Chap. 23). ASRTS is a national movement, initially developed in Denmark, dedicated to children's mobility, health, and overall wellness. The main goal revolves around promoting active school travel through a variety of community and school initiatives (Go for Green, 2003). ASRTS promotes healthier students, fewer emissions resulting in less air pollution, and overall safer school zones by reducing traffic volumes due to the focus on non-infrastructure and infrastructure measures (Active and Safe Routes to School [ASRTS], 2004). The program addresses a wide array of success factors and is a proven cost-effective intervention to get more kids active on their way to school. The ability of ASRTS to target and incorporate all four quadrants of the life-space model and be a proven success in intervention demonstrates an exemplar program for road safety prevention.

18.2.2.2 Age Related: Young Drivers

Young drivers represent a highly significant road safety concern in motorized countries. According to the World Health Organization, road traffic injury is the primary cause of death for young drivers worldwide (Peden et al., 2004). More specifically, in the United States, teenagers have motor vehicle collision rates that exceed those of drivers of any age, 16–17-year-olds being particularly risky (Williams, 2003). Quite interestingly, collision rates for 17-year-olds is 50% higher than that for 18-year-olds, and the rate for 16-year-olds is two and a half times higher than that for 18-year-olds, even though 18-year-olds have a higher collision rate than any older age (Williams, 1998). This poses an interesting dilemma regarding the age of onset of driving and associated problems.

California's graduated driver licensing (GDL; Chap. 24) program helps combat the disproportionately high rate of motor vehicle collisions and resulting traumatic brain injuries involving young drivers, particularly those under the age of 18 (Williams, 2003; Williams & Mayhew, 2004). By allowing new drivers the opportunity to gain experience through exposure of conditions that gradually increase in risk, drivers are better able to understand and learn how to curb some risks. Under graduated licensing, young drivers are initially granted partial driving privileges so that they may gain the necessary driving experience under conditions of reduced risk. As they gain experience and mature, they are awarded broader privileges until they finally receive a full license. The GDL model employed by California incorporates three stages and encompasses elements

that affect the individual and environmental factors of the road. When aspects of the program were implemented in Ontario, Canada, the Ministry of Transportation noticed a decrease in young driver motor vehicle collisions (Boase & Tasca, 1998; Ministry of Transportation, 2002). By incorporating aspects of the life-space model into an educational initiative, California's GDL exemplar program allows for safer roads by creating informed, experienced, and overall safer drivers.

18.2.2.3 Age-Related: Older Drivers

Similar to young children, an age group that remains vulnerable on the road are older adults, for a variety of reasons including greater health concerns. According to the World Health Organization (WHO), there were 193,478 older persons around the world, who were aged 60 and above, who died in 2002 due to road traffic crashes (Peden et al., 2004). Statistical data has shown that older adults are usually involved in crashes which occur at complex traffic situations, such as intersections (US Department of Transportation, 2004). Most studies have reported that aging affects a wide variety of skills that are crucial to driving safely. However, there is still a question regarding whether or not being of a certain age causes a person to be unfit to drive.

The research in this area has found that the older an individual is, the more prone they are to have an illness or health condition that can affect driving (Keall & Frith, 2004). With a developmental and ecological perspective in mind, human life involves continuous change (Volpe, 2004). Therefore, even the most competent and skilled drivers can be affected by the aging process. The initiatives aimed at older adults are unique by their own right and focus on promoting safe driving for this age group by targeting different areas of the problem, and not creating a stigma regarding this age group and the road.

The DriveABLE Assessment Centers (Chap. 25) is a safe driving initiative committed to keeping older and medically susceptible drivers safe on the road based on scientific research to provide in-office and in-car assessments for drivers who suffer from medical conditions that can affect their driving competence. DriveABLE has been working with physicians, licensing authorities, neurology clinics, and various healthcare organizations as a reimbursable service, providing a collaborative system. The system allows for the evaluation of the cognitive fitness of drivers with medical conditions or those returning to driving following an injury or illness. By focusing expressly on the internal state of individuals by assessing their health status, DriveABLE encompasses exemplar practices to combat the dangers that medical conditions or aging can pose on road safety through collaborative measures.

18.2.2.4 Capability: Drunk Drivers

A driver's blood alcohol concentration (BAC) remains the single most important independent variable for measuring the extent of the alcohol-crash problem (Jones, 2000). Research over the past two decades has definitively established that human performance at driving-related tasks is significantly impaired in the majority of people with BACs of 0.10 and higher. Techniques for testing and measurement have improved in recent years, resulting in an overall increased sensitivity to degradations of behaviors due to alcohol through laboratory experiments and using tests of actual driving performance (Beirness, 2001). Studies show increased impairment of many driving-related behaviors, even at a BAC level of 0.05 (Hingson, Heeren, & Winter, 1998). Furthermore, research continues to show that young drivers are more often involved in alcohol-related crashes than any other comparable age group (CDC, 2001). Rates of involvement, share of the problem, and risk of alcohol related crashes all reach their peaks with young drivers, including peak for fatal crashes (which occurs at an age of 21 years; Hingson, Heeren, & Winter, 1994).

The idea of a car that can be driven by someone impaired by alcohol consumption is a daunting thought. The Alberta Ignition Interlock Program (IIP; Chap. 26) aims to reduce excessive drinking and resultant alcohol-related collisions by cutting impaired individuals off from being able to start a car. The system requires the driver to breathe into a small breath-testing device linked to the vehicle ignition system in order to start the car, as well as keep the ignition running. This program allows individuals who have been convicted of impaired driving, as long as no injury or death have been caused, to get back on the road under cautious conditions (Beirness & Simpson, 2003). The interlock is installed for a minimum of 6 months or until the end of the court-ordered suspension period (Beirness & Simpson, 2003). The Alberta IIP can be directly linked to decreases in gross drunk driving offenses and decreases in minor, major, and fatal traffic injuries (Beirness & Simpson, 2003). This program aims to connect and involve the four aspects of the life-space model to provide a collaborative injury prevention program.

18.3 For What Follows

Road safety is essential in this increasingly vehicle-dependent world, especially given that road-related incidents are extremely prevalent and serious. The physical, emotional, and economic costs of subpar road safety are detrimental, especially when some incidents can plausibly be prevented. The prevention programs described in this section are exemplar as they tend to be holistic, multi-leveled, as well as sustainable—providing policy and program creators an opportunity to learn and incorporate beneficial, successful aspects for new worldwide implementations.

Evidently, the road is a complex system; however understanding risk factors and major influences of road-related incidents help determine the areas in need of support. Approaching road trauma prevention to combat nonfatal injuries, traumatic brain injury, or death is vital and proves to be difficult.

This chapter will comprehensively discuss the previously mentioned exemplary programs pertaining to road safety. The cases reviewed here provide a comprehensive and much needed overview of some unique and exemplar practices and programs in transportation-related prevention. More often than not, understanding the road system holistically allows for exemplary programs to target prevention efforts in intricate ways.

The aim is to offer policy-makers and organizations the ability to incorporate aspects of tested and evaluated practices that can be used as a prototype when creating and implementing programs for injury prevention, as it pertains to road safety.

References

Active and Safe Routes to School [ASRTS]. (2004). *Resource guide*. Retrieved August 2, 2004, from http://www.saferoutestoschool.ca/index.php?page=asrtsrg

Beirness. (2001). *Best practice in alcohol ignition interlocks*. Ottawa, ON: Traffic Injury Research Foundation.

Beirness, D. J., & Simpson, H. M. (2003). *Alcohol interlocks as a condition of license reinstatement*. Ottawa, ON: Traffic Injury Research Foundation.

Boase, P., & Tasca, L. (1998). *Graduated licensing system evaluation: Interim report*. Toronto, ON: Safety Policy Branch, Ontario Ministry of Transportation.

Bureau of Transport Economics. (2001). *The Black Spot Program 1996–2002: An evaluation of the first three years*. Australia: Bureau of Transport Economics.

Business Sweden. (n.d.). *Vision Zero: Traffic safety by Sweden*. Retrieved January 10, 2018, from http://www.visionzeroinitiative.com

Canada Safety Council. (2004). *OECD child injury deaths—Is progress stalled?* Retrieved July 26, 2004, from http://www.safety-council.org/info/child/oecd.html

Canadian Institute of Child Health (CICH). (2000). *The health of Canada's Children* (3rd ed.). Ottawa, ON: Canadian Institute of Child Health.

Canadian Motor Vehicle Traffic Collision Statistics: 2015. (2017). Retrieved February 20, 2018 from http://tc.gc.ca

Centers for Disease Control and Prevention. (2001). *Evidence of effectiveness of 0.08% blood alcohol concentration (BAC) laws: Findings from the Task Force on Community Preventive Services*. Atlanta: Centers for Disease Control.

Centers for Disease Control and Prevention. (2015). *10 Leading causes of injury deaths*. Retrieved February 20, 2018 from https://www.cdc.gov/injury/wisqars/pdf/leading_causes_of_injury_deaths_highlighting_unintentional_injury_2015-a.pdf

Centers for Disease Control and Prevention. (2017). *Fatal injury mapping*. Retrieved from https://wisqars.cdc.gov:8443/cdcMapFramework/

City of Toronto. (2017). *Vision Zero: Toronto's road safety plan 2017–2021*. Retrieved February 9, 2018, from https://www.toronto.ca/wp-content/uploads/2017/11/990f-2017-Vision-Zero-Road-Safety-Plan_June1.pdf

Department for Transport. (2015). *Reported road casualties in Great Britain: Main results 2014*. Retrieved February 20, 2018, from https://www.gov.uk/government/uploads/system/uploads/attachment_data/file/438040/reported-road-casualties-in-great-britain-main-results-2014-release.pdf

European Commission. (2005). *Road safety country profile*. Retrieved May 22, 2007, from: http://ec.europa.eu/transport/roadsafety_library/care/doc/profiles/pdf/countryprofile_sv_e n.pdf

Go for Green. (2003). *A brief history of the National ASRTS Program*. Retrieved July 22, 2004, from www.goforgreen.ca/asrts/history_e.html

Haddon, W. (1968). The changing approach to the epidemiology, prevention, and amelioration of trauma: The transition to approaches etiologically rather than descriptively based. *American Journal of Public Health and the Nation's Health, 58*(8), 1431–1438.

Henley, G., & Harrison, J. E. (2015). *Trends in serious injury due to road vehicle traffic crashes, Australia: 2001 to 2010*. Retrieved February 20, 2018, from https://www.aihw.gov.au

Hingson, R., Heeren, T., & Winter, M. (1998). Effects of Maine's 0.05% legal blood alcohol level for drivers with DWI convictions. *Public Health Reports, 113*(5), 440–446.

Hingson, R., Heeren, T. & Winter, M. (1994). Lower blood alcohol limits for young drivers. *Public Health Reports, 109*(6), 738–744.

Hunt, C. (1998). *Active/safe routes to school*. Ottawa, ON: Health Canada, Canadian Institute of Child Health.

Joly, M., Foggin, P., & Pless, I. P. (1991). Geographical and socio-ecological variations of traffic accidents among children. *Social Science and Medicine, 33*(7), 765–769.

Jones, R. K. (2000). *State of knowledge of alcohol-impaired driving: Research on repeat DWI offenders*. Darby, PA: DIANE Publishing.

Keall, M. D., & Frith, W. J. (2004). Association between older driver characteristics, on-road driving test performance and crash liability. *Traffic Injury Prevention, 8*, 112–116.

Korpal, P. R., Rayman, C. A., & Masters, P. H. (1994). *Evaluation of the Highway 401 Freeway Traffic Management System: Summary report*. Ministry of Transportation of Ontario: Freeway Traffic Management Section: Ontario.

Liu, X., & Yang, J. (2003). Effects of vehicle impact velocity and front-end structure on dynamic responses of child pedestrians. *Traffic Injury Prevention, 4*(4), 337–344.

Ministry of Transportation. (2002). *Ontario road safety annual report 2002: Building safe communities*. Safety Education Policy Branch. Retrieved July 20, 2004, from http://www.mto.gov.on.ca/english/safety/orsar/orsar02/summary.htm

National Safety Council. (2015). *Injury facts, 2015 Edition*. Retrieved January 26, 2018, from http://www.nsc.org/Membership%20Site%20Document%20Library/2015%20Injury%20Facts/NSC_InjuryFacts2015Ed.pdf

Ontario Brain Injury Association. (2002). *OBIA review* (Vol. 3-1). Retrieved June 20, 2004, from http://www.obia.on.ca/or3_1.html

Ontario Road Safety Annual Report. (2001). Ontario: Ministry of Transportation of the Government of Ontario.

Organisation for Economic Co-operation and Development [OECD]. (2004). *Keeping children safe in traffic*. Paris: OECD Publication Service.

Parachute. (2015). *The cost of injury in Canada*. Toronto, ON: Author.

Peden, M., Scurfield, R., Sleet, D., Mohan, D., Hyder, A. A., Jarawan, E., Mathers, C. (2004). World report on road traffic injury prevention.. Retrieved June 5, 2004, from http://www.who.int/world-health-day/2004/infomaterials/world_report/en/

Rivara, F., & Barbar, M. (1985). Demographic analysis of childhood pedestrian injuries. *Pediatrics, 76*, 212–214.

Road Crash Statistics. (2018). Retrieved February 20, 2018, from http://asirt.org

Swedish National Road Administration [SNRA]. (2006). *Safe Traffic- Vision Zero on the move*. Retrieved May 10, 2007, from: http://publikationswebbutik.vv.se/shopping/ShowItem.aspx?id=1317

United States Department of Transportation Federal Highway Administration. (2004). *Older driver facts*. Retrieved July, 2004, from http://safety.fhwa.dot.gov/fourthlevel/pro_res_olderdriver_facts.htm

Vision Zero Canada. (n.d.). *Vision Zero Canada*. Retrieved November 5, 2017, from https://visionzero.ca/

Volpe, R. (2004). *The conceptualization of injury prevention as change in complex systems*. Toronto, ON: University of Toronto.

Williams, A. F. (1998). Risky driving behaviour among adolescents. In R. Jessor (Ed.), *New perspectives on adolescent risk behavior* (pp. 221–237). New York: Cambridge University Press.

Williams, A. F. (2003). Teenage drivers: Patterns of risk. *Journal of Safety Research, 34*, 5–15.

Williams, A. F., & Mayhew, D. R. (2004). *Graduated licensing: A blueprint for North America*. Arlington, VA: Insurance Institute for Highway Safety; Ottawa, Ontario, Canada: Traffic Injury Research Foundation. Retrieved July 1, 2003, from http://www.highway-safety.org/safety_facts/teens/blueprint.pdf

World Health Organization (WHO). (2004). *World report on road traffic injury prevention—Chapter 1*. Retrieved August 4, 2004, from http://www.who.int/world-health-day/2004/infomaterials/world_report/en/chapter1.pdf

Vision Zero

Negar Ahmadi

Vision Zero is an initiative created in Sweden aimed to create road systems where there are no (zero) deaths as a result of road transportation. The approach is comprehensive as it is an understanding of human fallibility but attempts to design a transportation system that caters to it. The program involves planning, designing, and building roads and infrastructure to increase safety and reduce accidents by also meeting capacity and environmental challenges. Internationally, many of these goals and practices are being implemented to the ultimate goal of zero road-related deaths (Business Sweden, n.d.).

19.1 Background

19.1.1 A History of Vision Zero

Sweden is currently recognized by many as having some of the safest roads in the world. Initial efforts to reduce traffic collisions were implemented by the Swedish government in the 1960s and 1970s through transition to right-hand traffic, introduction of speed limits, enforcement of seat belt laws for motor vehicles, and imposed helmet use for motorcycles. These interventions reduced the number of fatalities from motor vehicle crashes in the early 1980s from 1300 deaths per

year to less than 800 deaths per year (National Society for Road Safety, 2002). However, by the late 1980s and early 1990s, Sweden experienced a sudden increase in the number of crash fatalities (900 deaths per year). The increase was argued to have resulted from Sweden's growing economy and increased car ownership and was immediately identified to require intervention (National Society for Road Safety, 2002). To readdress the problem, a group of researchers from the Swedish National Road Administration (SNRA) were assigned to manage traffic safety in Sweden between 1992 and 1995. From 1995 onward, the SNRA and the Swedish Ministry of Transportation closely cooperated to develop a traffic safety policy called Vision Zero. In October of 1997, the Swedish parliament adopted Vision Zero as a national policy to reduce traffic injuries and fatalities (Government Bill, 1996/1997). According to the Vision Zero Government Bill, "the long-term goal of traffic safety is that nobody shall be killed or seriously injured as a consequence of traffic accidents" and that "the design and function of the transport system shall be adapted accordingly" (Government Bill, 1996/1997). The goal of Vision Zero was to reduce motor vehicle fatalities by 50% between 1997 and 2007 and further reduce this figure to zero. Vision Zero is also designed to specifically focus on drink driving, safer speed limits, the use of seat belts, safer car design, road infrastructure improvements, and pedestrian and cyclist safety.

N. Ahmadi (✉)
McMaster University, Hamilton, ON, Canada

© Springer Nature Switzerland AG 2020
R. Volpe (ed.), *Casebook of Traumatic Injury Prevention*,
https://doi.org/10.1007/978-3-030-27419-1_19

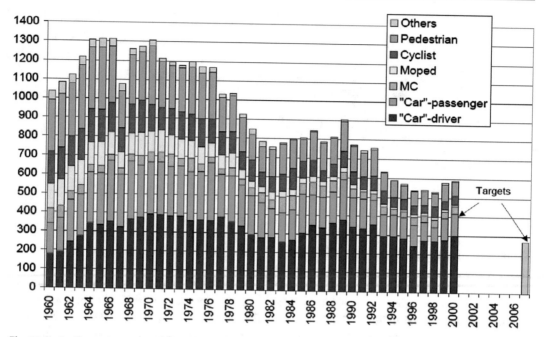

Fig. 19.1 An illustration of the fatalities as a result of road traffic in Sweden from 1960 to 2007 (National Society for Road Safety, 2002)

Figure 19.1 illustrates the number of fatalities before Vision Zero, after Vision Zero, as well as the projected goal of the policy in 2007. This figure illustrates the results intended to be achieved for the primary and secondary goals for each segment of the policy's target population.

The secondary or sub-goals of Vision Zero as noted in the Government Bill (1996/1997) are:

1. An accessible transport system
2. A high standard of transport quality
3. Traffic safety
4. A good environment
5. Positive regional development (Government Bill, 1996/1997)

Based on the primary and secondary goals, as well as the target population and key terms, Vision Zero clearly draws from an ecological framework, or a holistic approach, to structure an intervention for road safety. The policy ecologically frames the interventions and demonstrates its sustainability from the planning stages, that is, the implementing organizations studied in depth the problem to be addressed, explicitly outlined realistic primary

and secondary goals in the short and the long term, and clearly stated their conceptual understanding of the problem that recognizes the elements of an ecological framework. Sustainability exists because these goals and concepts emphasize the importance of understanding and modifying the person-person-environment interaction. For example, the main goal aims to protect road users (person) by adapting "the design and function of the transport system... accordingly" (environment; Government Bill, 1996/1997).

Box 19.1 Definition of *Relevant* Terms
In order to make Vision Zero a precise goal, the terms death, serious injury, and road traffic collision are clearly defined. The clarity of the following definitions is expected to make the goals of Vision Zero precise and easy to evaluate.

Death: defined by the medical definition of "brain death" and has to occur within 30 days of the collision.

Serious injury: defined as an injury leading to at least 3 weeks of hospitalization.

Road traffic collision: defined as an event that has happened on the road involving at least one motor vehicle and resulting in personal injury or material damage.

Note. Rosencrantz, Edvardsson, & Hansson (2007).

19.1.2 Elements of Vision Zero

Vision Zero is based on four elements: ethics, responsibility, safety philosophy, and creating mechanisms for change (World Health Organization [WHO], 2004).

Ethics. Vision Zero takes an ethical stance in its approach toward road safety by stating that "it is not acceptable that any people die or get seriously injured when utilizing the road transportation system" (Government Bill, 1996/1997). According to Lind and Schmidt (as cited in Rosencrantz et al., 2007), the ethical assumptions behind Vision Zero are the basis of the following five main principles:

1. If it is possible to prevent someone from being killed or seriously injured, then appropriate measures must be taken; human lives may not be traded for some other good.
2. Every project shall be done right from the start, i.e., every decision should be supported by scientific and empirical knowledge.
3. The best known solution should always be applied to any problem; time schedules or convenience may not excuse bad solutions when a better solution is known.
4. Both risk and the nature of damage should be taken into account in decisions whether to implement changes in any situation.
5. It should always be assumed that the responsibility for each loss of human life and health rests with those who design and implement the transport system.

Responsibility. Before Vision Zero, most of the responsibility for traffic collisions was placed on individual road users. However, in Vision Zero responsibility is shared by many different players involved in the road system. In other words, the politicians, road managers, car makers, and the police are as much responsible for the safety of the roads as the road users are responsible for following the rules of the road. According to Vision Zero, if the road users fail to follow the rules, it is then the responsibility of road designers to redesign the roads and govern road safety (WHO, 2004).

Safety philosophy. Vision zero is based on the principles that it is (1) inevitable to completely prevent human errors from occurring and that (2) beyond a certain threshold, recovery from a traffic collision is almost impossible for the victims involved. According to Vision Zero, the transport system should be designed in such a way to account for the human failings while preventing death or serious injury from happening. Vision Zero assumes that serious injuries or deaths due to traffic collisions are the result of chains of events, which should be interrupted or broken at any point. Therefore, car design, road infrastructure improvements, as well as the rules governing the safety on the road are among the factors that would help break the chain of events leading to deaths or serious injuries even when humans make mistakes and collisions happen (WHO, 2004).

Mechanisms for change. In order to govern the safety of the road users, change needs to take place. However, the process of change involves closely following the other three principles described earlier (Rosencrantz et al., 2007).

19.2 Resources

19.2.1 Stakeholders and Collaborators

Vision Zero employs human and fiscal resources adeptly and intensively to achieve its goals. Notably, the clear communication between professionals and nonprofessionals alike facilitates good long-term relationships that promote program sustainability. As mentioned earlier, Vision Zero shares the responsibility of road safety with many stakeholders, including the SNRA, municipal authorities, the Ministry of Transportation, the Swedish parliament, politicians, planners, police, community organizations, vehicle manufacturing companies, companies and organizations that purchase transport services, companies and organizations that transport both goods and people, and all the road users.

The SNRA is the main administration with national authority on the entire 98,300 km road system in Sweden. However, the municipal authorities are also responsible for the regulation and maintenance of 40,300 km of urban and rural roads in Sweden. The SNRA is responsible for providing the Ministry of Transportation with guidelines and road safety standards, while the Swedish parliament is mainly responsible for passing the legislations that are proposed by the Ministry of Transportation. Box 19.2 provides detailed description of the roles of the other stakeholders involved in Vision Zero (Swedish National Road Administration [SNRA], 2006).

Companies and organizations that purchase transport services: demand that transportation is carried out in a safe way in order for safety to become a competitive factor within the transport system.

Companies and organizations that transport goods and people: take initiative to include safety as a component in their travel policies. Companies can demand the employees to abide by all the rules and regulations of the road.

Road users: follow the rules and regulations of the roads.

19.2.2 Principles of Shared Responsibility and Sustainability

As previously discussed in this report, Vision Zero is based on the principles of shared responsibility between different stakeholders. This particular feature of Vision Zero contributes significantly to the sustainability of it. In fact, several definitions of sustainability have included close cooperation among various stakeholders as one of the main criteria for program sustainability. For instance, according to Volpe (2007), sustainable change requires "multi-disciplinary collaboration and coordination that employs trans-disciplinary concepts of prevention… to meet the changing and diverse needs of the population." Hence, as an element of sustainability, Vision Zero involves close collaboration of multiple disciplines from policy-makers to vehicle manufactures and road users. On the other hand, Johnson, Hays, Center, and Daley (2004) define sustainability as the process of integrating a prevention strategy and innovation into an ongoing practice to benefit diverse stakeholders. In this regard, Vision Zero has become integrated into the national policy of Sweden and is aimed not only to benefit the motorist but also to enhance the safety of cyclist, pedestrians, and all those using the roads.

Box 19.2 The Role of Stakeholders in Vision Zero

Politicians: involved in making decisions concerning community planning and traffic issues and the SNRA provides them with the guidelines and information necessary to make planning decisions.

Planners: responsible for implementing the political decisions concerning the design and the shape of the road transport system.

Police: enforce the traffic rules and regulations set by the Ministry of Transportation.

Community organizations: improve road safety in society and within each community.

Vehicle manufacturing companies: ensure all the necessary steps in improving vehicle safety are taken.

19.2.3 In-Depth Analysis of Collisions

According to Vision Zero, an understanding of what leads to fatal injuries or deaths due to traffic collisions is necessary to improve safety. Therefore, to meet this demand, the SNRA is made responsible to collect in-depth information from every collision that leads to fatalities or serious injuries in an approach called OLA (in Swedish). The acronym translates into English as objective/solution/accident. The OLA is carried out by the SNRA at both the local and the national level in Sweden (European Commission, 2005). Through this approach road designers and planners are encouraged to modify the road system in such a way that prevents similar crashes resulting in serious injury or death. The SNRA is notified by the police when a fatal accident has happened, and a team of investigators is sent by the SNRA to the scene to collect in-depth information. According to Stockholm Environment Institute (2006a, 2006b, 2006c), the in-depth information collected from the scene of the accident includes:

- The design of the road environment (e.g., road width, roadside ditches)
- The speed limit of the road
- Serious speed limit violations
- Model, year, and the safety specification of the vehicle
- Detail information of all the people involved in the collision (e.g., sex, age, use of safety equipment, drink driving, illness, suspicion of suicide)
- Details of human injury involved
- The police report
- Interview protocol

Once the details of the accident are compiled, the researchers assess the factors that caused the collision. According to SNRA (2006), the factors responsible for all fatal collisions are divided into the three following categories:

- *Excessive force*: when road users have followed all regulations and used all possible safety protection, but the error(s) made is too

due to the road environment in combination with the designated speed limit

- *Excessive risk*: when fatal collisions are due to insufficient use of personal safety protection such as not wearing seat belts or helmets
- *Beyond system restriction*: when fatal collisions are due to serious violation of the rules and regulations of the road, such as going beyond the speed limit

The information gathered from the collision by the SNRA is then used to create safety guidelines for road planners and policy-makers. The researchers at the SNRA further discuss the results of their investigation with the local road designers and propose suggestions to improve road safety. Furthermore, this information is used to increase awareness and improve enforcement of the rules, set by officials, for all stakeholders involved in the road system, including the road users (SNRA, 2006).

Therefore, according to Vision Zero, devising traffic safety interventions involves acquiring thorough understanding of the etiology of collisions including the contribution of the various factors and forces involved in collisions. Consequently, such a process of devising interventions makes Vision Zero very flexible as it becomes primarily based on the needs and shortcomings of the current road system. In other words, Vision Zero can be viewed as a cyclical process rather than a one-time sequential pattern. According to several researchers (e.g., Hanson & Salmoni, 2007; Johnson et al., 2004; Shediac-Rizkallah & Bone, 1998), the dynamic nature of a program and the cyclical process involved in devising implementations contribute significantly to the sustainability of that program. Thus, Vision Zero is a sustainable policy as it is dynamic in nature and involves a cyclical process when devising safety interventions.

On the other hand, as Hanson and Salmoni (2007) have proposed, the sustainability of a community-based program is facilitated when the program is defined and conceptualized within the context of an "ecological framework". Hence, the factors that are investigated when analyzing collisions in Sweden also align with understanding injury through an ecological framework. Within these factors, the policy identifies the need to modify road engineering but also targets the individual behaviors of the users of the roads in Sweden, including drivers, cyclists, and pedestrians. According to Volpe (2007), an ecological framework requires change to be envisaged holistically, that is, both individually/personally and communally/socially. In this regard, Vision Zero not only involves changing the behavior of individual road users but it also entails road infrastructure changes within the community. Therefore, Vision Zero clearly draws from an ecological framework to structure an intervention for road safety that contributes to its sustainability.

19.2.4 Funding

In order for the goals of Vision Zero to be met, certain modifications to the road system, as well as some policy changes, would have to take place. However, such modifications to the road system might involve changing the road infrastructure, which requires funding from the government. In fact, the Swedish government has allocated about SEK 4.9 billion between 2004 and 2015 (about $700 million US dollars) to construct new roads and modify the existing road system (European Commission, 2005). The nature of the source of funding has a great impact on the sustainability of a program (Scheirer, 2005). According to Hanson and Salmoni (2007), sustainable programs not only possess some degree of financial independence but also receive reliable financial assistance from it. In this regard, Vision Zero was first given a stable source of funding; however, throughout the years it has received more and more assistance from different funding bodies in Sweden. According to Mr. Johansson, the chief strategist from the SNRA (personal communication, April 19, 2007), within the past few years, traffic safety has become integrated within different organizations and therefore funding is provided by different organizations in Sweden. Therefore, through its financial commitment, the government has demonstrated a long-term commitment to Vision Zero and to ensure sustainability of the policy.

Since modifications to the road system might involve revisions to the rules and the regulations governing the roads (e.g., speed limits, the use of seat belts, or drinking and driving laws), financing and leadership from the Ministry of Transportation, the Parliament, and the SNRA, and commitment and cooperation from all other stakeholders are imperative for sustainability. However, in order to govern cooperation and in turn sustainability, an organization must be able to monitor, assess, and evaluate the tasks and objectives of the program and modify them to the best interest of all the stakeholders involved (Harris, Henry, Bland, Starnaman, & Voytek, 2003; Shediac-Rizkallah & Bone, 1998). To guarantee a strong level of participation and commitment for revised road rules, the Swedish government initiated a process called the National Coalition for Road Safety in 2002. The purpose of this process is to encourage the traffic stakeholders to better cooperate in making the roads safer (European Commission, 2005). Additionally, in 2003, the Road Traffic Inspectorate was established to monitor and analyze the safety developments taking place around Sweden.

19.3 Implementation

19.3.1 Road Infrastructure Changes

Since 1997, when Vision Zero was adopted as a national policy, the roads around Sweden have undergone major reconstructions in order to make them safer and reduce the likelihood of deaths or serious injuries. The major reconstructions in Sweden include roundabouts, steel cable guardrails, center guard rails, safe roadside areas, and roadside guardrails.

Roundabouts. One of the modifications made to the infrastructure of the Swedish roads has been the replacement of intersections with roundabouts. Since 1999, about 500 four-way intersections have been replaced with roundabouts (SNRA, 2006). In fact, roundabouts are known to have a calming effect and they are known to be particularly effective in reducing the seriousness of injuries (SNRA, 2006).

Steel cable guardrails. Cable guardrails are generally effective in catching the cars from falling down the bridges during an accident. Conventional guardrails deflect the cars back into the traffic, however by substituting conventional guardrails with steel cable guardrails, the car would be held and deflection into traffic would be prevented (SNRA, 2006).

Center guardrails. A center guardrail separates the two sides of traffic and thereby prevents head-on collisions. Since 1999 about 1300 km of center guardrails have been installed on the roads in Sweden (SNRA, 2006). The center guardrails are shown to be very cost-effective in preventing head-on collisions.

Safe roadside areas. Trees or any rigid obstacles along the roadside are known to be fatal in case of a collision. Therefore, steps have been taken to remove such fixed obstacles off the roadsides (SNRA, 2006).

Roadside guardrails. In places where removal of roadside obstacles is impossible, guardrails have been installed along the roadside (SNRA, 2006).

19.3.2 Non-infrastructure Changes

Right speed. Speeding has often been identified as the main cause of collisions leading to death or serious injury. Therefore, efforts have been taken to adjust the speed limits in roads around Sweden and further enforce those speed limits. Speed limits on the national roads, specifically rural roads, are currently being reviewed. Between 1998 and 2002, the speed limits were lowered from 110 to 90 km/h and from 90 to 70 km/h on 3000 km of national roads (European Commission, 2005). Furthermore, within buildup areas speed limits have been lowered to 30 km/h to ensure the safety of pedestrians and cyclists. It is important to note that speed limits are revisited every few years to assess their impact on traffic collisions.

Speed surveillance. Permanent speed surveillance cameras are places on the roads around Sweden. In fact, about 400 speed surveillance cameras were installed around Sweden between 1999 and 2005. The awareness of the presence of such cameras by motorists is known to have a traffic calming effect.

Use of seat belts. The seat belt has been shown to be extremely effective in reducing the risk of serious injury or death in traffic collisions. In 1999, the use of seat belts for all car occupants in Sweden became compulsory. Furthermore, it is mandatory for bus passengers to wear seat belts if their seats are equipped with one. All the new buses must be equipped with seat belts (European Commission, 2005). During December of 2002, the SNRA ran a campaign that promoted the use of seat belts, and in 2003 violation fines of the seat belt rules were doubled. In addition, seat belt reminders are being installed in about 60% of all the new cars, and they have shown to be very cost-effective in reducing deaths and fatal injuries resulting from collisions.

Safety standards of vehicles. The safety of the vehicle involved in a motor traffic collision is one of the factors that the SNRA will take into consideration when analyzing the crash scene. Since Vision Zero was adopted, several features of cars have been identified as problematic in serious collisions and efforts have been undertaken to enhance the safety of cars. For instance, analyses of whiplash injuries have shown that installing a whiplash protection system in the car can significantly reduce the risk of such injuries.

Drunk driving. Drinking and driving has been responsible for about 25% of all fatal crashes in Sweden. Therefore, efforts have been undertaken after Vision Zero was implemented to reduce drunk driving. In 1999 a pilot project with alcohol ignition interlocks was started in Sweden targeting people convicted of drink driving who had their license suspended. In this project, those who had their license suspended were given permission to drive again only if they had an alcohol ignition interlock installed in the car they were driving. Cars equipped with alcohol ignition interlocks will not be started until the alcohol level in the driver's breath has been checked. In 2003 the alcohol ignition interlocks project was expanded to include the whole country. See Chap. 26 of this volume for Alberta's alcohol ignition interlock program for more information about a drunk driving prevention program.

Furthermore, drunk driving is of particular concern among young people. To target young people between ages 18 and 24, in 2005 a national campaign called "Don't Drink and Drive" was started and was planned to run until 2007.

Cyclists and pedestrians. Vision Zero is based on the idea that the road system should be designed with a particular focus on what the human body can stand. Therefore, with regard to the safety of cyclists, helmet use is the main objective to be reached because it has shown to be particularly effective in reducing head injuries resulting from crashes. Since 2005, the use of helmets for children under the age of 15 has become compulsory. Furthermore, in spring of 2005 an extensive campaign was launched promoting the use of bicycle helmets. In an attempt to further increase the survival chance of pedestrians and cyclists in collisions, the speed limit in many built-up areas around Sweden has been dropped to 30 km/h.

19.4   Outcome

The Vision Zero policy has introduced a unique and radical way of looking at road safety, which is based on an ethical foundation and has demonstrated sustainability through its comprehensive ethical approach to policy implementation. Under the policy, the basic assumption is that humans make mistakes, but a safe transport system can help prevent these mistakes from happening. Vision Zero's long-term goal is to prevent death or serious injury from happening and to reduce the human and financial resources expended on unsafe roads; the policies in place are devised to adequately support the structural and non-structural measures being implemented.

At the most basic level, Vision Zero is evaluated by analyzing the number of fatalities due to road collisions in the years prior to and after the introduction of Vision Zero. According to Sweden's national statistics, the number of fatalities from motor accidents has gradually dropped from 537 (deaths per year, per 100,000) in 1996 to 445 (deaths per year, per 100,000) in 2006 (National Statistics of Road Traffic Accidents, 2006). According to Mr. Johansson, the chief strategist from the SNRA, the calculated effect of the activities of the SNRA (which are solely determined on the basis of Vision Zero) in the year 2006 was a reduction of 20 fatalities in total, which is better than any year before (R. Johansson, personal communication, April 19, 2007). With regard to the statistics on serious injuries, the observed trend is somewhat different. In 1996 the number of serious injuries was 3837, and this figure continued to increase even after Vision Zero was implemented to 4664 in 2003. However, since 2004 the number of serious injuries has been dropping, and in 2006 this figure was reduced to almost what it was in 1996 to 3959 serious injuries. Even though the number of serious injuries increased for a few years after Vision Zero was implemented, Vision Zero was successfully able to reduce this figure significantly in the following years by ensuring that appropriate modifications were made to the road system, yielding positive results in the longer term due to the program's research-intensive nature.

At a more complex level, however, the particular modifications made to the road system have all been evaluated individually and they have all shown to be very effective in reducing the number of fatalities and serious injuries resulting from traffic collisions. For instance, center guardrails are shown to be effective in reducing head-on collisions by 80% (R. Johansson, personal communication, April 19, 2007). Moreover, physical changes to the road system along with reducing speed limits to 30 km/h in some built-up areas (such as Gothenburg) have been shown to be effective in reducing the number of injuries by as much as 60–70% (European Commission, 2005). Below is an excerpt of a real-life experience of a Swedish citizen with the new and innovated steel cable guard rails, installed in roads around Sweden.

It was slippery, my car went into a skid and drove right into the cable guardrail. The car went sliding ahead along the rail before finally coming to a stop. I landed more gently than if I had driven into a normal guardrail and I was able to drive away myself. It was lucky for me that there was a guardrail because of the steep slope on the other side. If I had ended up there, I don't know what would have happened (SNRA, 2006).

According to Hansen and Salmoni (2007), "internally driven evaluations that account for individual experiences are more useful than externally driven evaluation methodologies, because the former method assesses and ensures a program's relevancy to the community" (Hanson, 2007; p. 45). Clearly, internally driven evaluations over the life of the project, that is, small ball evaluations, have been undertaken extensively for Vision Zero. Evaluators who assess the outcomes of the initiatives under Vision Zero have identified the conditions to be achieved in order to fulfill the goals of their policy. Externally driven small ball evaluations are also relevant to assess whether the objectives of the program are being met, how the program works, if any components of the program require adjustment, and whether there is potential for transportability.

Oxley, Corben, Fildes, O'Hare, and Rothengatter (2004), at the University Accident Research Centre, conducted additional evaluation into Vision Zero by assessing the vulnerability of older pedestrians and cyclists to traffic collisions. In their analysis, they referred to Vision Zero in Sweden as one of the "[exemplar] practices" around the world to reduce the risk of traffic injuries for older pedestrians and cyclists due to its innovative and effective philosophy.

According to Volpe (2007), passive engineered solutions tend to achieve the best results, particularly in injury prevention programs. As mentioned earlier, Vision Zero places enormous responsibility on road designers and engineers to design roads that prevent fatalities and serious injuries from occurring while simultaneously accounting for human errors. Notably successful road infrastructure improvements include conversion of the four-way intersections to roundabouts and installment of steel cable guard rails and center guardrails in the roads across Sweden.

Therefore, engineering, which is one of the contributing factors to sustainability of a program, is a significant component of Vision Zero. Moreover, evidence suggests that legislative intervention, as well as technological innovation, demonstrates increased effectiveness over active interventions that focus on educational or social programs, which attempt to solely modify existing behavior (Volpe, 2007).

Enforcement through legislation is a substantial component of any sustainable road collision prevention program. Vision Zero is no exception to this fundamental principle. Since 1997 the Swedish parliament has adopted Vision Zero as a national policy, with enforcement strategies in effect to ensure that the goals set by Vision Zero will be met (European Commission, 2005). However, the enforcements are designed not only for the road users but also for those who design the roads. Once a fatal accident has occurred and an assessment team from the SNRA has done full investigation of the accident, the SNRA provides the Ministry of Transportation with suggestions with regard to the road design. The road managers are required to implement the changes and presented by the ministry and further consult the SNRA about the process of modification. In cases where road changes involve modification of the rules and the regulations governing the safety of the roads, the road users are enforced to obey the new rules and regulations. In such cases, the law enforcement officials play an important part by monitoring the behavior of the road users. In fact, the National Police Board has prepared a national policy plan for traffic surveillance with a particular emphasis on offences against speed limits, non-use of seat belts, and drink driving (European Commission, 2005).

Since 1999, about 400 speed cameras have been installed across the country to better enforce speed limits (European Commission, 2005). The officials aim of to install 700 more cameras by 2007. The enforcement of seat belt laws in 2003 has involved doubling the fines for infringements, as well as enforcing seat belt laws for passengers on buses. The plan is to further increase the fines for infringement of the seat belt laws and dedicate 100% more law enforcement monitoring hours on seat belt controls (European Commission, 2005). In an effort to target drunk driving in 2004 alone, the law enforcement officials performed 1.56 million breath tests. The future goal is to increase breath tests to two million in 2007 (European Commission, 2005).

Training and educating new drivers are also an important part of the responsibilities of road safety administration in Sweden. Under Vision Zero, the changing face of the roads and the rules governing safety on the roads, such as changes in the speed limits, particularly signifies the importance of the role played by the SNRA in training new drivers. Vision Zero places emphasis on choosing professionals to train the new drivers, ensuring that they are well aware of the changes that have taken place within the system and are capable of conveying their knowledge about the current philosophy of road safety to the new drivers. According to the goals of Vision Zero, the process of training is to be changed from a driver simply acquiring the knowledge to control the vehicle to placing greater emphasis on gaining the ability to assess danger and risk and understand the causes and effects of traffic accidents.

In addition to training new drivers, educational sessions are provided for existing drivers to become familiar with the new philosophy on road safety that is adopted by Vision Zero. The educational programs are provided through local communities where the community members are made aware of the changes that occur to the roads at the local level. Such changes might include modification to the speed limits, installation of the center guardrails, or conversion of the four-way intersections into roundabouts. In 2005, wearing cycle helmets for all children and adolescents up to age 15 became mandatory. Since then, educational programs have been implemented in the schools and communities to promote helmet use among children and adolescents. In spring of 2005, an extensive campaign was held to promote the use of bicycle helmets for children and adolescents up to age 15 (European Commission, 2005).

The SNRA has also been very active in running various campaigns to inform the public about the road safety and the new standards set by Vision Zero. To address the issue of drunk driving, the SNRA is currently running a national campaign called "Don't Drink and Drive" directed at people of age 18–24, and it is expected to run till 2007. Furthermore, in 2002, the SNRA ran a campaign on speed limits, notifying the public of the new changes to the speed limits around Sweden as well as the dangers involved in breaking the limits. The SNRA ran yet another campaign during December of 2002, promoting more frequent use of seat belts (European Commission, 2005).

A fairly recent development of Vision Zero is a declaration called the "Tylösand Declaration" which entitles the Swedish citizens to certain rights regarding the road system. The five articles outlined in this declaration are as followed:

1. Everyone has the right to use roads and streets without threats to life or health.
2. Everyone has the right to safe and sustainable mobility: safety and sustainability in road transport should complement each other.
3. Everyone has the right to use the road transport system without unintentionally imposing any threats to life or health on others.
4. Everyone has the right to information about safety problems and the level of safety of any component, product, action, or service within the road transport system.
5. Everyone has the right to expect systematic and continuous improvement in safety: any stakeholder within the road transport system has the obligation to undertake corrective actions following the detection of any safety hazard that can be reduced or removed.

Empowerment is yet another factor that contributes significantly to the sustainability of Vision Zero. Since its adoption into the Swedish national policy in 1997, the concept of shared responsibility has materialized into both formal and informal collaboration between policy-makers, the road administration, law enforcement, as well as community members. In August 2002, the Swedish government formally instituted a National Road Safety Assembly with the aim to better coordinate stakeholders within initiatives regarding speed, protection systems, alcohol, and children safety (SNRA, 2006). This assembly has since developed into formal regional road safety assemblies that are dedicated to improving road safety at the local or regional levels. In sum, the close cooperation among the different players has provided the optimal condition for the goals of Vision Zero to be met.

At the administration level, the goals of Vision Zero are met through close cooperation between the SNRA and the Ministry of Transportation. The SNRA assesses road collisions and provides the ministry with potential improvements to the road infrastructure or modifications to the laws of the road. The ministry will then evaluate the suggestions set forth by the SNRA to reduce fatal or serious injuries, provide funding for changes to the roads, or review the laws and regulations in place for further improvements. Close ties between the law enforcement officials and the SNRA and the Ministry of Transportation is yet another effort to make the goals of Vision Zero a reality. Such close ties have resulted in better monitoring the roads as well as increasing the penalty for infringement of the laws of the road.

Since Vision Zero has been introduced, the SNRA and the Ministry of Transportations have been working closely with vehicle manufacturing companies to enhance the safety of new vehicles. About 60% of all the new cars are now equipped with seat belt reminders, and the Swedish Motor Vehicle Inspection now offers to install seat belt reminders for free (European Commission, 2005). Furthermore, newly built buses are now equipped with seat belts to enhance the safety of the passengers. The SNRA and the vehicle manufacturers have also begun to cooperate in identifying and analyzing areas of highest impact in vehicles that have been in accidents, and safety initiatives have been taken by the manufacturers to target such areas. Finally, Vision Zero has involved the entire municipality in its attempt to reduce fatalities and serious injuries caused by traffic collisions. In various municipalities, local residents work closely with the authorities to identify the location of death traps (points where most accidents occur) based on their personal experiences; they then discuss how road safety could be improved in their neighborhoods. Experience has shown that involving the entire community in the decision-making process results in safer roads (SNRA, 2006).

19.4.1 International Perspectives on Vision Zero

As mentioned earlier, external evaluations mean that Vision Zero can potentially be re-conceptualized and implemented by other organizations in a sustained manner and successfully transported and re-contextualized into their communities. In this regard, Vision Zero has been identified by various organizations to provide long-term effectiveness in other geographic contexts. In 2004, the World Health Organization (WHO) created a report on road traffic injury prevention and identified Vision Zero as an effective policy to prevent road traffic injury. According to this report, the systematic view of shared responsibility is an important component that has made Vision Zero an effective prevention program. Below gives the perspective of the WHO on Vision Zero in the World Report on Road Traffic Injury Prevention published in 2004.

> Vision Zero is relevant to any country that aims to create a sustainable road transport system, and not just for the excessively ambitious or wealthy ones. Its basic principles can be applied to any type of road transport system, at any stage of development. Adopting Vision Zero means avoiding the usual costly process of trial and error and using from the start a proven and effective method. (WHO World Report on Road Traffic Injury Prevention, 2004).

Stockholm Environment Institute (SEI) also conducted a comprehensive evaluation of Vision Zero in 2006. The evaluation was conducted for the Department of Transport of the United Kingdom, who is interested in adopting Vision Zero policy in the United Kingdom. To assess the effectiveness of Vision Zero, the SEI conducted interviews with the Swedish and the European stakeholders. Interviews in Sweden were conducted with nine representatives from the national government, academic institutions, and motor industry. The objectives of the interviews were to identify the key issues, concerns, and evidence that led to the adoption of Vision Zero as a national policy and the current perception of progress toward the goals set by Vision Zero (Stockholm Environment Institute, 2006a, 2006b, 2006c). Interviews with European stakeholders included six road safety policy stakeholders whose opinions were gauged about Vision Zero, its implementation, and its success.

Participants of the survey highlighted the benefits of Vision Zero and identified the advantages of shifting to an ethical foundation with regard to safety programs. For instance, when asked about Vision Zero, Brigitte Chaudhury, the Founder and President of UK charity RoadPeace and President (chair) of the European Federation of Road Traffic Victims, stated: "It is the only proper way of looking at deaths and injuries… we are offended by targets… they build into the planning that deaths and injuries will occur" (Stockholm Environment Institute, 2006a, 2006b, 2006c). Another participant of the study, Francesca Racioppi from the European office of the WHO, identified three important values of Vision Zero from a political and philosophical point of view:

1. Making explicit otherwise hidden trade-offs in societal values (e.g., trading speed for lives).
2. Shifting the paradigm of responsibility in a direction which is similar to what happened in the 1970s in environmental issues: moving from an approach of "educating" people to "behave safely" to making the providers of goods and services accountable for the safety of their products; this shift has already occurred in the area of chemical safety and other consumer products but has not yet fully materialized in the area of road traffic safety.
3. By making Vision Zero an overarching target because it may help push different stakeholders, with commonly diverging objectives, toward one common goal.

Similarly, Dimitrios Theologitis, the head of road safety at the European Commission (2005),
believes that Sweden's Vision Zero has made a substantial contribution to reducing deaths and injuries in Sweden. Although some responses obtained from the stakeholders also included some skepticism with regard to the achievability of Vision Zero, overall the report showed the majority of the opinions expressed support for Vision Zero, demonstrating the commitment in the attitude of the UK officials to develop a comprehensive strategy based on the principles and successes this program. It seems viable that Vision Zero can be translated into other European contexts as there is not only a willingness to learn about the policy but also researchers are keen to understand the specific geographic context in which the policy is successful.

As mentioned earlier, the Swedish government has committed approximately SEK 4.9 billion over 11 years to construct new roads or modify existing road systems. The SEI report analyzed the economic costs and benefits of Vision Zero and concluded that, if adopted, Vision Zero would lead to a stream of benefits valued at £111 billion for the United Kingdom. The economic benefits are far greater than the costs associated with the interventions. Therefore, adopting Vision Zero policy would not only help reduce the number of deaths and serious injuries but also reduce the economic costs associated with injury.

19.4.2 Global Initiatives

Due to the comprehensive and sustainable approach of Vision Zero, it can be classified as an exemplar practice that has the potential to be implemented in any country determined to reduce traffic injuries. Sweden's success of implementing and procuring favorable outcomes has received international recognition and has resulted in other countries, states, and municipalities to follow in the lead of the Sweden's Vision Zero initiative. The United Kingdom, Norway, and municipalities in Canada and the United States have adopted Vision Zero as their road safety initiatives.

After introducing the Vision Zero concept in 2015, Parachute—a Canadian injury prevention charity—formed the Parachute Vision Zero Network (www.visionzeronetwork.ca). This network comprises of key players across various sectors in order to bring them together and share current knowledge while providing access to valuable resources (Parachute, n.d.). Some examples of those involved in the network include road safety advocates, law enforcement, governments, municipalities, and businesses (Parachute, n.d.).

In addition to the resource and knowledge network made possible by Parachute, Vision Zero Canada (www.visionzero.ca) launched a national campaign in 2015 targeting individuals, groups, and governments. Vision Zero Canada employs the same principles of the Vision Zero initiative and aims to promote these principles and policies through typical media and social media efforts, promoting campaigns, and putting pressure on governments to change policies. Examples of campaigns Vision Zero Canada promotes include encouraging individuals to use more environmentally friendly alternatives to motor vehicle

transportation and the Love 30 Canada campaign, which is determined to make all urban and residential streets have a maximum speed limit of 30 km/h (Vision Zero Canada, n.d.).

So far, there are national, provincial, and municipal road safety plans either in place or in the process of being implemented following the Vision Zero policy. Notably, Edmonton (Alberta), Vancouver (British Columbia), Toronto (Ontario), and Ottawa (Ontario) have begun implementing Vision Zero efforts in Canada. As Canada's largest city, Toronto continues to experience serious injuries and fatalities as a result of the road. According to City of Toronto (2017), traffic fatalities have increased over the years, representing a 10-year high. See Fig. 19.2 for a visualization of Toronto's fatalities from 2005 to 2016 (City of Toronto, 2017).

As a result of this problematic situation in Toronto, the City of Toronto has released a road safety plan based on Vision Zero's exemplar policies. The City of Toronto aims to significantly reduce traffic fatalities by implementing a strategic, 5-year action plan (2017–2021), with the combined efforts of the city of Toronto and a

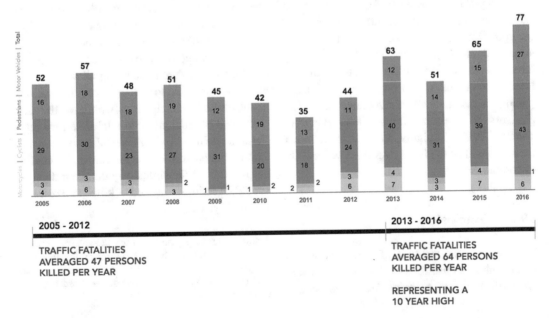

Fig. 19.2 Traffic fatalities in Toronto, Ontario from 2005 to 2016, color coded according to mode of transportation (City of Toronto, 2017)

variety of partner including Toronto Police Service; Toronto Public Health; the Disability, Access, and Inclusion Advisory Committee; the Canadian Automobile Association (CAA); and the Toronto District School Board (TDSB) to ensure the four major pillars of engineering, enforcement, technology, and education are collaborating (City of Toronto, 2017).

Toronto's Vision Zero Road Safety Plan addresses the following six emphasis areas determined through collision data analyses (City of Toronto, 2017):

- Pedestrians
- Schoolchildren
- Older adults
- Cyclists
- Motorcyclists
- Aggressive driving and distraction

Each emphasis area has its own action plan specific to the goal of eliminating fatalities or serious injuries to that specific area of the road. Importantly, existing safety measures are identified while also considering enhanced or new safety measures. For example, when focusing on increasing safety measures for pedestrians, a safety measure currently in place includes the incorporation of pedestrian countdown devices at signalized crossings. New or enhanced safety measures include reviewing street lighting at locations with high pedestrian volume and determining the effectiveness of automated pedestrian detectors to optimize intersections (City of Toronto, 2017). Similarly, more than 50 other measures will be the focus over the 5 years (City of Toronto, 2017).

19.5 Conclusion

The issue of road safety is of growing concern for all nations around the world. Roads in Sweden are built with safety prioritized over speed,

convenience, and superficial economic gain. Vision Zero is considered an exemplar practice based on a variety of factors. First, internal and external evaluators consider Vision Zero an innovative way of thinking about road safety by virtue of the principles that it is based on, namely, shared responsibility and a strong ethical philosophy. Second, Vision Zero has been institutionalized into the Swedish national policy; it maintains a sustainable source of funding and has already reported reduced incidences of collisions and injury rates. Third, Vision Zero policy educates the public about the various behavioral ways to prevent motor vehicle crashes. Fourth, it advocates for and implements improved engineering solutions, which are supported by legislation. Fifth, the goals of Vision Zero are met through active, strong, and close cooperation between the Ministry of Transportation, the SNRA, the Swedish parliament, and all stakeholders that are involved in the road system. Lastly, the Swedish government and community demonstrate clear leadership and coordination to make Vision Zero inherent in the way in which Sweden views and practices road safety. This leadership is only possible because the policy's operations are centralized to each level of government in an organized manner and because stakeholders make it a priority to buy in to the policy's goals and initiatives.

Sweden's approach to road safety by implementing Vision Zero policies has allowed for this exemplar practice to be executed by various countries and municipalities who have the ultimate goal of reducing road-related serious injuries and fatalities. Today, Vision Zero is known as a multinational traffic safety initiative and continues to promote the philosophy that no individual should be seriously injured or killed as a result of the road system.

Acknowledgments The author would like to express sincere appreciation to the key informant for this case study—Roger Johansson of the Swedish Road Administration in Borlänge, Sweden—whose consultation made this project possible.

BRIO Model: Vision Zero

Group Served: All road users.

Goal: To create a world with zero road-related injury or death.

Background	Resources	Implementation	Outcome
Developed in Sweden and as a result created some of the safest roads in the world Initial goal was to reduce motor vehicle fatalities by 50% between 1997 and 2007 and to further reduce it to zero Initiative to have zero road-related fatalities or injuries by putting the responsibility on the road system Draws from an ecological, holistic framework—focusing on the person-person-environment interaction	Vision Zero shares the responsibility of road safety with many stakeholders, including the Swedish National Road Administration (SNRA), municipal authorities, the Ministry of Transportation, the Swedish parliament, politicians, planners, police, community organizations, vehicle manufacturing companies, companies and organizations that purchase transport services, companies and organizations that transport both goods and people, and all the road users Swedish government has allocated about SEK 4.9 billion between 2004 and 2015 (about $700 million) to construct new roads and modify the existing road system	Since 1997, when Vision Zero was adopted as a national policy, the roads around Sweden have undergone major reconstructions in order to make them safer and reduce the likelihood of deaths or serious injuries Major constructions include roundabouts, steel cable guardrails, center guard rails, safe roadside areas, and roadside guardrails Specifically designed to focus on drink driving, safer speed limits, seat belt use, safer car design, road infrastructure improvements and pedestrian/cyclist safety	When appropriate modifications were made to the road system, yielding positive results in the longer term due to the program's research-intensive nature World Health Organization (WHO) created a report on road traffic injury prevention and identified Vision Zero as an effective policy to prevent road traffic injury Now is a successful multinational initiative: the United Kingdom, Norway, and municipalities in Canada and the United States have adopted Vision Zero as their road safety initiatives

Life Space Model: Vision Zero

Sociocultural: civilization/community	Interpersonal: primary and secondary relationships	Physical environments: where we live	Internal states: biochemical/genetic and means of coping
Provides safer road systems and drivers, understanding that holistic aspect of the road safety challenge	Changes how individual drivers respond to safety implements shared by all drivers (new signals, roundabouts, sealed shoulders, etc.)	Engineers evaluate the road network and bring about physical changes Changes include removing large tress, fixing bridge abutments, poles, sealing shoulders, increasing visibility	Removes the sole responsibility from the driver for casualty crashes to a marriage of driver/road condition Understands that humans make mistakes and tries to rectify that through other means

References

Business Sweden. (n.d.). *Vision Zero: Traffic safety by Sweden*. Retrieved January 10, 2018, from http://www.visionzeroinitiative.com

City of Toronto. (2017). *Vision Zero: Toronto's road safety plan 2017–2021*. Retrieved February 9, 2018, from https://www.toronto.ca/wp-content/uploads/2017/11/990f-2017-Vision-Zero-Road-Safety-Plan_June1.pdf

European Commission. (2005). *Road safety country profile*. Retrieved May 22, 2007, from http://ec.europa.eu/transport/roadsafety_library/care/doc/profiles/pdf/countryprofile_sv_en.pdf

Government Bill. (1996/1997). *137 Nollvisionen och det Trafiksäkra Samhället (Vision Zero and the Traffic Safe Society)*.

Hanson, H., & Salmoni, A. (2007). *The sustainability of the Stay on Your Feet demonstration project*. Ontario: University of Western Ontario.

Harris, D. L., Henry, R. C., Bland, C. J., Starnaman, S. M., & Voytek, K. L. (2003). Lessons learned from implementing multidisciplinary health professions educational models in community settings. *Journal of Interprofessional Care, 17*(1), 7–20.

Johnson, K., Hays, C., Center, H., & Daley, C. (2004). Building capacity and sustainable prevention innovations: A sustainability planning model. *Evaluation and Program Planning, 27*, 135–149.

National Society for Road Safety. (2002). *Fatalities in Swedish road traffic*. Retrieved May 10, 2007, from http://www.ntf.se/english/pdf/0209Killed%20in%20Sweden.pdf

National Statistics of Road Traffic Accidents. (2006). *Personskadeolyckor 1985–2006*. Retrieved June 27, 2007, from http://www.vv.se/templates/page-3wide_2068.aspx

Oxley, J., Corben, B., Fildes, B., O'Hare, M., & Rothengatter, T. (2004). *Older vulnerable road users—Measures to reduce crash and injury risk*. Retrieved March 15, 2007, from http://www.monash.edu.au/muarc/reports/muarc218.pdf

Parachute. (n.d.). *Parachute Vision Zero Network*. Retrieved December 19, 2017, from https://www.visionzeronetwork.ca

Rosencrantz, H., Edvardsson, K., & Hansson, S. O. (2007). Vision Zero—Is it irrational? *Transportation Research Part A, 41*, 559–567.

Scheirer, M. A. (2005). Is sustainability possible? A review and commentary on empirical studies of program sustainability. *American Journal of Evaluation, 26*(3), 320–347.

Shediac-Rizkallah, M. C., & Bone, L. R. (1998). Planning for the sustainability of community-based health programs: Conceptual frameworks and future directions for research, practice and policy. *Health Education Research, Theory & Practice, 3*(1), 87–108.

Stockholm Environment Institute. (2006a). *About Vision Zero*. Retrieved May 10, 2007, from http://www.sei.se/visionzero/moreinfo.htm

Stockholm Environment Institute. (2006b). *All fatal accidents investigated*. Retrieved May 22, 2007, from http://www.vagverket.se/filer/2586/Djupstudie%204%20s%20eng.pdf

Stockholm Environment Institute. (2006c). *Vision Zero: Adopting a target of zero for road traffic fatalities and serious injuries*. Retrieved May 24, 2007, from http://www.sei.se/visionzero/VZFinalReportMarch06.pdf

Swedish National Road Administration. (2006). *Safe Traffic- Vision Zero on the move*. Retrieved May 10, 2007, from http://publikationswebbutik.vv.se/shopping/ShowItem.aspx?id=1317

Vision Zero Canada. (n.d.). *Vision Zero Canada*. Retrieved November 5, 2017, from https://visionzero.ca/

Volpe, R. (2007). *The conceptualization of injury prevention as change in complex systems*. Unpublished Paper, University of Toronto.

World Health Organization. (2004). *World report on road traffic injury prevention*. Retrieved May 9, 2007, from http://www.who.int/world-health-day/2004/infomaterials/world_report/en/index.html

Black Spot Program: Australia

20

Susan Ball

Australia's Black Spot Program understands the holistic approach to road safety and aims to combat it by studying trends in driver and collision behavior. High-risk locations, referred to as high hazard, hazardous, or black spots, are identified. Accordingly, black spot projects are road improvement treatments that focus on reducing the number of casualties at these particular locations on a road network through the most cost-effective means. Typically, Black Spot Programs focus on reduction factors such as fixed roadside objects that infringe on traffic lanes (large trees, bridge abutments, poles, etc.), unsealed shoulders, high traffic volumes and minimal traffic control, poor visibility, and pedestrians (strip shopping centers, school crossings, school bus drop-off points, etc.).

20.1 Background

20.1.1 Road Safety, Road Engineering, and Holistic Function

Research shows that a majority of crashes are caused by human factors (Bureau of Transport Economics, 2001, p. 3). Theoretically, changing

the driver attitude and behavior could substantially reduce the incidence of crashes. Engineering improvements offer a strategy to target the worldwide problem of high crash rates because more is known about how to actually achieve sustained improvements in road systems than sustained changes in human behavior. This being said, no one problem operates in isolation and as such must be treated from within many disciplines to offer the most effective long-term results (BTE, 2001, p. 3). Injury prevention, including road-related injury prevention, is most effective when it meshes legislative, educational, behavioral, technological, and economic practices (Volpe, 2004). Specifically, passive (engineering and enactment) versus active (education and economic incentives) prevention seems to produce more effective results (Volpe, 2004). Most roads were planned and designed with motor vehicles in mind, but traffic (human) safety is rarely explicitly considered at this stage (Persaud & Lord, 2004). A consequence of the "mixed road" reality is that those relying on non-motorized transport are being put at increasing risk. What might be considered good planning for motorized transport may not be good planning for non-motorized transport.

At this level, road trauma prevention initiatives generally fall under three categories: safety-conscious design of roads, safety audits, and remedial action at high-risk crash sites. The description of the program to follow considers

S. Ball (✉)
The Mabin School, Toronto, ON, Canada

© Springer Nature Switzerland AG 2020
R. Volpe (ed.), *Casebook of Traumatic Injury Prevention*,
https://doi.org/10.1007/978-3-030-27419-1_20

301

each of the above listed initiatives. Recognizing that it is more difficult to change human behavior than it is to modify physical conditions and environments makes engineering alternatives more appealing. Engineering-based traffic calming measures, defined as physical measures to eliminate the negative consequences of motorized vehicle use, alter driver behavior, and improve the situation for non-motorized street users, are among the most effective means of reducing traffic death according to the Institute for Transportation and Development Policy (ITDP). ITDP is an American-based agency that has, since 1985, advocated for environmentally sustainable and equitable transportation policies and projects across the world. Other viable solutions in reducing traffic casualties include designing roads specific to their function, executing traffic calming measures such as speed bumps and roundabouts, and through informing and educating the public (World Health Organization [WHO], 2004). These suggestions from WHO speak directly of Volpe's passive and active initiatives. Volpe describes passive prevention as dependent upon enactment and engineering, while active prevention uses education and economics in its execution. As well, WHO offers that "a wide range of effective interventions exist, and experience in countries with long histories of motorized travel has shown that a scientific 'systems approach' to road safety is essential to tackling the problem. This approach addresses the traffic system as a whole and looks at the interactions between vehicles, road users, and the road infrastructure to identify solutions." The holistic nature of this approach acknowledges the interconnectedness of any problem and applies it to road safety. The life-space model within the complex systems approach (Volpe, 2004) recognizes the humanistic qualities of preventative efforts, including not only the persons involved but also those systems and environments used by people. Sociocultural, interpersonal, and physical environment and internal states are considered using the life-space model weaving the working elements of individual daily functioning within a larger working system of multiple and whole communities. As stated by Volpe (2004), "Injury

prevention is about culture and society, communities and neighborhoods, families and friends, life styles and ways of thinking. The assumption we begin with is that injuries are preventable, not chance occurrences."

20.1.2 Human, Vehicle, and Road Interactions

The causes of road crashes are explained by many factors but are rooted in the inconsistency between the driver behavior and road environments and/or vehicle characteristics (BTE, 2001, p. 5). The performance level of a driver varies as it is impacted by factors such as fatigue, drowsiness, illness, and lack of concentration. In turn, the road environment varies due to factors such as traffic flow rates, geometric features of the road, and road type. To accommodate this, the driver must adapt his/her performance based on demands of the road system. A crash happens when there is a discrepancy between the driver's performance and his/her adaptability to the demands of the road environment (BTE, 2001, p. 5). The safety margin between the driver's performance level and the demands of the road environment can be increased through engineering improvements in the road design. Mr. Greg Moxon, manager of the National Black Spot Program, recognizes that it is more effective to change roads than it is to change driver behavior. Inevitably drivers will make errors, but engineering improvements on a road network can reduce the performance demands on a driver thereby reducing the likelihood of a crash (BTE, 2001, p. 5). Users of the road will make mistakes; however, when several users are making the same mistake, chances are that elements of the road are misleading and are worthy of further investigation (Morgan, personal communication, July 13, 2004). The Bureau of Transport Economics offers substantial theoretical and empirical evidence that support beliefs that engineering improvements to a road network alone may not significantly decrease the number of crashes if driver behavior compensates for these structural safety changes (BTE, 2001, p. 5). "It has been suggested that the most effective treatments make the traffic system objectively safer while simultaneously increasing subjective risk, thus motivating drivers to maintain high performance levels" (BTE, 2001, p. 6). They offer that road engineering aims should target the road environment and ensure that low performance demands are made on the driver while protecting drivers from underestimating the dangers posed by the road environment (BTE, 2001, p. 6).

20.1.3 The Federal Black Spot Program

Austroads Road Facts 2000 reports that Australians drive further and longer than any other nation. In 2000, Australians drove 180.7 billion kilometers on a national road network stretching 805,836 km. Austroads is an association consisting of the Australian and New Zealand road transport and traffic authorities. Members are made up of the road transport and traffic authorities of the six Australian states and two territories, the Commonwealth Department of Transport and Regional Services (DOTARS), the Australian Local Government Association (ALGA), and Transit New Zealand. The role of Austroads is to contribute to the process of improving Australian and New Zealand transport by conducting national research on behalf of Australian road agencies, advocating better practice by road agencies, facilitating communication between road agencies, and providing expert advice to the Australian Transport Council (ATC) and the Standing Committee on Transport (SCOT) (http://www.austroads.com.au). Australia has recorded deaths due to road crashes since 1925, and since then as many as 164,190 people have lost their lives on the road. Recorded statistics between 1925 and 1970 show a consistent increase in road fatalities except during significant times in history such as the Great Depression and the Second World War. Since 1970 the number of road fatalities has decreased, especially during the 1980s and 1990s. Road fatalities in 1999 represented less than half of the 1970 rate. Significant reduction in fatal road accidents can be attributed to a heightened public awareness about road safety as well as improvements to roads and vehicles, road safety legislation, public education, and police enforcement technology. As a consequence of joint forces of action, Australia's roads have become much safer and have emphasized the effectiveness of a coordinated effort by the government (Australian Bureau of Statistics, 2002).

The federal government of Australia has operated target programs for over a decade dealing with specific road hazards including physical conditions and management of dangerous locations with crash histories involving death or serious injury. The largest programs specific to reducing the social and economic costs of road trauma are the federal government's Black Spot Programs. The first Black Spot Program began on July 1, 1990, and currently operates as the Capital Funding for Black Spots Roads Program more commonly known as the Federal Road Safety Black Spot Program. Although there is not a universal definition of a black spot, it can be defined as an area where at least three or more casualty crashes within 3 years have occurred. Casualty crashes involve those where one or more people are injured or die. The relative risk of a crash on a road network varies but tends to concentrate in high-risk locations. These locations can be referred to as crash concentrated, high hazard, hazardous, or black spots. Black spots are complicated by many factors that include degree and type of risk, road characteristics, traffic exposure, and crash severity. Black spot projects are road improvement treatments that focus on reducing the number of casualties at a particular location on a road network through the most cost-effective means. Typically, Black Spot Programs focus on reduction factors such as fixed roadside objects that infringe on traffic lanes (large trees, bridge abutments, poles, etc.), unsealed shoulders, high traffic volumes and minimal traffic control, poor visibility, and pedestrians (strip shopping centers, school crossings, school bus drop-off points, etc.). The most hazardous black spots are often treated first, followed by those less dangerous sites, as funding becomes available. Inevitably new black sites emerge as traffic patterns and roads change over time, as new roads are developed, and as unidentified hazards are reported. At any given time, there are many black spot locations throughout Australia (BTE, 2001, p. xiii).

20.2   Resources

20.2.1 Stakeholders and Collaborators

The Federal Office of Road Safety (FORS) administers the Black Spot Program on behalf of the federal government as a part of the Commonwealth Department of Transport and Regional Development. It is the state road and transport agencies that manage individual programs within their area. The Federal Minister for Transport and Regional Development organizes the Black Spot Consultative Panel in each state comprising of the Parliamentary Secretary to the Minister for Transport and Regional Development, representatives of related state and road transport authorities, municipal governments, community, and road users. This panel involves all interested and involved authorities and persons who then consider and address each nomination for black spot treatments within a state. Throughout the duration of the program, all governments, transport authorities, and community road users have been a collaborative part of its execution and maintenance. Without multiple partnerships it would not meet its critical goals of reducing countrywide road trauma.

20.2.2 The Victoria Black Spot Program

VicRoads estimates that 24,000 Victorians are killed or injured in road crashes each year. During the past 6 years, more than 30,000 people were seriously injured and sent to hospitals because of road crashes. The annual economic cost of road trauma for Victorians is around $1.8 billion.

Victoria was first to implement a Black Spot Program in 1979 and demonstrated an impressive performance considering its low level of expenditure per person up until 2000–2001 (BTE, 2001, p. 53). In Victoria there are currently three Black Spot Programs: a federal program, an ongoing state program funded from the state budget, and a statewide program funded from the Transport Accident Commission (TAC). VicRoads implements the program and Monash University Accident Research Centre (MUARC) evaluates the program (BTE, 2001, p. 14). As of 2001, the Victorian Government was the only state to conduct a large-scale evaluation of state-funded black spot treatments. The main objective of the program is reducing the social and economic cost of road trauma through the targeting of road sites with poor crash history for the purpose of improving the physical conditions and management. As well, the most recent program aims at reducing rural road trauma (BTE, 2001, p. 137). As many as 60% of fatal crashes and 50% of serious injury crashes happen outside of metropolitan areas (population of more than 100,000). As a result of this, approximately half of all black spot funds in each state are designated for non-metropolitan projects under the current program (BTE, 2001, p. 139). The Bureau of Transport Economics identifies that although less accidents happen in regional areas as compared to urban areas, regional crashes tend to have more severe consequences (BTE, 2001, p. 13). The 2000 National Road Safety Strategy claimed, "Improving the safety of the roads is the single most significant achievable factor in reducing road trauma."

20.2.3 Allocation of Funds

The federal government spent $145 million in the first 4 years of the Black Spot Program (BTE, 2001, p. 9). Some $36 million per year from 1996–1997 until 1999–2000 was allocated for the Federal Black Spot Program, expanding to $40.8 million in 2000–2001 and $41.7 million in 2001–2002. The federal government provides funding for treatments of crash sites that meet the designated criteria and this funding works to assist existing expenditures of the states. What makes the allocations of funds particularly interesting and unique from other prevention programs is how they are distributed at various levels. The federal government's expenditure on Black Spot Programs directly trickles into state and territory governments for distribution into their black spot expenditure conditional upon meeting designated criteria for treatment (BTE, 2001, p. 10). This allows state and territory governments to allocate the external federal grant money to the treatment of black spots thereby freeing up their budget for other necessary spending (Rome, personal communication, August 3, 2004).

Ms. Liz de Rome, a road safety specialist, clarified the roles of state and federal governments: 80% of the roads are local responsibilities and 20% of the roads are federal responsibilities. She states, "It is the road authority that really drives the program." Since July 1, 1996, when the current program was introduced, federal funding for black spot treatments has remained stable in real terms (BTE, 2001, p. 10). National rates of road trauma are addressed through regional and urban areas in all states and territories (BTE, 2001, p. 13). Funds are allocated between states and territories according to the average population and number of casualty crashes in each area 3 years prior to the start of the program. Of these funds, regional and urban locations each receive an equal amount to be allocated to each jurisdiction (BTE, 2001, p. 13). As of the end of June 1999, there have been 983 black spots projects put in place through the Australian Transport Safety Bureau totaling approximately $59.5 million (BTE, 2001, p. xiii).

In recent years, the Australian government has continued to support the program by investing $684.5 million from 2013/2014 to 2020/2021 (Australian Government, 2017). Furthermore, the government has decided to extend the program even more and will continue to financially support it by providing $60 million per year from 2021 to 2022 (Australian Government, 2017).

20.3 Implementation

20.3.1 Identification and Treatment (Road Safety Audit, Cost-Benefit Analyses)

Working from a cost-effectiveness strategy, funding is made available for those black spot sites with a proven crash history. The proof is often in the road safety audit, a process that looks at the factors that contribute to crashes and assesses the road system in terms of, in the case of rural roads, for example, the alignment, the conditions of shoulders, and the location of hazards. A project proposal must demonstrate a benefit to cost ratio of at least 2 to 1 (BTE, 2001, p. 138). It is a proactive process in conjunction with Austroads of not only identifying potential crash sites before they happen but also assessing those sites that have in the past been identified but perhaps over time have not met the threshold because of the random nature of crashes (Veith, personal communication, July 12, 2004).

Beyond crash history, local knowledge and opinion and statistical data are used to identify and prioritize black spots (BTE, 2001, p. 138). Projects with an estimated federal cost of less than $500,000 are given preference (BTE, 2001, p. 140). Benefit-cost analyses done prior to the start of a project help determine whether or not a project should go ahead (BTE, 2001, p. 115). Benefit-cost analysis done at the end of the project help determine if expectations were met, whether or not it is worthwhile to continue or whether or not to initiate a similar project in the future (BTE, 2001, p. 115). Within each jurisdiction databases are analyzed in a process of marking dangerous sites. Of these marked sites, some are chosen for treatment as black spot sites. Most sites in the Federal Black Spot Program are nominated through state and territory governments (BTE, 2001, p. 95). Nominations of sites are derived through state and local governments, community groups, clubs and associations, road user groups, and industry. A consultative panel meets to consider all nominations for black spot treatments for a particular state (BTE, 2001,

p. 141). The consultative panel must prepare a submission to the federal minister listing those nominated black spot proposals with comments.

After submissions from consultative panels, the minister will decide on programs for each state. The combination of factors that cause traffic accidents are managed using a matrix specifying traffic engineering solutions. These crashes are then analyzed in terms of the pattern of accident types, called Definitions for Coding Accidents [DCA code], as well as other factors that are repeated. The matrix is used to guide particular application of treatments and provides an estimated outcome from a range of associated treatments. The matrix is divided into two tables: table one relates to intersections and table two relates to road sections not related to intersections. Emphasis is put on the movement of road users leading up to a crash so that appropriate treatments are put in place to best prevent the same crash (http://www.dotars.gov.au/transprog/road/blackspot/index.htm).

The Federal Black Spot Program outlines four basic approaches to reducing the number of road crashes using engineering treatments, although only the two addressed by the federal government are listed below:

- Black spots or single sites—whereby specific sites or short sections of the road are treated
- Route action—executing familiar treatments on routes with unusually high crash rates

Collection of road crash data is managed by each state and territory based on police crash reports. Reports are compiled from police at the site of the crash or resulting from individuals reporting the crash to the police station (BTE, 2001, p. 55). Most jurisdictions maintain crash site records for a minimum of 20 years, although in recent years, there has been a push toward less record keeping, especially of less severe crashes. Although the probability of a crash is impacted by a multitude of influences, a treatment will likely only reduce the risk of one influence. Choosing an appropriate treatment will become considerably difficult if one cannot access particular types of crashes at particular types of

sites: the very information that establishes a site as dangerous. Black spot crash reduction factors are the result of specific treatments that are applied to intersections, road pavement widening, grade separation, rail crossings, barriers, curve treatment, fixed roadside hazards, pedestrian/bicyclist access, and street lighting. Listed below are the specific treatments used by Victoria that have shown a reduction of casualty crashes as a result of their implementation and are similar to those used by other states (Table 20.1).

20.3.2 Information Management

Data storage is often formatted in a three-tier system that deals separately with crash details, vehicle details, and casualty details thereby requiring minimal memory capacity. The manner in which data is entered as recorded by police is also specific to each jurisdiction. Vital to a successful Black Spot Program is the ability to identify where crashes happened. This process involves correctly identifying the crash location and accurately recording the location of the crash into the database so that information can be easily accessed (BTE, 2001, p. 59).

20.3.3 Alternative Assessment Tools

The road safety risk manager, produced by the Australian Road Research Board (ARRB) and funded by Austroads, is a computer-based method of determining the relative risk associated with different situations and the relative risk associated with treatments. The software produces a risk score of a particular area using determined risk factors, as well as a risk score to show what implementation of a particular treatment might mean. This derives an estimate of benefit and ranking, although not considered a benefit/cost analysis (Veith, personal communication, July 12, 2004). Technological tools such as this could potentially be used as a function of the implementation process for local governments in determining how to best treat the problem but is not currently a function of the Black Spot Program.

Table 20.1 Black spot treatments, Victoria

Intersection	Road pavement widening	Curve treatment	Grade separation	Rail crossing facilities	Barriers	Fixed roadside hazards	Pedestrian/bicyclist	Street lighting
New roundabout New Signal Fully controlled right turn phase Roundabout replacing signals Mount signal heads on mast arms Channelization, turning lanes Sheltered turn lanes (urban) Sheltered turn lanes (rural) Additional lane at intersection Skid resistant overlay Red light camera Staggered T Splitter islands (rural, low volume)	Add lane Add median strip Bridge widened or modified Bridge replaced Widen shoulder Seal shoulder with painted edge line Seal shoulder with tactile edge line Reconstruct highway Overtaking lane Right turn lane Left turn lane	Delineation Reflectorized guide post Raised reflectorized pavement markers Tactile edge line marking Barrier line Shoulder seal plus reseal, inside of curve Shoulder seal, reseal plus delineation, inside of curve Reshape, shoulder seal, reseal plus delineation, inside of curve Realignment plus delineation Warning/advisory signs Improve super elevation Improve transition curves Lane widening Paved shoulder widening Unpaved shoulder widening Side slope flattening	Intersection grade separation (of existing signalized intersections) Pedestrian overpass	Warning signs upgrade to flashing lights Warning signs upgrade to boom barriers Flashing lights upgrade to boom barriers	Upgrade median barriers Guardrail (other than for bridge end post)	Tree removal (rural) Pole removal (lighting poles, urban) Replace rigid poles with frangible poles Extend culverts Embankment treatment Guardrail for bridge end post Impact attenuator	Refuges, channelization, curb extension Pedestrian signals Bicycle paths, threshold treatments	Provision of street lighting

20.4 Outcome

20.4.1 Evaluation and Review Results

Improving road safety through Black Spot Programs is just one of several means. Despite success of previous Black Spot Programs ongoing evaluation is critical to examine whether further expenditure is warranted. The question then is, "do black spot treatments produce a statistically significant decrease in the number of crashes in an area?" Overall, those sites with crash histories involving death or serious injury showed very strong evidence of improved safety. Very strong evidence is indicated by the probability of a crash which is less than 1 in 1000 (BTE, 2001, p. xv). The Bureau of Transport Economics completed the Black Spot Program 1996–2002: an evaluation of the first 3 years in August 2001. The evaluation was based on a before and after assessment of black spot treatment effectiveness. It compares the history of a crash site after treatment with the expected crash history if no treatment was applied. Using the cost-benefit standard, the Black Spot Program generated a net value of $1.3 billion. For every taxpayer dollar invested, there was a $14 return in lives saved, injuries prevented, and related cost savings. Precisely because of the higher amount of traffic flow through capital city black spots, the program operating in these areas produced significantly greater benefits than regional areas. Evaluations of the Victorian Black Spot Program implemented in 1994–1995 and 1995–1996 by VicRoads demonstrated an average reduction of 11 casualty crashes per annum per million dollars invested. This means that for each $100 million invested (in 1995 dollars), there would be 26 lives and significant number of injuries saved each year into the future.

The review of the first 3 years by the Bureau of Transport Economics showed strong evidence that sites with crash histories involving death and serious injury indeed improved. A weakness evidenced by the program was that it did not consistently reduce the number of casualty crashes in urban and non-urban areas. Specifically, in non-urban areas traffic islands on intersection approaches, indented right and left turn lanes, non-skid surfaces, and pedestrian facilities had no statistically significant impact on road safety. There was strong evidence however that signs and new traffic lights with turn arrows did improve safety in non-urban areas. Strong evidence is indicated by a probability of less than 1 in 100 (BTE, 2001, p. xv). Moderate evidence supported increased safety in the same areas due to medians, shoulder sealing, edge lines, and improved lighting. Moderate evidence is indicated by a probability of less than 1 in 50 (BTE, 2001, p. xv).

Overall, the program is estimated to have prevented 32 deaths and 1539 serious injuries due to crashes spanning 3 years. This translates into reduction of casualty crashes by 31% in capital cities and 48% in regional areas. The national fatality rate in 2002 was 8.75 deaths per 100,000 people: the lowest recorded rate in a decade and continues on the downward trend. These numbers, however, don't reflect the 40% reduction target set by the federal government. Assuming the reduction is met by a linear downward rate, it is still higher than what should be expected. The evidence does support continuing the Black Spot Program with few modifications for increased effectiveness. Accordingly, for the 2003–2004 financial year, the federal government allotted $180 million for roads over the next 4 years and about $45 million per year for the National Black Spot Program. During the 4-year period of analysis, spending related to the Black Spot Program totaled $116 million. Even with what can be considered a relatively small amount of spending, the financial expenditure bill was reduced by about $1.3 billion. The argument of how to best spend money on identified areas of need can potentially infringe on the statistical benefits of the Black Spot Program. Upon close examination however, the initial objective of reducing the number of casualties via the most cost-effective means has clearly been met. Engineering-based programs such as black spot treatments mean that once a problem is fixed, it's fixed, and the site doesn't require the resources, effort, or support that it once did. Concise monitoring of the treatment site is necessary, however, to judge its effectiveness (Morgan, personal communication, July 13, 2004). The effectiveness of Black Spot Programs in both developing and developed countries is rooted in the prioritization of funds. If a government is able to link the program to the greatest need of the roads for that particular situation, it can offer the systematic benefits evidenced in Australia (Rome, personal communication, August 3, 2004).

20.4.2 Gaps and Future Directions

Systematic preventatives and interventions such as the Black Spot Program are solid examples of advancements in organized networks that aim at reducing road traffic injuries. An upcoming technological arena for exploration is the Global Positioning System (GPS). This system takes advantage of computerized technology that appeals to society's ability to move forward with innovation. If used in conjunction with Black Spot Programs, GPS receivers would help to identify crash sites thereby giving accuracy to crash site locations. They also provide clear and reliable information instantly and are affordable and simple to use (BTE, 2001, p. 60). This type of innovation might have the potential to dramatically assist current systems of tracking accidents. Limited trials and, therefore, limited success mean that GPS investigation is largely an unexplored area with potential for breakthrough implementation. In the event that the initiation of a Black Spot Program is made elsewhere, it would prove beneficial to acknowledge and adjust those few weak areas. Beyond the specific use of GPS for identifying crash locations, it is worth exploring the wealth of possibilities connected to all aspects of road design, maintenance, and prevention of road-related injuries set within the goals of the Black Spot Program.

Common with large amounts of data is the problem of processing and managing its bulk. With regard to road injury, the organization of this data includes post-crash information, specifically fatal injury and hospitalization. Hospital admission or treatment specifies that a person has been in the hospital for at least 24 h. Records such as these are important because they provide injury statistics leading to preventative injury measures. In Australia the police recording of this information is often inconsistent and complicated because not all of those dispatched in ambulances are actu-

ally admitted to hospitals. A system for tracking casualties via ambulance transport and treatment is also a deficiency. Consequently, the reliability of the data depends on whether or not police follow through at the hospitals as well as how thoroughly this is done (BTE, 2001, p. 61). In Victoria, the most recent and successful location of a Black Spot Program, the closest definition within the federal definition of hospital admission or treatment is the sent to hospital category. This is misleading because it refers only to those dispatched to the hospital in an ambulance directly from the scene of a crash and neglects anyone deviating from this limited definition. Data management is an issue in many locations.

Another recognized problem is that not all individuals who are sent to hospitals due to road trauma actually show up on police reports or database records (BTE, 2001, p. 62). Australia lacks a clear system of identification for individuals admitted to hospitals because of road trauma, therefore making it very difficult to align the records so that information on multiple admissions of the same individual can be gained. It also roadblocks gathering of information on average hospital stay, average cost incurred, and on specifics to individuals and their crash details (BTE, 2001, p. 62). The incongruence between reported crash statistics and hospital records creates a gap that, if not filled, leads to incomplete post-crash data and lagging prevention. A key area that needs future targeting is a system of information management that offers concise and accurate post-crash data so that preventative crash initiatives best serve a deficit.

Standing alone the Black Spot Program provides a strong example of excellence as evidenced by satisfying criteria specific to communities, individuals, local and federal governments, and physical environments. Australia prevented an estimated 32 deaths and 1539 serious injuries due to crashes spanning 3 years because of Black Spot Programs.

Acknowledgments The author would like to express sincere appreciation to the key informants for this case study: Greg Moxon of the Department of Transport and Regional Services in Canberra, ACT, Australia; Gary Veith of Australian Road Research Board in Port Melbourne, VIC, Australia; and Robert Morgan, a Road Safety Engineer in Surrey Hills, VIC, Australia—whose consultation made this project possible.

BRIO Model: Black Spot Programs

Group Served: All individuals on the road (motorists, bicyclists, and pedestrians).

Goal: To identify hazardous (black spot) road locations that have resulted in collisions and improve roads to reduce the number of casualties.

Background	Resources	Implementation	Outcome
Understands that changing driver behavior is implausible and therefore engineering improvements must be made for injury prevention efforts Adopts a holistic approach to road safety—in that many aspects of human behavior and the environment interact in order to create dangerous roads First Black Spot Program in Australia started in 1990—now known as the Federal Road Safety Black Spot Program "Black spot" defined as an area where at least three or more casualty crashes within 3 years have occurred	The Federal Office of Road Safety (FORS) administers the Black Spot Program on behalf of the federal government State road and transport agencies manage individual programs with specific areas First 4 years of the program, the federal government spent $145 million From 2013 to 2022, the federal government will spend approx. $800 million	Identification of black spots is successful by understanding crash history, statistical data, and local knowledge from individuals Black spot programs focus on reduction factors in order to reduce the number of casualties at a particular location through the most cost-effective means Factors including fixed roadside objects, high traffic volumes, poor visibility, and pedestrians and are combated through funding measures like traffic signals and roundabouts to reduce risk of collision	The program continues to be implemented and funded by the Australian federal government for 30 years In the first 3 years, it is estimated 32 deaths and 1539 serious injuries were prevented

Life-Space Model: Black Spot Programs

Sociocultural: civilization/community	Interpersonal: primary and secondary relationships	Physical environments: where we live	Internal states: biochemical/genetic and means of coping
Federal initiative yet community-based intervention through reporting of potential black spots Involvement of government and legislative bodies (the Bureau of Transport Economics, federal, state, and territory governments)	Changes how individual drivers respond to safety implements shared by all drivers (new signals, new roundabouts, sealed shoulders, etc.)	Engineers evaluate the road network and bring about physical changes These changes include removing large trees, fixing bridge abutments, poles, etc., sealing shoulders, increasing visibility	Removes the sole responsibility from the driver for casualty crashes to a marriage of driver/road condition

References

Australian Bureau of Statistics. (2002). *Australia: A history of road fatalities in Australia*. Commonwealth of Australia: Australian Bureau of Statistics.

Australian Government. (2017). *Department of Infrastructure, Regional Development and Cities. Black Spot Program*. Retrieved March 1, 2018, from http://investment.infrastructure.gov.au/infrastructure_investment/black_spot/index.aspx

Bureau of Transport Economics. (2001). The Black Spot Program 1996–2002: An evaluation of the first three years. Canberra: Bureau of Transport Economics.

Persaud, B., & Lord, D. (2004). Estimating the safety performance of urban road transportation networks. *Accident Analysis and Prevention, 36*(4), 609–620.

Volpe, R. (2004). *The conceptualization of injury prevention as change in complex systems*. Toronto, ON: Life Span Adaptation Projects, University of Toronto.

World Health Organization. (2004). Media Centre. Retrieved August 12, 2004, from http://www.who.int/mediacentre/releases/2004/pr24/en/

Vera Roberts

The Institute for Transport Studies at Leeds University, piloted the implementation of External Vehicle Speed Controls (EVSC) and Intelligent Speed Adaptations (ISA) to control traffic flow and improve road safety. EVSC/ISA works by combining Global Positioning Satellite (GPS) technology with digital road maps complete with posted speed limits to prevent vehicles equipped with EVSC/ISA devices to be driven faster than posted limits.

21.1 Background

The Institute for Transport Studies (ITS) at the University of Leeds is composed of five research groups:

1. Safety
2. Network modelling
3. Traffic and statistics
4. Economics and behavioural modeling
5. Transport policy and appraisal

These groups work on an individual and coordinated basis to develop new research initiatives in the field. This case will focus on work by the Safety research group that lists its main goal as:

To improve fundamental understanding of road user behaviour in interactions with the road environment, the vehicle, traffic systems and information systems. To use that understanding to develop and assess new systems for road user safety (ITS, 2002).

To that end, the Safety research group examines not only systems to enhance safety but also the negative impact of new technologies. One ITS project that utilizes technology for improved vehicle safety is the Intelligent Speed Adaptation (ISA) project with the earlier research referred to as the External Vehicle Speed Control (EVSC) project. This research has yielded predictions that suggest EVSC/ISA could be eight times more effective at preventing injury and fatality from vehicle accidents in the UK than the implementation of compulsory front occupant seatbelt wearing, the most effective road safety measure in the UK to date (ITS, 2002). EVSC/ISA works by combining Global Positioning Satellite (GPS) technology with digital road maps complete with posted speed limits to prevent vehicles equipped with EVSC/ISA devices to be driven faster than posted limits.

21.1.1 Description of Consumers

The initial target population for the EVSC/ISA project are citizens of Great Britain who may be drivers or passengers of motor vehicles and who

V. Roberts (✉)
Inclusive Design Research Centre, Ontario College of Art and Design University, Toronto, ON, Canada
e-mail: vroberts@ocadu.ca

© Springer Nature Switzerland AG 2020
R. Volpe (ed.), *Casebook of Traumatic Injury Prevention*,
https://doi.org/10.1007/978-3-030-27419-1_21

may be road users. The EVSC/ISA research was carried out under contract to the Department of Environment, Transport and the Regions (DETR; Now renamed Department for Transport [DFT]), and the target population was naturally the population of Great Britain.

In 2001, there were 313,046 road casualties in Great Britain. Of these casualties, 37,094 were serious injuries (Department for Transport, Local Government and the Regions [DTLR], 2001). These injury statistics cross all age levels, socio-economic status and road uses. In the United States, 38.5% of the spinal cord injuries (SCI) reported since 1990 were caused by motor vehicle crashes, and motor vehicle crashes are the leading cause of SCI in the US (National Spinal Cord Injury Statistical Center [NSCISC], 2001). It may be expected that SCI causation rates in the UK will be similar to that of the US as well as in other western countries. Indeed, Headway, a brain injury association in the UK, estimates that 40–50% of all head injuries are caused by road traffic accidents and that road traffic accidents are most commonly associated with severe injuries (Headway the Brain Injury Association, 2002).

Development of methods for speed control is particularly important as a roads injury prevention method. The Parliamentary Advisory Council for Transport Safety (PACTS) in the UK finds that not only is excess or inappropriate speed a main or contributory factor in one third of all collisions, but also that Impact speed determines the severity of injury, e.g. 5% of pedestrians hit at 20 mph [32 kph] are killed, at 30 mph [48 kph] 45% are killed and at 40 mph [64 kph] 85% are killed (PACTS, 2002).

21.1.2 History and Development

The Institute for Traffic Studies was founded in 1966 at the University of Leeds and became an autonomous entity in 1971. The institute has been recognized for research quality and received the highest rating for research quality in the HEFC Research Assessment Exercises for the years 1996 and 2001. Furthermore, in 1995 ITS

was the first University department in the UK to achieve ISO 9001 accreditation for research. Two thirds of ITS activity are research.

The EVSC/ISA research carried out by ITS took place from February 1997 to February 2000. The research into EVSC/ISA continues at the institute, and the current project will conclude in 2005. This case will focus on the concluded research project but will provide information about the current project.

If implemented, EVSC/ISA will help to prevent injury as well as to reduce the severity of injury. Because excess motor vehicle speed is implicated not only in causing accidents but also increasing the severity of injury, programs such as EVSC/ISA, which seek to confine motor vehicle speed to posted speed limits, have the potential to prevent injury at the primary and secondary levels in that they will have an impact on both the pre-event and event phase of injury as outlined by Haddon (1980). Furthermore, EVSC/ISA affects all three factors involved in injury: host, agent and environment, such that the host or driver cannot ignore posted limits in the environment, and as such the energy of the vehicle or agent to cause injury is reduced.

The development of this prevention strategy at ITS began several years ago when ITS applied for and received funding from a UK research council to begin research on use of EVSC through simulator trials. Around the same time, researchers in Sweden were investigating driver acceptance of ISA and were utilizing one test vehicle. The ITS team next worked on an EU project investigating ISA and, in this project, carried out all of the simulator work as well as investigating user acceptance and applications of ISA for rural roads and dangerous curves. The remaining ISA projects carried out by ITS were funded by the DETR through a tender and bid process in which ITS succeeded. Each consecutive EVSC/ISA project builds on knowledge gained from the previous project.

The core prevention strategy of EVSC/ISA is to reduce the top speed of vehicles. ITS researchers reviewed more than 120 studies regarding speed and traffic accidents and found that while the degree of the relationship between speed and accident risk is not linear, there is a definite and unmistakable correlation between the two variables. Furthermore, the studies showed overwhelmingly that increased speed is associated with increased severity of injury for both occupants and vulnerable road users.

While ISA research has been carried out for about 20 years, the impetus for the development of the current ISA strategy was in part formed by a 1996 UK Department of Transport report suggesting EVSC/ISA as speed control. At this time the DETR issued a tender for ISA research in the UK.

The ITS researchers set the following criteria for the EVSC/ISA from the outset: (1) cost effective, (2) acceptable to the driver, (3) logistically feasible and (4) safe. Furthermore, the ITS team reviewed previous work carried out in speed control as well as formed links with other projects both within and outside the UK. A chief concern for the researchers was to find ways to maximize the benefits of ISA. From the beginning the researchers had hypothesized a strict system. To date, no one else has operationalized the system so strictly. For example, researchers in Sweden were investigating a haptic throttle that would become stiffer as speed limits were exceeded. This system, however, may be overridden by the driver in a variety of ways and is only relevant when the foot is on the accelerator. The ITS team was interested in different technology that would prevent drivers from exceeding appropriate speed levels rather than provide feedback that speeds were inappropriate for the road or road conditions.

The objectives of these strategies are: to reduce the number of injuries and deaths due to speeding in the sense of speeding as exceeding the speed limit and speeding in terms of excessive speed for road conditions; to facilitate compliance with speed limits; and to inform policy decisions about implementation of EVSC/ISA or EVSC/ISA within the UK. The safety benefit of the EVSC/ISA system is always the paramount objective of the system, and it is largely through this increased safety and reduction in injury that significant cost to benefit ratios are achieved.

21.1.3 The EVSC/ISA Model

The EVSC/ISA model can be conceptualized as an autonomous system that utilizes GPS information and a digital road map to track the posted speed limit for a given car position and convey that limit to the driver and vehicle. There are several variants of the system that have been investigated by the ITS researchers. The variations are of two dimensions of the system: (1) its level of intervention or permissiveness, and (2) the currency of the speed limit. For the former aspect, three models have been developed and are described as follows:

1. Advisory: display the speed limit and remind the driver of changes in the speed limit.
2. Voluntary ("Driver Select"): allow the driver to enable and disable control by the vehicle of maximum speed.
3. Mandatory: the vehicle is limited at all times.

(Carsten & Tate, 2000, p. 12)

The researchers hypothesized a further variant that would be a combination of (2) and (3) in that it would be a mandatory system that would allow limited excursions for the purpose of overtaking. Variations in the currency of speed dimension have been conceptualized in three ways:

1. Fixed: the vehicle id informed of the posted speed limits.
2. Variable: the vehicle is additionally informed of certain locations in the network where a lower speed limit is implemented. Examples could include around pedestrian crossings or the approach to sharp horizontal curves. With a Variable system, the speed limits are current spatially.
3. Dynamic: additional lower speed limits are implemented because of network or weather conditions, to slow traffic in fog, on slippery roads, around major incidents, etc. With a Dynamic system, speed limits are current temporarily.

(Carsten & Tate, 2000, p. 12)

A third dimension involves the strictness to which EVSC control is applied. This dimension applies only to mandatory and voluntary EVSC and relates to the method of control exercised in the vehicle. The ITS researchers find that the standard method of haptic throttle (pedal becomes stiffer as car exceeds speed limit) has shortcomings and instead favors a combination of dead throttle and active breaking where the initial intervention is not a communication to the driver but rather an intervention between accelerator position and engine control. In this way the vehicle speed control system cannot be overcome by the driver.

21.2 Resources

21.2.1 Stakeholders

The Department for Transport is a major stakeholder in the project as are groups such as PACTS and the European Safety Council. Enactment is an integral part of an effective injury prevention program, and these groups could have a bearing on this aspect. Other stakeholders include road users and manufacturers. Potentially important stakeholders are fleet managers who bear responsibility for safety of their vehicles in relation to other road users as well as to their drivers. Fleet managers who request ISA technology from manufacturers for their vehicles could play an important role in uptake of the safety program.

Stakeholders needed to consider a variety of issues at the time the initial EVSC/ISA project was developed. While a review of available research confirmed that speeds were a contributing factor to severity of injuries sustained in motor vehicle accidents, a practical and safe way to limit vehicle speeds was not as clear. The researchers were required to develop not only a system for limiting vehicle speeds but also a plan for implementation of such a system. Furthermore, the researchers needed to determine the optimum system for implementation, driver compliance, cost-benefit of system and application to different road types and road users. Politicians, vital for the support and enactment of such a system, are sensitive to public opinion in this area so driver acceptance and public support is a great issue for the system developers.

Indeed, at the politician level, the senior level has been very nervous about the research and does not have plans for implementation just doing research. Also, the benefits of implementation of ISA will be most obvious about 15 years after implementation, and this time frame does not help to reduce political concerns about public opinion. The political position may change as implementation of the system is gaining momentum in Europe. In particular, Sweden is attempting to have fitment of an ISA system mandatory in all new cars from 2010 onward. Furthermore, the researchers found that the public does support some kind of speed control provided concerns about driver control may be allayed.

In the past, car companies had been hostile to EVSC/ISA fitment; however, several of the major European automobile manufacturers are showing more acceptance of the ISA system. Indeed, in France, Renault and Peugeot are participating in an ISA study, and the technology branch of Volvo has indicated its support for ISA publicly as well. Daimler-Chrylser has also shown some interest in ISA technology. The most noticeable "hold-outs" have been German automobile manufacturers.

There is evidence of public support for some kind of speed limiting system; however, there is also concern for cost and driver control. Cost concern will become less and less with mass production, especially since the necessary technology (i.e. GPS, navigation systems, electronic engine control) will be in cars already for purposes other than ISA.

The first phase of the EVSC/ISA project was exploratory and had project goals and objectives that reflected this exploratory nature. The second phase of EVSC/ISA that will continue to 2005 builds on the findings of the first phase and proceeds with greater field testing of the developed EVSC/ISA models. There is a need for the UK to continue to collaborate with EVSC/ISA trials that are ongoing in EU countries as well as to develop a program of informed public debate, cooperation of manufacturers and national policy that will enable EVSC/ISA to be developed and implemented sooner than the target year 2020.

The big issues for participating countries are to develop digital road maps that are accurate and then to make a decision about how the speed limits will be delivered to the system. An essential requirement of the system is that speed limits be updated frequently and automatically. Another issue for EU-wide implementation is development of standards. While the degree of control of the system may be determined at a national level, all of the EU countries must participate in developing standards for implementation such as fitment, system requirements, manufacturer requirements and other practicalities.

21.2.2 Collaborators

The DETR/DfT has had an extensive role in the project by providing interest in and funding for the research. There has been extensive collaboration between researchers across Europe, and twice each year these researchers come together to discuss their ISA research findings and ideas. There is also collaboration at the authority level of the EU. Ministers have a high-level group on speed management who also meet to discuss and exchange information. Other collaborators include PACTS as a vehicle to the members of parliament and other safety lobby groups. In future, the researchers expect that safety organizations will have a large role in helping others to learn about and understand ISA.

21.2.3 Resources to Implement Prevention Strategies

The UK EVSC/ISA researchers have always been able to obtain funding for the different phases of research into the safety initiative. Originally, the project was funded through a grant from the Engineering and Physical Sciences Research Council. The second phase (the EU collaborative project) of research was funded by the EU. Since 1996, the project has been funded by the DETR. ITS has always provided the physical resources necessary to carry out a program of research, while the funding agencies have provided the financial support for the research and technology development.

21.2.4 Inputs to the Prevention Model(s)

The system architecture has settled on a GPS-based infrastructure. The project research has shown that, for safety reasons, a driver-select type system is the system of choice for implementation rather than a mandatory, driver override system until a significant level of vehicles in the UK is equipped with an EVSC/ISA system. The researchers also note that technology has moved on to such an extent that it is easier to modify a car now than it was even 4 or 5 years ago.

This initiative followed a logical progression of development. The initial research started on a small scale through literature review, survey and simulations in the lab and has progressed to in-vehicle road trials. The data from these investigations provide input for cost-benefit analysis of the EVSC/ISA system.

Indeed, benefit analysis has been a part of the EVSC/ISA project from the outset. Several aspects of the EVSC/ISA have been analyzed:

- Predicted accident savings
- Expected travel time increase
- Fuel consumption savings
- Cost-benefit analysis of the entire system
- Public acceptance

This benefit analysis has enabled researchers to work from predictions to provide a solid case for various levels of ISA control and levels of system responsiveness to changing road conditions.

While there are many EVSC/ISA trials currently in place in the EU (France, Belgium, Sweden and The Netherlands), none of these projects have had a large influence on development of the UK project. The researchers do feel that it was researchers in Sweden who brought attention to the possibility of EVSC/ISA systems for road safety, but since then the development of the different projects has been parallel and complementary.

21.3　Implementation

EVSC/ISA is still at the pilot stage although the ITS researchers have developed a plan for implementation of the system in the UK. The implementation plan spans 19 years and is outlined in Table 21.1.

The course to full implementation necessarily spans more than a decade due to the complexities of the proposed system, legal implications, need for international cooperation and requirement of political will.

21.3.1　Effective Practices

The researchers were interested in determining the maximum reduction in accidents and the resulting maximum benefit-to-cost ratio. To that end, the researchers considered three different levels of intervention of the system as well as responsiveness of the system. The results showed that regardless of level of intervention, the greatest benefit was seen in a dynamic system that would have the capability of responding to changing road and weather conditions. For this

reason, the most effective system to implement would be a dynamic ISA system and would prevent the most injuries from occurring.

Encouragement to adopt this system is found in the impressive benefit-to-cost ratios and reductions of injury predicted from the model. The interest in the system is growing at the national level in several EU countries and is also being addressed at the EU level. This growing political will may produce a stepped-up implementation plan. For example, Sweden is already interested in seeing mandatory fitment of vehicles by 2010, 3 years earlier than the projected date of the UK researchers (O. Carsten, personal communication Nov. 2002).

Implementation across all of the EU countries will certainly have complexities related to national difference. There are regions where drivers are more likely to engage in negative driving behavior, and resistance to ISA will likely be great. This resistance, however, can be overcome, and planning and negotiations between the countries should enable an implementation plan that is suitable for each member country. At the EU level, it is necessary for the countries to agree upon fitment and other practicalities of the system. Each country, however, may have the option of how to implement the system. For example, some countries may choose to implement voluntary use of the system, while others may implement mandatory use of the system. Cooperation among the countries, however, will see that all cars will be able to utilize the system should the driver want to use it or be required to use it.

A full implementation of the strategy will require political support and leadership. Public support and adoption of the system is also key. The system is viewed by researchers as similar to seatbelt implementation: a measure that has great potential for reduction of injury but will require time, public trust and enactment of laws in order to realize this potential.

The system raises three main concerns in some groups: (1) loss of driver control and subsequent increase in driver risk, (2) loss of personal freedom to control one's vehicle and (3) increased cost to the consumer. Through further testing and fitment of different types of vehicles

Table 21.1 Path to full implementation of ISA

Year	Step
2000–2005	Further research including larger scale trials
2005	Decision to move forward toward full implementation
2005–2010	Preparation and enactment of standards
2010–2013	Preparations for production on new vehicles
2013	Mandatory fitment on new vehicles
2013–2019	Voluntary usage
2019	Requirement for mandatory usage

Note. This table outlines the implementation plan across 19 years as developed by ITS researchers (Carsten & Tate, 2000)

(e.g. motorcycles), the ITS researchers believe that they will be able to further demonstrate that drivers will not be endangered by the system due to loss of control. Furthermore, technology developments have enabled the system to be implemented in a cost-effective manner. Issues of personal freedom will likely have to be considered at a legislative level such that undue loss of freedom or privacy do not result through implementation of this safety measure that will force compliance with posted speed limits.

Ongoing development of the system will require that developers keep abreast of technologies as they improve. The Motor Industry Research Association (MIRA) and ITS have an interest in these issues and will consider technological developments on an ongoing basis. The key concern of the researchers is that the system under development not be frozen to the current technology.

21.3.2 Actors in Decision Making and Planning

Researchers funded by governments play a key advisory role in the planning and data support for implementation of ISA. Eventually, it will be governments and car industries that will have to negotiate and agree on standards for vehicle fitment. Car fitment could be a cooperative endeavor between manufacturers and governments or, should the industry show a great deal of opposition to mandatory vehicle fitment, then government directives may be required for compliance with the endeavor. There is some political support for ISA in the UK, for example from the House of Commons select committee on transport; also, there will be support and lobbying by the safety community for the implementation of ISA.

21.3.3 Ongoing Evaluation of the Prevention Strategy

Over the next couple of years, researchers will conduct more in-vehicle trials. These trials will provide opportunity to look for safety benefits,

examine driver behavior while using the system and evaluate and problems that could occur as a result of using the system. These trials will enable the researchers to confirm or refute the impressive safety benefits predicted from simulator trials.

Each EVSC/ISA project has involved evaluation, and each subsequent project builds on the findings and lessons learned from the previous project. In this way, an iterative approach to development of ISA has been carried out and continues to be an integral part of the project. Also, the researchers continue to monitor the related technologies and other research. It was this vigilance that enabled the ITS researchers to move from a hardware-intense beacon system for ISA to the GPS system now proposed.

21.4 Outcome

21.4.1 Evaluation

The EVSC/ISA project focused on evaluation as a key factor in planning implementation. For this reason, a number of evaluations were conducted before any implementation of the actual program. The evaluations spanned all three phases of the project and are outlined in Table 21.2.

While the EVSC/ISA intervention is large scale and requires careful planning, the evaluation process of phase one is relevant for any planned intervention. A thorough review of speed-related accident literature enabled the project team to understand the effect of different levels of speed reduction in a variety of road conditions on both vehicle occupants and other road users. Thus, the team established not only the link between speed and accident injury rates but also the degree of average speed reduction that would bring about a reduction in accident and injury rates. Furthermore, the review enabled the team to establish values for estimation of benefit of the proposed intervention.

The survey, focus group and analysis of technical approaches to implementation employed in phase one helped the team to anticipate a variety of issues that may arise from implementation

Table 21.2 Evaluations and key findings for Phase One (February–October 1997) of EVSC/ISA project

Evaluation	Key findings
Review and meta-analysis of existing vehicle speed accident literature	Reduction of mean speed necessary to reduce accident rates 10K speed reduction on urban roads has significant reduction in fatalities to vulnerable road users
Review of studies of speed limited vehicles	Conventional speed limiting measures do not prevent large proportion of drivers from speeding Driver compensatory behavior could reduce safety benefit of speed limiters Control method must be acceptable to driver and have no increase in mental load
Review of existing programs Nationally and in EU	Other countries are working toward implementation of similar systems
Analysis of technical approaches to implementation	Potential hazards at every level of intervention considered Safety objectives set as basis for validation of program
Household survey of speed, speed limiting applications and costs	Some level of speed control welcome Maintenance of vehicle control important to drivers
Focus group of EVSC/ISA concept	General resistance to concept due to concern for adaptability to changing road conditions Speed control welcomed
Cost/benefit analysis	Benefit may be greater than any other intervention to date Benefit will vary with level of operation (advisory or mandatory)

Note. This table is created by summarizing findings from Carsten and Fowkes (1998)

of the EVSC/ISA system. The ITS Safety Researchers conceptualized the system in terms of the following:

- Means of implementation
- Level of intervention
- Potential hazards at every level of intervention
- Evaluation with safety objectives as basis of validation of EVSC and necessary features

This analysis forms an iterative evaluation of the system in which a feedback loop informs further development and planning of the system.

Conception of the model was further informed through survey and focus groups where drivers were able to express concerns and beliefs about speed limiters. While speed control was a welcome concept, the data showed drivers were concerned about potential decrease in driver safety if the system was not able to adapt or allow the driver to control for changing road conditions.

Finally, the encouraging results of the cost-benefit analysis enable the project team to move confidently to the next phase of planning and implementation. Phase two of the project

incorporated simulations and field tests into the evaluation process. Table 21.3 outlines the evaluations and key findings for the second phase of the EVSC/ISA project.

The second phase builds on the findings of the initial research into EVSC and moves forward from modeling and review to driver simulations. In these simulator trials, data collection about driver response to the system variants could be collected, and the researchers were able to look for negative compensatory driver behavior that could reduce the overall safety benefit of the system. Indeed, drivers unable to overtake vehicles were inclined to follow more closely, increasing their risk of collision. Other observations enabled through simulator trials include driver attitude toward the system after exposure, and the response to the system was positive.

Simulations enable the research team to plan for implement in-vehicle trials. One significant finding for the in-vehicle trial was that no negative compensatory behavior such as following too closely was observed in driver participants. Further findings from the in-vehicle trials show potential for increased safety benefit to drivers through awareness of potential hazards and decreased number of critical incidents.

Table 21.3 Evaluations and key findings for Phase Two (January 1998–May 1999) of EVSC/ISA project

Evaluation	Key findings
Simulator trials (mandatory, driver select and variable)	Drivers unable to overtake followed more closely and decreased minimum time to collision gap Little change in journey time due to EVSC/ISA Drivers show improved attitude toward EVSC/ISA after trial especially in driver select group
Test vehicle (mandatory and driver select)	Slow drivers did not speed up Negative compensatory behaviors not evident Decreased number of conflicts or critical incidents Initial increase in workload that later decreased with familiarization Concern about overtaking or accelerating out of danger Some frustration with system due to other drivers following too closely (i.e. Unable to keep up with traffic flow) Drivers with mandatory system report increased awareness of potential hazards
Relevant estimates (time, fuel, emissions)	Slightly longer driving time Reduced fuel consumption Decrease in emissions on motorways Slight increase in emissions in rural networks
Evaluation of potential implementation issues and plan	Motorcycles present implementation difficulty Required components will be in average passenger car by 2010 for purposes other than EVSC/ISA
Evaluation of implementation approaches (system variants)	GPS with in-vehicle display preferred Need to consider further maximization of cost-benefit ratio

Note. Summarized from Carsten and Fowkes (2000a)

Table 21.4 Predicted accident reduction by dimension of EVSC/ISA system

How intervening	Fixed speed limit (%)	Variable speed limit (%)	Dynamic speed limit (%)
Advisory	10	10	13
Driver select	10	11	18
Mandatory	20	22	36

Note. Carsten and Fowkes (2000b)

Further evaluation in this phase include estimates of journey time, fuel consumption and emissions with the system variants, evaluation of implementation issues, development of a plan of implementation and evaluation of effectiveness of system variants. These predictions and plans provide a solid foundation for the next phase of EVSC/ISA research.

The third phase of the project builds on the findings of the first two phases. Costs and benefits of the project were reviewed in light of the project findings, legal and production issues were considered and a strategy for implementation was constructed.

The proposed system could have three levels of intervention (shown in Table 21.4) and could have speed limit information provided in three different ways. To review, a fixed system would be based on posted limits, a variable system would also include speed changes for some geographic features and the third system would have the additional feature of responding to current road conditions. The most significant reduction is expected from a mandatory system that updates speed limit information dynamically.

In every case, the dynamic system produces the greatest benefit in terms of accident reduction. This difference is largely due to the ability of a dynamic system to adapt speed not only according to posted limits but also to darkness, adverse geometry, adverse weather and adverse road surface. Mandatory systems also produce the greatest safety benefit; however, for driver safety, a mandatory system is not reasonable until a critical mass of road vehicles are equipped with the EVSC/ISA system.

The EVSC/ISA system will realize the majority of its benefits when penetration of the system is 60% of vehicles. At this point, non-equipped vehicles would be sufficiently constrained by equipped vehicles. For this reason, any benefit beyond this level of penetration will be less significant.

The researchers propose a plan of implementation in the UK that would see voluntary usage of the system begin in 2013 with mandatory usage implemented by 2020 based on a decision to implement the system in 2005. This implementation plan allows time for further research (large-scale trials), development of standards (preferably written at the EU level), development of digital maps, preparation for vehicle fitment of new vehicles and mandatory fitment of new vehicles with the EVSC/ISA system (Carsten & Tate, 2000).

The researchers were diligent in hypothesizing both the potential negative and positive effects of the system. Since safety is of paramount importance to the researchers, they considered how the proposed system might compromise safety and sought to ameliorate these issues. In this way, there were no significant unanticipated positive or negative outcomes of the trials. The data did show that in the on-road trial, there was no significant difference in journey time—a result that was not expected by the research team—however, it is expected that this result would not hold up across all road conditions. The result did cause the researchers to adjust the model for the journey time category with the expectation that for some categories of road, there would be no difference in journey time with use of the system.

Cost–benefit analysis is an important component of any injury prevention program evaluation. The analysis is particularly important for an initiative like ISA since implementation would be nation-wide, require manufacturing changes and possibly legislation. The system must be shown to be of clear benefit without undue costs in order for the system to gain public and political support for implementation. The following tables (Tables 21.5 and 21.6) outline the costs and benefits associated with implementation of an EVSC/ISA system.

The higher cost associated with the mandatory rather than advisory system relates to the additional vehicle fitments related to controlling the maximum speed via electronic engine control.

Table 21.5 Discounted costs of an advisory EVSC system 1998 (in million pounds)

Cost item	Fixed	Variable	Dynamic
Infrastructure (Digital maps and sensors)	4.87	7.30	26.17
Maintenance (Digital maps and sensors)	13.62	13.62	27.44
In-vehicle equipment (new vehicles)	3694.15	3694.15	3694.15
Cost of annual map updates	116.71	116.71	116.71
Total	3829.35	3831.78	3864.47

Note. Carsten and Fowkes (2000a, 2000b)

Table 21.6 Discounted costs of a mandatory EVSC system 1998 (in million pounds)

Cost item	Fixed	Variable	Dynamic
Infrastructure (Digital maps and sensors)	4.87	7.30	26.17
Maintenance (Digital maps and sensors)	13.62	13.62	27.44
In-vehicle equipment (new vehicles)	5231.02	5231.02	5231.02
Cost of annual map updates	116.71	116.71	116.71
Total	5366.22	5368.65	5401.34

Note. Carsten and Fowkes (2000a, 2000b)

Table 21.7 Discounted benefits of EVSC 1998: fuel savings (in million pounds)

	Low GDP fuel savings	High GDP fuel savings
Advisory system	1460	1625
Driver select system	1826	2032
Mandatory system	3651	4064

Note. Carsten and Fowkes (2000a, 2000b)

The benefits of the systems as shown in Tables 21.7 and 21.8, however, show an increased value in benefit with a mandatory system over an advisory system.

Table 21.9 illustrates that a large part of the benefits relates to savings from accident reduction although fuel savings are also a significant factor particularly as environmental concerns over burning of fossil fuels continues to rise. The overall cost-benefit ratios based on these projected figures are shown in Table 21.9.

Table 21.8 Discounted benefits of EVSC 1998: accidents (in million pounds)

	Fixed: low GDP savings on accidents	Fixed: high GDP savings on accidents	Variable: low GDP savings on accidents	Variable: high GDP savings on accidents	Dynamic: low GDP savings on accidents	Dynamic: high GDP savings on accidents
Advisory system	17,816	24,673	18,772	25,997	25,534	35,361
Driver select system	17,987	24,909	19,626	27,179	31,046	42,994
Mandatory system	35,973	49,818	39,252	54,358	62,092	85,989

Note. Carsten and Fowkes (2000a, 2000b)

Table 21.9 Benefit-cost ratios (assuming in-vehicle capability for mandatory system)

	Low GDP growth: fixed	Low GDP growth: variable	Low GDP growth: dynamic	High GDP growth: fixed	High GDP growth: variable	High GDP growth: dynamic
Advisory system	3.6	3.8	5.0	4.9	5.1	6.8
Driver select system	3.7	4.0	6.1	5.0	5.4	8.3
Mandatory system	7.4	8.0	12.2	10.0	10.9	16.7

Note. Carsten and Fowkes (2000a, 2000b)

The potential for accident injury and fatality reduction with the EVSC/ISA system is significant and worth pursuing. Indeed, as is illustrated in Table 21.9, the calculated benefit ratio for all versions of a mandatory system is 7 or more with mandatory dynamic systems having much higher ratios than the other variants. Furthermore, the system would allow for rapid implementation of speed limit changes such as traffic calming measures without the usual road reconstruction requirements.

Indeed, the target system suggested by the ITS Safety researchers is a dynamic mandatory ISA system. Although the dynamic system has a cost 2.9 times more than a fixed system, the projected benefits from injury prevention seem to justify the additional cost. Furthermore, it is expected that broadcast technology improvements already becoming available will enable reliable broadcasting of dynamic speed messages to vehicles (Carsten & Tate, 2000). Also, with the full implementation date for the proposed system not until 2019, it is reasonable to assume technology advancements and prudent not to harness decision making to current technologies only.

21.4.2 Current ISA Project Evaluation

The current ISA project will have masses of data from the in-vehicle trials such as position, speed and system usage. Additionally, the researchers will conduct interviews with and surveys of participants in order to gain feedback about the system as well as monitor for changes in attitude/system acceptance after exposure to the system.

The short-term outcome of the current project is the wealth of data that will be collected, while the long-term outcome is expected to be increasingly accurate prediction of overall safety changes if everyone had the technology. These measures will be crucial in moving the system forward from trial usage to implementation.

21.4.3 Dissemination of Information

The researchers utilize a number of means to disseminate project findings to stakeholders. Foremost is the preparation of a significant number of report deliverables and final reports to the funding agency. The researchers also utilize standard methods for dissemination such as publications and conference presentations. In addition to these methods, the researchers consult with interested groups and government, as well as with other researchers in the field. Finally, ITS maintains a website (http://www.its.leeds.ac.uk/) with information about the projects, and copies of project deliverables are made available to the public through this site.

As has been noted earlier, there have been a number of ISA projects and trials throughout

Europe. The largest trial is currently in place in Sweden, while other trials and projects are running in the Netherlands and France.

21.5 Conclusion

The implementation of External Vehicle Speed Controls (EVSC)/Intelligent Speed Adaptations (ISA) to control traffic flow and improve road safety yields predictions that utilizing it is eight times more effective at preventing injury and fatality from vehicle accidents in the UK than the implementation of compulsory front occupant seatbelt wearing, the most effective road safety measure in the UK to date (Carsten & Fowkes, 2000b). The technology allows for the speed of cars and other motorized vehicles to be presented road-side while driving for the benefit of the driver. EVSC/ISA works by combining Global Positioning Satellite (GPS) technology with digital road maps complete with posted speed limits to prevent vehicles equipped with EVSC/ISA devices to be driven faster than posted limits (Carsten & Fowkes, 2000b). Being distracted or zoning out regarding one's speed while driving is common, and therefore having visual reminders of staying within the speed limits has proven to be helpful (O. Carsten, personal communication, November 13, 2002). When these reminders are already part of the vehicle, the effectiveness of road safety is increased further.

Acknowledgments The author would like to express sincere appreciation to the key informant for this case study: Oliver Carsten of the Institute for Transport Studies, University of Leeds in Leeds, West Yorkshire, England—whose consultation made this project possible.

BRIO Model: External Vehicle Speed Controls/Intelligent Speed Adaptation

Group Served: All individuals.

Goal: To prevent road related injury by providing visual reminders of important aspects of the road.

Background	Resources	Implementation	Outcome
In the UK, 40–50% of all head injuries are caused by road traffic accidents and that road traffic accidents are most commonly associated with severe injuries Core prevention strategy of EVSC/ISA is to reduce the top speed of vehicles Objectives are to reduce the number of injuries and deaths due to speeding, to facilitate compliance with speed limits and to inform policy decisions about implementation of EVSC/ISA or within the UK	Since 1996, the project has been funded by the DETR GPS-based infrastructure	Researchers determined the maximum reduction in accidents and the resulting maximum benefit to cost ratio Currently, researchers funded by governments play a key advisory role in the planning and data support for implementation of ISA	Focus on evaluation as a key factor in planning implementation. Therefore, a number of evaluations were conducted before any implementation of the actual program Team established not only the link between speed and accident injury rates but also the degree of average speed reduction that would bring about a reduction in accident and injury rates In-vehicle trials show potential for increased safety benefit to drivers through awareness of potential hazards and decreased number of critical incidents

Life Space Model: External Vehicle Speed Controls

Sociocultural: civilization/community	Interpersonal: primary and secondary relationships	Physical environments: where we live	Internal states: biochemical/genetic and means of coping
Advocacy at international level (EU) to implement safety initiative	Changes how drivers interact with each other in terms of following, over-taking and aggression	Sets traffic speed to posted limits (removes current need to "keep up with traffic" that moves faster than posted limits)	Removes responsibility from driver for maintenance of posted speed limits

References

Carsten, O., & Fowkes, M. (1998). *External vehicle speed control, phase I: Executive summary.* Leeds, UK: Institute for Transport Studies, University of Leeds.

Carsten, O., & Fowkes, M. (2000a). *External vehicle speed control, phase II: Executive summary.* Leeds, UK: Institute for Transport Studies, University of Leeds.

Carsten, O., & Fowkes, M. (2000b). *External vehicle speed control: Executive summary of project results.* Leeds, UK: Institute for Transport Studies, University of Leeds.

Carsten, O., & Tate, F. (2000). *Final report: Integration.* Leeds, UK: Institute for Transport Studies, University of Leeds.

Department for Transport, Local Government and the Regions. (2001). *Transport statistics bulletin: Road casualties in Great Britain, main results: 2001 (Provisional).* London, UK: Crown.

Haddon, W. (1980). Advances in the epidemiology of injuries as a basis for public policy. *Public Health Reports, 95*(5), 411–421.

Headway the Brain Injury Association. (2002). *Statistics and common causes.* Retrieved November 2002, from http://www.headway.org.uk/default.asp?step=4&pid=38

Institute for Transport Studies. (2002). *Safety studies.* Retrieved November 2002, from http://www.its.leeds.ac.uk/research/index.html

National Spinal Cord Injury Statistical Center. (2001). *Spinal cord injury facts and figures at a glance: May 2001.* Birmingham: University of Alabama.

Parliamentary Advisory Council for Traffic Safety. (2002). *Fifteen key facts about road safety.* Retrieved November, 2002, from http://www.pacts.org.uk

COMPASS Program

22

David Gentili

Ontario's COMPASS program focuses on critical areas concerning traffic congestion that threaten safety on the road. COMPASS is an empirically proven method of reducing accidents on freeways cited as primary locations for transportation-related injury, in and around major urban areas, such as Toronto, Canada (Ontario Road Safety Annual Report [ORSAR], 2001).

22.1 Background

The portion of Highway 401 (Ontario) that traverses the northern section of the Municipality of Metropolitan Toronto was originally conceived and designed as a bypass providing an east/west route for through traffic without entering the urban area. However, the unprecedented growth of the Greater Toronto Area (GTA) starting in the 1950s saw increases in traffic volumes that increasingly exceeded the design capacity. By 1958—before construction of Highway 401 was even completed—it became apparent that a major expansion had become necessary. What followed was a period of expensive expansion projects that aimed to alleviate the increasingly apparent deterioration of conditions of travel. The result of these projects is the existing 12-line

express/collector configuration of the highway (completed by 1972).

Although costly, these expansions improved accessibility to Highway 401 and stimulated both residential and industrial development along the corridor. By the late 1970s, Highway 401 no longer served as a bypass but as a major urban freeway for commuting traffic within the GTA. Second to only the Santa Monica Freeway in Los Angeles, California, Highway 401 has been one of the busiest highways in North America since this time—with an average daily traffic volume exceeding 320,000 vehicles per day as of 1994 (ORSAR, 2001).

However, over the past 25 years the traffic volumes on Highway 401 have still been steadily increasing by an estimated annual rate of 4.7% (Korpal, Rayman, & Masters, 1994). This increasing travel demand within a fixed capacity system has again begun to result in an overall deterioration of the level of service and, subsequently, in increasing congestion and safety levels: over the last 15 years the annual number of motor-vehicle accidents on Highway 401 grew faster than traffic volumes (Korpal et al., 1994).

22.1.1 History and Development: COMPASS

With the potential for congestion relief from new or expanded roadway facilities decreasing, the rationale for the Highway 401 COMPASS

D. Gentili (✉)
Toronto, ON, Canada

© Springer Nature Switzerland AG 2020
R. Volpe (ed.), *Casebook of Traumatic Injury Prevention*,
https://doi.org/10.1007/978-3-030-27419-1_22

Freeway Traffic Management System (FTMS) was established by the mid 1970s (Public Works and Government Services Canada [PWGSC], 1999).

Based on successful FTMS programs in Los Angeles and Detroit, COMPASS was initially designed to facilitate the management of both recurring and non-recurring congestion. Recurring congestion occurs when demand exceeds available capacity, most often during the morning and afternoon periods of peak traffic flow. Non-recurring congestion results from temporary capacity reductions due to incidents such as accidents or stalled vehicles. These two forms of congestion are not mutually exclusive; in fact, incidents are more frequent—and more severe—during periods of recurring congestion (Korpal et al., 1994).

Initially a research project funded by the Government of Ontario during the mid-1970s that targeted the Queen Elizabeth Way (QEW) freeway around Mississauga, COMPASS was designed to smooth the flow of traffic between Erin Mills Parkway and Hurontario Street, where a large number of vehicles entering the freeway during morning rush hours created stop-and-go driving conditions (Korpal et al., 1994). However, by the 1980s the project had been successfully sold to provincial decision makers as a cost-effective solution to the increasingly salient congestion problem in Southern Ontario (i.e., in and around urban regions like the GTA).

COMPASS has been expanded to include three more target areas:

- Burlington (1986) on the Burlington Bay James N. Allan Skyway
- Toronto (1991) through the 16 km of Highway 401 passing through the center of Toronto between Martin Grove Road and Yonge Street
- Ottawa (1997) through 21 km of Highway 417 from Highway 416 in the west to Regional Road 174 in the east.

This case study focuses on the Toronto COMPASS System (which now includes the initial component on the QEW). This is primarily for three reasons: it is undoubtedly the most comprehensive and far-reaching program, it has the most rigorous empirical support for its effectiveness, and it takes road safety into greater consideration than any of the other variants (P.H. Masters, personal communication, 2004; Korpal et al., 1994).

On January 30, 1991, 13 Changeable Message Signs (CMSs) on Highway 401 between Yonge Street and Martingrove Road went into operation, marking the first day of full system operation of the Toronto COMPASS System. This marked the culmination of more than 13 years of FTMS efforts in Ontario. Since then, the system has been continuously monitored, enhanced, and expanded through extensive studies, design efforts, and capital investments in infrastructure. The Toronto COMPASS has resulted in an improvement of not only mobility, but traffic safety along this key transportation corridor (Korpal et al., 1994).

22.1.2 Project Aims

The Highway 401 Corridor Traffic Systems Management Study (1980, through Korpal et al., 1994) recommended a FTMS with electronic vehicle detectors in the pavement, closed circuit television, and CMS as major system elements of a comprehensive program for Highway 401 in and around Toronto. The system philosophy included an emphasis on:

1. Intensive information control
2. Improving safety and incident management
3. Increasing cooperation between agencies responsible for traffic management on Highway 401
4. Improving collection, quality, and quantity of traffic data

Following a series of approvals, the recommendations of the study were accepted, and subsequent design and implementation stages of the Highway 401 FTMS followed immediately thereafter. The Preliminary Design Report (1986, through Korpal et al., 1994) of an FTMS initially proposed along Highway 401 between Renforth Drive and Neilson Road established the following specific project aims:

1. A reduction of vehicular delay and accident risk due to non-recurring congestion through rapid detection of, response to, and removal of incidents on the freeway and through efficient management of traffic during incidents.
2. A reduction of vehicular delay due to recurrent congestion through efficient management of traffic using the freeway.
3. An improvement of safety levels for motorists using the freeway by advising motorists of traffic and roadway conditions.
4. A reduction in energy consumption by achieving improved traffic conditions with vehicular delay.

In order to achieve the above objectives, the Highway 401 FTMS was designed to incorporate a number of control strategies, initially including incident management, inter-agency coordination, management of construction and maintenance activities, traffic information dissemination to the public, and data collection components. However, within 2 years of initial system operation, management of recurring congestion was introduced—the objective being to achieve a new goal of balance between traffic flow of the express and collector lanes.

With the implementation of these strategies, the Toronto FTMS (today called COMPASS) now effectively targets all areas outlined in the Preliminary Design Report and incorporates all system elements of the 1980 Highway 401 Corridor Traffic Systems Management Study (through Korpal et al., 1994). Additionally, today there are two cited primary program aims—congestion reduction and accident reduction (P.H. Masters, personal communication, 2004).

22.2 Resources

22.2.1 Stakeholders and Collaborators

The primary stakeholder in the program has been the Ministry of Transportation of the Government of Ontario (MTO). Additionally, commuters and the media at large are considered stakeholders because of their reliance on the COMPASS program for traffic updates (P.H. Masters, personal communication, 2004).

The primary collaborators, understood as those who play a key role in implementation of the program, consist of the MTO, the media, the Municipality of Toronto, the Municipality of Mississauga, various universities (like the Engineering Faculty of the University of Toronto), and various Emergency Services (such as Paramedic, Firefighting, and Law Enforcement Agencies).

The COMPASS System has existed largely within the legislative framework. The Highway Traffic Act of the 1970s reaffirmed governmental jurisdictions and responsibilities for road safety, alleviating earlier points of friction between the FTMS programs of the municipalities and those of the provinces (such as an ambiguity over whether ramp monitoring was a provincial or municipal responsibility). As mentioned, in the case of the Toronto COMPASS, the Municipality of Toronto is considered a collaborator with the MTO.

Although the COMPASS System philosophy has consisted of a broad approach to the problem of congestion, the disciplines of the engineering sciences have undoubtedly played the largest role in the implementation of the program. That being said, COMPASS has relied heavily on an informational component since the very first stages of the project to achieve its goals. As the program has taken on accident reduction as not simply a positive side effect, but as a primary aim, the health sciences are beginning to play an additional role. COMPASS targets the individual (electronically giving information to drivers on automated highway signs) and the community at large (supplying information to media). Additionally, it both prevents accidents from occurring and minimizes the impact and severity of incidents after the fact (by both decreasing the time of response of Emergency Medical Services and altering flow patterns such that secondary accidents are decreased).

The Minister of Transportation of the Ontario Government has been the traditional supporter of the COMPASS System—this is cited as true regardless of the changes of government over the past decade (P.H. Masters, personal communication, 2004). Now, the MTO plays less of a decision-making role than in the initial stages; however, its support of the program has not decreased (P.H. Masters, personal communication, 2004).

Professionals (in this case, mostly engineers) and small community contacts have additionally been cited as important supporters of the program. Yet, what started as close knit relationships with personal contacts has grown into a network of national and international relationships between universities, governments, communities, and consultants (Intelligent Traffic System Strategic Plan: Halton Region [ITSSP:HR], 1999). Additionally, many of those who work on the program now were those who played an important role in the implementation of COMPASS at its earliest stages. This has resulted in a group of individuals with an unprecedented amount of expertise in FTMS programs—making them an experienced and marketable population (P.H. Masters, personal communication, 2004). Over five consulting companies make use of this population of engineers whose services are in demand all over the world (ITSSP:HR, 1999).

The implementation of the previously defined strategies has been accomplished by a series of high-technology components and techniques with close inter-agency coordination procedures for on-road service. It is the effective integration of these elements that contributes to the successful outcomes (discussed in later sections). These components include the:

- Traffic Operations Centre:
  - The central facility to which all information from the COMPASS system is transmitted and from which all traffic management strategies are directed. It is located at the MTO complex in Downsview and contains the traffic operations room, the central data processing and communications equipment, and other central equipment for the FTMS.
- Field Equipment:
  - Consisting of inductive loop vehicle detectors, 170 local traffic controllers who

monitor traffic conditions and gather traffic data, closed circuit TV cameras to provide full visual coverage of Highway 401 for traffic management activities, and CMSs to provide advisory driver information.
- Communications System:
  - Provides the linkage between the traffic operations center, the FTMS field equipment, and the interface with other agencies.
- Interface with Incident Management Agencies:
  - Ensures a high degree of coordination of activities with the OPP, Emergency Patrol, fire departments, towing community, and others during incident management.
- Interface with Public Information:
  - Interfaces with the news media and the MTO, Ontario Provincial Police (OPP), and metropolitan Toronto public information offices for the dissemination of up-to-date traffic information.

The costs of the COMPASS program have been steadily decreasing over the past decade, attributed to the expertise of those individuals involved in the program and a steady increase in the effectiveness of technology coupled with just as steady a decrease in costs associated with that technology. Initially, costs of the program were approximately $1 million for each kilometer of operation. The cost–benefit ratio has now changed such that costs are now approximately $500,000 for each kilometer of operation (P.H. Masters, personal communication, 2004).

As will be discussed in Sect. 22.3, due to the results of the program and the good relationship with the MTO (which burdens the costs associated with the program), costs for continual maintenance are always available. However, today there are some $100 to $200 millions of highlighted needs; these include needs at expanding and updating the system and continued research on better and cheaper ways of implementation (P.H. Masters, personal communication, 2004). However, it has been stressed by program officials that although these are important needs, the system as it exists today works (P.H. Masters, personal communication, 2004). The primary reason for this lack of money at expansion is cited to be the result of "significant competition" faced by those trying to have their funding increased by the MTO (P.H. Masters, personal communication, 2004).

22.3 Implementation

The traditional decision makers of the COMPASS program have been the internal staff of the COMPASS program and the MTO. The successful interaction between these groups and consultants has been highlighted as a key factor in the success of the program (P.H. Masters, personal communication, 2004).

However, the MTO has had a decreasing role in decision making. According to contacts, this is the result of a general acceptance in the effectiveness of the program among government officials and the capabilities of the senior administrators of COMPASS (P.H. Masters, personal communication, 2004). Decisions are made primarily on a cost–benefit ratio—this is because the technology behind the program allows decision makers to accurately predict the benefit of expansion of the program in any given area, e.g., the volume decrease for implementation in a given kilometer (Hellinga, Baker, Van, Aultman-Hall, & Masters, 1999; Korpal et al., 1994).

Historically, technical risk and public support were additional important factors in implementation decision making. Early on in the design process, the implementation of the key strategies (outlined in Sect. 22.1) occurred in progressive stages dependent on relative weightings of all of the above three factors. However, as the program methodology has become increasingly entrenched and trusted, the latter two no longer play a significant role (P.H. Masters, personal communication, 2004).

Although the senior management of COMPASS has gained a considerable amount of independence in deciding when and where expansions are needed, the role of the MTO in expansion cannot be underestimated—politicians still decide on the funding envelope and therefore limit what expansions are plausible (P.H. Masters, personal communication, 2004). This has been primarily the result of the government in viewing the program as a simple highway expansion,

rather than taking into consideration the additional benefits such as the safety component (P.H. Masters, personal communication, 2004). Although funds are always allocated for maintenance of the problem as it exists, governments can significantly differ in the amounts of money allocated for expansions in any given year (P.H. Masters, personal communication, 2004).

The structural relationship of the various program administrators is such that, internally, administrators sometimes come into conflict over money for expansion in their areas (P.H. Masters, personal communication, 2004). However, this being said, accurate cost–benefit predictions and the expertise at smooth coordination between program administrators make this a minor problem (P.H. Masters, personal communication, 2004).

Although both the aims of the project and the major systems elements of COMPASS have not changed, some of the strategies and philosophies have. For example, within engineering, the initial civil and electrical engineering strategies have been replaced by computer programming and design strategies (P.H. Masters, personal communication, 2004). Additionally, a health perspective is playing an increasingly prominent role in the overall program philosophy. However, as will be discussed in Sect. 22.4, health workers currently play a supportive rather than fundamental role in the program—the COMPASS staff is still primarily made up of engineers.

22.3.1 Program Components

Incident Management is one of the key roles identified for the COMPASS system. The primary aspects of incident management are incident detection, verification, and response. Incident detection is the first step of incident management and is accomplished by COMPASS in using both automatic and manual methods. Automated incident detection is provided through vehicle detection stations (consisting of detector loops embedded in the highway pavement and spaced 600–700 m apart) that measure traffic characteristics on an ongoing basis. The COMPASS software monitors the detector data and alerts the operators of unusual conditions. The operators may also detect potential problems by manually monitoring the closed-circuit television monitors providing live video coverage of traffic operations in the Highway 401 corridor.

Once either the system or the operators have detected an incident, the incident verification process follows using the closed-circuit television system. For valid incidents, operators determine if the event warrants a response. If the event does not warrant a response, it is internally logged, and operators return to the monitoring process. When a response is required operators initiate appropriate inter-agency incident coordination response procedures and FTMS system responses as required.

Inter-agency incident coordination response procedures focus on the role of various agencies in responding to an incident. Depending on the nature of the incident several agencies may be involved in this process, including:

- The Ministry's emergency patrol service
- The Ontario Provincial Police
- Private towing trucks
- Ambulance services
- Fire departments
- MTO maintenance staff themselves

Coordination and management of response activities by the various agencies is of primary importance in order to achieve a safe and quick removal of incidents. This is facilitated from the Traffic Operations Centre.

FTMS system response focuses on the dissemination of traffic information. Given the operator-entered information, the system produces a recommended response plan consisting of CMS messages. There are 13 CMSs located in advance of diversion points and connecting roadways. They provide information to motorists, warning them of traffic problems ahead and enabling them to make decisions regarding possible route diversions.

Media messages are produced through the Traffic and Road Information System (TRIS), which is also operated from the Traffic Operations Centre. Both scheduled and non-scheduled

incident information is entered into a database, and reports are automatically faxed to approximately 20 media subscribers on a regular or emergency basis. In some cases, video images are also disseminated to the media. Additionally, TRIS now includes an online component.

Confirmed incidents are monitored by COMPASS operators to detect any changes that may require an upgraded response. When incidents have been cleared, CMS messages are returned to normal, the media is informed, and operators resume the regular monitoring process.

Congestion management was implemented approximately 2 years following initial system operation in an effort to meet the objective of managing recurring congestion. This is accomplished by monitoring traffic flow in both the express and collector lanes. The system software detects differences in operating speeds between the two facilities and then informs the driver of the traffic conditions ahead in each of the parallel roadways. This provides the driver with information on how well traffic ahead is operating and provides him or her with the opportunity of selecting the roadway with the least congestion. This strategy also provides a balancing effect between the two facilities and optimizes the utilization of both roadways.

The congestion management strategy is an automated process with the system software monitoring vehicle detector data and selecting the appropriate CMS messages. No operator intervention is required.

22.3.2 Ongoing Evaluation

As part of the MTO's constant efforts to improve traffic safety and traffic circulation on provincial freeways, an evaluation of the effectiveness of the FTMS on Highway 401 was conducted in 1994 (Korpal et al., 1994). This study, referred to as "Evaluation of the Highway 401 Freeway Traffic Management System," focused on a performance analysis of the system with emphasis on the initial system between Yonge Street and Martingrove Road. The evaluation objectives were:

1. To evaluate the effectiveness of the initial phase of the COMPASS system
2. To identify areas for further system improvements
3. To provide a framework for the ongoing assessment of system performance
4. To compile a database of system performance parameters for future reference and comparison

The effectiveness of the initial phase of COMPASS was evaluated by examining how well the system met its objectives, as set out in the original Preliminary Design Report (PDR). This was achieved through the use of a number of measures of effectiveness which were defined based on the PDR objectives and calculated "before" and "after" COMPASS to develop both a quantitative and qualitative analysis of the impacts of the program.

Since the above objectives were achieved by the implementation of both incident management and congestion management strategies, to evaluate the performance of these traffic management strategies with respect to these objectives, the following measures of effectiveness were selected:

- Incident duration
- Vehicular delay
- Secondary accidents
- Quality of traffic flow
- Driver responses to CMS messages

Reductions in vehicular delay due to non-recurrent congestion result directly from reductions in incident duration. A reduction in the duration of an incident results from a rapid detection, an appropriate and prompt response, and a coordinated removal of the incident. For this reason, incident duration and vehicular delay were selected as the measure of effectiveness for objectives (1) and (4).

Secondary accidents are, by definition, the result of previous primary incidents and should be reduced by the implementation of effective incident management strategies. Reductions in secondary accidents are the combined effect of reduced incident duration and availability of timely motorist information on traffic and roadway conditions through CMSs. A reduction in secondary accident rates would therefore indicate that COMPASS is meeting, at least partly, both objectives (1) and (3). Thus, secondary accident rates were selected as the measure of the effectiveness for those objectives.

With the implementation of congestion management strategies through the use of CMSs, motorists are advised of the congestion ahead and can reduce delays by diverting from express to collector lanes and vice versa. For the purpose of congestion management, Highway 401 has been divided into congestion management zones. The operational speed within each one of these zones was selected as the measure of effectiveness for objective (3).

The provision of information on traffic and roadway conditions to motorists is referred to in objective (3). Through the use of CMSs COMPASS provides incident and congestion messages. A driver behavioral survey was used as the measure of effectiveness to evaluate how useful these messages are and how motorists use the information provided.

22.4 Outcome

The results of Korpal et al. (1994) showed that incidents on Highway 401 are quickly detected and confirmed through the use of traffic detectors and CCTV cameras. Inter-agency coordination allows a prompt and appropriate response. Efficient on-site traffic management procedures allow fast and safe removal of incidents. On average, COMPASS reduces the average duration of incidents, from 86 to 30 min, from occurrence to clearance.

The longer an incident remains on the highway, the longer the delay experienced by vehicles upstream of the incident. By reducing incident durations from 86 to 30 min, COMPASS reduces the average delay per incident by 537 vehicle-hours. Over 300,000 h of vehicle delay are saved each year through faster identification of incidents as a result of the COMPASS system between Yonge Street and Martin Grove Road and through swift responses to the incidents resulting from effective Incident Management Plans. Such a large decrease in vehicular delay can be directly associated with significant savings in travel time, fuel consumption, air pollution, and operating costs of the vehicles for the road users.

Secondary accidents are accidents caused, directly or indirectly, by a previous incident— referred to as primary incident or primary event. The risk of secondary accidents can be reduced by rapidly removing primary incidents from the roadway and by promptly informing motorists upstream from the primary incident of the occurrence of an event ahead. Approximately 200 accidents per year are prevented by displaying incident messages on CMSs when incidents occur.

The congestion management system provides a mechanism by which traffic demand can be effectively balanced between the express and collector lanes during times of congested traffic flow. The system also improves traffic safety by enabling motorists to take the necessary precautions when approaching congested areas. The implementation of congestion management has resulted in improving the quality of peak period traffic flow. In addition to increasing the average speed between 7% and 19%, the severity of congestion has been reduced.

Drivers' responses to CMS messages were evaluated by conducting a survey of 624 drivers. A large majority of drivers (80%) find CMS messages helpful, easy to read and understand. Reductions in both accidents and travel time were the personal benefits most frequently identified by drivers. The survey concluded that the CMS system is an effective moderator of driver behavior.

COMPASS generates real resource savings in accident costs, travel time costs, and vehicle operating costs which amount to over $10 million per year. The investment on the initial portion of COMPASS yields significantly high returns to the overall economy. The rate of return on the investment is 18%; the payback period is 3½ years. The above real resource savings

include 1.8 million liters of fuel saved per year. Other indirect or non-quantifiable benefits are also significant. They include: reduced air pollution (over 400 tons of air pollutants per year), enhanced data collection and analysis capabilities, research and export potential, and future productivity gains.

The potential worldwide market for advanced traffic management systems is valued in excess of $50 billion over the next 10 years. As a result of their work with COMPASS, both manufacturers and consultants in the province of Ontario are already key players in the international market. The export of goods and services amounted to $20 million in 1993 and will likely exceed $60 million in 1994.

Korpal et al. (1994) also highlighted several critical areas where COMPASS needs to be improved. According to them the program needed:

1. Improved Automatic Incident Detection—the existing incident detection algorithms are currently detecting less than 50% of those incidents identified by the System. Improvements to this automatic detection rate must be investigated along with the associated benefits. Such benefits will include more freedom for the operators to concentrate on jobs other than scanning the roadway with the CCTV cameras.
2. Increase CMS Use—more use of the changeable message signs will help to strengthen driver's confidence that the system is working. New areas to be investigated include winter maintenance operations such as snow plowing.
3. Automated Dissemination to Media—the provision of better information to drivers has been shown to reduce accidents. Better systems with more automation are required to provide traffic information to the media. The present system largely is a manual operation with the related delays and errors. The provision of a system to automatically disseminate the congestion monitoring information would be a good preliminary step. Today,

this goal is largely seen to have been achieved with the introduction of a comprehensive Internet component to COMPASS—where information is reliably updated through automatic processes at regular, 10-min intervals (COMPASS, 2001).

4. Communications with Responders—The link between the control center and the emergency services on the road also merits investigation. Better links between these authorities will further improve the clearance times for future incidents.

22.5 Conclusions

Ontario has become the standard bearer in Advanced Traffic Management Systems over the past decade (P.H. Masters, personal communication, 2004; ITSPC, 1999). COMPASS is proven effective at all of its goals and has made an increasing attempt at broadening its scope and philosophy.

This being said, there is room for improvement beyond the engineering needs outlined by Korpal et al. (1994). Not only are there some highlighted areas of expansion (such as the Gardiner Expressway and Don Valley Parkway), COMPASS needs to increasingly cooperate with other organizations if it wishes to increase its impact. Specifically, there is an initial issue of communications with responders (mentioned above) so that more and better information gets from operators to responders in less time. Additionally, coordination of COMPASS with counterparts in other jurisdictions (like the mentioned separate FTMS of the Municipality of Toronto) is needed such that benefits are shared, and costs minimized. This is not simply an issue of "COMPASS moving off the ramps and into municipalities" (P.H. Masters, personal communication, 2004), but of facing some potentially serious organizational changes so that the provincial and municipal systems can share information to optimize both the system overall and increase the responsiveness of each component in the case of an incident (e.g., in the case of an motor-

vehicle collision on the Highway 401 in Toronto, COMPASS should share information much more quickly with the FTMS of the Municipality so that the traffic volume of the main arterial roads can be modified).

Additionally, COMPASS requires increasing participation by those in disciplines other than engineering. Although program officials now value the positive impact of COMPASS on accident reduction (to the point where it is today considered one of the two fundamental goals of the program along with congestion reduction), there is not as yet a significantly active role of health professionals in the decision-making process. This comes when administrators have cited a problem in selling COMPASS as a health initiative (P.H. Masters, personal communication, 2004). Administrators have no doubt made serious and honest attempts to broaden the role themselves, including health workers' and researchers' promises to increase the weight of their claim, broaden the scope and philosophy of the project still further, and tap the additional funding resources that program administrators cite as vital for their continued expansion (P.H. Masters, personal communication, 2004).

Despite this, COMPASS is undoubtedly an empirically proven method of reducing accidents on freeways in and around major urban areas such as Toronto, which is cited as one of the primary locations for transportation related injury (ORSAR, 2001). Additionally, it is cited as one of the best such examples of FTMS programs in the world (Hellinga et al., 1999; ITSPC, 1999; Korpal et al., 1994; PWGSC, 1999). Although the initial stage along the QEW in and around Mississauga relied heavily on FTMS programs elsewhere (primarily Los Angeles and Detroit), the current COMPASS System in Toronto has effectively reversed this relationship—FTMS programs in Atlanta, Salt Lake City, Kansas City, Portland Oregon, and even the originally cited program in Los Angeles now incorporate components of COMPASS. Additionally, the Municipality of Toronto has incorporated many of the elements, strategies, and aims of COMPASS for its own FTMS systems—such as in downtown Toronto (P.H. Masters, personal communication, 2004;

Intelligent Transportation Systems Plan for Canada [ITSPC], 1999). It is therefore considered an ideal example of an exemplar practice in road safety for this casebook.

Acknowledgments The author would like to express sincere appreciation to the key informant for this case study: Philip H. Masters of the Ontario Ministry of Transportation in Toronto, ON, Canada—whose consultation made this project possible.

BRIO Model: COMPASS Program

Group Served: Drivers in areas with high levels of traffic congestion, specifically in the Greater Toronto Area (GTA) of Ontario, Canada.

Goal: To minimize and manage traffic congestion (recurring and non-recurring) in critical areas.

Background	Resources	Implementation	Outcome
Based on successful Freeway Traffic Management Systems (FTMS) in Los Angeles and Detroit Toronto FTMS (now known as COMPASS) incorporates a number of control strategies, including management of recurring and non-recurring traffic, effectively targeting all areas outlined in the Preliminary Design Report and all system elements of the 1980 Highway 401 Corridor Traffic Systems Management Study	Primary stakeholder is the Ministry of Transportation of the Government of Ontario (MTO) Primary collaborators who play a key role in implementation consist of the MTO, media, Municipality of Toronto, Municipality of Mississauga, various universities, various emergency services (paramedics, fire, law enforcement) Initial costs per kilometer of operation were $1 million, now is approx. $500,000	COMPASS is relied upon by the media and commuters for traffic updates Employees today are those who played an important role in the implementation of COMPASS early on—resulting in individuals with an unprecedented amount of expertise (this has allowed a steady decrease of costs) Decisions are made primarily on a cost–benefit ratio Aspects include congestion management and incident management which consists of incident detection, an incident verification process, and inter-agency incident coordination	COMPASS targets the individual, by electronically providing information to drivers on automated highway signs, and the community, by supplying information to media about congestion and accidents Both prevents accidents from occurring and minimizes the impact and severity of incidents after the fact (by decreasing time of emergency response) FTMS programs elsewhere now incorporate components of COMPASS (including Los Angeles)

Life Space Model: COMPASS Program

Sociocultural: civilization/community	Interpersonal: primary and secondary relationships	Physical environments: where we live	Internal states: biochemical/genetic and means of coping
Government support for a community-based intervention for traffic congestion, to prevent primary and/or secondary accidents Provides the community with knowledge of traffic congestion and any accidents to ensure a smoother flow of traffic for commuters Allows emergency vehicles to arrive with less travel time and disturbances	Individuals can react and plan their travels knowing travel times due to congestion, and travel safety due to accident identification All drivers are better able to handle any accidents or congestions while on the road due to information being presented accurately and efficiently By conveying traffic information through media outlets, such as television and radio, motorists have better knowledge of the traffic	Road network and routes are constantly being monitored Road conditions are being communicated to motorists, and information is being conveyed on the road itself through visual messages	Provides motorists a sense of security regarding road safety, travel conditions, and commute times

References

COMPASS. (2001). *COMPASS Highway 401 traffic camera home page*. Toronto, ON: Ministry of Transportation of the Government of Ontario.

Hellinga, B., Baker, M., Van, A., Aultman-Hall, L., & Masters, P. (1999). *Overview of a simulation study of the Highway 401 FTMS*. Kingston, ON: Transportation Systems Research Group, Queen's University.

Intelligent Transportation Systems Plan for Canada. (1999). *En Route to intelligent mobility. TP 13501E*. Ottawa, ON: Transport Canada.

Korpal, P. R., Rayman, C. A., & Masters, P. H. (1994). *Evaluation of the Highway 401 Freeway Traffic Management System: Summary report*. Ministry of Transportation of Ontario: Freeway Traffic Management Section: Ontario.

Ontario Road Safety Annual Report. (2001). Ministry of Transportation of the Government of Ontario, Ontario.

Public Works and Government Services Canada. (1999). *GHG reduction benefits of the deployment of intelligent transportation systems on Canada's road/Highway network*. T8013-8-0205/W.

Aleeza Janmohamed

Active and Safe Routes to School (ASRTS) is a national movement dedicated to children's mobility, health, and overall wellness. The main goal revolves around promoting active school travel through a variety of community and school initiatives. ASRTS promotes healthier students, fewer emissions resulting in less air pollution, and overall safer school zones by reducing traffic volumes due to the focus on non-infrastructure and infrastructure measures. The program addresses a wide array of success factors and is a proven cost-effective intervention to get more kids active on their way to school.

23.1 Background

23.1.1 Safe Routes to School: What Is It?

Active and Safe Routes to School (SRTS) describes a community-based road safety program that aims to make a child's journey to and from school safer. It may also encompass other goals such as reducing child pedestrian injuries, promoting safety, creating a cleaner environment by reducing traffic congestion, and promoting a healthy and active lifestyle. The program utilizes a multidisciplinary approach that can be modified for the needs of specific communities, and it is for this reason that the promotion perspective of the program varies from community to community. The program works to embrace the definition of security by first identifying community risks, whatever they may be, and utilizing this knowledge to foster motivation and intention to deal with the risks and associated consequences (Volpe, 2004). The definition of safety is also considered as the program works with the local community to increase social capital and create a culture of care (Volpe, 2004). The success of the program is that it works within a community at the local level to systematically identify needs, create partnerships for a stakeholder group, and disseminate information through a public education campaign. Community members are empowered to promote the development of a sustainable program in order to reclaim neighborhoods and motivate further engagement toward change (O'Brien, 2004; J. Kennedy, personal communication, August 5, 2004). Experts in the field of child pedestrian safety have identified Safe Routes to School as an exemplary practice currently in existence (M. Vegega, personal communication, July 21, 2004; O'Brien, 2004). The main strengths are that it uses a multifaceted approach based on a collaborative and participatory planning process, and it works to build on the diverse knowledge of community

A. Janmohamed (✉)
The Sterling Hall School, Toronto, ON, Canada

© Springer Nature Switzerland AG 2020
R. Volpe (ed.), *Casebook of Traumatic Injury Prevention*,
https://doi.org/10.1007/978-3-030-27419-1_23

members while fostering a sense of ownership and responsibility. The program is efficient, scalable, flexible, draws on experience, and is extremely proactive (Institute for Transportation & Development Policy, 2004; O'Brien, 2004). SRTS falls within the Pre-Crash phase of the Haddon matrix and involves both human and environmental factors. It will be demonstrated that the target area of reducing the risk of injury can be achieved through better planning and design of school catchment areas. In addition, there is potential to reduce exposure to the risk of road traffic through changes in land-use and transport policy.

23.1.2 History of Safe Routes to School

The preliminary model for the Safe Routes to School program was developed in Denmark. In the mid-1970s, Denmark was cited as having the worst child pedestrian accident rate in Western Europe. This drove the municipality of Odense in 1978 to start up a program where they would make dangerous routes to schools safe by identifying and improving specific road dangers that needed to be addressed (ATKINS, 2002). The project included an extensive planning process where parents and children were surveyed and consensus-building sessions were held. The measures that were taken included creating a network of traffic-free pedestrian and bicycle paths, establishing slow speed areas for certain roads, and complementing these with traffic calming measures (speed humps and traffic circles). The program was successful in reducing the number of serious pedestrian injuries for both children and adults (ATKINS, 2002; Transportation Alternatives, 2001). In 3 years, the annual accident rate was reduced by 85% (Go for Green, 2003). The success in Denmark led to the implementation of slightly modified Safe Routes to School programs in the United Kingdom, Australia, New Zealand, Japan, France, the United States, and Canada. However, it is the Scandinavian countries who are exemplars as they have a remarkable reputation for sustainable

transportation where the car is secondary to the cyclist and the pedestrian (J. Kennedy, personal communication, August 5, 2004).

When a group called Sustrans in the UK initiated ten Safe Routes to Schools pilot projects in 1995 (Sustrans, 2004), it served as the inspiration for two Canadian programs. The Green Communities Association (GCA) Active and Safe Routes to School (formerly Greenest City) program in Ontario and the Way to Go! School Program in British Columbia (J. Kennedy, personal communication, August 5, 2004).

23.1.3 General Components

Safe Routes to School programs bring together key stakeholders to collaborate in addressing road safety issues using a specific method. These stakeholders may include some or all of the following: school board representatives, school trustees, school administrators, parents, students, local councilors (other politicians), traffic engineers, traffic police, community members, crossing guards, nonprofit organizations (concerned with the environment, sustainable transportation, children's safety, injury prevention, etc.), and local government (ministry of education, health, transportation). The specific method followed in Canada, which is similar to that in Europe, New Zealand, and Australia, includes three distinct phases utilized to visualize the components of the program (Safekids Aotearoa, 2015; ASRTS, 2004):

1. *The Set-Up Phase*: the key stakeholders are identified and enrolled into the program.
2. *The Data Collection and Action Planning Phase*: hazardous environments and behaviors are addressed through data collection; action is planned to address the identified issues using a combination of engineering, education, enforcement, and policy strategies.
3. *The Implementation and Monitoring Phase*: the planned action is implemented and monitored.

In addition to the common components, each SRTS program can be generally classified into four broad approaches: The Traffic Calming Model, The Funding Model, the Encouragement Model, and the Enforcement Model. Individual programs may mix various aspects of these models or they may coexist in a single province or community. The models can be used to reflect methodically about what programs are doing and why they are doing it (Transportation Alternatives, 2001).

The Traffic Calming Model is "fundamentally based on changing the behavior of motorists through changes in street design" (Transportation Alternatives, 2001, p. 6). Some examples include programs in Denmark (Odense), Britain, Germany, Holland, The Bronx (New York), and Arlington Virginia. These programs also utilize education and enforcement strategies. The main goal is to measurably reduce crashes, injuries, and deaths involving child pedestrians or cyclists near schools. The program also aims to create safe routes to and from school in order to increase the number of children participating in active transportation (Transportation Alternatives, 2001).

The Funding Model includes programs that win funding for districts to create engineering, education, and enforcement campaigns. The goals are similar to the previous model; however, it means that legislation is passed at the federal, state, or local level in order to guarantee significant levels of funding for SRTS programs. For instance, in California, one third of federal Surface Transportation Safety funds are dedicated to local SRTS programs (Transportation Alternatives, 2001).

The Encouragement Model describes programs that have limited funding and work to direct public and political attention to active transportation to school. Marketing and behavioral change methods are frequently used. "Encouragement campaigns can be developed into a consensus building and marketing tool to win increased community, political, and governmental support for traffic calming and increased police enforcement and engineering changes" (Transportation Alternatives, 2001, p. 8). This is the model that best describes Ontario's Active and Safe Routes to School Program.

The Enforcement Model usually depicts short-term programs which are responsive to a child pedestrian injury or death. Police enforcement is assigned to high crash schools, and police visits provide safety education. These campaigns are not sustainable and become more effective if they are part of a broader traffic enforcement strategy (Transportation Alternatives, 2001).

23.1.4 History of Ontario's Active and Safe Routes to School Program

In Canada the early 1990s was a time of interest and action in the field of Active Transportation. There was a call to establish projects that would allow Canadians to try to become more active in their forms of transportation. A call to action was made to 50,000 communities, workplace, and school leaders across Canada (Go for Green, 2003). Action Plans on Active Transportation were made in every province and territory in 1993. Schools were identified as one of the three areas that required action.

In 1995, Jacky Kennedy was volunteering at The North Toronto Green Community, a non-profit organization interested in promoting conservation through grassroots action and the development of sustainable, self-supporting, long-term initiatives to improve the community for residents and their children. It was at this time that she began researching the Sustrans Safe Routes to School program and worked to create a strategic plan and a model for a pilot project for Toronto. In 1996, severe government cuts to the environmental sector led to a loss of funding for all "Green Communities" (J. Kennedy, personal communication, August 5, 2004). Green Communities are locally based non-profit organizations that help to build sustainable communities through activities that conserve resources, prevent pollution, and protect green space and natural ecological processes; the Green Communities Association (GCA) is the national network of these community-based organizations that deliver these innovative and environmental programs and services (Green Communities Association, 2003;

J. Kennedy, personal communication, August 5, 2004). These activities included supporting alternative and active modes of transportation. Since 1991, Green Communities have constructed a successful model which provides cost-effective services and activities that benefit the environment, the economy, and the quality of life in the communities in which they operate (North Toronto Green Community, 2004).

In 1996, despite the cuts, the Toronto Atmospheric Fund provided the funding to create a new organization called Greenest City, a community-based non-profit environmental organization. The first Safe Routes to School program in Canada was implemented in Toronto at this time with the support of the Toronto District School Board. The project was called Active and Safe Routes to School (ASRTS). A pilot study was started with three Toronto public schools. The program was easily established as there was a lot of initial interest from the communities and the program grew quickly through media promotion. The program began with three main components: Walking School Bus, No Idling at School, and Classroom Mapping using Blazing Trails Through the Urban Jungle (J. Kennedy, personal communication, August 5, 2004; Informa, 2001; ASRTS, 2004). These components will be further explained below.

In 1997 there were some initial write-ups in two of the largest daily newspapers, the Toronto Star and the Globe and Mail. During this same time period, on the other side of the country, the Greater Vancouver Regional District decided to fund The Way to Go! School Program to develop a model to promote alternative transportation for elementary schools, which was very similar to Toronto's program. The main difference between the programs was that The Insurance Corporation of British Columbia, a public insurance board, incorporated the safe routes initiative as part of their traffic safety and awareness program and helped to disseminate it across the province. Throughout 1997, the Toronto and British Columbia programs were working closely as they shared ideas and collaborated on resources (J. Kennedy, personal communication, August 5, 2004).

Toward the end of 1997 it became clear that the program did not have the capacity to meet all the demand. Go for Green, a national non-profit, charitable organization that encourages Canadians to pursue healthy, outdoor physical activities while being good environmental citizens, was approached (Go for Green, 2003). With funding from Health Canada, a "National Working Group on Active Transportation" meeting was organized, and it was decided that a national safe route to school initiative should be put into action. A steering committee of which Jacky Kennedy was a member identified nine initial components for the Safe Routes to School program. They were as follows:

- A communications plan
- Resource materials
- Pilot projects
- Classroom curriculum support resources
- Walking school bus and other active transportation modes
- Legislation and policy development
- Physical environments/infrastructure
- Leadership development and human resource support
- Recognition program

For the first 2 years Jacky Kennedy (Ontario) and Bernadette Kowey (British Columbia) were contracted for Go for Green and extremely active producing all the resources that currently exist. In 1999–2000 Ontario and BC were removed from the national program leaving them to function autonomously (J. Kennedy, personal communication, August 5, 2004). Although a variety of organizations promote and coordinate the programs in the rest of the Canadian provinces and territories, they are maintained nationally by Go for Green (2003).

In December 2003 the Green Communities Association assumed responsibility for the Ontario ASRTS project. And in the same way that ASRTS drew its inspiration from the European Safe Routes to School programs, New Zealand, Australia, and the United States have utilized Ontario's program as a model (J. Kennedy, personal communication, August 5, 2004).

In Ontario, the Active and Safe Routes to School program is under Green Communities Canada. Green Communities Canada is part of the Active School Travel Canada working group formed in 2016 to connect the leading organizations for active school travel across Canada. Like this foundation, other provinces including British Columbia, Quebec, Alberta, Nova Scotia, Manitoba, and Saskatchewan have their own active school travel programs. Within each province are additional communities and hubs to coordinate efforts, which may include schools, school boards, public health boards, municipalities, and other representatives.

23.2 Resources

23.2.1 Human Resources

Human resources are perhaps the most important contribution to this program. The successful implementation, sustainability, and longevity of the program largely depend on the participation and support of the entire community. Staff members provide the majority of the assistance required in the first few years of a new community's program. After that it is up to the local program collaborators to take a leadership role.

Partnerships with various organizations also help to build a strong foundation for the projects. Past partners include The Clean Air Champions, Ontario Physical Health and Education Association (OPHEA), and Way to Go! School Program (J. Kennedy, personal communication, August 5, 2004).

23.2.2 Financial Resources

In 2004, the program required $200,000 per year to maintain the level of support and increase participation across Ontario. This included two full-time staff salaries with benefits, seed funds for new communities, program resources (IWALK, Walking School Bus, No Idling at School campaign, Cross Canada Walking Challenge Maps, etc.), provincial communications and promotion, and research opportunities. The estimated average value of annual cash and in-kind contributions in these communities today is $150,000.

Current Ontario supporters include the Heart and Stroke Foundation, Canadian Automobile Association—South Central Ontario (CAA-SCO), Metrolinx, and Ottawa Student Transportation Authority/City of Ottawa. In addition, the Ontario Ministry of Tourism and Recreation became a new funding partner in September 2004. In-kind support is provided by The Cooperators, The Printing House, Way to Go! School Program, Go for Green, and Natural Resources Canada (No Idling at School campaign). Some of the past funders have included the Laidlaw Foundation, the Toronto Atmospheric Fund, Toronto Heart Health, and Toronto Public Health.

The most substantial grant for the program has been a 3-year grant from the Ontario Trillium Foundation, which began in 2001. The funding was mainly used to test the stakeholder model and attempt to establish a sustainable program within the given timeframe. Numerous communities have found ways to match the funds to ensure that they were not completely reliant on the grant. This is important, as communities need to learn how to institutionalize their program at the local level. Just as the ASRTS program reflects individual communities, the decisions about distribution of funds have been unique to each community as well. Some communities used the money to pay the salary of an individual to work on transportation/air quality issues; others used it for leverage in their community or even as part of a general fundraising plan to raise more contributions.

23.2.3 Curriculum and Promotional Resources

Ontario's Active and Safe Routes to School program and B.C.'s Way to Go! School Program have developed a number of successful resources that are widely used across Canada. The first resources were used for the pilot schools in 1996 and were reproduced by Toronto Public Health.

The Walking School Bus (WSB) is a major part of the ASRTS program and is a concept that was first presented by Australian, David Engwicht, in his book entitled "Reclaiming our Cities and Towns: Better Living with Less Traffic" (Engwicht, 2003). A WSB is two or more families walking to school together for safety. Some schools have organized pickup destinations where children meet a parent who acts as a WSB driver. ASRTS has made comprehensive resources available describing the specifics about starting a WSB. This includes mapping the school catchment area, getting parents involved, helping families to get to know one another, and utilizing local police, local councilor, and traffic engineer to help promote safer routes (ASRTS, 2004).

Blazing Trails Through the Urban Jungle Classroom is a guide that was developed in 1994 by Transportation Options in Toronto (Go for Green, 2003). It provides teachers with the tools to implement mapping techniques in the classroom based on safety and sustainable transportation.

A revised version of the Green Communities ASRTS Resource Guide, supported by MOST, and an updated promotional brochure, have been created and are available. Of the 1000 guides and 3000 brochures that were printed, over 600 guides and 2500 brochures have already been distributed. The Resource Guide provides detailed information on how to implement all the aspects of ASRTS such as International Walk to School Week, Cross Canada Walking Challenge, Neighborhood Walkabout, No Idling at School campaign, and the WSB. In addition, there are resources that link ASRTS to the Ontario curriculum, themes, and celebrations that can be used throughout the school year, as well as evaluation tools.

In the spring of 2000, the Green Communities province-wide No Idling at School campaign was launched as part of ASRTS. Over 1000 toolkits were distributed to schools and were extremely well received. The toolkit is easy to use and comprehensive, providing schools with innovative ways to reduce vehicle idling in their community.

ASRTS does not have a steady budget so they efficiently make use of existing resources from other programs around the world. For instance, although French resources are available on their website, French immersion students may use the Go for Green website to register in French if they wish. Also, additional IWALK teaching resources are provided online for schools and are adapted from Dorset County in the UK, as they are deemed to be a good fit for the Canadian context. The site is also an important aspect of the program because it allows schools and communities to share success stories and ideas which serve to build a social capital network. This component of sharing is in the spirit of the capacity and knowledge building that ASRTS authenticates.

23.3 Implementation

23.3.1 History of ASRTS Implementation

The Green Communities Association Active and Safe Routes to School Ontario dissemination model was first piloted in the Greater Toronto Area (GTA). Through this mode, the program has seen rapid growth. In Toronto alone almost 200 elementary schools participate. In September 2004, Toronto Public Health in partnership with the City of Toronto's Transportation Services department assumed responsibility for the Toronto program, thereby moving it to a more locally sustainable level and a step closer to the program's institutionalization. Support and consulting expertise are still available to them through Green Communities.

This came about after the initial pilot phase with three Toronto schools during 1996. Toronto Public Health helped to expand the pilot through the involvement of their Scarborough office and six new schools came on board. After the amalgamation of the City of Toronto, the public health role was expanded across the new city. School site safety was in the interest of Toronto Police Service and the Toronto's Transportation Department. Gradually, as these organizations became involved through neighborhood walkabouts, they became convinced of the relevance of SRTS to address child pedestrian safety issues in schools. The involvement of these important stakeholders is significant as it allowed the program to expand beyond the realm of environmental and health groups. Interest in the program continued to spread from Toronto to areas outside the city, including York and Durham Regions. More pilots were initiated, including Peel Region, and by 2000 most of the GTA was involved (J. Kennedy, personal communication, August 5, 2004).

In 2001 a grant was awarded to the Green Communities Association by the Ontario Trillium Foundation to disseminate the GTA's ASRTS program model across Ontario.

23.3.2 ASRTS Community Selection and Program Implementation

An Ontario Trillium Foundation funded project begins by identifying a local champion, preferably a Green Community member, as defined by the Green Communities Association. Typically, Green Communities already have developed strong partnerships with the key stakeholders needed for ASRTS. An initial 2-h presentation/meeting is held in the community by the Green Communities Association in order to introduce the program, discuss community needs, and address issues. If there is sufficient interest and commitment from all stakeholders to establish a local pilot program, a stakeholder committee is established. The GCA provides $10,000 per year for 3 years, all resources at no cost, and consulting time. Based on the experience that has been gained working in the GTA, the GCA feels that is takes up to 3 years to establish a potentially sustainable program in a community.

> …It takes a long time. First of all, scheduling the meeting, getting people to report back. It's a very long process; you can't do these projects in a year. It is a long haul. You are suggesting something new, you're working with policy makers, decision makers and bureaucracies, and it's very slow. And you want it to work! You're actually setting the groundwork or the foundation for building what you only hope will be a sustainable program (J. Kennedy, personal communication, August 5, 2004).

There are nine suggested components of the ASRTS program, and they are presented as part of a school year calendar (ASRTS, 2004) (Fig. 23.1).

The program can be implemented into a school at the community's own pace and does not necessarily follow the model above. However, the components introduced in the given time frame are purposeful, and success has been demonstrated in most school settings. For instance, ASRTS is introduced to schools in June so that teachers and administrators can plan for successful implementation of the program the following school year. In the first year of the program implementation, the primary event suggested is for the school community to participate in October's International Walk to School week (IWALK). This initial step is small yet vital because it is what concretely determines participation level and commitment from the school, parents, and students. It also provides the opportunity for some media and promotional work around the issue of child pedestrian safety, the environment, and children's health (J. Kennedy, personal communication, August 5, 2004).

In the second year of the program three pilot schools are chosen within the community. Each school is carefully chosen to represent different dynamics. All the stakeholders work closely with each school to identify barriers that may exist and come up with strategies to deal with them. These may differ from school to school. After IWALK, at the school level, families are now encouraged to participate in Walking/Wheeling Wednesdays on the first Wednesday of every month or every Wednesday. This activity may be tied into the school curriculum persuading teachers to incorporate it into class time. For instance, resources such as the Cross Canada Walking Challenge allows students to earn points each time they walk to school and win the Golden Shoe Award. This provides enjoyable and educational opportunities to extend healthy living and safety messages to the students as well as the larger community. Around this time, it is a good idea to encourage schools to conduct a Neighborhood Walkabout to track safety issues and collect baseline data. Parents, children, and teachers are surveyed as part of this needs analysis process to gather data on setting goals, identifying volunteers, and uncovering barriers. Existing pedestrian facilities, dangerous locations, safe routes,

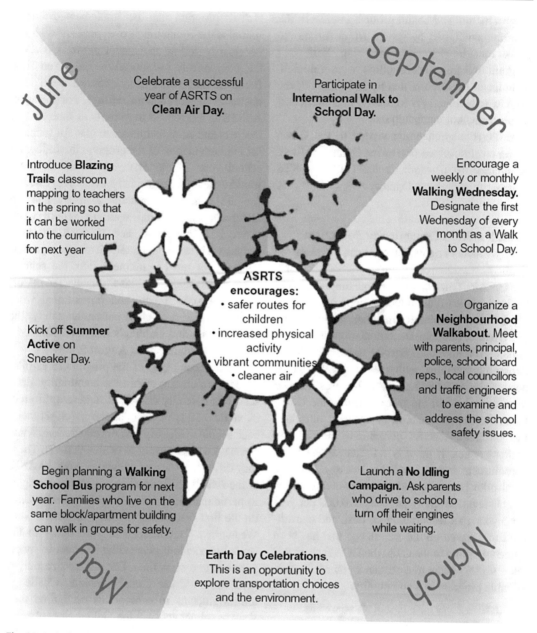

Fig. 23.1 A description of campaigns and implementations of ASRTS over the course of a year

and police data on traffic accidents in the area are all mapped. The flexibility of ASRTS and the collaborative planning practice has a chance to excel as partners and stakeholders meet to decide what components of the program work for them. Next, a timeline is established, and alternatives are sought. For instance, if students are unable to walk to and from school due to distance or if they are bussed, a kilometer club can be started during recess and lunch. The scope of the ASRTS resources and activities truly demonstrate their suitability for schools as they are synchronized with curriculum, provide linkages to safety education, and promote students to be physically active (J. Kennedy, personal communication, August 5, 2004).

The No Idling at School campaign is usually implemented in the spring because it has been shown that people make a greater connection to air pollution in the spring and are more willing to participate. In schools with a high percentage of vehicle trips and very resistant parents, a No Idling at School campaign can be the motivator toward gradually changing attitudes and can lead to the creation of an exclusion zone around the school and even toward implementing Walking School Buses (J. Kennedy, personal communication, August 5, 2004).

A crucial component of the ASRTS program is to keep motivation levels high especially among students. This means that the program should be fun. ASRTS highly values celebrating successes; hence, celebrations are included as components of the program (J. Kennedy, personal communication, August 5, 2004). It is important to include stakeholders in the celebrations as well. "When your local mayor, councilor, traffic engineers, and police officers are invited to a fun event at the school it makes all the difference in the world. Most changes will take place during a celebration because they see everyone being active" (J. Kennedy, personal communication, August 5, 2004).

After a year and a half, the ASRTS program manager in conjunction with the main collaborators conducts an assessment. At this time a number of factors are examined: the participation rate, which aspects of the program are working, the identification of support needs, how stakeholders and collaborators feel. At this stage it is usual to find schools needing assistance and requesting ideas to keep families motivated to meet their intended school travel plans (J. Kennedy, personal communication, August 5, 2004).

23.4 Outcome

Due to the diverse nature of the Safe Routes to School programs, rating the effectiveness of the program and the evaluations is a difficult task (M. Vegega, personal communication, July 21, 2004). In Ontario, ASRTS has not had the capacity to track neurotrauma injuries. In addition, baseline data of child pedestrian injuries specifically tracking age, day of the week, and time is not readily available (J. Kennedy, personal communication, August 5, 2004). The Safe Routes Program facilitates numerous other ways of tracking outcomes which are based on the goals of the individual communities. As noted in the previous casebook, "Many programs provide services potentially relevant to prevention but with no demonstrated connection to injury prevention. Thinking contextually allows these undertakings to be considered as resources to the prevention effort." (Volpe, 2004, p. 6). With this in mind we can begin to examine how Ontario's various communities define success. According to Jacky Kennedy (personal communication, August 5, 2004):

> Each community will have different issues that they are involved in so things that may excite the people in Ottawa will just be a bomb in London. So, when you sit back to look at all this work it's just incredible to see the diversity of projects that we have on the ground now and each can be seen as a success.

23.4.1 Evaluation of ASRTS Goals

The main goal of ASRTS is to assist school communities in encouraging safe and active travel to and from school. One of the main ways to measure this is to look at the participation rate. The Active and Safe Routes to School program in Ontario is growing steadily over the years and the demand for the program remains high. From 2001 to 2003 the program grew from 400 schools in nine communities to over 850 schools in 19 communities. In just 2 years the program participation has increased from the Greater Toronto Area (population 5 million) to an additional 19 communities encompassing 4.5 million people. As of 1999, Ontario had a population of 11.5 million, and ASRTS reached a total of 9.5 million people. During 2003, 21% of Ontario elementary schools participated in at least one ASRTS activity. This is approximately 330,000 students, their families, and school staff. In addition, 67 of the

106 Ontario school boards participated. Ontario has the highest level of participation in North America (J. Kennedy, personal communication, August 5, 2004; ASRTS, 2004).

Active and Safe Routes to School also aims to teach children the pleasures of walking and encourage healthy, lifelong habits. According to surveys of children in schools, students are "voting with their feet" and say they would rather walk to school than be driven; 75% of Ontario's elementary school children would prefer to walk or cycle to school (O'Brien, 2004). From May 2000 to June 2001 three research projects were conducted to address the barriers that exist and strategies to overcome them. One of these is York University's Centre for Sustainability's Ontario Walkability Study which examined and validated children's experiences and aspirations. It was conducted by Greenest City with the support of the Laidlaw Foundation and the Ontario Ministry of the Environment. Over 6369 surveys were completed by students and data on students' usual travel mode, preferred travel mode, and the walkability of children's routes. A huge gap exists between 3.5% of students who regularly use active transportation versus 72.2% who desire more active transportation (York University's Centre for Sustainability [YUCS], 2001).

ASRTS strives to create a sustainable program in each community. It is clear that parental involvement is key in addition to the children's motivation. Hence, the second study was a "Parent Attitudes and Travel Behavior Regarding the Trip to School" report (O'Brien, 2001). The results demonstrate that parents and educators who had already participated with ASRTS had reduced their car trips to school and also changed other travel behavior. Parents who had not participated in ASRTS were unaware of any options regarding opportunities to change their travel behavior with respect to the school trip and had never considered driving less (O'Brien, 2001).

The third study, Small Steps/Large Rewards: A community-based social marketing research project (Informal Market Research, 2001), carefully examined a number of issues such as the problems associated with walking to school, the variables that influence participation, the benefits of the program, the views of the program organizers, and ways to promote the program more successfully. This research was important for the progress of ASRTS as it touched on another goal. In order to increase safety by creating a culture of care and building social capital, the issues need to be fully understood and information needs to be continually disseminated to community members.

ASRTS has also touched on the goal of increasing physical activity levels of children because it has been shown that students participating in 15 days of ASRTS-related activities are walking about 675,000 km (ASRTS, 2004). In addition, environmental goals are being met as collectively during 2003; Ontario ASRTS schools participating in the No Idling at School campaign reduced climate change CO_2 emissions by approximately 210.5 tons. This is the equivalent to 26,600 h of idling or running ten cars for 24 h a day, 7 days a week for almost 4 months (ASRTS, 2004).

If we reflect momentarily on the evaluations conducted in Odense, Denmark, success of the program was originally clearly defined as a reduction in children's injuries. This was the main focus of the program. They examined the overall effect of the program in terms of accidents and personal injuries, also as a breakdown of personal injuries in regard to type of age, type of transport, and the school route project initiative. The method of the evaluation consisted of an assessment of accidents before and after the program, balanced against a control group consisting of six similar municipalities to correct for the general accident trends (ATKINS, Road Traffic and Safety, 2002). The results indicate that the school routes projects significantly reduced the number of accidents registered with the police by 18%, which corresponds to 17.7 accidents a year. Also, there was a falling trend in personal injuries by 20% or 8.8 personal injuries a year. Furthermore, the safe routes project evaluation reported to have especially reduced serious accidents. Overall the Odense safe routes program saved society DKK 15.7 million per year in costs of accidents (ATKINS, 2002). The decreases are mainly attributed to the traffic-calming, low-speed roads, speed bumps, raised surfaces, and signal changes that were made.

However there has been a shift in the definition of injury prevention. It has expanded to focus on social conditions or mechanisms that support health and well-being (Volpe, 2004). This is a change that has been seen in SRTS programs and can most clearly be seen in Odense. According to Troels Andersen, an engineer who has been involved with SRTS since its inception, in Odense, injury prevention is no longer the main focus (T. Andersen, personal communication, August 10, 2004). In fact, he stated that Ontario's program which includes health and the environment as outcomes is ahead of Odense as this is the direction that they are moving toward (T. Andersen, personal communication, August 10, 2004). According to Dr. Vegega of the NHTSA, another reason that it is difficult to compare the outcomes of various programs is that, except for Odense, all other Safe Routes to School programs are fairly recent. Odense began a comprehensive evaluation 10 years after its initiation, and the evaluation was conducted for 13 years (1986–1999). Unfortunately, other programs do not have the luxury of this longevity (M. Vegega, personal communication, July 21, 2004). A final indicator of success in ASRTS is that Jacky Kennedy has been trying to release herself from the ownership of the Toronto program. From now on the Toronto program will be no different than any other program in Ontario and that is significant because communities in Ontario have true ownership of their own programs (J. Kennedy, personal communication, August 5, 2004). Hence, in the upcoming years the measure of success will not be a singular aspect of safety, but the program as a whole. Sustainability, community ownership and commitment, secure funding, and even the joy of active travel will come to the forefront (M. Vegega, personal communication, July 21, 2004; O'Brien, 2004).

In summary, the ASRTS program is successful as it incorporates all aspects of the Life Space model within the Complex Systems approach.

23.4.2 Future Directions

Ontario's program encompasses a wide range of disciplines; however, the ASRTS program has been dominated by the environmental sector. There is a great need for involvement from the angle of injury prevention (J. Kennedy, personal communication, August 5, 2004; M. Vegega, personal communication, July 21, 2004). The most important direction for ASRTS is to secure funding in order to continue to provide seed money for new communities and support for existing projects. For instance, in Denmark, Netherlands, the UK, and the United States, SRTS programs have a place in the ministry of transportation and have a budget from the government. If Ontario can embrace a Funding Model, ASRTS can achieve security, credibility, and allow opportunities for the program to advance and take on new challenges. Jacky Kennedy feels that:

> although there is an awful lot of work to do...we are making a good start and we are heading in the right direction...The more communities that become involved and the more traffic engineers, politicians, and public health units that start to grasp this project—they say 'yes, this really works for us"—then we can hopefully move closer to the day when we can have some serious funding and really institutionalize the program, not just in Ontario, but across Canada (personal communication, August 5, 2004).

Go for Green and the Canadian Institute of Child Health conducted 20 key informant interviews with Canadian experts regarding child and youth risk factors associated with active transportation to and from school (Hunt, 1999). Their recommendations for SRTS programs in general, in addition to those of Dr. Maria Vegega (personal communication, July 21, 2004), Dr. Catherine O'Brien (personal communication, August 4, 2004), Jacky Kennedy (personal communication, August 5, 2004), and Troels Andersen (personal communication, August 10, 2004), provide a summative conclusion to this exemplary practice case study.

- Public Policy Changes
  - Fiscal measures where each municipality sets priories and budgets for changes in the

physical environment through traffic calming and traffic reducing technology (speed limits, speed humps, red light cameras)
- Police cycle patrols for routes to school
- Nationally reduce speed limits in front of school zones
- Priority snow clearance for all routes to school
- By-laws to reduce wait times in school parking zones to decrease traffic volume
- Reimbursement of low-income families for child safety equipment such as helmets
- School-based Policy Changes
  - Create designated drop-off/pickup points to keep pedestrians and traffic separated, with eventually an exclusionary zone around the school
  - Create Safe Routes to School handbook and regular enforcement of school safety policy
  - Establish staggered dismissal so that smaller children receive more attention from crossing guards and parents and there is less chaos
  - Promote the supervision of young children to/from school
  - Assess the need for before and after school care
  - Supply reflectors for children to wear (by school)
  - Involve parents and children throughout all planning for SRTS
- Physical Changes
  - Establish multipurpose traffic calming measures (Esthetic islands with vegetation), wider sidewalks, refitting school entrances, elevated crossings (children have a shorter distance to travel, increased visibility), corner bulges (children can see traffic from behind parked cars at an elevation)
  - Create colorful, fluorescent street signs to identify school zones that are refreshed intermittently to prevent desensitization
  - Establish Parent Parking Patrols to reinforce security of a school drop-off zone
  - Paint colorful footprints along the chosen safe routes

- Strengthen Community Action
  - Establish community partnerships
  - Recognize the unique dynamics in each school community (ethnic diversity, socio-economic status)
  - Encourage all community members to be a good role model in traffic
  - Establish surveillance systems to collect and evaluate community traffic data
  - Recruit more Block Parents in urban neighborhoods
  - Advocate a paradigm shift to active transportation, for instance, build a critical mass of walkers, "eyes on the street" to increase safety, and celebrate active transportation
- Develop Personal Skills
  - Teach children traffic safety skills
  - Teach parents skills
  - Teach driver skills

23.5 Conclusion

Active and Safe Routes to School is a national movement dedicated to children's mobility, health, and overall wellness. The main goal revolves around promoting active school travel through a variety of community and school initiatives (Go for Green, 2003). ASRTS promotes healthier students, fewer emissions resulting in less air pollution, and overall safer school zones by reducing traffic volumes due to the focus on non-infrastructure and infrastructure measures (ASRTS, 2004). The program addresses a wide array of success factors and is a proven cost-effective intervention to get more kids active on their way to school. The ability of ASRTS to target and incorporate all four quadrants of the life-space model and be a proven success in intervention demonstrates an exemplar program for road-safety prevention.

Acknowledgments The author would like to express sincere appreciation to the key informants for this case study: Jacky Kennedy of the Green Communities Association in Toronto, ON, Canada and Catherine O'Brien of the Centre for Sustainable Transportation in Eaganville, ON, Canada—whose consultation made this project possible.

BRIO Model: Active and Safe Routes to School

Group Served: Elementary school students.

Goal: Promoting active school travel to improve children's mobility, health, and create safer school zones.

Background	Resources	Implementation	Outcome
The worst child pedestrian accident rate in Europe was found in Denmark, where the preliminary model for SRTS was developed—being successful in reducing the number of injuries Four models exist: Traffic calming model, designed to change motorists' behaviors; Funding model, to create education campaigns; Encouragement model, for programs that work directly with the public and politics; and the Enforcement model, to respond to child pedestrian injuries and death In Ontario, ASRTS is under the Green Communities Canada and started in 1999 to implement the program	Seven provinces have implemented an ASRTS program, with a variety of communities and hubs required to coordinate efforts—including schools, school boards, municipalities Ontario supporters include the Heart and Stroke Foundation, CAA, and Metrolinx ASRTS lacks a steady budget—but has received two substantial grants in 2001 and 2017 ASRTS has a popular website that allows schools and communities to share success stories and ideas to build a social capital network	More than 200 elementary schools participate in Toronto ASRTS program provides suggested components as part of the school year calendar A variety of programs and campaigns are implemented across the country for a variety of different goals including walking school busses, creating safer school zones, and motivating students and parents to be more active on their way to school	The results indicate that the school routes projects significantly reduced the number of accidents registered with the police by 18%, which corresponds to 17.7 accidents a year Also, there was a falling trend in personal injuries by 20% or 8.8 personal injuries a year ASRTS has also increased physical activity levels of children

Life Space Model: Active and Safe Routes to School

Sociocultural: civilization/community	Interpersonal: primary and secondary relationships	Physical environments: where we live	Internal states: biochemical/genetic and means of coping
Participatory, collaborative planning process involving the whole school community in program goals and delivery Dissemination of knowledge to community about a multitude of issues: child pedestrian safety, childhood obesity, benefits of active living, joy of sustainable transportation, environmental damage, over-reliance on cars Community involvement at different levels: civil engineers, police, municipal government, teachers, parents, and students working together to make roads to school safe Community advocacy is promoted	Increased driver-pedestrian awareness Neighborhood cohesion through programs like WSB Closer school-family relations	Neighborhood walkabout, safety audit Traffic technology measures Traffic calming measures	Empowerment of children, teachers and parents and other members of the community to become advocates of their health, the environment, and road safety Development of long-term appreciation for sustainable transportation

References

Active and Safe Routes to School. (2004). *Resource guide*. Retrieved August 2, 2004, from http://www.saferoutestoschool.ca/index.php?page=asrtsrg

ATKINS. (2002). *Evaluation of projects regarding routes to schools in the Municipality of Odense*. Retrieved May 17, 2004, from http://www.saferoutestoschools.org.uk/?c=5000&t=freepublist.htm

Engwicht, D. (2003). *Reclaiming our cities and towns: Better living with less traffic*. Philadelphia: New Society Publishers.

Go for Green. (2003). *A brief history of the National ASRTS program*. Retrieved July 22, 2004, from www.goforgreen.ca/asrts/history_e.html

Green Communities Association. (2003). *Mission and values*. Retrieved July 28, 2004, from http://www.gca.ca/indexcms/index.php?mission

Hunt, C. (1999). *Active/safe routes to school*. Ottawa: Health Canada. Canadian Institute of Child Health.

Informal Market Research. (2001). *Small steps/large rewards: A Community based social marketing research project*. Toronto, ON: Greenest City.

Institute for Transportation & Development Policy. (2004). *Safe routes to schools fact sheet*. Retrieved July 7, 2004, from http://www.itdp.org/PR/factsheet_srts.pdf

North Toronto Green Community. (2004). *What is a green community?* Retrieved August 10, 2004, from http://www.ntgc.ca/green_C.html

O'Brien, C. (2001). *Parent attitudes and travel behavior regarding the trip to school: Opportunities for sustainable mobility* (Doctoral Thesis). www.saferoutestoschool.ca

O'Brien, C. (2004). *Child-friendly transport planning*. Mississauga, ON: The Centre for Sustainable Transportation.

Safekids Aotearoa (2015). Child Unintentional Deaths and Injuries New Zealand, and Prevention Strategies. Auckland, NZ: Safekids Aotearoa.

Sustrans Safe Routes to School. (2004). Retrieved May 12, 2004, from http://www.saferoutestoschools.org.uk/?c=5000&t=freepublist.htm

Transportation Alternatives. (2001). *The 2001 summary of safe routes to school programs in the United States*. New York City: Surface Transportation Policy Project.

Volpe, R. (2004). *The conceptualization of injury prevention as change in complex systems. Life Span Adaptation Projects*. Toronto: University of Toronto.

York University's Centre for Sustainability. (2001). *Ontario walkability study: Trip to school: Children's experiences and aspirations*. Toronto: Greenest City.

Graduated Driver Licensing: California Program

24

Sophie Kiriakou

California's Graduated Driver Licensing (GDL) program helps combat the disproportionately high rate of motor vehicle collisions and resulting traumatic brain injuries involving young drivers, particularly those under the age of 18. By allowing new drivers the opportunity to gain experience through exposure of conditions that gradually increase in risk, drivers are able to understand and curb some risks. Certain conditions include having a nighttime driving component, highway driving age restrictions, and supervisions while driving. Under graduated licensing, young drivers are initially granted partial driving privileges so that they may gain the necessary driving experience under conditions of reduced risk. As they gain experience and mature, they are awarded broader privileges until they finally receive a full license.

24.1 Background

There is a great need to prevent the disproportionately high rate of motor-vehicle collisions (MVC) and neurotrauma that young drivers, particularly those under the age of 18, experience (Williams, 2003; Williams & Mayhew, 2004). The graduated driver licensing (GDL) system

was developed to provide these new drivers with the opportunity to gain gradual driving experience under conditions that minimize the exposure to risk (Simpson, 2003; Williams & Mayhew, 2004). The first GDL model that was introduced was developed by the National Highway Traffic Safety Administration (NHTSA) in the late 1970s in the United States but was debated and largely rejected by the public (Simpson, 2003). At this time, the Insurance Institute for Highway Safety (IIHS) published promising research supporting GDL but was accused of an "insidious attack" on adolescents and their lifestyles (Yaksich Jr., 1982). An important feature of GDL, the nighttime driving component, was regularly rejected as "anti-teenager," whereas today such restrictions are considered reasonable and exist in numerous jurisdictions based on their effectiveness in reducing MVCs for teens (Williams, 2001). Following the United States' initial attempt, New Zealand pioneered the first truly GDL system in 1987. Following close behind New Zealand to introduce the system was Canada in 1994, and then the United States in 1996 (Simpson, 2003). Since 1994, 58 jurisdictions (47 US states, the District of Columbia, 9 Canadian provinces, and 1 territory) have implemented one or more elements of graduated licensing (Williams & Mayhew, 2004).

Many sources have documented the success of the GDL system on decreasing the high MVC rates, injuries, and fatalities among new drivers,

S. Kiriakou (✉)
Toronto, ON, Canada
e-mail: sophiekiriakou@gmail.com

© Springer Nature Switzerland AG 2020
R. Volpe (ed.), *Casebook of Traumatic Injury Prevention*,
https://doi.org/10.1007/978-3-030-27419-1_24

particularly young drivers (Simpson, 2003; Williams & Mayhew, 2004). Although this is true, a GDL system's level of effectiveness may vary depending on a number of factors (D. Mayhew, personal communication, July 2004; Simpson, 2003), including the number and strength of the components that are implemented (Mayhew, Simpson, & Pak, 2003; Simpson, 2003; Williams & Mayhew, 2004). The following section will describe a model or "exemplar practice" GDL system in more detail and indicate what the optimal components of the system should consist of, based on a report entitled "Graduated Licensing: A Blueprint for North America" (Williams & Mayhew, 2004). This report was developed to assist jurisdictions that are considering adopting a GDL system or changing their current GDL system to be more comprehensive and effective in reducing young driver MVCs. The recommendations are primarily based on scientific evidence and also on what GDL systems are intended to accomplish (D. Mayhew, personal communication, July 2004; Williams & Mayhew, 2004). Furthermore, this report contains ratings of all GDL systems in North America as of December 2003, according to the degree to which they meet these optimal requirements. Those jurisdictions that had a GDL system in place were rated as "good," "fair," "marginal," or "poor," which reflect the strength and likely effectiveness of the systems in reducing injuries (Williams & Mayhew, 2004).

Based on the known risk factors associated with the over-representation of young drivers in MVCs as discussed in the literature review, optimal GDL systems, according to Williams and Mayhew (2004), should consist of several elements within a three-stage system. The first stage is the supervised learner's period that should have a minimum entry age of 16, a mandatory holding period of 6 months, and a minimum amount of supervised driving by a parent or guardian of 30–50 h. The second stage consists of receiving an intermediate license (once the driving test is passed) which should limit unsupervised driving conditions, including a restriction on nighttime driving (preferably between 9 pm and 5 am), and the number of passengers in the

vehicle (no more than one teenage passenger). Finally, the full-privilege driver's license becomes available after the first two stages are completed. An additional recommendation for strengthening a GDL system, although not fully supported yet by evidence, includes developing stronger parental involvement in the licensing process (Williams & Mayhew, 2004).

Despite the demonstrated effectiveness of this system in Canadian jurisdictions (e.g., Boase & Tasca, 1998; Simpson, 2003), several provinces including Ontario were only given a "marginal" rating, indicating that much more could be done to enhance the systems' effectiveness. In particular, Ontario does not yet include a passenger or nighttime driving restriction, which, according to Williams and Mayhew's (2004) report and numerous other studies, is crucial in reducing MVCs fatalities for young drivers (Chen, Baker, Braver, & Li, 2000; Lin & Fearn, 2003). According to the Ontario Ministry of Transportation (2002), passenger restrictions are already in effect in 31 jurisdictions across North America, including California, and have been in effect in New Zealand since 1987. In response to the evidence demonstrating the effectiveness of passenger restrictions in other jurisdictions and an analysis of the 2002 collision records in Ontario, the Ontario Minister of Transportation, Harinder Takhar, is proposing to introduce this restriction in legislation to further increase the success of the current GDL system in the province (Takhar, 2004).

Although the enhanced California GDL system that was implemented in 1998 contains many, but not all, of the optimal qualities of the model GDL system as described earlier, it was still given the highest rating, "Good," for the strength of its system (Williams & Mayhew, 2004).

24.1.1 History

In 1983, California was one of the first jurisdictions to implement a few basic elements of a preliminary GDL model that was developed by the NHTSA in 1977 (Simpson, 2003). Although this partial GDL system (called provisional licensing) in California was shown to be effective in reducing MVCs among young drivers (Hagge & Marsh, 1988), the current case will report on a more comprehensive and rigorous GDL law that California implemented July 1, 1998 based on a model crafted by the Automobile Club of Southern California (ACSC; S. Bloch, personal communication, August 26, 2004). California's GDL Senate Bill (SB) 1329 was entitled "Brady/Jared Teen Driver Safety Act of 1997" after two teenagers, Brady Grasinger and Jared Cunningham, who were killed in separate MVCs in California (A. Drumm, personal communication, August 2004).

24.1.2 Consumers

Although some jurisdictions target novice drivers of all ages (e.g., Canada and New Zealand), California's GDL system (and other US jurisdictions with GDL) targets only young novice drivers. In a report by the IIHS and NHTSA (2004), the rationale for only targeting young drivers is due to the fact that in the US 16-year-old drivers have higher collision rates than drivers of any other age, including older adolescents (IIHS & NHTSA, 2004). Furthermore, in the US, young people make up the majority of the beginning drivers; therefore, the GDL system focuses on this age group (IIHS & NHTSA, 2004).

24.1.3 Primary Goal of System

The primary goal of the enhanced GDL system was to reduce the number of teen deaths and injuries caused by MVCs as teenagers were found to be disproportionately more likely to be involved in collisions, especially at night (A. Drumm, personal communication, August 2004; California State Senate, 1997). The alarming statistics demonstrating the over-representation of young drivers in MVCs in California were a large motivating factor to implement the GDL law. Not only are MVCs the leading cause of death among teenagers in the United States, but in California nearly

18,000 teen drivers are injured or killed every year (American Automobile Association, 2004). Furthermore, the need to implement the new GDL system was based on the following startling statistics about young drivers (American Automobile Association, 2004):

- Too many young driver crashes:
  - Although teenagers 15–19 years old make up only 4% of licensed drivers in California, they comprise the drivers in 9% of fatal car crashes, and 10% of injury crashes.
- Too many young driver nighttime crashes:
  - Less than 4% of the miles driven by 16 and 17-year-olds nationally occur between midnight and 5 am, but 13% of the teenagers' fatal crashes take place between these hours.
- Too many teen passengers at risk:
  - Two-thirds of all teenage passengers killed and injured nationally are passengers in cars driven by other teens. In California, 18,000 teen passengers are injured or killed annually in vehicles driven by teenagers.

Finally, although the prevention of neurotrauma was not an explicit goal of the GDL bill, by reducing the number of MVCs it can be expected that the number of neurotrauma cases will also decline. This is based on the evidence that one of the leading causes of both head and spinal cord injuries for young drivers are MVCs as discussed previously in the literature review (Canadian Paraplegic Association, 2000; SMARTRISK Foundation, 1998).

24.1.4 Secondary Goal

According to the chief lobbyist and legislative representative involved in promoting and generating a strong coalition supporting California's GDL system, the secondary goal of GDL was to educate the legislature and the public, especially parents, about the severity of the young driver problem, and accordingly, to encourage support for the proposed new requirements (A. Drumm, personal communication, August 2004).

24.1.5 California's GDL Model

The following model contains all of the components within the three-stage licensing system proposed in SB 1329.

Stage 1: Learner's permit (Be at least 15½ years old and under age 18)

- Have completed a basic driver education course or be enrolled in driver education and training.
- Pass the DMV traffic law, road sign, and vision tests and pay $15 fee.
- Hold the instruction permit for at least 6 months (previously the law specified 30 days).
- Complete 50 h of supervised driving (an increase of 20 h), including 10 h at night.
- Parent/guardian must certify in writing that these hours have been completed.
- Complete both classroom driver education and formal behind-the-wheel training.
- Maintain a clean driving record. Not drink and drive. Even a 0.01% concentration of alcohol in blood—less than one drink—will result in a 1-year license suspension for drivers under age 21.

Stage 2: Provisional/intermediate license (Be at least 16 years old, but less than 18)

- Pass a behind-the-wheel driving test.
- For the first 6 months (or until age 18), no passengers under age 20 allowed unless a licensed driver age 25 or older is present. Exceptions permitted for school, employment, family, and medical need (licensees must carry a statement from the appropriate school official, employer, doctor, or parent/guardian).
- For the first 12 months (or until age 18), no driving permitted between midnight and 5 am, unless accompanied by licensed driver age 25 or older (exceptions same as for passenger restrictions). Violation of passenger or nighttime driving restrictions results in either court-ordered community service or a fine ($35—first fine, $50—second fine).

- A teen driver must be stopped for another violation such as speeding or failing to wear a safety belt before a ticket is written for violating conditions.
- One citation or at-fault crash within 12 months results in a DMV warning. Two or more result in license restrictions and suspensions.

Stage 3: Full license (Become 18 years old)

- Drivers under 21 are still subject to a 1-year license suspension if their blood alcohol concentration exceeds 0.01% when driving (Department of Motor Vehicles, 2004).

24.1.6 Haddon and Complex Systems Approach

California's GDL system not only addresses the pre-event phase of injury prevention as defined by Haddon (1980), but more importantly it applies to all four quadrants of a young driver's life space model within the complex systems approach to injury prevention (Volpe, 2004). In terms of the Haddon matrix, both the human and environment factors that interact during the pre-event phase are being addressed by California's comprehensive GDL system. First, the elements of the GDL system that affect the human factor include secondary police enforcement of restrictions, compulsory driver education and training courses, and parental enforcement of supervised driving hours during the learner's permit stage. In terms of the environment factor, young drivers are restricted from driving during risky nighttime hours and with any passengers under the age of 20 when not supervised. Both of these human and environment factors that are addressed with GDL will help in reducing the likelihood of MVCs occurring.

Based on the complex systems approach (Volpe, 2004), many elements of California's GDL system fit easily into the four quadrants of a young driver's Life Space model. According to the theoretical framework, since these four areas of the life space are being affected by the GDL system, it is likely that a stronger injury prevention effort is taking place (Volpe, 2004).

24.2 Resources

24.2.1 Collaborators and Stakeholders

The primary collaborators of the California GDL system leading up to the passing of SB 1329 were the Automobile Club of Southern California (ACSC) and the California State Automobile Association (A. Drumm, personal communication, August 2004). After the GDL law came into effect, the California Department of Motor Vehicles (DMV) was responsible for a portion of the implementation. Despite this, a representative from both the DMV and a primary member of the coalition supporting the new GDL program indicated that the DMV continue to receive support from original members of the coalition in the form of public statements supporting the California GDL system, traffic safety updates, and research efforts (e.g., from the ACSC research department; J. Curranco, personal communication, August 2004; A. Drumm, personal communication, August 2004).

The entire coalition of stakeholders and supporters of the California GDL law consisted of over 50 different traffic safety groups, parent and teacher associations, injury prevention groups, law enforcement officials, and medical professionals. Notable among this coalition was the Trauma Foundation of the San Francisco General Hospital, whose mission is to reduce the number of injuries and deaths through prevention, improved trauma care, and improved rehabilitation (Trauma Foundation, 2004). As the coalition continued to grow in numbers over the course of a year, the passion and drive to ensure the passing of the GDL SB 1329 was evident among all supporters involved. According to Drumm (personal communication, August 2004), the GDL legislation "could not have happened in California if it were not for the strength and the sheer numbers of the coalition."

24.2.2 Educational Materials

The ACSC developed the GDL model components for California from an evaluation of the GDL research literature (S. Bloch, personal communication, August 26, 2004). At the time the ACSC began evaluating research components, there was no overarching GDL model available for implementation, so they examined the various components that researchers and policy experts were talking about and developed a model based on what they wanted for California (S. Bloch, personal communication, August 26, 2004). This model was then modified during the legislative process, but the fundamental model of specific implementable proposals was developed by ACSC (S. Bloch, personal communication, August 26, 2004). In terms of educating the public and the legislature about the proposed GDL system in California, educational materials and folders were prepared for handing out to parents, teachers, etc., during legislative hearings and outreach presentations (A. Drumm, personal communication, August 2004).

After the GDL law came into effect, the California Department of Motor Vehicles (DMV) had to make changes to the California Driver Handbook which is an educational resource containing all of the information regarding the requirements teenagers need to qualify for a license. Also requiring modification was the Parent-Teen Driving Aid handbook that was developed to aid the parents of teenagers about how they can help provide their teenagers with additional driving practice (J. Curranco, personal communication, August 2004; National Conference of State Legislatures [NCSL], 2000).

24.2.3 Financial Costs (Licensing and Operations Division Pre-licensing Policy Section)

Since California already had a provisional license before the more comprehensive GDL plan was adopted, the DMV did not change many of the basic procedures to obtain the license, which cut down on costs. Furthermore, according to the DMV's pre-licensing policy section, a portion of the funds generated by the licensing fees helps to cover the cost of implementation and ongoing delivery of the system (J. Curranco, personal communication, August 2004). The costs connected with implementation were estimated by the legislature to be $41,520 in Fiscal Year 1997–1998 and $102,155 in the next fiscal year (NCSL, 2000). Funding was to be provided by the State General Fund to the Department of Motor Vehicles for implementation of the GDL program. This includes costs in changing the system programming and creating forms and written materials. According to a review of GDL systems by the National Conference of State Legislatures (2000), Walt Steuben, the chief of the DMV Justice and Government Liaison Office, believes these costs are "minimal, for the saving of teen lives" (NCSL, 2000).

24.3 Implementation

24.3.1 Effective Practices

24.3.1.1 Pre-implementation of GDL Legislation

After the legislation was introduced, the coalition of GDL law supporters set out to educate the public about the risks facing young drivers (e.g., nighttime driving, teen passengers) and about how the new GDL requirements being proposed could help save lives (A. Drumm, personal communication, August 2004). The coalition accomplished this through press releases, visits to high schools and parent teacher associations. Parents who had lost teenagers in MVCs testified before the legislature about the need for the new law, and their testimony was very meaningful and profound (A. Drumm, personal communication, August 2004).

The greatest challenge to the proposed GDL bill was the implementation of the nighttime driving restriction (A. Drumm, personal communication, August 2004). For example, some parents were concerned about their son or daughter not being able to drive home alone from work

late at night (after 11 pm). Other parents expressed concerns about school activities and questioned whether the legislation would prohibit, for example, their teen from driving to swim practice very early in the morning (before 5 am)—which fell within the restricted driving period. The bill was amended to address some of these concerns. Originally the bill was set to have a nighttime driving restriction from 11 pm to 5 am, but there was an amendment made that changed the restriction to start 1 h later at midnight (A. Drumm, personal communication, August 2004). Furthermore, exceptions were permitted for school, employment, family, and medical need as long as the young driver carried a statement from the appropriate school official, employer, doctor, or parent/guardian. A similar exemption was made for the passenger restriction component of the bill (A. Drumm, personal communication, August 2004).

While not compromising the overall safety benefits of the bill, these changes addressed concerns from some parents/guardians who were faced with transportation circumstances whereby the provisions of the bill could have been problematic (A. Drumm, personal communication, August 2004). The new law had to be workable for all parts of the state, including some of the unique rural California communities. Without public acceptance, this important public safety law could have been jeopardized (A. Drumm, personal communication, August 2004).

24.3.1.2 Post-implementation of GDL Legislation

After the GDL law came into effect, the California Department of Motor Vehicles (DMV) also set out to educate the public about the new requirements through press releases, visits to high schools and parent teacher association, and changes to the California Driver Handbook and the Parent Teen Driver Handbook (J. Curranco, personal communication, August 2004; NCSL, 2000).

Based on the SB 1329, the DMV was not only responsible for the process of licensing young drivers under the GDL law, but also for inspecting, licensing, and regulating state Driving

Schools and setting criteria for them to include in their lesson plans. Whenever the DMV receives new legislation relating to driving standards, they are required to then inform the driving schools about the new curriculum content so it can be included in programming (J. Curranco, personal communication, August 2004). Furthermore, whenever a new bill is passed and the DMV are responsible for implementing it, they have to change all of the driver handbooks and information on the websites to encompass the new information, which according to the DMV can be somewhat costly (J. Curranco, personal communication, August 2004).

Although politicians and traffic safety groups are normally the leaders in proposing changes to the legislation, on some occasions the DMV is proactive and proposes legislation to change components of the licensing system. When this occurs, the pre-licensing policy section of the DMVs licensing and operations division develops a proposal which then has to be approved by the immediate management, followed by the director of the division, and finally to the agency secretary who oversees the entire department. If it is approved at this level, then it is prepared into a proposal for legislation (J. Curranco, personal communication, August 2004). The evidence to support their proposals come from feedback and suggestions from the public in the form of letters or phone messages, internal (DMV Research and Development Division) and external research reports and national studies, or just based on their general observations and monitoring of the system over time (J. Curranco, personal communication, August 2004).

An example of a change to the GDL system that the DMV were responsible for concerned the age at which teenagers could take their first drivers education course. Originally, they were able to take a course at 15 years old, but that was changed to 15½, because that is the age teenagers are able to receive their learner's permit. The DMV felt that the teenagers would forget what they learned and find it difficult to apply the knowledge with the 6-month delay between education and permit to drive (J. Curranco, personal communication, August 2004).

24.3.2 Ongoing Evaluations

In addition to the general monitoring of the GDL system by the frontline workers and employees of the licensing and operations division and pre-licensing section of the DMV in charge of running the GDL system, the Research and Development Division of the DMV along with other public and private traffic safety research groups (e.g., ACSC, IIHS) are involved in ongoing evaluations of the effectiveness of the California GDL system. These research groups have studied not only the effectiveness of the California GDL system in saving lives, but also how well teenagers and parents (two main consumers of GDL) support and comply with the system requirements.

24.4 Outcome

The impact of California's GDL system on young drivers will be examined based on three evaluations that were conducted by separate traffic safety research groups in California including the IIHS, the Research and Development Branch of California's DMV, and the Southern California Injury Prevention Research Centre. The first study examines parents' and their teenagers' opinions regarding the California GDL system (Williams, Nelson, & Leaf, 2002); the second and third studies focus on determining how effective the system is in reducing injuries, fatalities, and overall MVCs for young drivers affected by the law (Masten & Hagge, 2003; Rice, Peek-Asa, & Kraus, 2004).

According to Williams, the senior vice president of the IIHS and chief scientist, it is important to examine how teens and their parents adjusted to California's rigorous new GDL law, because "safety benefits of graduated licensing will be limited if compliance isn't widespread" (IIHS, 2001, p. 4). Also, because California's system is one of the toughest in terms of its restrictions (e.g., no passengers under the age of 20 for first 6 months), the potential to inconvenience parents and young drivers is greatest due to the delay of mobility that was previously available to teens (IIHS, 2001). With these important factors in mind, Williams et al. (2002) investigated how families adjusted to California's tougher GDL law. Surveys were conducted to learn what teenagers and their parents thought about the new components and whether they reported any behavior change. There were two groups of beginning California license holders who were surveyed three times during the first year of licensure with their parents being interviewed twice. One group ($n = 543$) was subject to the new GDL requirements, while the other ($n = 814$) was not.

In general, the results indicated that parents strongly approved of the new GDL system. A large majority endorsed the new 6-month learning permit requirements, the nighttime restrictions, and slightly less for the passenger restrictions. Among parents whose teenagers were faced with the new requirements, 79% were strongly in favor of the GDL system and only 4% were neutral or opposed (Williams et al., 2002). Although teenagers were less approving of the new requirements, most accepted the new learner's permit rules, and the majority of teenagers favored the night restriction. Approximately one-third endorsed the passenger restriction. Despite compliance not being fully universal, the new requirements resulted in young drivers holding their learner's permits longer and accumulating more practice driving before licensure, as well as decreasing the amount of reported driving after midnight and the transportation of teenagers when drivers were initially licensed (Williams et al., 2002). Most teenagers subject to the new rules said they were able to do the activities they wanted despite the changes. Almost three-quarters said they were not affected much by either the nighttime or passenger restriction. An important factor to note is that the post-GDL group surveyed was the first group to go through a GDL system that may have appeared to take away some mobility that was previously available to young people. Therefore, in succeeding years, when the new rules have become the norm, they are likely to become even more acceptable than what this study demonstrated (Williams et al., 2002). A few limitations of the study should

be noted for their possible effects on the results: (1) since the survey was primarily based on self-reported data and involved the recollection of past events, both these factors can produce incorrect reporting, including the possibility that parents and teens may have overstated compliance with the new rules; (2) although every DMV region in California was included, the samples were not necessarily representative of teenagers getting licensed during these periods (Williams et al., 2002). Overall the results indicate that the new licensing system is favorably accepted by teenagers and their parents and has substantially increased the types of behaviors that collectively are expected to lead to MVCs and injury reductions (Williams et al., 2002). These reductions in MVCs, injuries, and fatalities have been found and will be examined next.

A study by the DMV's Research and Development Branch (Masten & Hagge, 2003) analyzed several different crash types and age groups (notably the 15–17 age group), using time series analysis and flexible intervention start points to determine whether the enhancements made to the California's teen licensing program in July 1998 resulted in MVC reductions for teen drivers. Furthermore, the collision rates for adult drivers aged 24–55 were used as a control series in a few of the analyses to account for history-related factors that would have affected collisions for both age groups. What are notable among the findings are the significant reductions in injuries and fatalities specific to the introduced nighttime driving and passenger restrictions. In particular, the 12-month nighttime restriction was associated with a sudden-permanent 0.44% reduction in total crashes happening during the hours of midnight to 5 am for 15–17-year-olds starting 1 year following the implementation of the nighttime restriction. The results also suggested a significant sudden-permanent 0.45% reduction in teenage nighttime injury/fatal MVCs starting 1 year following the program implementation. These effects translate into savings of 153 total collisions and 68 injury collisions annually for 15–17-year-olds (Masten & Hagge, 2003).

In terms of the 6-month passenger restriction, it was associated with a marginally significant sudden-permanent 2.52% reduction in 15–17-year-old total teen passenger collisions, and a significant gradual-permanent reduction stabilizing at −6.43% in fatal/injury passenger collisions when using an intervention date 1 year following the program start date. These effects translate to savings of 878 total collisions and 975 fatal/injury collisions annually for 15–17-year-olds (Masten & Hagge, 2003).

Although these reductions in fatalities and injuries were found regarding nighttime and passenger restrictions, the researchers did not find a significant decrease in overall MVCs or fatalities and provided a number of reasons for this finding (Masten & Hagge, 2003). For instance, they suggest that conducting an analysis using a more sensitive measure might have captured the nighttime and passenger restriction effects among the total reductions in MVC (R. A. Hagge, personal communication, July 2004). Furthermore, since a significant reduction in young driver MVC was found when the first provisional licensing program was implemented in 1983 (including some components of the current system), the authors suggest that it is possible that the pre-GDL collision rates already reflected the influence of collision reductions associated with the original teen licensing program evaluated by Hagge and Marsh (1988). Despite this, the researchers believe that California's GDL system is currently an exemplar practice in preventing young driver fatalities and injuries but should be continually improved upon in order to become more effective in saving lives (R. A. Hagge, personal communication, July 2004).

A study by Rice et al. (2004) evaluated the effectiveness of California's rigorous GDL system using a pre-post design and found large reductions in injury and fatal MVCs for young drivers. The researchers used fatal and injury collision data of 16- and 17-year-old drivers for 1-year pre-GDL (1997) and for 2 years post-GDL implementation (2000–2001). The control group consisted of young adult drivers aged 25–34. The researchers chose this age group as the control because of similar influencing factors affecting their lives and the lives of young drivers (Rice et al., 2004). Across the pre- and post-GDL time periods, overall trends in young driver MVC rates were examined by estimating and comparing per-capita collision rates. Pre-GDL rates were compared individually with rates from each of the two post-GDL time periods, and an adjusted rate ratio method was used to estimate the change in teenage driver rates compared to the control group between time periods (Rice et al., 2004).

The results of the analyses demonstrate that the implementation of California's GDL law was followed by significant decreases in both severe/fatal and minor injury collisions for 16- and 17-year-old drivers (Rice et al., 2004). For instance, the overall fatal/severe injury collision rates significantly decreased by 28% from 1997 to 2000 and by 17% between 1997 and 2001 for young drivers. Based on the adjusted rate ratios, the researchers were able to estimate that in both the 2000 and 2001 post-GDL periods, the expected number of fatal/severe injury collisions was reduced by 400 with the expected number of minor injury collisions reduced by more than 3000 (Rice et al., 2004).

Also notable among the findings is that the biggest reduction in fatal/severe collision rates (35–36%) was observed during the GDL night driving restriction between midnight and 5 am. Similar to Masten and Hagge's (2003) study, Rice et al. (2004) have also demonstrated the success of California's nighttime restriction in reducing teenage driving during these high-risk hours and ultimately reducing fatal/severe injury collisions. In terms of the effectiveness of the passenger restriction, the number of 16-year-old drivers in the sample who were only carrying passengers dropped by more than a third in both of the post-GDL years. This finding suggests that the GDL system had a beneficial effect on the unsupervised carrying of teenage passengers (Rice et al., 2004).

Overall, based on the examination of these three studies evaluating the effectiveness of California's GDL system, it is evident that the primary goals for implementing California's SB 1329 were met.

24.5 Conclusions

Although the risks associated with the young driver issue are complex in nature, California's multi-staged, GDL system contains many important elements that target the known risk factors associated with the overrepresentation of young drivers in MVCs (e.g., age, inexperience, night-time driving, and teenage passengers) and has been regarded as one of the strongest GDL systems to date (D. Mayhew, personal communication, July 2004; Williams & Mayhew, 2004). In addition, this multifaceted system targets all four quadrants of the young driver's life space as discussed earlier, which in theory creates a more effective intervention strategy in reducing injuries (Volpe, 2004).

The California GDL program evaluated in this report is considered to be one of the strongest in North America; however, there are additional features that could be added or improved that may help to strengthen the program (Masten & Hagge, 2003; Rice et al., 2004). In addition to beginning the nighttime restriction at an earlier time and finding ways to raise compliance with the nighttime and passenger restrictions, the program could be improved by making a teenager's advancement from one stage of licensure to another reliant upon sustaining a collision- and violation-free driving record (Masten & Hagge, 2003). Furthermore, it has been suggested that compliance with the nighttime and passenger restrictions could be elevated by allowing law enforcement officers to stop teenagers because they believe they are violating these limits (i.e., primary enforcement) instead of waiting for another violation to occur first (secondary enforcement; R. A. Hagge, personal communication, July 2004; Masten & Hagge, 2003). Also, to increase compliance of these restrictions, it is suggested that stronger penalties be imposed by the DMV. Presently, teenagers who violate their licensing laws in California only receive a small fine or community service duty through the courts and are not subjected to losing demerit points or their license by the DMV. This latter consequence has been suggested to be an action that would further deter teenagers from driving in riskier situations (Masten & Hagge, 2003). Despite these criticisms, California's GDL system remains one of the strongest in North America.

Acknowledgments The author would like to express sincere appreciation to the key informants for this case study: Anne Drumm of the American Automobile Association in Sacramento, CA, USA and Juanita Curranco of the California Department of Motor Vehicles in Sacramento, CA, USA—whose consultation made this project possible.

BRIO Model: Graduated Driver Licensing Program, California

Group Served: Young novice drivers.

Goal: To help combat the high rate of collisions involving young novice drivers.

Background	Resources	Implementation	Outcome
California was one of the first jurisdictions to implement a few basic elements of a preliminary GDL model (provisional licensing) in 1983, which was shown to be effective in reducing MVCs among young drivers July 1998 a more comprehensive and rigorous GDL law was implemented, entitled "Brady/Jared Teen Driver Safety Act of 1997" after two teens who were killed in MVCs in California	Primary collaborators before the law was passed were the Automobile Club of Southern California (ACSC) and the California State Automobile Association After the law came into effect, the California Department of Motor Vehicle (DMV) was responsible for a portion, with an entire coalition of stakeholders and supporters consisting over 50 different traffic safety groups, parent and teacher associations, injury prevention groups, law enforcement officials, and medical professionals Costs were minimal as the DMV did not have to change many of the basic procedures of obtaining the license	The model consists of 3 stages: learner's permit, provisional/intermediate license, full license After the law came into effect, supporters set out to educate the public through press releases, high school visits, and parent–teacher associations Greatest challenge was the implementation of the nighttime driving restriction, which was successfully compromised on after much debate DMV responsible for licensing young drivers as well as inspecting and regulating state driving schools and setting criteria, as well as implementing and communicating any changes in law Evaluations continue to occur	Separate traffic safety research groups examined the impact of California's GDL system Results from the studies generally indicate that parents strongly approved Significant reductions in injuries and fatalities specific to the introduced nighttime driving and passenger restrictions were witnessed

Life Space Model: Graduated Driver Licensing Program, California

Sociocultural: civilization/community	Interpersonal: primary and secondary relationships	Physical environments: where we live	Internal states: biochemical/genetic and means of coping
Overall support and compliance for CA's GDL by parents and teens, safety groups, politicians, and others within the CA communities Parents and police will be the primary enforcers of this legislation in order to ensure teenagers are following the restrictions	Young drivers will have to learn to say no to their teenage peers who want to drive around with them while unsupervised by an adult Teenagers are being trained and supervised while driving with their parents or guardian during the learner's permit stage and the intermediate GDL stage	Teenagers will not be allowed to drive when it is nighttime unless supervised by an adult	Teenagers, passengers, and parents will understand the importance of complying with the passenger and nighttime restriction for their safety and well being

References

American Automobile Association. (2004). Teen drivers: A guide to graduated driver license.: Retrieved August 12, 2004, from http://www.csaa.com/global/articledetail/0,1398,1004040000%257C1274,00.html

Boase, P., & Tasca, L. (1998). *Graduated licensing system evaluation: Interim report.* Toronto, ON: Safety Policy Branch, Ontario Ministry of Transportation.

California State Senate. (1997). Legislative Council Digest: Senate Bill 1329 Introduction.: Retrieved August 1, 2004, from http://info.sen.ca.gov/cgi-bin/postquery?bill_number=sb_1329&sess=9798&house=B&site=sen

Canadian Paraplegic Association. (2000). *Spinal cord injury in Canada.* Ottawa. Retrieved August 1, 2004, from www.canparaplegic.org

Chen, L. H., Baker, S. P., Braver, E. R., & Li, G. (2000). Carrying passengers as a risk factor for crashes fatal to 16- and 17-Year-old drivers. *Journal of the American Medical Association, 283,* 1578–1582.

Department of Motor Vehicles. (2004). Driver License and Identification Card Information: How to apply for a provisional permit if you are under 18. Retrieved August 13, 2004, from http://www.dmv.ca.gov/dl/dl_info.htm#PERMINOR

Haddon, W. Jr. (1980). Advances in the epidemiology of injuries as a basis for public policy. *Public Health Reports, 95*(5), 411–421.

Hagge, R. A., & Marsh, W. C. (1988). *The traffic safety impact of provisional licensing* (Report No. 116). Sacramento: California Department of Motor Vehicles.

Insurance Institute for Highway Safety. (2001). *Status Report, 36*(6), 4–5.

Insurance Institute for Highway Safety & National Highway Traffic Safety Administration (2004). *Questions & answers: Teenagers: Graduated driver licensing.* Online report. Retrieved July 21, 2004, from http://www.iihs.org/safety_facts/qanda/images/grad_lic.pdf

Lin, M. L., & Fearn, K. T. (2003). The provisional license: Nighttime and passenger restrictions. *Journal of Safety Research, 34*(1), 49–51.

Masten, S. V., & Hagge, R. A. (2003). *Evaluation of California's graduated driver licensing program.* California Department of Motor Vehicles, Report RSS 03-205.

Mayhew, D. R., Simpson, H. M., & Pak, A. (2003). Changes in collision rates among novice drivers during the first months of driving. *Accident Analysis Prevention, 35*(5), 683–691.

National Conference of State Legislatures. (2000). *NCSL transportation review: Graduated Licensing for Teen Drivers.* Retrieved July 21, 2004, from http://www.ncsl.org/programs/transportation/trgradli.htm

Ontario Ministry of Transportation. (2002). *Ontario road safety annual report 2002: Building safe communities.* Safety Education Policy Branch. Retrieved July 20, 2004, from http://www.mto.gov.on.ca/english/safety/orsar/orsar02/summary.htm

Rice, T. M., Peek-Asa, C., & Kraus, J. F. (2004). Effects of the California graduated driver licensing program. *Journal of Safety Research, 35*(4), 375–381.

Simpson, H. M. (2003). Evolution and effectiveness of graduated licensing. *Journal of Safety Research, 34,* 25–34.

SMARTRISK Foundation. (1998). *The economic burden of unintentional injury in Canada.* Toronto, ON: SMARTRISK Foundation.

Takhar, H. (2004). *Introduction of an act to enhance the safety of children and youth on Ontario's roads.* Statement by the Ontario Minister of Transportation, Queen's Park, Toronto. Retrieved June 20, 2004, from http://www.mto.gov.on.ca/english/news/statements/stat040504.htm

Trauma Foundation. (2004). Making change happen: Over 25 years of injury prevention. Retrieved August 13, 2004, from http://www.tf.org/tf/images/TFOverview.pdf

Volpe, R. (2004). *The conceptualization of injury prevention as change in complex systems. Life Span Adaptation Projects.* Toronto: University of Toronto.

Williams, A. F. (2001). Barriers and opportunities in reducing motor vehicle injuries. *Injury Prevention, 7,* 83–84.

Williams, A. F. (2003). Teenage drivers: Patterns of risk. *Journal of Safety Research, 34,* 5–15.

Williams, A. F., & Mayhew, D. R. (2004). *Graduated licensing: A blueprint for North America.* Arlington, VA: Insurance Institute for Highway Safety. Retrieved July 1, 2003, from http://www.highwaysafety.org/safety_facts/teens/blueprint.pdf

Williams, A. F., Nelson, L. A., & Leaf, W. A. (2002). Responses of teenagers and their parents to California's graduated licensing system. *Accident Analysis and Prevention, 34*(6), 835–842.

Yaksich Jr., S. (1982). Teenagers under attack. *Journal of Traffic Safety Education, 29,* 7–11.

DriveABLE Assessment Centers Inc.

25

Daniella Semotok

The DriveABLE Assessment Program began by targeting the vulnerable driver population of older adults. DriveABLE targets all ages that may have cognitive impairments as a result of medical conditions or medications. By combining technology and research, the DriveABLE Assessment program aims to aid those who suffer from medical conditions, often brought on by aging which influences driving competence. The program is exemplar in the way it targets a wide variety of medical conditions, and its comprehensive approach of including physicians as the basis of referrals and implementing assessment programs that allow for older drivers to continue driving. DriveABLE provides service, software, and hardware solutions for commercial fleets, governments, insurers, and the medical community to help determine if medical conditions have affected one's driving competence and ability, also described as "driver risk assessment" (J. Brown, personal communication, 2018).

25.1 Background

25.1.1 Description of Consumers

The target population for the DriveABLE Assessment Program are drivers who suffer from a medical condition that can affect their driving competence. Such medical conditions can include cardiovascular and cerebrovascular disease, stroke, dementia, long-standing diabetes, neurological disorders, sleep disturbance, head injury, and psychiatric disorders, in addition to certain medications (DriveABLE, n.d.). Although the DriveABLE Assessment program is essentially for an individual of any age with a medical condition which can interfere with driving, a high proportion of individuals referred to DriveABLE are over the age of 65. The high proportion of older drivers is because of the strong association between age and having one or more medical conditions that can affect driving abilities. As mentioned earlier, there are a high proportion of older adult collision fatalities and injuries as well as a number of individuals driving who have medical conditions which can affect their driving ability. Nevertheless, the demographic characteristics of the target population vary because a medical condition may affect an individual regardless of age or status. What does make this population specific is that they are road users and have a medical condition that puts them at-risk for being unsafe to drive.

D. Semotok (✉)
Toronto District School Board, Oakville, ON, Canada
e-mail: daniella.semotok@tdsb.on.ca

© Springer Nature Switzerland AG 2020
R. Volpe (ed.), *Casebook of Traumatic Injury Prevention*,
https://doi.org/10.1007/978-3-030-27419-1_25

25.1.2 History and Development of DriveABLE

The DriveABLE Assessment Centre was originally started as a research endeavor to assess fitness to drive of an individual whose competence to drive is questionable due to the onset or progression of a medical condition. Because scientifically justifiable assessments were not available, a research program was initiated in 1991 by Dr. Allen Dobbs, who was the Director of the Neurocognitive Research Unit within the Northern Alberta Geriatric Program. Dr. Dobbs had an established interest in cognitive impairment in association with executing daily activities. This research commenced with a scientific approach, unlike other previous research in this area. The approach used was to first establish the driving errors of healthy drivers, in order to have a starting point for determining driving errors due to medical impairments (A. Dobbs, personal communication, 2004). The reasoning behind this is that normal, healthy drivers often make mistakes while driving. Thus, persons with medical disabilities should not be penalized for making driving errors typical of the general driving population. However, the errors made by cognitively impaired and unsafe drivers are likely to be different from those made by healthy drivers. That knowledge was thought to be basic to being able to identify medically impaired drivers and protect the healthy competent drivers from being inappropriately evaluated as unsafe and unfit to operate a vehicle. The researchers believed that a defensible driving evaluation must be able to justify with scientific evidence why specific errors are taken as competence indicators. Although errors made by healthy drivers are not justified through this process, it is the necessary beginning point in identifying driving errors signaling the driver is medically impaired. The medically impaired criterion could be assigned when the driver made driving errors that are beyond those of healthy drivers.

The next step in this process was to develop a road course that would reveal the driving errors specific to cognitively impaired, unsafe road users. Scientific data derived from the research was used to identify where on the road course the competence-defining driving errors occurred. The attributes of those locations (number of lanes, speed, controlled/uncontrolled intersection, visual sight lines, and clutter, etc.) were then analyzed to identify the road-course attributes needed to reveal the critical driving errors. These road course attributes were defined in a way that effective road courses could be replicated in multiple locations (DriveABLE, 2003a).

The first study conducted by Dr. Dobbs and his researchers was to determine the driving errors of healthy drivers and those of cognitively impaired drivers. Through a comparison of these driving errors, the goal was to identify the driving mistakes that differentiate the medically impaired drivers. The healthy driver samples consisted of a group of young drivers aged 30–40 years old and an older group of drivers aged 65 and over. This research study also included a sample of drivers who were cognitively impaired. In the first study nearly all of the drivers suffered from dementia but were licensed and currently driving. This group was established as the "unsafe driving" group, because the literature showed high crash rates among persons with dementia. All participants completed visual, motor, balance, mental testing by the Rehabilitation Medicine department of an Edmonton Hospital, and a domain approach defined set of neuropsychological tests administered by the Neuropsychology department of that hospital. The Rehabilitation Medicine testing was designed by occupational therapists. The neuropsychology testing was developed by selecting tests from different domains of mental abilities relevant for driving. The participants in the study also were engaged in a number of research tests that were selected or designed by the research team. Instead of following the domain approach, these tasks recognized the complexity of the driving task. The selected tasks were complex and required the concurrent use of mental abilities from different domains or shifting among domains (A. Dobbs, personal communication, 2004).

After the in-office testing, all participants were assessed through the use of a carefully planned road evaluation. All driving errors were recorded using the provincial licensing standards and criteria. Using the provincial standards, 28% of the healthy drivers failed the road test. This confirmed the research team's suspicions that not all driving errors are competence defining errors. Some are just bad-habit errors of competent drivers (A. Dobbs, personal communication, 2004).

The errors committed by the three groups were compared to identify the type, frequency, and severity that are associated with cognitively impaired unsafe drivers and those that are the driving errors of healthy competent drivers. The results of this study provided the researchers with a base of knowledge regarding the driving errors of unsafe drivers suffering from medical impairments (DriveABLE, 2003a).

The next step in this process was to discover the road course attributes necessary to reveal the driving errors that are associated with declines in driving competence due to a medical condition. Scientific data derived from the research was used to define the critical driving errors. The attributes of the road course associated with high frequencies of these critical errors were studied. Based on the findings, criteria were developed for laying out a road course that would have elements known to reveal competence-defining errors. In addition, the road course criteria had to be developed in a way that they could be used to replicate effective road courses in multiple locations (DriveABLE, 2003a; A. Dobbs, personal communication, 2004).

In addition to producing a road course assessment, the team developed a cognitive evaluation. This process was also based on scientific data and was representative of driving performance. The approach focused on assessing the cognitive abilities that are associated with driving that require different domains and abilities. This was executed as an in-office evaluation and is computer presented and scored. The computer testing is presented in a touch-screen fashion and is easy to use, regardless of computer experience. There were over 500 participants who assisted in testing the in-office evaluation (DriveABLE, 2003a).

Validation research for the computer presented cognitive assessment test and the road test was also conducted using a sample of over 400 participants. This sample included individuals with varying medical conditions resulting in cognitive decline, and with a wide age range. The results of the study showed that the criteria that had been developed for the road test were valid. As well, the computer screen test was an excellent predictor for actual driving performance. The researchers found that there was 95% accuracy in identifying impaired drivers in comparison to safe drivers (A. Dobbs, personal communication, 2004). It has been noted that DriveABLE has utilized the largest sample that has ever been tested for cognitive ability, physical capabilities, and driving patterns in any other study worldwide (DriveABLE, n.d.; A. Dobbs, personal communication, 2004).

25.2 Resources

25.2.1 Collaborators During the Developmental Research

There were a number of individuals who assisted during the developmental research. The research team from the Neurocognitive Research Program, first of the Edmonton General Hospital and later the Neurocognitive Research Unit of the Glenrose Rehabilitation Hospital consisted of the following members: Allen Dobbs, PhD Director and Research Psychologist, Donald Schopflocher PhD Biostatistician, Robert Heller PhD Cognitive Psychologist, Bonnie Dobbs PhD Gerontologist, and Barbara Carstensen RN, BSc the Research Coordinator. As well, Medical, Rehabilitation Medicine, Neuropsychological evaluation expertise, and Hospital Administration support was provided by personnel from the Edmonton General Hospital and the Glenrose Rehabilitation Hospital. This included the following individuals: Peter McCracken, MD, FRCPC (Chief of Geriatric Medicine, Chair of the Division of Geriatric Medicine), Jean Triscott, MD, CCFP, FAAFP (Family physician, head of the Memory Clinic), Ivan Kiss, PhD Neuropsychologist (Neurocognitive Research Unit and Neuropsychology Department), Denise Walters, Executive Director, Edmonton

General Hospital, Nancy Renolds, Vice President, Special Initiatives, Edmonton General Hospital, Debora Cartwright, OT, Head Rehabilitation Medicine, Edmonton General Hospital, Linda Barrett, Director of Northern Alberta Geriatric Program, and Sandra Chaley, OT (A. Dobbs, personal communication, 2004). In addition, the Alberta Government provided assistance during the development of the program: Catarina Versaeval, Executive Director, Seniors Directorate, Ministry Responsible for Seniors; convened government group, and Representatives from Alberta Transportation, Solicitor General, Alberta Health and Wellness. There were many other individuals who took part in the collaboration process of the research. Supplementary support was provided by Alberta Motor Association (CAA Alberta), driving evaluators during the developmental and validation phases, the nursing staff from the Memory Clinic, neuropsychology test administrators, rehabilitation medicine assessors, and research assistants for the in-office test development and validation and closed course driving evaluation,

The resources for the DriveABLE program fall into two categories: Initial support for the research phase and the post research phase when DriveABLE was founded and began delivering driving assessments (A. Dobbs, personal communication, 2004).

25.2.2 Initial Support for the Research

25.2.2.1 Financial Support

The grant funding for the research phase was provided by Alberta Mental Health Research Fund ($80,000), Alberta Health Services Research Innovation Fund ($302,397), Alberta Heritage Foundation for Medical Research ($40,000), Alzheimer Society of Canada ($99,905), and the Canadian Aging Research Network (Network of Centers of Excellence Program: $246,165; A. Dobbs, personal communication, 2004). As well, the following provided in-kind funding and support: Department of Psychology at the University of Alberta, Edmonton General Hospital, Glenrose Rehabilitation Hospital, and

the Alberta Motor Association. Additionally, the National Research Council IRAP commercialization grant ($23,800) and the Alberta Heritage Foundation for Medical Research Technology Commercialization Phase II ($150,000) and Phase III ($500,000) funds have been awarded to enhance the evaluation and quality assurance software and to further the development and expansion of DriveABLE Assessment Centers.

25.2.2.2 Supporters of the Research

Physicians such as Peter McCracken and Jean Triscott as well as other physicians were instrumental in requesting the development of a driving assessment program. These physicians, along with 50 community physicians and the Alberta Transportation Driver Records, provided the referrals for the research project (A. Dobbs, personal communication, 2004). Letters of support were also provided by The Alberta Council on Aging, Alberta Motor Association (CAA Alberta), Chair, Medical Advisory Board of Alberta Transportation, and the Northern Alberta Regional Geriatric Program, Capital Health Authority (A. Dobbs, personal communication, 2004).

25.2.3 Post-Research: The Founding of DriveABLE Assessment Centers Inc.

In 1998 when the research process was complete, there was overwhelming support toward the development of an assessment process based on the research results and means of delivering that assessment. This was recognition of need for taking the research information to the next level in creating an assessment process (A. Dobbs, personal communication, 2004). The unique situation of DriveABLE is that it is a program which stemmed out of a validated and scientific research process. The University of Alberta encouraged the development, and thus, DriveABLE was established as a spin-off company from the University (DriveABLE, n.d.).

The establishment of DriveABLE required equipment, software development, and training of personnel. The end result was a DriveABLE center which conducted computer-based competency tests in addition to road tests for drivers whose abilities were questionable. The DriveABLE centers that were in operation were licensed to use the DriveABLE system, and receive equipment, software, training, and road course setup from the company. In 2004, DriveABLE had 20 Assessment Centers in Canada, five in Florida, and New York and Colorado also have licensed centers (A. Dobbs, personal communication, 2004).

25.2.4 Support for the DriveABLE Assessment

Encouragement for the DriveABLE Assessment Centers was provided by many organizations. These include: Regional Chairs Committee, Alberta Health Regions; Alberta Council on Aging; John Eberhard, PhD, Senior Research Psychologist and Chair, Transportation Research Board Older Driver Program, National Highway Traffic Safety Administration, US Department of Transportation; John Arnold, Chief Scientist, National Research Council; Palliser Health Authority, Alberta; Lakeland Regional Health Authority, Alberta; Provincial Health Authorities of Alberta, College of Physicians and Surgeons, Alberta; Alberta Medical Association, Minister of Health and Wellness, Alberta Health and Wellness, Minister of Transportation, Alberta Transportation, Florida Atlantic University, Boca Raton, Senior Resource Alliance, Area Agency on Aging, Orlando, Florida, and the Parker Jewish Geriatric Institute, New York (A. Dobbs, personal communication, 2004). The number of supporters continues to grow as DriveABLE continually expands throughout Canada and the United States.

25.3 Implementation

25.3.1 Effective Practices

DriveABLE centers use the same evaluation process, which has two components: a computer-based cognitive assessment and a road evaluation.

The purpose of the in-office testing is to increase the safety of the evaluation by identifying the most dangerous drivers without the need for a road test (DriveABLE, n.d.). If the road test is necessary, it is administered by specialized driving evaluators who have received training from DriveABLE. As well, the vehicle that is used for the road evaluation is equipped with dual-brake for additional safety.

The computer-based cognitive assessment is referred to the DriveABLE Cognitive Assessment Tool (DCAT). The DCAT consists of six tasks that measure cognitive processes that are essential for safe driving and predict on-road performance. Thus, the aim is to identify—through hardware and software—medically at-risk drivers (DriveABLE, 2016a). Specifically, this tool uses a "plug-and-play system" that comprises a touch screen and a three-button base (DriveABLE, 2016a). It accurately measures the following aspects of driving: motor speed and control, speed of attentional shifting, span of attentional field, coordination of mental abilities, identification of driving situations, and spatial judgment and decision making (J. Brown, personal communication, 2018; DriveABLE 2016a). Refer to Box 25.1 for a detailed description of the six tasks (J. Brown, personal communication, 2018).

Box 25.1 Tasks of the DriveABLE Cognitive Assessment Tool (DCAT)

1. Reaction time: Client is asked to hold down a button until a shape appears on the screen, then reach up and touch it as quickly as possible.
2. Attentional field: Client is asked to make a decision about shapes in a box seen in the middle of the screen while trying to identify the location of a dot somewhere around the periphery of the box. This task measures possible narrowing or deficit areas in the peripheral field
3. Spatial judgment: A series of lines run up and down the screen, and the client is asked to move a box safely through

(continued)

(continued)

the lines at the first opportunity. This is representative of judgment being made at intersections which happens to be one of the largest areas of concern with cognitively impaired drivers

4. Attentional shifting: This measures the clients' ability to react to cued and mis-cued information being presented and the speed of processing or delays. The client is asked to touch a button on the side where a number sign (#) appears in a box. Cues include: central, where an arrow points to a box and peripheral, where one of the boxes lights up

5. Executive decision making: This task looks at how a client can store memory while still performing tasks. In the baseline, the client is simply asked to track X's as they appear in boxes. In the second level, the client is asked to touch the box where the X just appeared. This task has a number of relevant measures for driving, including disengagement, focus, working memory, and executive decision making

6. Identification of hazardous situations: The client watches a driving scene and chooses the best of four answers presented after the scene. The client has limited time to make the decision, which is similar to real life driving, where you must make the best decision possible in the quickest time

The DriveABLE road course is referred to as the DriveABLE On-Road Evaluation (DORE). This is a scientifically developed on-road evaluation that tests specifically for decline in cognitive skills. Unlike other road tests, the DORE tests for cognitive impairment—not bad-habit errors that are common among experienced drivers (DriveABLE, 2016a). It compares the driving errors of healthy drivers against drivers that are otherwise cognitively impaired. It set out to evaluate driving characteristics which are specific to drivers with cognitive impairments. No penalties are given for errors which would be characteristic of normal, healthy drivers.

The results are discussed with the driver, as well as sent to the physician involved (typically a family physician), and to driver licensing bureaus in some locations and depending on the referring physician's directive. The DriveABLE assessor often asks that a family member remain present during the explanation of the process. This is to ensure that another individual, besides the person being assessed, is present to understand the process that is occurring.

25.3.2 Actors in the Decision Making

The purpose of DriveABLE Assessment Centers is to be a widely available injury prevention program for individuals of all ages who suffer from a medical condition which can impair driving ability (DriveABLE, n.d.). Physicians value this program because of the scientific basis on which it was developed and also because it allows them to refer an individual to be assessed, rather than make that judgment decision on their own (A. Dobbs, personal communication, 2004). In many ways the DriveABLE program helps to protect the physician-patient relationship. This can occur when a patient's license is revoked, and there may be strong implications on the relationship between the patient and the physician (DriveABLE, 2003a).

Referrals for DriveABLE are accepted from Physicians, Licensing Authorities, and Insurance Agencies and from family members and friends of the driver in question. When an individual is referred from a family member or friend, it is asked that a physician be notified and be involved in the decision-making process (DriveABLE, n.d.). A driving evaluation is often needed when medical conditions result in impairments that negatively affect driving. Some of the identified "red flag" medical conditions are as follows (DriveABLE, 2003a):

- Cardiovascular disease, if associated with cerebral ischemia
- Cerebrovascular disease

- Head trauma, including traumatic brain injury
- Chronic respiratory diseases
- Cognitive impairments and dementia
- Psychiatric disease, including schizophrenia, personality disorder, and chronic alcohol abuse
- Certain medications, including anti-depressants and anti-histamines
- Neurological diseases, including multiple sclerosis and Parkinson's disease

25.3.3 Execution

DriveABLE currently receives no government funding and is currently a for-profit business (J. Brown, personal communication, 2018). However, there is reimbursement available for clients.

In Ontario, the Ministry of Transportation (MTO) has licensed sites. The MTO requires mandatory reporting by physicians when they come across any "red-flag" medical conditions or individuals who have any driving-related cognitive difficulties (J. Brown, personal communication, 2018). If a physician was not to report this to the MTO, they would be found liable and fined (J. Brown, personal communication, 2018). Once reported to the MTO, there is a review of the individual, and subsequently, they are sent to the appropriate testing, which may be DriveABLE. If it is DriveABLE, the client is responsible for paying for the testing, which is approximately $700.00 (J. Brown, personal communication, 2018). After being evaluated, those results are sent back to MTO and a board of MTO medical officers review the results and determine any next steps. At this point, the MTO is who determines how long individuals are cleared to drive or have to be retested or reviewed—not DriveABLE (J. Brown, personal communication, 2018).

Conversely, in British Columbia and Alberta, DriveABLE is no longer used as a primary tool. Instead, if a doctor was to refer someone to a DriveABLE licensed site, the results would go to the doctor. Moreover, in Manitoba, DriveABLE is provided through public insurance, who also pays for testing. The provincial driving licensing

organizations are not involved in this process (J. Brown, personal communication, 2018).

In the United States, the system is different because Medicare and Medicate pay for the testing. DriveABLE does offer the physicians reimbursement codes for providing and implementing assessments, which has proved to result in a large growth in the United States because of this incentive and lack of burden on individuals (J. Brown, personal communication, 2018). Unfortunately, medical authorities in Canada have yet to find a way to implement DriveABLE into their provincial health plans as it is not seen as a necessary aspect (J. Brown, personal communication, 2018).

25.3.4 Ongoing Evaluation

DriveABLE has been involved in performing ongoing evaluation in several ways:

25.3.4.1 Equal Testing for Urban and Rural Road Users

There was an ongoing evaluation conducted for determining equal fairness of the DriveABLE assessment process for both urban and rural drivers. In order to assess this, DriveABLE compared the outcome of the evaluation for urban and rural drivers who had been to DriveABLE for an assessment. The sample of rural and urban drivers was closely matched on diagnosis, age, sex, and their score on a test regarding cognitive abilities (MMSE). After the individuals in the sample completed the DriveABLE assessment, the results were evaluated. The findings showed that there was essentially no difference in the pass and fail rates of the matched rural and urban samples. Thus, the evidence indicates that there is scientific confirmation that the procedures are equally fair for both urban and rural drivers who are assessed by DriveABLE.

25.3.4.2 Standardization and Quality Assurance Procedures

DriveABLE is involved in ensuring standardization and quality assurance in three ways (DriveABLE, 2003b):

1. Setup and training for DriveABLE Assessment Centers
   (a) All individuals involved in administering the DriveABLE in-office assessment and road evaluation are certified after receiving personalized, on-site training from DriveABLE personnel.
   (b) The design of the road course is also critical to ensuring standardization. Each road course is set out by DriveABLE personnel based on specified elements. Although it is true that no two road courses are completely alike, the elements that are sought after for the design of the course are those that have been shown by research to disclose driving errors.
2. Final standardization of the road course is also achieved across DriveABLE licensed centers by calibrating the fail criterion to match the difficulty of the road course. As well, the competence screen assessment is the same at all locations, and the outcomes are sent to the main DriveABLE location in Edmonton for scoring.
3. Quality assurance is monitored in several ways:
   (a) Authenticating the known relationship among cognitive assessment tasks at each site over time.
   (b) Re-confirmation of calibration for standardization of the road test at scheduled times.
   (c) Assessing road test evaluators by validating that expected errors occur in specific areas which the research identified as being associated with specific types of driving errors.
   (d) Also, there are evaluations of road test examiners scoring results by comparing his or her rating of driving with scores given for the driver errors.

DriveABLE takes pride in their level of standardization and ongoing monitoring and evaluation. It is felt that with a high level of standardization, physicians and driver licensing agencies should feel confident in their assessment practices (A. Dobbs, personal communica-tion, 2004). In addition, DriveABLE is currently updating the software they use to provide more automated quality assurance procedures (DriveABLE, n.d.).

The DriveABLE program has made efforts to have a variety of meetings with physicians in different provinces regarding the usability of the DriveABLE report forms. Suggestions and feedback made by physicians and reviewing officers within licensing authorities have been taken into consideration, and forms have been modified into the most usable way (A. Dobbs, personal communication, 2004).

A survey was also conducted by DriveABLE with 117 people and their caregivers who had completed the driving assessment process. This sample represented individuals who were asked to stop driving due to an unsafe level of errors from the DriveABLE evaluation. The survey found that 27% of these individuals continued to drive, with their caregivers reporting incidences of a crash or close call by these drivers (A. Dobbs, personal communication, 2004).

25.4 Outcome

The outcome of DriveABLE licensing has been overwhelmingly positive. One way of defining the success of DriveABLE is by its acceptance throughout Canada, as well as the United States (A. Dobbs, personal communication, 2004). In recent years, DriveABLE Head Office has stopped providing assessment services. Instead, DriveABLE provides the technology and training to licensed and certified organizations in order to create licensed assessment providers. This is for a variety of reasons, most notably that each province, state, or country can have different rules pertaining to driver fitness, and it would be inefficient for DriveABLE to have multiple centers all over North America when such variables exist. Licensed assessment providers are available across Canada, across the United States of America, and in Auckland, New Zealand. For a complete list of current licensed sites, visit https://driveable.com/index.php/get-an-assessment/licensed-sites (DriveABLE, 2016b).

Because of its scientific basis, DriveABLE was selected by Jansan-Ortho as the criterion in a multi-center study of the effects of RR on the driving competence of treated Alzheimer patients. Several other research projects in Canada and elsewhere have adopted the DriveABLE Assessment process as their driving competence criterion in studies of stroke, the value of rehabilitation using simulators, and other topics. In partnership with the Ontario Safety League, there are assessment sites in Toronto, Brampton, Barrie, Hamilton, Kitchener, St. Catharine's, Owen Sound, Oakville, Sudbury, Waterloo, and Whitby (DriveABLE, 2016b). Centers also are located in British Columbia, Alberta, New Brunswick, Quebec, Nova Scotia, Yukon, and Saskatchewan, and in 25 states (US) as well as Puerto Rico (DriveABLE, 2016b).

25.4.1 Florida

Florida has been encountering a unique situation where a large segment of its population is 65 years of age and older. More specifically, of these older adults, almost one half will be 75 and older (Florida Department of Transportation, 2004). In addition, there are added elder drivers killed or injured in traffic collisions in Florida than in any other state. According to The Road Information Project, 268 older drivers in Florida were killed in 2001 (The Road Information Program [TRIP], 2003). The Florida Department of Highway Safety and Motor Vehicles (DHSMV) selected DriveABLE as their criterion in a multi-center research project to evaluate brief driver screening procedures. The Florida DHSMV subsequently selected DriveABLE as the driver evaluation process to be used in their Safety Resource Centers. There are currently eight locations across Florida in Boca Raton, Brooksville, Clearwater, Fort Myers, Pompano Beach, Sunrise, Stuart, and Tallahassee (DriveABLE, 2016b).

Along with this program, Florida has employed the Elder Roadway User Program, a safe driving initiative committed to keeping older drivers safe on the roads. This specific program focuses on improving roadways in order to compensate for the natural effects of aging, primarily visual acuity and allowing additional time for decision making. The Elder Roadway User Program has been established since 1992 and is continuously committed to making roadway designs that assist older drivers. The proposed solution incorporates a complex system approach to accommodate older drivers by focusing on the physical environment and the internal states. In order to effectively implement the road design changes, the improvements were separated into two categories:

25.4.1.1 Short-Term Improvements

These were improvements which could be conducted by maintenance forces or specialty contracts in a short amount of time. These improvements began immediately and were completed throughout the state of Florida.

- Reflective Pavement Markers:
  - The Reflective Pavement Markers provide increased delineation for the intended road being traveled during dark or rainy conditions. The Department of Transportation requires 40-ft spacing on all areas of the State Highway System. As well, there is RPM spacing of 20 ft for areas where there are sharp curves.
- Wider Pavement Markings:
  - The reason for providing wider pavement markings is to clearly delineate the roadway while driving at night. Pavement markings are required to be 6-in. wide, for all state roads.
- The Use of Advance Street Name Signs:
  - Advance street name signs provide the older driver with additional time for decision making. At the initial stage advance street name signs were installed at major intersections; however, now they are installed wherever needed.
- Improved Pedestrian Features at Intersections:
  - The improvements made at pedestrian crossings are essential to safe mobility. Often the alterations made to roadways affect pedestrian crossings. For example, adding roadway lanes affects pedestrians by increasing

the distance that must be traveled safely across an intersection. Due to the fact that pedestrian crossings are used frequently by older adults, it is imperative to ensure that there are varying walking speeds and to increase the number of refuge islands.

- Increase Emphasis on Effective Traffic Control Through Work Zones:
  - A work zone is one of the most hazardous areas an older driver can experience. There are several practices which have been implemented to ensure safe traveling through work zone areas. These improvements include temporary reflective pavement markers to increase the delineation of the road, advance warning signs of an upcoming work zone area, and well-maintained signs and barricades for effective visibility.

25.4.1.2 Long-Term Improvements

The goal of the long-term improvements is to enhance the traffic control device visibility, in addition to providing advance notice and visibility along roadways.

- New lettering and sign sizes for stop, yield and all standard warning signs throughout the state.
  - A 20/70 vision was selected as the design acuity. This was chosen because it is the minimum corrected visual acuity allowed in Florida for attaining a driver's license. This improvement had been altered from a 20/40 vision which was the previous standard.
- Installing more advance notice signs for stop signs and lane assignment signs for freeway entrance ramps.
  - These signs help reduce last minute decisions made by drivers. The advance lane assignment signs provide additional reaction time for lane changes just before an intersection or entrance ramp. The advance lane assignment signs should be used on six-lane approaches to intersections to delineate the turn/through lanes and on all approaches to freeway entrances where a left turn is required.

- Enhanced pavement markings and sign sheeting to provide increased visibility.
  - These pavement markings are used in accordance with advance notice signs. Lane assignment pavement arrows and messages are used in association to improve effectiveness of advance notice signs. These are to be installed as far back from the intersection or ramp as possible.
- Improved intersection design elements:
  - Given that older adults are most frequently involved in intersection crashes compared to other age groups, it has been an important task to simplify intersection operation. There are two types of intersection improvements that have been made:
- Offset left turn lane:
  - There is a high involvement of left turn crashes among older adults. This is because visual and cognitive abilities begin to diminish with age. Difficulty is found with judging speed of oncoming vehicles and choosing appropriate gaps in which it is safe to travel. The implementation of offset left turn lanes hopes to accommodate for safer travel through intersections.
- Offset right turn lane:
  - The purpose of an offset right turn lane is to enhance visibility. Moving the turn lane farther to the right will provide a larger separation between the turn lane and the through lanes.

It has been an efficient approach to implement the roadway design alterations in both a short-term and long-term process. Through this process there have been gradual roadway improvements which have had the opportunity to be evaluated through effectiveness studies (Traffic Engineering Manual, 1999).

25.4.2 Additional Acknowledgements

Dr. Dobbs was awarded The Claude P. Beaubien Award of Research Excellence by the Alzheimer Society of Canada's Research Panel for the research underlying the DriveABLE assessment (A. Dobbs, personal communication, 2004; DriveABLE, n.d.). In 1998 Dr. Dobbs was selected as an Alberta Innovator of the Year for the development of DriveABLE Assessment Centers Inc. (A. Dobbs, personal communication, 2004; DriveABLE, n.d.).

25.4.3 Newer Projects

There are several new projects that DriveABLE is conducting (A. Dobbs, personal communication, 2004; DriveABLE, 2004):

- Funding has been received for a project entitled: "Driving competence in patients with ophthalmic conditions." The goal is to determine the appropriateness of the DriveABLE procedures, or extensions needed, for evaluating drivers with three common visual conditions of older drivers: (1) primary open angle glaucoma of varying visual field deficit severity, (2) proliferative diabetic retinopathy (PDR) requiring pan retinal laser photocoagulation treatment (PRP) in one or both eyes, and (3) clinically significant macular edema (CSME) requiring focal laser photocoagulation treatment in one or both eyes.
- Funding has been received for a project entitled: "Development of a roadside protocol for law enforcement officers to identify drivers who may be medically impaired."
- Funding has been received for a project entitled: "The development of a physician screen for identification of medically-at-risk drivers." The goal is to further validate and possibly extend a short, physician friendly screening tool for physicians to use when making decisions about which patients need to be evaluated for driving competence.
- Funding has been received for a project entitled: "Development and assessment of psycho educational group interventions": (1) for individuals with Alzheimer disease who have lost

their driving privileges, and (2) for their primary caregivers.

DriveABLE concerns itself with four major industries:

1. **Neurology**. DriveABLE aims to help patients help themselves by allowing clients take a hands-on approach to going in the right direction about their driving capabilities.
2. **Student transportation**. DriveABLE aims to keep the community safe by promoting assessments for school bus drivers to measure potential declines in driving ability.
3. **Healthcare**. DriveABLE aims to promote physicians to check driving ability during healthcare checkups.
4. **Fleet**. DriveABLE provides a product that allows for screening for success. This allows companies that hire drivers to pre-screen new employees to determine cognitive driving ability.

25.5 Conclusion

DriveABLE is an injury prevention program that deals with the complex, yet sensitive, issues surrounding mental ability and driver competence. DriveABLE has received tremendous positive response for the development of a driving evaluation procedure that is grounded in a strong research base, spanning countries. Injury prevention for older adult drivers needs to be thought of in terms of the whole context or situation. The concerns relating to older adult drivers are clearly multifaceted and require a combination of strategies which concentrate on different areas. With the implementation of the exemplar program of DriveABLE, these concerns can be helped and roads as well as drivers can be safer.

Acknowledgments The author would like to express sincere appreciation to the key informants for this case study: Allen R. Dobbs of the DriveABLE Assessment Centers Inc. in Edmonton, AB, Canada and Mark C. Wilson of the Florida Department of Transportation in Tallahassee, FL, USA—whose consultation made this project possible.

BRIO Model: DriveABLE Assessment Program

Group Served: Older driver; Individuals with cognitive/medical conditions.

Goal: Combining technology and research to provide a driver risk assessment program that determines driving competence as a result of medical conditions.

Background	Resources	Implementation	Outcome
Clients are typically over the age of 65 and have one or more medical conditions that can affect or have affected driving abilities. The program was developed by Dr. Allen Dobbs after empirical studies that identified both healthy driver behavior and cognitively impaired driver behavior A road course assessment and a cognitive evaluation was produced	During development, the Alberta Government provided assistance, as well as other supporters DriveABLE had assessment centers across Canada and the United States In recent years, DriveABLE has stopped providing assessment services—instead provides technology and training to licensed and certified organizations, creating licensed assessment providers	Clients with medical conditions or on certain medications are referred to DriveABLE sites through physicians, licensing organizations, or family/friends All centers use the same evaluation process involving a computer-based cognitive assessment (DCAT) and a road evaluation (DORE) DCAT involves tasks that measure aspects of driving, including attention, spatial judgment, and reaction time DORE is scientifically developed for on-road evaluations that test for cognitive impairment, by comparing results against healthy driver habits	Licensed centers exist across Canada—in seven provinces and one territory, the United States—in 25 states and Puerto Rico, and in Auckland, New Zealand Dr. Dobbs was awarded "The Claude P. Beaubien Award of Research Excellence" by the Alzheimer Society of Canada for research underlying DriveABLE assessment Dr. Dobbs was selected as Alberta Innovator of the Year in 1998 for the development of DriveABLE assessment centers Now, DriveABLE concerns itself with neurology, student transportation, healthcare, and fleet—providing products for a variety of aspects of cognitive and driving ability assessment

Life Space Model: DriveABLE Assessment Program

Sociocultural: civilization/community	Interpersonal: primary and secondary relationships	Physical environments: where we live	Internal states: biochemical/genetic and means of coping
Advocacy for a valid and scientific assessment Multi-disciplinary approach which involves researchers, physicians, occupational therapists, government agencies, insurance companies as well as others Use of community services to bring awareness to medical conditions which can interfere with driving	Involving family members, caregivers, and physicians as part of the referral process Protects the physician/patient relationship because physician no longer has to make a judgment decision	Use of on-road evaluation to identify unsafe driving. Road course is designed to reveal errors made by drivers who are unsafe, while allowing healthy drivers to pass Equal testing for urban and rural road users	Assessing unsafe driving due to the onset of a medical condition such as Alzheimer's disease, neurological disease, heart disease, head injury, stroke, diabetes, and other conditions affecting mental ability Use of computer-based tests which assess mental and motor skills relevant to driving Support group studies underway to help the individual and their family members deal with the stress of no longer being able to drive

References

DriveABLE. (n.d.). *Home*. Retrieved from http://www.driveable.com

DriveABLE. (2003a). *Research-based assessments for medically at-risk drivers*.

DriveABLE. (2003b). *Standardization and quality assurance procedures*.

DriveABLE Assessment Centers. (2004). Retrieved June 14, 2004, from http://www.driveable.com

DriveABLE. (2016a). *Industries*. Retrieved January 20, 2018, from www.driveable.com

DriveABLE. (2016b). *Licensed sites*. Retrieved February 19, 2018, from https://driveable.com/index.php/get-an-assessment/licensed-sites

Florida Department of Transportation. (1999). *Traffic engineering manual. Florida's elder road user program*.

Florida Department of Transportation. (2004). *Traffic Operations Office: elder roadway user program*. Retrieved May, 2004, from http://www.dot.state.fl.us/trafficoperations/elderoad.htm

The Road Information Program. (2003). *Designing roadways to accommodate the increasingly mobile older driver: A plan to allow older Americans to maintain their independence*. Washington, DC: Author.

David Gentili

The Alberta Ignition Interlock Program (IIP) aims to reduce excessive drinking and resultant alcohol-related collisions by cutting impaired individuals off from being able to start a car. The system requires the driver to breathe into a small breath-testing device linked to the vehicle ignition system in order to start the car (M. Fuhr, personal communication, July 2004). This program allows individuals who have been convicted of impaired driving, as long as no injury or death have been caused, to get back on the road under cautious conditions (Beirness & Simpson, 2003). In addition to requiring the driver to blow into the device to start the car, the program requires the individual to randomly blow into the device each hour after that to keep the vehicle running. The Alberta IIP can be directly linked to decreases in gross drunk driving offenses and decreases in minor, major, and fatal traffic injuries (Beirness & Simpson, 2003).

26.1 Background

Although first prototyped in the 1960s, Dr. Douglas Beirness (2001) reports that the development of a reliable in-car alcohol screening device proved to be a challenging, decades-long exercise. The development of portable and accurate breath testing devices for law enforcement in the late eighties changed things. Alcohol Ignition Interlocks—based on the technology of breath-alcohol concentration (BAC) measurement devices still commonly used by law enforcement agencies today, allowed researchers to explore new avenues of practical research (Beirness, 2001). While concerns about the prospect of individuals circumventing the device persist, technological innovations have led to practical and reliable devices that can prevent the operation of a motor vehicle if its driver has a BAC over a predetermined threshold value.

Modern Alcohol Ignition Interlock systems are directly linked to the vehicle ignition system and use a sensor to measure BAC. In order to operate the car, the driver is required to give a breath sample at every attempt to start the vehicle. The alcohol sensor detects if the driver of the vehicle has a BAC above the pre-set level and prevents the vehicle from starting if this is the case. There are a variety of devices available that rely on a number of technological innovations to prevent tampering and circumvention—this can include temperature and pressure sensors (to identify the driver), a periodic re-test feature (to stop the driver from drinking after ignition), and a data recorder (to log all activities associated with the device).

After more than a decade of use by various agencies in several jurisdictions, Alcohol Ignition

D. Gentili (✉)
Toronto, ON, Canada

© Springer Nature Switzerland AG 2020
R. Volpe (ed.), *Casebook of Traumatic Injury Prevention*,
https://doi.org/10.1007/978-3-030-27419-1_26

Interlock devices are now recognized as one of the few methods available for effectively combating the "hardcore drunk driver problem" (Century Council, 2003). Specifically, IIPs have become a popular means to prevent persons convicted of a previous drunk driving offense from repeating the behavior (Beirness & Simpson, 2003; Coben & Larkin, 1999; Raub, Lucke, & Wark, 2003; Sweedler, 2003). When used in conjunction with effective legislation, Alcohol Ignition Interlock systems can provide offenders with an alternative to a full license suspension—allowing offenders to use their vehicles for necessary driving, including with respect to employment. In other words, an effectively structured IPP can provide a bridge between full suspension and full license reinstatement, allowing offenders to drive their cars legitimately within the statutory driver licensing system of the jurisdiction in question, while at the same time providing assurance to the public that their health and safety has been protected (Beirness, 2001).

In 2001, it was reported that five Canadian provinces, not including Alberta, had at least established a statutory framework to allow the establishment of an IIP for drunk driving offenders. As reported by Beirness (2001), these decisions have been encouraged by the Federal government, such as the 1999 amendments to the *Criminal Code of Canada* which gave provinces the ability to reduce the mandatory period of driving prohibition for a first drunk driving offense if the offender participates in an IIP.

Today, IIPs are established and respected tools that aid in the re-integration of drunk-drivers into society and have a proven track record of protecting the public. This was not the case mere decades ago! As the Province of Alberta took the first serious steps in Canada at implementing a comprehensive IIP (referred to hereafter as the Alberta Ignition Interlock Program, or Alberta IIP) their role in pioneering this technology deserves to be recognized in this case study. It remains one of the best standards of such programs worldwide (M. Fuhr, personal communication, July 2004; Beirness & Simpson, 2003; Voas, Marques, Tippetts, & Beirness, 1999; Weinrath, 1997).

26.1.1 Exemplar Practices in Alcohol Ignition Interlocks

According to Beirness, Simpson, and Robertson (2003), to identify an "exemplar practice" of an AII program, two predominant issues must be considered: the first being the implementation of programs where interlock devices are able to work under real-world conditions (i.e., prevent consumers from operating a vehicle while intoxicated), and the second being the ability of interlock programs to prevent subsequent occurrences of impaired driving among program participants (i.e., prevent previous IIP consumers from driving while intoxicated in the future).

As mentioned, the initial concerns about interlock devices were of the first category—there were many questions as to the accuracy and reliability of the technology and the ease with which the device could be circumvented by drivers (Beirness, 2001). After years of research and development and collective field experiences of programs worldwide, these concerns have mostly been alleviated (M. Fuhr, personal communication, July 2004). The literature overwhelmingly supports the proposition that current AII systems are able to reliably identify individuals who have consumed too much alcohol and prevent them from operating the vehicle. This is, again, primarily due to the development of a variety of systems that prevent virtually all attempts at circumventing them. Experience with AII devices over the past decade show that, alone, they perform exceptionally well and do the job for which they were designed—i.e., to prevent those with elevated BACs from operating their vehicles (M. Fuhr, personal communication, July 2004; Beirness, 2001; Beirness & Simpson, 2003; Voas et al., 1999; Weinrath, 1997).

Unfortunately, the literature also suggests that, by themselves, AII devices do not provide a residual effect in preventing impaired driving after the device is removed from the vehicle (Beirness, 2001; Marques, Voas, Tippetts, & Beirness, 1999; Voas et al., 1999). Although these findings do not reflect the efficacy of interlock programs, they do show that AII programs have positive effects at reducing recidivism while installed and therefore on gross recidivism rates (Voas et al., 1999). Studies suggest that in solely engineering-based AII programs, recidivism rates will sharply rise after the device is removed such that there is no comparable difference to those who did not have AII devices installed (Marques et al., 1999; Voas et al., 1999). However, this should come as no surprise to those familiar with the literature on solely engineering-based solutions to complex, far-reaching problems. In this case, since AII devices are really only designed to prevent someone who is intoxicated from operating a vehicle, it does not necessarily follow that the target behavior of drinking would be at all affected. For example, since many drunk-driving recidivists suffer from clinical diagnoses of alcoholism, it should not be expected that the installation of an AII device would, by itself, effectively prompt a change in this underlying pattern of alcohol abuse (Marques et al., 1999). This stresses that AII programs must rely on more than the device itself if they are to have a more durable impact. Studies of programs that incorporate broader, more multidisciplinary approaches suggest a more durable effect (Beirness, 2001).

In summary, the collective findings of empirical studies have allowed researchers to identify a set of criteria, or "exemplar practices," for interlock programs (Beirness, 2001; Beirness et al., 2003).

These elements are:

- A perspective that considers AII programs as coordinated set activities designed to ensure that the program participants do not drive after drinking (i.e., as more than the device itself)
- Backed by strong, clear legislation
- An AII device that has been certified to meet or exceed established performance specifications
- A reliable service provider that understands and is committed to dealing with the DWI offender population
- Mandatory participation of all convicted DWI offenders with the option of voluntary early entry into the program by low risk offenders

- Authority monitoring of offenders, including a review of interlock data records
- Regular monitoring of offenders, including a review of interlock data records
- Duration of program participation linked to the success of the individual in the program
- Integration of the interlock program with other DWI sanctions and programs, particularly rehabilitation (Beirness, 2001).

These are, of course, of particular value in helping researchers identify an "exemplar practice" of an AII program in general and are therefore of incredible value to us. Although we will return to these criteria at the conclusion of this case study, keeping them in mind while reading subsequent sections may help further illustrate our chosen AII program as an exemplar practice.

26.1.2 History and Development: Alberta IIP

By the late 1980s, Alberta's booming economy—mixed with its increasingly transient workforce—was resulting in a road safety crisis (M. Fuhr, personal communication, July 2004). The Alberta IIP was initially conceived as part of a comprehensive package of impaired driving initiatives presented to the Solicitor General's Department in 1988. The focus of these initiatives was the introduction of new—and further exploration of old—tools to help alleviate the role of drunk driving in the road safety crisis. It was not until April 1990, however, that Alberta's Driver Control Board formally introduced Canada's first IIP. In what is referred to as the "pilot study," the Royal Canadian Mounted Police (RCMP) ran a program restricted to repeat offenders, many of whom were ordered by the Driver Control Board to have an Alcohol Ignition Interlock installed as a condition of license reinstatement. It was report that only 48 cases were considered during this phase of the project.

By May 1994 the program was deemed to have sufficiently passed established testing standards and was expanded into the beginnings of the comprehensive, province-wide program that we see today (M. Fuhr, personal communication, July 2004). Drunk driving offenders are now given the opportunity to volunteer for the interlock program if they meet certain criteria. Those who elect to participate in the program are allowed to drive with the device on their vehicles for 6 months, or until the end of their first year of suspension, at which time under normal conditions their license would be reinstated (Voas et al., 1999; Weinrath, 1997).

26.1.3 Project Aims

The target population of the Alberta IIP is drivers convicted of an impaired driving offense under the *Criminal Code of Canada* and provincial statutes. The primary goal of the program a is to prevent participants from driving while intoxicated throughout the period the device is installed, and to reduce the likelihood of subsequent impaired driving after the device is removed (Beirness, 2001; Beirness & Simpson, 2003). The Alberta IIP has secondary, more broad goals: to protect other road users from previously convicted impaired drivers, to allow suspended impaired drivers to prove that they are now safe drivers (i.e., in order to get their license fully reinstated), to facilitate employment, to reduce the impact on the families of drunk driving offenders, to use the device as a behavior modification tool by reinforcing the message that "drinking and driving do not mix," to determine other needed remedial actions such as addiction counseling, and as an early warning system to identify potential recidivists and direction them into treatment before they re-offend (M. Fuhr, personal communication, July 2004).

26.2 Resources

26.2.1 Stakeholders and Collaborators

The primary stakeholders in the program have been the Solicitor General, the Alberta Ministry of Transportation and the Alberta Transportation Safety Board, various government services, law enforcement agencies and the courts, Guardian Interlock Systems (Alberta IIP developer), and the Alberta Alcohol and Drug Abuse Commission (AADAC). Offenders themselves are considered stakeholders because subsequent offenders due to the changes to the *Criminal Code of Canada* that allows the option of driving earlier than would otherwise be the case. Of course, the public is also considered a stakeholder given the problem of drunk driving (recidivist drunk driving especially) and its physical, economic, and social damages (M. Fuhr, personal communication, July 2004; Century Council, 2003; Voas et al., 1999).

The initial collaborators, understood as the primary leaders in implementation, were the Driver Control Board (DCB), Solicitor General's Department, Alcohol Countermeasure Systems, the Alberta Research Council, and the impaired driver education programs of Alberta Alcohol and Drug Abuse Commission (AADAC). Additional collaborators were various municipal affairs (i.e., Registries) and several non-governments, non-profit organizations like People Against Impaired Driving (PAID).

The primary collaborators were the Alberta Transportation Safety Board and the Transportation Department of the Alberta Provincial Government, various government services, special interest groups like Mothers Against Drunk Driving (MADD), Guardian Interlock Systems and Guardian Interlock Services (new companies which stem out of the larger Alcohol Countermeasures Systems, Inc.), and the Alberta Motor Association and its impaired driver education program.

Each discipline has had a role throughout the implementation of the Alberta IIP, yet it is important to once again stress the two primary purposes of the program: to stop offenders from re-offending while the device is installed; and to decrease the rates of offenders re-offending in the future. The first goal is obviously primarily reliant on successful engineering and applied science initiatives. By themselves, these have had very little proven effect in successfully achieving the second, more far-reaching goal. The Alberta

IIP has had to rely on other disciplines, most prominently applied psychology, in achieving this second goal. In many ways, the Alberta IIP can be used as a prime example at the limitations of a single disciplinary approach in achieving broad, long-term goals. Even when the device was proven effective, an increasing consideration of personal, sociocultural, and economic variables helped enhance the effectiveness of the program. This is a prime example of the benefits of the Complex Systems Approach and the Life Space Model as outlined by Volpe (2004). Only when the Sociocultural, Interpersonal, Internal States, and Physical Environment are considered "equal" and in "relation" to each other do programs become most effective at alleviating a far-reaching and complex problem.

The Alberta IIP is managed by the Transportation Safety Board (previously the Driver Control Board), a quasi-judicial agency that acts "in the interest of public safety" (Alberta Transportation Safety Board, 2018; Minister of Transportation for the Province of Ontario, 2018). The Transportation Safety Board has been given the authority by law to remove unsafe drivers from the road; at the time of writing it consisted of two full-time civil servants and 30 community members appointed by the Legislative Assembly of Alberta. Section 22 of the *Traffic Safety Act* (2000) created the Board and granted it the authority to suspend the operator's licenses of people referred to it for a definite or indefinite period of time, prescribe any measure or course of remedial education, mandate treatment as a condition of possession of an operator's license, and/or prescribe terms and conditions for the possession of an operator's license. The operational specifics of continuing management of the Alberta IIP will are discussed in the Implementation section.

Maintenance of the Alcohol Ignition Interlock devices is provided by Guardian Interlock Services (the service division of Guardian Interlock Systems, the primary interlock manufacturer for North America), which operates two interlock service centers in the Province of Alberta—one located in Calgary, the other in Edmonton (Marques et al., 1999). In Alberta, the Alcohol Ignition Interlock devices have had to meet a special Qualification Test Specification for use in the province since 1992—this is considered one of the best such standards, worldwide (M. Fuhr, personal communication, July 2004, National Highway Traffic Safety Administration [NHTSA], 1999). Additionally, the Alberta IIP has relied on a fuel cell sensor unit since 1994, which has the added benefit of allowing a critical rolling retest requirement (i.e., periodic retesting while the vehicle is underway), and the inclusion of a data recorder (for tracking BAC levels and failed attempts at starting the vehicle).

As mentioned, the expansion of the Alberta IIP was the result of a successful, but limited, pilot phase conducted by the RCMP from 1990 through 1994. During this phase some of the unique components of the program were implemented, such as the Qualification Test Specification, but also the specified lockout BAC level of 0.04, opposed to the common 0.025 (NHTSA, 1999).

Installation costs are charged to the driver ($133.75), followed by monthly maintenance fees of $101.65. Due to the method of controlling expenses where offenders pay the costs of installation and maintenance of the device throughout the period it is installed, the program has been pitched as cost neutral. This appears to be true; with a private firm burdening the continuing costs of development and offenders paying for their own participation. The program is cost effective compared to its counterparts (M. Fuhr, personal communication, July 2004). The cost of additional services (such as participation in educational programs) is also burdened by the offender (M. Fuhr, personal communication, July 2004; Beirness, 2001). While this may seem like a benefit, particularly when pitching the program to decision makers, it also includes drawbacks that potentially limit the effectiveness of the program. This will be discussed under Outcomes.

26.3 Implementation

As outlined, responsibility for the administration of the Alberta IIP falls to the Transportation Safety Board which, by way of Section 30(1) of the *Traffic Safety Act*, have certain offenders reported to it by either the Minister of Transportation (Alberta), a Judge, or Registrar. The Board decides on a candidate's eligibility for the program. Although the Ministry of Transportation (Alberta) decides official policy, the Board has the authority to determine the extent to which candidates are "a threat to public safety." It also reviews the case and then on the decision of how to proceed (M. Fuhr, personal communication, July 2004). People find out the specifics of the program, primarily through third party Registry Agents who provide information to their communities and, additionally, are responsible for getting official application forms to offenders (again, at cost to the offender),

Alberta IIP participants are drunk driving offenders who have elected to take part in the program as a requirement for license reinstatement. Participants volunteer because of the possibility at having their licenses returned earlier than would otherwise be the case (Weinrath, 1997). To be eligible for the program, drivers must meet the following criteria:

- Only drivers convicted under sections 253, 254, or 255 of the Criminal Code of Canada can apply—Drivers convicted of impaired driving causing injury or death are not eligible to apply to the Ignition Interlock Program.
- The driver must have served the court-ordered driving prohibition period.
- The court order must authorize that the driver is eligible to participate in the Ignition Interlock Program.
- If the driver is a repeat offender, he/she must attend a hearing in person, with the Board.
- The driver must have served all other non-alcohol-related suspensions such as driving while a license is suspended and have paid all overdue motor vehicle fines.
- The driver must participate in the program a minimum of 6 months (Weinrath, 1997).

To be eligible, first time offenders have to complete a short period of license suspension (typically 3–6 months) and attend a short educational program (Voas et al., 1999; Weinrath,

1997). Second offenders serve at least 2 years of full suspension (while completing a weekend intervention program) before they are eligible for the program. Third-time offenders must serve all 3 years of license suspension and complete an intense educational program before being eligible. Participation is not always voluntary. In some situations, participation in the Alberta IIP is a mandated requirement for license reinstatement for those deemed to be especially serious cases (which due to the discretionary powers of the Board can even include first offenders and/or consist of a lifelong condition on licenses).

Participating in the program essentially means that the driver must breath into the Alcohol Ignition Interlock device (usually mounted on the dash board) to start their vehicle, and to re-test each hour after that to keep the vehicle running. Any reading over .04 BAC prevents the vehicle from starting or continuing to operate. The interlock is installed for a minimum of 6 months or until the end of the court-ordered suspension period.

At first, the Alberta IIP was an independent project and not overtly tied into other governmental efforts at combating drunk driving recidivists. However, the Transportation Safety Board did realize the implications of several early outcome measures, which mirrored the more comprehensive evaluations of programs elsewhere in that only short-term (while the device was installed), rather than long-term (after it was removed) recidivism reduction was actually being reliably achieved (M. Fuhr, personal communication, July 2004). Before having passed out of its initial pilot phase, the Alberta IIP had become progressively more integrated with other, non-engineering-based efforts offered in the province. Eligibility for participating in the Alberta IIP became dependent on the successful participation in other, similarly mandated programs (like the educational IMPACT Program, an addiction assessment and education program for repeat drunk drivers). Yet for some time the Alberta IIP itself remained quite one-dimensional in method. A continuous stream of possible engineering solutions promised a better, more reliable device better protected against circumvention and human error (Beirness, 2001).

The first expressed concerns of the Alberta IIP were no different than those expressed elsewhere—there was skepticism that the devices would live up to manufacturers' claims when used under real-world conditions (M. Fuhr, personal communication, July 2004). Reports coming out of other jurisdictions, primarily in the United States, showed that the early interlock devices were relatively easy to bypass (Beirness, 2001). However, with the integration of the newer generation of devices built on the early experiences of other IIPs, these concerns have been largely alleviated (Beirness, 2001; Collier, 1994). Modern devices include not only sensors and systems designed to prevent circumvention, but additional technology that could reliably detect and record all attempts to bypass the system (Beirness, 2001; Voas et al., 1999).

This last point is a fairly important caveat; it is generally accepted that a motivated individual will undoubtedly be able to circumvent any system (Beirness, 2001). However, with the added electronic recording of all events associated with the device and the reliable recording of attempts at circumvention (successful or not), the possibility of subsequent decision making based on this information with respect to specific cases was an added feature (M. Fuhr, personal communication, July 2004). The Traffic Safety Board took advantage of this and decided that all drivers should be monitored on an ongoing basis and that they must have demonstrated positive use of the device before being permitted to remove it. The Traffic Safety Board has the authority to suspend any drivers whose readings show a continual pattern of alcohol abuse.

An additional early experience with interlocks was the difficulty in having offenders install the device (M. Fuhr, personal communication, July 2004). Even with those who were deemed eligible to volunteer for the program—where participation in the interlock program the most desirable, and sought-after course of action—many offenders simply passed up the opportunity or failed to comply with the requirement after volunteering (M. Fuhr, personal communication, July 2004; Beirness, 2001). Even those who were mandated to use the Alcohol Ignition Interlock would often not have the device installed—a direct violation the conditions placed on their licenses (Beirness, 2001). For some time, there was no reliable system in place to ensure compliance; the very first generation of devices required constant calibration and maintenance, thus allowing continued monitoring of compliance, but the newer devices didn't require this "tinkering" and added this concern. Again, these were largely alleviated with the introduction and use of extensive monitoring systems in the program (M. Fuhr, personal communication, July 2004).

Most of these implementation issues were common to all IIPs—problems identified and/or solved in one region were quickly incorporated in another (M. Fuhr, personal communication, July 2004; Beirness, 2001). Government had the added benefit of one corporation (Alcohol Countermeasures, Inc., the parent corporation of Guardian Interlock Systems, Inc.) manufacturing and maintaining most of the offered Alcohol Ignition Interlock devices across the continent. In the case of Alberta, however, there were unique concerns at getting the devices to operate in practice (M. Fuhr, personal communication, July 2004). Firstly, the role of geography meant that in the case of breakdowns, participants could suddenly find themselves stranded in an isolated geographical region! Secondly, the intense temperatures of some regions in winter meant a special strain on the technology. All of these problems were largely solved by: (a) the continual incorporation of newer, more reliable, more durable technologies in the construction of the device (Beirness, 2001), and (b) the stringent qualifications laid down by Province of Alberta in 1992 (Electronics Test Centre).

With regard to Alberta IIP participants themselves, a most commonly reported problem is trouble starting the vehicle when sober—referred to as false positive. The extent that this was a real problem is unknown, although research does suggest that early devices could respond to other, non-impairing, substances (Beirness, 2001). Regardless, the introduction of the fuel sensor cell technology in alcohol detection sufficiently eliminated this threat (M. Fuhr, personal communication, July 2004). The cases of false positives that remain are largely believed to be attributable to non-metabolized alcohol that remains in the body many hours after consumption has ceased. In an analysis of records from Alcohol Ignition Interlock recorders, Marques et al. (1999) found failed breath-tests to be common on Saturday and Sunday mornings. Since an elevated BAC on Saturday or Sunday mornings is often evidence of a heavy drinking episode the previous evening, it is reasonable that these findings were indicative of the usual pattern of excessive consumption in cases of people with an alcohol abuse problem. This can be seen as a benefit as a skilled program monitor or case manager can use this data to illustrate the metabolism of alcohol and focus on the extent of the individual's consumption and additional needs for rehabilitation (M. Fuhr, personal communication, July 2004; Century Council, 2003; Beirness, 2001).

Alberta IIP participants are not always pleased with the system. There have been reports of embarrassment and inconvenience at having to constantly provide a breath sample to drive (M. Fuhr, personal communication, July 2004; Beirness, 2001). Additionally, the cost of the system is also a common complaint and may well be a legitimate concern (Beirness, 2001; Beirness & Simpson, 2003; Voas et al., 1999; Weinrath, 1997). It is reported that positive comments are also common; participants can speak favorably about the system that prevents them from driving after drinking, of being reminded that they have consumed too much alcohol to drive, and of forcing them to take responsibility prior to an episode of drunk driving (M. Fuhr, personal communication, July 2004; Beirness, 2001).

The remaining issues of implementation were primarily of a logistical nature. First, members of the Traffic Safety Board were originally reluctant to either mandate or offer participation to offenders—a consequence of inadequate knowledge of the existence of such programs and/or a personal belief that such programs were not effective (M. Fuhr, personal communication, July 2004). Second, the initial poor communication between program administrators, providers, and the board played a large factor in failing to capture cases

where the device was not installed, or circumvented (M. Fuhr, personal communication, July 2004; Beirness, 2001). With over a decade of experience, the various agencies involved in implementation have learned to work together in such a way as to deal with these issues effectively (Beirness, 2001). However, there is ample room for growth of the program.

26.3.1 Behavioral Intervention

There is no one set of established programs that is used in conjunction with participation in the Alberta IIP, and the specifics of educational and/or behavioral programs linked in with the program can differ significantly from jurisdiction to jurisdiction. The Outcomes section will be using a case study of one such set of complementary programs and comparing participants to those not receiving such an additional intervention. The specifics of that program will be described here, but one must be cautious of generalizing its effectiveness with the effectiveness of similar programs offered elsewhere in the province. For our purposes, we are not attempting to imply it is the best of such programs, we are simply illustrating the potential of the multidisciplinary approach of the Alberta IPP in better achieving its goals, and as such, being an exemplar program.

From the beginning, the research model presumed that the Alcohol Ignition Interlock device would impact road safety by improving the motivation of offenders to separate their drinking behavior from driving (Marques, Tippetts, Voas, Danseco, & Beirness, 1998). The idea was that a simple "behaviorist effect" would lead participants to separate the two activities and thus provide an effect even after the device was removed. However, this effect did not materialize as intended. Decision makers behind the Alberta IIP began to look for ways to incorporate other disciplines within the program so that a more "durable effect" would be achieved.

The City of Calgary was the focus of an empirical study aiming to gauge the ability of a four-element, multidisciplinary intervention at changing alcohol abuse behavior in conjunction with the Alberta IIP (Marques et al., 1999). On monthly or bimonthly service visits, the interventions occurred during the interlock-service waiting period. Over 1 year, depending on the length of the interlock assignment in question, there were seven to 12 occasions when the offenders came in. The elements, while not delivered in a structured format, consisted of educational support (e.g., the pragmatics of living with an interlock and helping users to avoid warnings and failures, staying in the program, avoiding the costs of further drunk driving offenses), case management support (to assist in finding and using community resources relevant to various needs, such as family counseling, job counseling, grief counseling, and addiction treatment), motivational enhancement therapy (to enhance a sense of responsibility toward self-change and to being movement along the change-readiness continuum), and protective planning support (assisting in planning for activities during the high-risk post-interlock period) (Marques et al., 1999).

The Alberta IIP in this case takes into consideration the Sociocultural, Interpersonal, Physical Environments, and Internal States components of the Life Space Approach (Volpe, 2004). We see an additional bias toward active use of the community and available help networks through the management support therapy component, an additional drive at getting offenders to take responsibility for their actions and change their norms and values through the motivational enhancement therapy component, an active attempt at trying to lessen the economic stress that many of those who participate in the Alberta IIP acutely feel through the educational support component, and a focus on how living, play space, and language in the protective planning component. Throughout all these components we see a drive to increase the self-efficacy, health, and quality of life of participants. When added to the obvious engineering effects of the device itself, the Alberta IIP becomes a prime example of an impressive technological innovation that incorporates a well-rounded, complex system approach to the problem of recidivist drunk driving offenses.

26.3.2 Process and Outcome Evaluation

26.3.2.1 Process

In the case of the Alberta IIP, process is largely a question of "whether the IIP is able to reliably stop recidivism while installed in the car" and "whether issues of circumvention and/or error can be continuously monitored and dealt with" (Beirness, 2001). The monitoring of specific cases by the Board, coupled with the joint international enterprise of AII device manufacturing, has resulted in a continuous stream of useful information regarding better ways the Alberta IIP can achieve these goals (M. Fuhr, personal communication, July 2004; Beirness, 2001). Cases are constantly monitored, and due to the nature of data recording, a constant stream of information is given out by the device to those in a position to directly influence both general policy and specific cases themselves (M. Fuhr, personal communication, July 2004).

26.3.2.2 Outcome

The objective of outcome evaluation studies is, in this case, a question of determining "the extent to which interlock programs reduce the incidence of subsequent DWI [drunk driving] behavior among participants" (Beirness, 2001). With the case of the Alberta IIP, stakeholders and collaborators have had the benefit of being the focus of several major empirical studies conducted by experts in the field (M. Fuhr, personal communication, July 2004; Marques et al., 1999; Voas et al., 1999; Marques et al., 1998; and Weinrath, 1997). These reviews, discussed specifically in the following section, allow the formation of a broad picture of how the program started, evolved, and where it is going in the future.

26.4 Outcome

26.4.1 Pilot Phase: 1990–1994

Michael Weinrath (1997) conducted the first comprehensive evaluation of the effectiveness of the Alberta IIP in 1997. In the study, a disproportionate stratified random sample of license-suspended Alberta impaired drivers was selected from computer files covering the years 1989–1994. The sample comprised 994 offenders of age 20 and older, including all female drunk drivers from those years (125), a random selection of 701 male drivers (sampling frame of 4394), and 189 ignition interlock cases (sampling frame of 441) from the years 1990–1994. Subsequent reclassification resulted in a final breakdown of 168 ignition interlock program cases and 826 impaired drivers in the comparison group. Because of the given time period, the following results give us an insight into the program's effectiveness during its pilot phase.

For the Alberta IIP, even when controlling for the effects of other risk factors, participation in an ignition interlock program reduced the likelihood of recidivism from impaired driving, high-risk driving, and injury collisions. When compared with a group who received only license suspensions, ignition interlock program participants were twice as likely to successfully avoid repeat drunk driving. Ignition interlock cases were 4.4 times less likely to record a new serious driving violation and 3.9 times less likely to be involved in an injury collision. Similar program effects were observed to a sub-sample of chronic impaired drivers.

Survival rates for drivers with their licenses reinstated displayed additional evidence of the program's effectiveness, even after the ignition interlock device was removed. A difference of 10% in drunk driving recidivism at the 24-month mark indicated the overall program effectiveness, whereas a 5% difference at the 15-month mark for after-interlock cases showed evidence of post-program treatment effects.

Due to these results, Weinrath concluded that the ignition interlock had succeeded as both a vehicle-based and individual-based sanction by itself—warranting "continued operation of the program in Alberta" (Weinrath, 1997, p. 57). Importantly, the results of this study showed that, right from the beginning, the Alberta IIP was more successful than many of its counterparts, "the results ... were more supportive of ignition

interlock than evaluations conducted in Ohio and California and much more consistently positive than outcomes observed in Oregon" (Weinrath, 1997, p. 57).

It was reported that comparisons of program effectiveness studies are extremely difficult due to the many uncontrollable factors affecting road safety that vary among jurisdictions. Even so, Weinrath concluded that the nature of the Alberta IIP was responsible for this outcome:

> Ignition interlock was (and remains) part of a larger assessment process by the DCB, which can vary the length of program assignment for more serious cases and requires offenders to take driver education and alcohol/drug programs. As mentioned, drivers who continue to drink and fail their ignition interlock BreathalyzerTM test too often may be suspended and have their program length extended. Put simply, the success of Alberta's program likely was due to more individualized management of impaired drivers ... (1997, p. 57).

26.4.2 The Alberta IIP, Province Wide: 1996–1998

In 1999, Voas and colleagues conducted a study of the effectiveness of the Alberta IIP among participants who took part in the program between 1996 and 1998. Records of 35,132 drivers convicted of DUI (driving under the influence) between July 1, 1998 and September 30, 1996 were analyzed. Repeat DUI offenses were measured during and after the interlock period. The results showed that while offenders had interlocks on their vehicles, drunk driving recidivism was substantially reduced. However, once the interlock had been removed and the participants had had their licenses fully reinstated, their DUI rate was the same as other offenders. What this study suggests is that while the device itself is effective at decreasing recidivism while installed in an offender's vehicle, the other aspects of the program were not effective at bringing about a desired, durable effect. This may have been due to the fact that the Traffic Safety Board was unable to offer the personalization it had during the pilot phase with a large population, relying on established guidelines rather than extensively monitoring each, individual case.

Even more concerning was the finding that only 8.9% of eligible drivers elected to participate in the interlock program—therefore not significantly increasing the overall effectiveness of the province's overall management of DUI offenders! In the end, the program was found to have produced a small (5.9%) overall reduction in the recidivism rate of all drunk driving offenders during this period. The reasons for this, as well as current and needed efforts in fixing this problem, are thoroughly discussed in this case study's conclusions.

26.4.3 Alberta IIP and Co-coordinated Multidisciplinary Interventions: 1994–1997

In 1999, Marques et al. conducted a preliminary study of the patterns of BAC and driving logged on ignition interlock records and to assess whether this event record proved to be a useful outcome measure for a behavioral intervention. There were 1309 first-time, second-time, and third-time drunk driving offenders who agreed to participate during interlock installation and who took part in a human-services (supportive guidance) intervention based on motivational interviewing and pragmatic counseling. These offenders were measured and compared to those who were not offered the intervention. After controlling for prior offenses, demographics, and reported drinking levels, offenders at the intervention site (Calgary) were less likely to have recorded failure BAC tests than were offenders at the control site (Edmonton). These patterns mimic the high-risk periods for DUI arrests and alcohol-involved fatal crashes. In the end, the interlock was found to successfully block drinking and driving during high-risk periods, and the data suggests that the services intervention was affecting DUI behavior itself. This strongly suggests that the Alberta IIP is most effective when it is used in conjunction with other, multidisciplinary techniques. However, it remains to be seen whether the intended "durable effects" of the program are now being achieved (or re-achieved).

26.4.4 Alberta IIP and Identification as an Exemplar Practice

It is now time to go back and see how the Alberta IIP rates on the "best [exemplar] practice criteria" that were originally outlined (Beirness, 2001; Beirness et al., 2003). First, the Alberta IIP has definitely evolved into a program that combines and incorporates other programs into its successful implementation and is becoming increasingly multi-dimensional in approach. Second, it is considered successful practice of the Alberta IIP to be more than the device itself. Third, certification standards are among the highest in the world. Fourth, the Alberta IIP makes use of a reliable service provider, Guardian Interlock Services, which is the oldest and most established Alcohol Ignition Interlock device manufacturer and service provider to our knowledge. Fifth, regular monitoring of offenders is an integral part of the program. Finally, it was the very studies from Alberta that stressed the impact program length had on outcome.

Despite the above, it was reported that there is room for improvement. Firstly, it has been noted by many involved in the program that extra participation by trained police officers is needed (M. Fuhr, personal communication, July 2004). This includes a greater role in monitoring participants, enhancing their ability to identify interlock participants who are not in compliance with the interlock restriction. Secondly, despite the fact that the Transportation Safety Board has received acclaim for its individualized treatment of participants, particularly in the earlier phases of the program, additional research could ascertain how legislation can be changed to make the program more effective. This is primarily an issue of looking more deeply into expanding, and increasing the effectiveness, of mandatory participation legislation.

26.5 Conclusions and Future Directions

The evaluations of the Alberta IIP have had many benefits. They have shown that the interlock devices have had to undergo and pass rigorous testing standards to gain wide acceptance. Also, those upgrades to the interlock device were necessary to address practical application issues. The introduction of data loggers was critical to support ongoing monitoring of users, and the interlock device substantially lowers repeat drunk driving offenses while the offender is using the device. Furthermore, the client's' use of the device must be monitored, and sanctions imposed for incorrect use. Extended use of the interlock device may be warranted for those individuals who can't regulate their proper use of the device. Here, authority rests with the agency responsible for driver licensing and control, and regular monitoring should include a review of data from the recorder. Length of participation is linked to participation success, and the proof exists that the program should be integrated with other drunk driving programs, including sanctions, rehabilitation, and education (M. Fuhr, personal communication, July 2004).

The issue of the program participation (or lack thereof) is a very important and concerning issue to those directing the program (M. Fuhr, personal communication, July 2004; Beirness, 2001; Weinrath, 1997). Some have attributed this mainly to the extensive costs burdened by participants. While some argue that one who is able to afford to drink should be able to afford the relatively small costs of the program, drunk driving offenders are usually faced with extensive fines and are also expected to burden any treatment costs in addition to the costs associated with Alberta IIP participation. Future studies must ascertain the level to which this is indeed a factor—if it is, it may illustrate at how not taking into consideration economic aspects can actually hurt an otherwise promising, engineered solution, and adds further support for Complex Systems Approaches like the Life Space Model (Volpe, 2004).

In an effort to increase participation rates, program coordinators need to increase distribution of information about their program to those eligible to participate (e.g., sending brochures out to vehicle registration centers). However, according to program officials, participation rates remain at less than 15% of the total eligible population (M. Fuhr, personal communication, July 2004). An important future direction is the need for more research on drunk driving recidivists, and how better to reach individuals to participate in the program (M. Fuhr, personal communication, July 2004). Additionally, the impact of tougher and expanded mandatory participation legislation, as previously mentioned, may help to play a role in fixing this problem (Beirness, 2001).

The Alberta IIP is a clear illustration that a well-intentioned, single-discipline approach can be enhanced, significantly, by consideration and effective incorporation of a broader, multidisciplinary perspective. While based on a simplistic premise, the current, effective iteration of the Alberta IIP takes more into account than the simple act of starting and operating a vehicle while intoxicated. It considers underlying patterns of abuse and the various, sociocultural, economic, and personal problems faced by drunk driving offenders, which help broaden and lengthen the effects of the program. This case study also highlighted engineering achievements, and these deserve due credit—the device excelled at preventing drunk driving while installed and had a tangible effect on recidivism rates throughout the province. The decision makers guiding the Alberta IIP do not appear to be considering the issue of which method works best, but rather which methods, used together, can work better. Although there is certainly an ongoing question of how better and more standardized multidisciplinary approaches can be incorporated into the program, the Alberta IIP clearly illustrates the effectiveness of the Complex Systems Approach in reaching broad goals while targeting immediate ones.

The Alberta IIP is considered exemplary. Although the program can be improved further, studies suggest that Alcohol Ignition Interlock programs remain one of the best ways to deal with the increasingly prevalent hardcore drunk driving problem. The Alberta IIP can be directly linked to decreases in gross drunk driving offenses and decreases in minor, major, and fatal traffic injuries. This program aims to connect and involve the four aspects of the life space model to provide a collaborative injury prevention program.

Acknowledgments The author would like to express sincere appreciation to the key informants for this case study: Mitch Fuhr of the Alberta Transportation Ministry in Edmonton, AB, Canada and Tammy Merenick of the Transportation Safety Board in Edmonton, AB, Canada—whose consultation made this project possible.

BRIO Model: Alberta Ignition Interlock Program (IIP)

Group Served: Drivers convicted of an impaired driving offense.

Goal: To prevent participants from driving while intoxicated, and to reduce the likelihood of subsequent impaired driving.

Background	Resources	Implementation	Outcome
Impaired driving as a result of alcohol consumption is a major area of road safety and injury prevention Alcohol Ignition Interlocks (AII) programs are popular as a means to prevent persons convicted of previous drunk driving offenses from repeating behavior In 1990 Alberta's Driver Control Board introduced Canada's first AII program	A number of studies and results have been conducted in reference to alcohol ignition interlock programs—the data and results have helped Alberta develop their program Maintenance of the AII devices is by Guardian Interlock Services—provides two interlock service centers in Alberta The Alberta IIP has been tested and had to meet a number of qualifications and specifications for use in the province Installation costs the driver around $130, and a monthly maintenance fee of about $100, and development costs are handled by a private firm—which allows it to be sold to corporations and governments as "cost-neutral"	Responsibility for administration falls to the Transportation Safety Board (Alberta) Majority of Alberta IIP participants are drunk driving re-offenders who have elected to take part in the program as a requirement for license reinstatement Participating in the program means that the driver must blow into the AII device to start the vehicle and to blow randomly each hour to keep the vehicle running—any reading over .04 BAC inhibits the vehicle from starting or continuing to operate The interlock is installed for a minimum of 6 months or until the end of the court-ordered suspension period	Even when controlling for the effects of other risk factors, participation in an ignition interlock program reduced the likelihood of recidivism from impaired driving, high-risk driving, and injury collisions—AII cases were 4.4 times less likely to record a new serious driving violation, 3.9 times less likely to be involved in an injury collision (1997) Combines and incorporates other programs into successful implementation, being multi-dimensional has led to Alberta IIP to be an exemplar program Participation rates remain at less than 15% of the total eligible population (2004)

Life Space Model: Alberta Ignition Interlock Program

Sociocultural: civilization/community	Interpersonal: primary and secondary relationships	Physical environments: where we live	Internal states: biochemical/genetic and means of coping
Offenders take responsibility for their actions and future behavior. Offenders are able to use their cars and participate in the highly transient Alberta economy. Police and courts have a better way at monitoring offenders when they are out in the community. Economic problems sometimes addressed by programs used in conjunction with program.	Some programs used in conjunction with program help provide help networks. The public can be assured that recidivist offense will be avoided or detected. Better identification of hardcore drunk drivers (through data recorder analysis).	The physical barrier to drunk driving re-offense while the device is installed. Some programs used in conjunction with program help identify activities to avoid recidivism after device is uninstalled.	Increases in self-efficacy due to successful participation. Constant reminder to participants that they have drunk too much and reduction in stress at feared "slipups" due to assurance.

References

Alberta Transportation Safety Board. (2018). Policy statement. Retrieved from http://atsb.alberta.ca/AboutUs.htm.

Beirness, D. J. (2001). *Best practice in alcohol ignition interlocks*. Ottawa, ON: Traffic Injury Research Foundation.

Beirness, D. J., & Simpson, H. M. (2003). *Alcohol interlocks as a condition of license reinstatement*. Ottawa, ON: Traffic Injury Research Foundation.

Beirness, D. J., Simpson, H. M., & Robertson, R. D. (2003). International symposium on enhancing the effectiveness of alcohol ignition interlock programs. *Traffic Injury Prevention, 4*, 179–182.

CanLII. (2000). *Traffic Safety Act RSA 2000*. Ottawa, ON: Author.

Century Council. (2003). *The national agenda: A system to fight hardcore*. Washington, DC: Author.

Coben, J. H., & Larkin, G. L. (1999). Effectiveness of ignition interlock devices in drunk driving recidivism. *American Journal of Preventive Medicine, 16*(1), 81–87.

Collier, D. W. (1994). *Second generation interlocks lead to improved program efficacies*. Paper presented at Transportation Research Board 73rd Annual Meeting, Washington, DC.

Marques, P. R., Tippetts, A. S., Voas, R. B., Danseco, E. R., & Beirness, D. R. (1998). *Support services provided during interlock usage and post interlock repeat dui: Outcomes and processes*. Landover, MD; Ottawa, ON: Pacific Institute for Research and Evaluation; Traffic Injury Research Foundation.

Marques, P. R., Voas, R. B., Tippetts, A. S., & Beirness, D. J. (1999). Behavioral monitoring of dui offenders with the alcohol ignition interlock recorder. *Addiction, 94*(12), 1861–1870.

Minister of Transportation for the Province of Alberta. (2018). *Memorandum of understanding between the Minister of Transportation for the province of Alberta and the Alberta Transportation Safety Board*. Retrieved from http://atsb.alberta.ca/AboutUs.htm.

National Highway Traffic Safety Agency. (1999). *Traffic safety facts 1998. DOT HS 808 806*. Washington, DC: Author.

Raub, R. A., Lucke, R. E., & Wark, R. I. (2003). Breath alcohol ignition interlock devices: Controlling the recidivist. *Traffic Injury Prevention, 4*, 199–205.

Sweedler, B. M. (2003). Preventing alcohol crashes: The role of ignition interlocks. *Traffic Injury Prevention, 4*, 177–178.

Voas, R. B., Marques, P. R., Tippetts, A. S., & Beirness, D. J. (1999). The Alberta interlock program: The evaluation of a province-wide program on dui recidivism. *Addiction, 94*(12), 1849–1859.

Volpe, R. (2004). *The conceptualization of injury prevention as change in complex systems. Life span adaptation projects*. Toronto, ON: University of Toronto.

Weinrath, M. (1997). The ignition interlock program for drunk drivers: A multivariate test. *Crime & Delinquency, 43*(1), 42–59.

Part IV

Traumatic Injury Prevention Programs Within Complex Systems

Overview of Traumatic Injury Prevention Programs Within Complex Systems

27

Chelsi Major-Orfao

Community programs offer an exceptional approach to prevention as they are implemented within an individual's life space, catering to the needs of their specific environment. These programs intend to create a positive safety culture that prevents serious injuries among its community members. To do so, prevention programs should strive to establish community competence, the ability of a community to build resilience in its members (Cohen, Chavez, & Chehimi, 2010). With a focus on community resilience, the blame for individual victims is often lifted, producing community responsibility for prevention and building on community strengths that may have been previously overlooked (Cohen et al., 2010). However, sustainable change can only occur when individuals participate within their community programs, generating that resilience. In order to promote this buy-in, community values such as collaboration and respect should be reflected within the prevention program.

For some time, unintentional injury has been a major focus of community programs, as it represents the leading cause of premature morbidity and mortality in most of the world's industrialized nations (Volpe, Lewko, & Batra, 2002). Worldwide, unintentional injury-related deaths totaled approximately 3,600,000 in 2011, resulting in a death rate of 52 per 100,000 population (National Safety Council, 2015). Table 27.1 breaks down some countries to create a picture of the magnitude of unintentional injury for these industrialized nations. Specifically, within the United States, unintentional traumatic brain injury (TBI)—injuries caused by a bump, blow, or jolt to the head that disrupts the normal function of the brain—is a major cause of disability and death, contributing to approximately 30% of all injury deaths (Centers for Disease Control and Prevention, 2017). There are a variety of independent social variables that can have influence on the burden of unintentional injuries. Such variables that have an impact and need to be taken into account by community programs are race (Table 27.2), gender (Fig. 27.1), age (Fig. 27.1), and social economic status.

Unintentional injuries also create detrimental costs for societies—resources that would be better dedicated to community prevention services. Within community programs, it is vital to have an overview of the direct and indirect costs that traumatic unintentional injuries can have on an individual's life space. For example, not only might finances have a direct impact on an individual's acute health and/or rehabilitation process, but further the injured individual's family may be required to provide financial or emotional support, in which their education or employment may be affected by loss of wages, promotions, or hours. Therefore, good public health should not be seen through the eyes of treatment, but from a

C. Major-Orfao (✉)
Sunnybrook Research Institute, Toronto, ON, Canada

© Springer Nature Switzerland AG 2020
R. Volpe (ed.), *Casebook of Traumatic Injury Prevention*,
https://doi.org/10.1007/978-3-030-27419-1_27

Table 27.1 Unintentional injury-related deaths and death rates by gender and age

Country	Year	Deaths (% males)	All ages (deaths per 100,000 population)
Argentina	2010	10,187 (73%)	24.6
Australia	2011	5898 (60%)	26.1
Egypt	2011	12,213 (81%)	15.2
France	2010	25,414 (55%)	40.4
Japan	2011	61,517 (55%)	48.8
Netherlands	2011	3985 (49%)	23.9
United Kingdom	2010	14,143 (56%)	22.7
United States	2010	121,053 (63%)	39.1

Note: This public data represented in this table is from the National Safety Council [NSC] (2015)

Table 27.2 Unintentional injury-related deaths and death rates by race per 100,000 population, U.S., 2011

Race and sex	Rank	Number	Rate
All races	5	126,438	40.6
Males	3	79,257	51.7
Females	6	47,181	29.8
White	4	109,751	45.1
Males	3	68,123	56.5
Females	6	41,628	33.9
Black	5	12,531	30.7
Males	3	8387	43.1
Females	7	4144	19.5
Not white or black[a]	4	4156	15.1
Males	3	2747	20.6
Females	5	1409	10.0

Note: Rates are deaths per 100,000 population in each race/sex/Hispanic origin group. Total column includes 399 deaths for which Hispanic origin was not determined (NSC, 2015)
[a]Includes American Indian, Alaskan Native, Asian, Native Hawaiian, and Pacific Islander

science-based and prevention-oriented lens, in order to create community benefit and lessen the burden on the individual (Cohen et al., 2010). Although good public health may reduce morbidity and mortality, save money, and improve quality of life, it requires an investment of time and effort that communities will have to prepare for in order to see tangible results (Cohen et al., 2010). Thus, the burden of direct and indirect costs, which can be seen from different levels of an individual's life, can be prevented if a community program implements strategies within those same levels.

Due to the different needs of individual nations, the structure of a community prevention program must depend on the diverse needs of the community members they serve, whether it is a policy-based level or a micro level intervention. It is also important to note the transferability of programs between communities. Although communities might have the same prevention needs, replication of a program may require adaptations to serve the different populations in order to build that community resilience.

27.1 Section Chapters

The Community Intervention section is divided by the different environments within an individual's life space and proves to demonstrate essential elements of exemplary practice within community-based programs, serving as a foundation for other program prevention strategies. Illustrating themes of modeling, communication, as well as the dissemination of knowledge and education, these programs are distinguished examples for future prevention endeavors.

27.1.1 Residential-Based Interventions

Residential injuries are defined as injuries that occur in and around houses, boarding homes, apartments, and the immediate surrounding areas (National Committee for Injury Prevention and Control [NCIPC], 1989). Young children are particularly vulnerable to residential injuries that could result in mortality. This is due to the extensive time young children spend within their residential environment, combined with their developmental stage that necessitates their physical exploration, especially in cases where parents do not provide adequate surveillance. Children, who are under the age of 5 years, experience approximately two-thirds of unintentional injuries when at home (Laflamme & Eilert-Peterson, 1998). This high rate of injury draws attention to

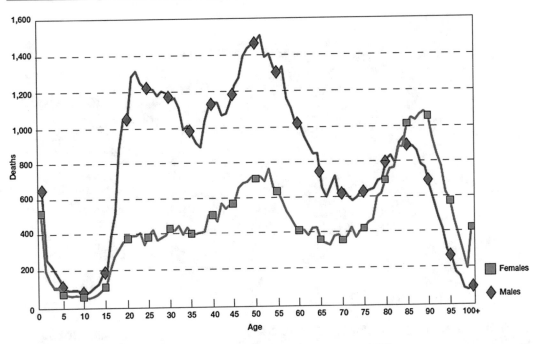

Fig. 27.1 Unintentional injury-related deaths by sex and age, U.S., 2011 (NSC, 2015)

the need of safety prevention methods that have a residential focus.

The Nurse Family Partnership (NFP) and the University of California Los Angeles (UCLA) Parent-Child Health Wellness Program both employ prevention strategies that target individuals within their intimate living environment. The Nurse Family Partnership (Chap. 28) has registered nurses deliver intensive, comprehensive home visitations to first-time mothers from disadvantaged backgrounds and promotes effective, competent caregiving. During these visits, children and their families engage in activities congruent with the objectives of the program associated with the child's stage of development (Nurse Family Partnership [NFP], 2007). This program follows families from the 14th week of gestation until their children turn 2 years old, providing continuous support within their residential environment through different parts of their child's upbringing. In order for this program to replicate effectively in a different community, randomized controlled trials with two different state populations were conducted upon first

implementation of NFP. Not only were similar results found in both (decrease childrearing beliefs associated with child maltreatment, decrease in child abuse and neglect, as well as decreases of child injury incidents); studies conducted decades later with the same participants showed a reduced number of females entering the criminal justice system, receiving Medicaid, and participants being less likely to die from preventable causes when compared with their control group counterparts. In addition, according to the NFP program, per dollar invested in NFP, state and government cost savings average $2.90 and the total benefits to society equal $6.40 (NFP, 2017). Since the replication of the program in 1996, there have been 269,311 families served in 42 states in addition to the US Virgin Islands (NFP, 2017).

Similarly, the UCLA Parent-Child Health Wellness Program (Chap. 29) targeted health and safety strategies within the home. However, this program specifically supported low-income young parents with intellectual disabilities and/or difficulties. While many parents are knowledgeable

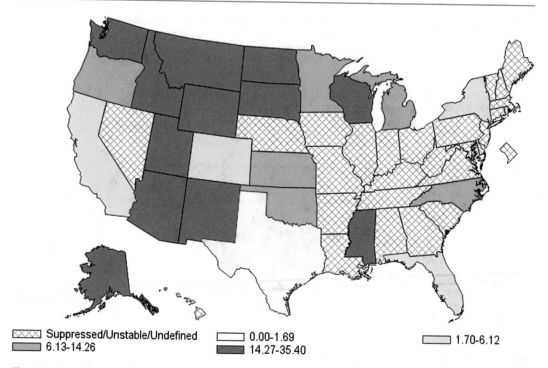

Suppressed/Unstable/Undefined   0.00-1.69   1.70-6.12
6.13-14.26   14.27-35.40

Fig. 27.2 Unintentional TBI of AI/AN individuals within the United States from 2008 to 2014, death rates per 100,000 population. From "Fatal Injury Mapping" by the Centers for Disease Control and Prevention (2015)

about injury risks in the home, some parents tend to be unable to apply that knowledge to practice. Thus, families headed by parents with intellectual disabilities or learning needs are often considered the most vulnerable in the community (Tymchuk, Lakin, & Luckasson, 2001). By entering a parent's home to provide real-life examples of how to improve their space and supervision, it was shown that maternal knowledge outcome variables were greater than mothers who received interventions outside the home (Tymchuk et al., 2001).

These residential-based programs are the essence of community interventions as they explore the most intimate of environments, allowing for the enhancement of interactions within families with the goal of injury prevention in mind.

27.1.2 School-Based Interventions

School-based interventions are unique environments for prevention programs as they target a wide range of individuals while incorporating community members for sustainability and practicality. For populations that have isolating environments, schools can be a good vessel to implement specific prevention methods that cater to a population's milieu.

The Indian Health Services Injury Prevention Program (Chap. 30) is set within a unique community, mostly with aboriginal individuals who are disproportionately at risk for specific types of injury. American Indian/Alaska Native (AI/AN) individuals die from accidental injury at a rate that is three times that of other races, as shown through Fig. 27.2 (Indian Health Service, 2000). These greater morbidity and mortality rates not only create emotional suffering and economic burden but also result in the loss and delay of opportunities to build healthy, local cultural communities. Therefore, this program furthers the education of AI/AN individuals by providing pre-service and in-service training to community members in the field of injury prevention. With the goal of raising the health status of AI/AN individuals, this program strives to increase the prevention knowledge and ability of tribes to address their own incidences of severe injury and death. Due to this, numerous individual fellowship programs, training projects, and prevention articles/programs have been developed. Thus, the Indian Health Services Injury Prevention Program creates sustainability and the potential for modeling opportunities to others within the community.

School-based prevention programs can also educate children and youth on potentially traumatic situations they may encounter and how to become advocates within their community spaces. The National Brain and Spinal Cord Injury Program (Chap. 31) provides school-based programming, alongside general public awareness and education, to create brain-friendly spaces within their community. Young people specifically between the ages of 5 and 24 are the most at risk for brain and spinal cord injuries, with estimates over 100,000 young people admitted to hospitals per year for these injuries (ThinkFirst National Injury Prevention Foundation, 2006). It was found that the curriculum implemented in schools significantly improved knowledge in students from first to third grade. Therefore, the need for a curriculum that challenges children and youth to help make practical safe choices that lower their risk and operates in an all-encompassing school environment is imperative.

Likewise, the UCLA Labor Occupational Safety Program (Chap. 32) provides a similar service focused on informing young people about potential harmful situations. Young workers (14–24 years of age) experience workplace injuries at higher rate than other workers, due to physical limitations, psychological elements, and environmental factors within the job (Delp, Runyan, Brown, Bowling, & Jahan, 2002). In response, this program developed a curriculum based on an empowerment education model that focused on educating young people about hazards they may encounter in the workplace. In addition, this curriculum informs youths about their rights and responsibilities, provides an array of resources, and teaches them the skills they need to advocate for themselves. The curriculum focuses on building critical consciousness and provides real opportunities to create change in the community. Beyond targeting schools, the UCLA Labor Occupational Safety Program also targets community centers with the intention of reaching youth who have dropped out of school.

27.1.3 Hospital-Based Interventions

Hospitals are generally regarded as treatment centers for injuries; however, they can also be a vessel for prevention interventions. Hospital-based interventions often focus on receiving the best treatment or on receiving educational information when getting discharged. The MOREOB program (Chap. 33) strives to improve existing moments of care with a preventive lens. In 2004, it was found that 1 in 81 newborns experienced traumatic birth injury that occurred unintentionally while patients were under medical care, management, or supervision (Baker et al., 2004). This cause for concern allowed the MOREOB program to update current obstetrical unit culture in order to create a more communicative environment that embraces a holistic approach, focused on patient safety. Figure 27.3 demonstrates a downward trend curve for the obstetrical services in terms of average cost per liability claim compared to all other departments within the hospital, since the pilot phase of the MOREOB program was launched in 2002 (Milne & Salus Global Corporation, 2010). This data demonstrates support for the fundamental premise of this hospital-based program; when knowledge and communication is increased, a patient safety culture can be achieved, translating to better baby outcomes. Therefore, by integrating professional practice standards with updated guidelines, this program reduces the traditional hierarchy, thus ensuring the use of teamwork in obstetric environments and preventing injury.

Not only do hospital-based interventions aim to improve the quality of care given to their patients, but they also provide an opportunity for prevention information to be administered. The Safe Babies New York, previously known as the Upstate New York Shaken Baby Syndrome

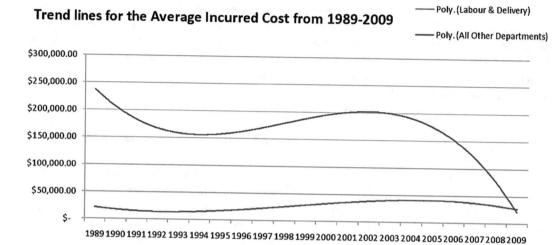

Fig. 27.3 Trend lines for the average cost per claim incurred from 1989 to 2009. HIROC data taken from 39 participating MOREOB hospitals (Milne & Salus Global Corporation, 2010)

Education Program (Chap. 34), has provided parents with educational materials within a hospital setting. This program started due to the alarming amount of head injuries seen in infants under the age of 1 (Billmire & Myers, 1985; Blumenthal, 2002; Fulton, 2000). Shaken baby syndrome (SBS), a constellation of inflicted head injuries sustained by infants and young children after being violently shaken, was deemed a potential cause of this trauma. This shaking often occurs in response to a baby crying or other factors that can trigger the person caring for the baby to become frustrated or angry. Figure 27.4 displays the "crying curve," in which infants' crying begins to increase around 2–3 weeks of age and peaks around 6–8 weeks. Therefore, this program aims to educate parents about infant crying as a phase of infant development and methods to manage that stress in order to decrease SBS.

The program's impact on annual incidence rates of SBS for the pilot program in Upstate New York was unprecedented. From 1998 to 2005, the rate of SBS decreased from 8.2 to 3.8 cases per year (from 41.5 cases per 100,000 live births to 22.2 cases per 100,000 live births; Dias et al., 2005). These remarkable results encouraged other environments to implement this program. Dias et al. (2005) found the Western

New York project experienced a 47% drop in SBS incidences whereas the Finger Lakes Region experienced a drop by 41%. The SBS curriculum is operational in several states, including Canada, and will continue to deliver this exemplary prevention program across regions in North America. However, it is important to keep in mind that the program may need stages of implementation to ensure that it fits within the community it caters to. Two key factors were identified for successful replication: finding capable project coordinators and maintaining a manageable pace of program implementation. With this in mind, due to the hospital setting of this program, integration and distribution of prevention materials is efficient as well as trackable.

27.1.4 Policy-Based Interventions

Among the benefits to developing a national injury prevention strategy through policy-based changes are the enormity of lives saved from harm or death, reduced expenditures for hospital care, and a diminished economic burden borne by taxpayers (Insurance Canada, 2005). The New Zealand Injury Prevention Strategy (NZIPS) aims to create injury-free, safety cultures and

Fig. 27.4 Development of infant crying as a teaching method to educate parents on SBS (CDC, n.d.)

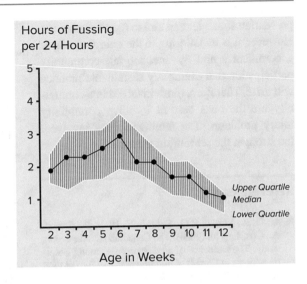

environments by increasing awareness as well as updating harm-reduction policies. The strategies that are implemented by policy interventions are catered to the individuals within the specific environment that is being targeted by the policy and address the area's pressing injury matters at that time. For instance, the New Zealand Injury Prevention Strategy (Chap. 35) focused on six national priority areas for injury prevention which included drowning, workplace injuries, motor vehicle crashes, suicide and self-harm, injuries from falls, and finally, assault specific to community and/or sexual violence—as they were discovered to be the most pressing needs of the community. To monitor performance from a national level, NZIPS released the Chartbook of the New Zealand Injury Prevention Strategy: Serious Injury Outcome Indicators, to determine progress and improvement within those specific injury areas. This demonstrates a type of community prevention program that deals with all facets of injury under one umbrella, with a collaborating effect toward injury prevention on a grand scale.

27.2   For What Follows

Injury prevention is an international important public health issue. The World Health Organization published a report in 2002 estimating that injuries accounted for 12% of global ailment (even greater than that of cardiovascular 10%, or respiratory disease 5%), road traffic accidents at 23%, falls around 11%, and violence, drowning, poisoning, and fires at 5–7% (World Health Organization, 2002). These injuries carry an inherent risk for neurotrauma which can manifest into a lifetime of disabilities or even fatality. Beyond the cost for individuals, there are also major financial repercussions for societies. Therefore, preventing these injuries from happening in the first place, as opposed to treating injuries once they have occurred, is a worthwhile investment as demonstrated by the aforementioned programs.

These exemplary injury prevention programs are provided here as foundations and examples for other prevention endeavors to learn from and/or expand on. The residential-based programs feature families and caregivers as a vessel for injury prevention, while school programs highlight the value of making use of existing community resources to create holistic environments that support sustainability. Hospital programs within the community sector focus on care practices and dissemination of information to patients to continue the prevention strategies outside of a medical environment, while policy programs highlight the bird's-eye view of community prevention by targeting the general area from the perspective of that society's members. In essence, multiple prevention strategies can aim to modify behavior. However, it is by tailoring to the unique needs of a community and by encouraging community participation that exemplary sustainable practice will arise. Therefore, those involved in a community are the ones best fit to solve community injury problems. The more members involved, the stronger the prevention message.

References

Baker, G. R., Norton, P. G., Flintoft, V., Blais, R., Brown, A., Cox, J., et al. (2004). The Canadian adverse events study: The incidence of adverse events among hospital patients in Canada. *Canadian Medical Association Journal, 170*(11), 1678–1686.

Billmire, M. E., & Myers, P. A. (1985). Serious head injury in infants: Accident or abuse? *Pediatrics, 75*(2), 340–342.

Blumenthal, I. (2002). Shaken baby syndrome. *Postgraduate Medical Journal, 78*(926), 732–735.

Centers for Disease Control and Prevention. (2015). *Fatal injury mapping*. Atlanta, GA: Author. Retrieved from https://wisqars.cdc.gov:8443/cdcMapFramework/mapModuleInterface.jsp

Centers for Disease Control and Prevention. (2017). *TBI: Get the facts*. Atlanta, GA: Author. Retrieved from https://www.cdc.gov/traumaticbraininjury/get_the_facts.html

Centers for Disease Control and Prevention. (n.d.). *Preventing shaken baby syndrome: A guide for health departments and community-based organizations*. Atlanta, GA: Author. Retrieved from https://www.cdc.gov/violenceprevention/pdf/preventingsbs.pdf

Cohen, L., Chavez, V., & Chehimi, S. (2010). *Prevention is primary: Strategies for community well-being*. Oakland, CA: Prevention Institute.

Delp, L., Runyan, C. W., Brown, M., Bowling, M., & Jahan, A. S. (2002). Role of work permits in teen workers' experiences. *American Journal of Industrial Medicine, 41*, 477–482.

Dias, M. S., Smith, K., DeGuehery, K., Mazur, P., Li, V., & Shaffer, M. L. (2005). Preventing abusive head trauma among infants and young children: A hospital-based parent education program. *Pediatrics, 115*, 470–477.

Fulton, D. R. (2000). Shaken baby syndrome. *Critical Care Nursing Quarterly, 23*(2), 43–50.

Indian Health Service. (2000). *Trends in Indian health, 1998-1999*. Rockville, MD: Author.

Insurance Canada. (2005). *Insurance Bureau of Canada joins SMARTRISK in calling for a National Injury Prevention Strategy*. Toronto, ON: Author. Retrieved from http://www.insurance-canada.ca/consinfogeneral/IBC-injury-prevention-510.php

Laflamme, L., & Eilert-Peterson, E. (1998). Injuries to pre-school children in a home setting: Patterns and related products. *Acta Paediatrics, 87*, 206–211.

Milne, J. K., & Salus Global Corporation. (2010). *Performance improvement in patient safety and risk reduction with participation in the MOREOB Program. A review of the national data from hospitals participating in the Salus MoreOB obstetrical patient safety program*. Mississauga, ON: Salus Global Corporation. Retrieved from http://www.moreob.com/images/pdfs/en/july2010impactofmoreob.pdf

National Committee for Injury Prevention and Control. (1989). *Injury prevention: Meeting the challenge*. New York, NY: Oxford University Press.

National Safety Council. (2015). *Injury facts*. Ottawa, ON: Author. Retrieved from http://www.nsc.org/Membership%20Site%20Document%20Library/2015%20Injury%20Facts/NSC_InjuryFacts2015Ed.pdf

Nurse Family Partnership. (2007). *Home visit experience*. Hamilton, ON: Author. Retrieved from http://www.nursefamilypartnership.org/content/index.cfm?fuseaction=showContent&contentID=47&navID=46

Nurse Family Partnership. (2017). *Nurse Family Partnership Snapshot*. Hamilton, ON: Author. Retrieved from https://www.nursefamilypartnership.org/wp-content/uploads/2017/11/NFP_Snapshot_Sept2017.pdf

ThinkFirst National Injury Prevention Foundation. (2006). *Home*. Retrieved from www.thinkfirst.org

Tymchuk, A., Lakin, K. C., & Luckasson, R. (2001). Life at the margins: Intellectual, demographic, economic, and social circumstances of adults with mild cognitive limitations. In A. Tymchuk, K. C. Lakin, & R. Luckasson (Eds.), *The forgotten generation* (pp. 21–39). Baltimore, MA: Paul H. Brookes.

Volpe, R., Lewko, J., & Batra, A. (2002). *A compendium of effective, evidence-based best practices in prevention of neurotrauma*. Toronto, ON: University of Toronto Press.

World Health Organization. (2002). *Global burden of diseases attributable to injuries, 2000 estimate*. Geneva: Author. Retrieved from http://www.who.int/violenceinjuryprevention/main.cfm?p=0000000079

Nurse-Family Partnership

28

Keren Epstein-Gilboa and Tanya Morton

The Nurse-Family Partnership (NFP) is an evidence-informed, community health program that serves mothers in their first pregnancy with possible risk factors that may impair parenting. Each new mother is partnered with a registered nurse during the early prenatal stage. The nurse conducts multiple home visits from pregnancy into early childhood with the aim of identifying risks and facilitating healthy interactions between parents and their children (Nurse Family Partnership [NFP], 2017).

28.1 Background

The Nurse Family Partnership (NFP) is based on model created by Olds and colleagues and is based on work with children in a daycare center in Baltimore during the 1970's (Olds, Kitzman, Cole, & Robinson, 1997). The center serviced a community with low socioeconomic status, inadequate housing and play areas, and high rates of unemployment and crime low (Columbia Broadcasting System [CBS] Evening News, 2007). Olds noted the negative impact of risk fac-

tors such as caregiver substance abuse and maltreatment on young children. The researcher decided to create a program that would reduce risks and enhance developmental outcomes from an early age (CBS Evening News). Olds model is influenced by a program that was in place in Elmira, NY in the 1970's that screened young children for developmental problems but that lacked a valid and reliable scientific design. Olds improved the design of the program to include rigorous scientific scrutiny (Goodman, 2006).

28.1.1 Creating a Model

An important early influence on Olds' design was Bronfenbrenner's work on human ecology (Goodman, 2006). Bronfenbrenner's (1979) ecological model implies that multileveled and mutually influential systems impact child development. Children are part of family microsystems that are influenced by and interact with the mesosystem. Their mesosystem may include healthcare organizations, schools, and other intervening agencies, including but not limited to community, corporate, and government structures. The impact of the sociocultural macrosystem is felt at all levels of the mutually contingent system. Therefore, an ecological understanding of children's health and social outcomes implies that one may provide varied levels of intervention,

K. Epstein-Gilboa (✉)
Private Practice, Toronto, ON, Canada

T. Morton
Catholic Children's Aid Society of Toronto, Toronto, ON, Canada

© Springer Nature Switzerland AG 2020
R. Volpe (ed.), *Casebook of Traumatic Injury Prevention*,
https://doi.org/10.1007/978-3-030-27419-1_28

including individual, family and community strategies.

Olds' original model used ecological concepts, was flexible, and evolved over time to reflect novel concepts and feedback from front-line staff (P. Hill, personal communication, August 14, 2007). With each successive randomized control trial (RCT), additional theoretical concepts were examined and incorporated. Concepts associated with attachment as well as self-efficacy theories were increasingly emphasized due to the growing need for theory. Resulting program models that would promote adaptive behavior change (Olds et al., 1997). The inclusion of attachment theory (Bowlby) promoted the use of interventions that enhanced clients' abilities to competently read and respond to their babies' communicative signals. Parental capacity to understand children and their developmental needs as well as limitations reduces the risk that they will abuse and neglect their children and contribute to associated unintentional injury (Peterson & Gable, 1998). Several theories guide the model, enabling interventions

to reach diverse components of clients' inner and outer world (Kitzman, Olds, et al., 1997). In Table 28.1, the empirical and theoretical underpinnings of the program and their practice implications with respect to injury prevention are summarized.

These models served as a foundation for the development of objectives. There are three Nurse-Family Partnership goals set out:

1. Improve pregnancy outcomes by helping women engage in good preventive health practices, including prenatal care from their healthcare providers, improving their diets, and reducing their use of cigarettes, alcohol, and illegal substances
2. Improve child health and development by helping parents provide responsible and competent care
3. Improve the economic self-sufficiency of the family by helping parents develop a vision for their own future, plan future pregnancies, continue their education, and find work (NFP, 2017).

Table 28.1 Theoretical underpinnings of the program and practice implications

Model	Empirical underpinnings	Main contributions	Domain targeted by the NFP	Practice implications
Human ecology theory	Bronfenbrenner's person-process-context model (1979)	Emphasize the influence of social context on human development	Clients' formal and informal social support system and other social networks	Enhance the clients' physical and social environment by drawing on the support of partners and family members and connect clients to social and material resources and services
Self-Efficacy theory	Bandura (1977)	Suggests that individuals' behavior is based on their beliefs about (1) the outcome of that behavior and (2) the likelihood that they can successfully accomplish these behaviors	Participants' sense of self-efficacy and control over their lives	Educate clients about the effects of their behavior on self and family and promote the achievement of small realistic goals that will incrementally build clients' confidence, independence, and control over their lives
Attachment theory	Bowlby (1969)	Attests that the attachment between caregivers and infants is biologically designed to keep infants safe from threats of harm	The attachment (i.e., behaviors that promote positive interactions) between the client and her baby	Assist clients' in reflecting upon their own attachment-related experiences. Promote and model sensitive, responsive caregiving relationships

Note: Olds et al. (1997), Olds (2002)

28.1.2 Preliminary Studies

The original model and curriculum for the program was polished by Olds and colleagues in the mid-1970s. Olds accepted funds from the US Public Health Service for the first 2 years of the study only when the curriculum, pilot study, and other program components were in place. Subsequently, the first RCT was underway by 1978 in Elmira NY in a semirural community with multiple socio economic disadvantages (Goodman, 2006). An RCT (a study where half the participants are randomly assigned to a treatment group and half are assigned to a control group) is the most rigorous research method for measuring the effectiveness of a program due to its capacity to control for the influence of confounding factors on a program's outcomes. The Robert Wood Johnson foundation provided a grant for continuation of the program approximately 2 years after it was launched. Funding was also offered by the Carter Administration (Goodman, 2006).

Funding was also offered by the Carter Administration (Goodman, 2006). However, Olds refused this funding due to his concern that fidelity to the model would be compromised by the Carter administration's proposal to replace professional nurses with paraprofessionals. Olds wanted the original program standards to be empirically well-tested before any changes were made (Goodman, 2006). The development of program standards, such as the required education and training levels of staff, is a quality assurance mechanism that promotes sustainability (Johnson, Hays, Center, & Daley, 2004; Nutter & Weiden, 1988).

28.1.2.1 Transportability and Sustainability

The second RCT was conducted in a different settings with a diverse populations in order to test the model's transportability. The trial was conducted with a largely African-American population in the urban inner city of Memphis TN that differed from the Caucasian, semirural community of Elmira, (Olds, 2005). Both Elmira and Memphis were communities with low socioeconomic status and with the typical correlates of poverty: poor social and health outcomes including low birth weight and high infant mortality and morbidity (Goodman, 2006). The nature and design of the home-visiting services were essentially the same in both Elmira and Memphis (Olds, 2002). However, Olds and colleagues refined the program model in Memphis for African-American families. The researchers consulted the scholarly literature, a national program advisory committee, a local community advisory committee, and participants via focus groups and individual feedback (Kitzman, Olds, et al., 1997). Therefore, there was an understanding of how the community and cultural context of the program may influence program delivery and effectiveness. This understanding of contextual influence was essential. Without it, similar programs implemented in different communities may produce different results, with little direction on how to interpret diverse findings (Nilsen, 2005).

Results of the Memphis trial suggested that the model was transportable to different cultural and community contexts. The children who had received the intervention children experienced significantly fewer injuries and less serious injuries than the control children. Olds was reluctant to replicate trials in various communities due to the risk that the program could be "watered down" in an effort to cut costs and become less effective. For example, higher caseloads or shortening a program's length may have decreased the program intensity. Moreover, in several proposed replications of the NFP, paraprofessionals who did not possess formal training in the helping professions were considered as the home visitors, instead of registered nurses (Goodman, 2006). Watering down of program components in the name of cost containment, although well intentioned, is a common threat to the sustainability of effective prevention programs (Jones & Offord, 1991).

Olds conducted a third RCT to investigate treatment results of services provided by nurse home visitors versus paraprofessionals as a means of ensuring consistency in future programs. The researcher included a control group that received no extra service as a baseline comparison. The RCT occurred in Denver in 1994 and was funded by The Colorado Trust. About half the sample population were Hispanic, and 87% of the sample population were unmarried (Olds, 2005). Similar to the planning of the Elmira trial, the model was reviewed by members of the cultural community before implementation (Olds et al., 1997). The results of this trial suggest that paraprofessionals did not elicit the same positive results as the nurses in the key domains of maternal and child functioning and child development (Olds, 2005).

Rates of unintentional child injury and child abuse were not a focus in the Denver trial, due to the diverse settings in which participants receive healthcare in Denver and the low rates of state-substantiated child maltreatment in the target population. However, the Denver trial added credibility to the model's transportability to a range of community and cultural contexts. Following this trial, the researchers also concluded that registered nurses would be the front-line workers (Olds et al., 2004; Olds, Henderson, Phelps, Kitzman, & Hanks, 1993). Olds et al. (2002) suggest that one reason why nurses had more success than paraprofessionals in promoting enduring mothering behaviors is due to the apparent expert stance. The authors explain that the target population appears to regard nurses as more authoritarian than paraprofessionals and the target population internalizes novel concepts better when they are promoted by authoritarian figures.

28.1.3 Taking the Program to Scale

In 1996, efforts began to replicate the program in communities across the USA. Research and consultation undertaken by Olds and his team suggested that it would be better to obtain funding from state governments and to marshal community interests in a state-based approach to national implementation rather than a site-specific expansion. For example, the Colorado-based nonprofit organization Invest in Kids advocated for the NFP throughout the state and gathered grassroots support (Howard, Husain, & Velji, 2005). The efforts of Invest in Kids and those of program

champion Senator Norma Anderson led to the passing of Colorado's Nurse Home Visitor Act in 2000 where the program was enshrined in legislation (NFP, 2007e; Goodman, 2006). Some key elements of the Nurse Home Visitor Act (2000) included:

- Earmarks $75 million from Medicaid and the State Children's Health Insurance Program funds over 10 years to support the program in Colorado
- A secured $300 million in state tobacco settlement funds
- Increase in funding each fiscal year in order to support expansion up to 2011–2012
- The Colorado Department of Public Health and Environment (CDPHE) administering the program
- Local communities applying to the CDPHE for funds with which to implement the program (Invest in Kids, n.d.)

To consolidate the planning process for the expansion, a national head office was established in Denver. The national office responsibilities for program management included recruiting and training new sites, quality control, program monitoring, and reporting procedures. In 2000, the team enlarged and became an initiative of the National Centre for Children, Families, and Communities (NCCFC). The program was incorporated as a nonprofit agency in 2003 and was entitled the Nurse-Family Partnership.

A web-based clinical information system (CIS) was established by the national office for the ongoing monitoring and evaluation of local sites. The local site data are benchmarked against objectives gleaned from the clinical trials and national data. This data can help local sites identify areas of strength, areas for change, and lessons learned (O'Brien, 2005). Both process and outcome data are collected from nurses and delivered to the national office. Nurses submit process data on the respective amount of time they spend teaching each of the domains of the program. Data is also collected on a set of core outcome variables, including rates of childhood injuries and child abuse/neglect (O'Brien, 2005;

Olds, 2002). Although these outcome variables are based on the results of the RCTs, the NFP only has the capacity to collect information on injuries, ingestions, and abuse by maternal report (P. Hill, personal communication, September 20, 2007). Child abuse registries and medical/hospital records cannot provide data for the community replications due to confidentiality and privacy laws.

The NFP is implemented in 42 states, serving over 260,000 families, with a five-time return (NFP, 2017). The program is also being evaluated in Canada and is available in several locations throughout the country (Children' Health Policy Centre, 2019). Additional foundations and corporations have joined the Robert Wood Johnson Foundation in supporting the central program. Expansion has occurred according to careful planning on the part of Olds and colleagues, and the marshaling of stable and adequate funding has continued to be integral to expansion of the program.

The review of the background and development of NFP suggests it was mounted by a truly committed individual with a vision—David Olds. Program features that subscribe to the principles of sustainability (e.g., Johnson et al., 2004; Jones & Offord, 1991) include the presence of an influential and proactive individuals in the program, careful planning of program development evaluation and administration, and consideration of the needs of each community.

28.2 Resources

28.2.1 Stakeholders and Collaborators

The analysis of the resources of the NFP demonstrates the important role that stakeholders play in the sustainability of the program. A review of the literature and key informant information demonstrate that central features associated with the sustainability of NFP are the careful selection of appropriate stakeholders, accurate task definition, ensuring stakeholders' perceptions of the program are realistic, and the dissemination of positive program results. The resources also emphasize that systemic mutuality and communication are important features of the program (NFP, 2007b; P. Hill, personal communication, August 14, 2007).

Olds was the original stakeholder in this program. As a researcher, he firmly believed that preventive interventions must be based on evidence, as well as consequently an established, firm research basis to the program. Olds gathered data demonstrating the association between poverty, parenting difficulties, unintentional injury, child abuse, and later criminal behavior. This data helped Olds gain the support of interested parties, including the US Public Health Service and the Robert Wood Johnson Foundation, as discussed previously, which facilitated the establishment and maintenance of the program in earlier years.

Olds and several of the original stakeholders remain actively invested in the present NFP program. Stakeholder interests and roles are reinforced by systemic communication which strengthens and sustains the program. The interdependence between the levels of the system of stakeholders is demonstrated by their contingent roles and tasks (P. Hill, personal communication, September 20, 2007). Stakeholders at the research level of the NFP include Olds and his team. The research and clinical program is affiliated with the NCCFC, based at the University of Colorado Health Sciences Center (NFP, 2007e). The implementation of longitudinal studies allows NFP to measure short- and long-term outcomes in the program. However, the NFP National Service Office maintains a close association with the Prevention Research Center; the two remain professionally independent (NFP, 2014). Research is influenced by the decisions at the administrative level which is inclusive of a board of directors, foundation supporters, and administrative employees. The role of these stakeholders is to oversee the financial aspects of the program, to allocate funding, and to make decisions about the implementation of the program in various areas. Research and financial decisions affect the clinical work that takes place at the various sites (NFP, 2007a).

Stakeholders in each site include the agencies, supervisors, front-line workers, and participating women and their families. The employees uphold the program by implementing it with actual families and collecting process and outcome data (NFP, 2007e). Families contribute to the program through their willingness to participate and by internalizing messages advancing their lifestyle. Their stories of success, such as the prevention of child abuse and unintentional child injury, gratify local stakeholder, ensuring that they continue to support the program (P. Hill, personal communication, September 20, 2007).

Qualitative and quantitative data are used to influence child welfare and law enforcement agencies, the judicial system, as well as early childhood education and healthcare agencies. These agencies refer clients, create conditions conducive to the NFP in local community centers and agencies, devise facilitative policies, include the NFP in their local budget, and provide funding to the program. Public donors such as municipal governments or private donors including corporations are examples of stakeholders who support the work of diverse agencies by providing funding that sustains the program. Corporations have donated materials and provided funding for small- and large-scale events at local sites (NFP, 2007a). A continuum of stakeholder support is facilitated when stakeholders perceive that the program meets their needs.

28.2.2 Collaborators

Systemic interaction sustaining the stakeholder component of the program is also evident in the interactions between the collaborators in this program. The first professionals to collaborate with Olds were other researchers who helped him design and implement the program as a research project. Together with administrative professionals, the researchers helped Olds and his team initiate and implement RCTs in three locations. Various collaborators also helped facilitate taking the program to scale. Additional politicians and legislators collaborated with the

NFP as stakeholders providing funding and supportive legislation (NFP, 2007a).

All agencies and families collaborate with the program on a voluntary basis. The central office willingly participates with all interested agencies following an examination of their goals and their ability to implement the program according to the existing philosophy. Similar to other aspect of this program, the collaboration between various levels of the system, such as the national office, the research department, and the implementing agencies, is sustained by a clear communication style and fidelity to the program's model (NFP, 2007a).

28.2.3 Resources to Implement Prevention Strategies

The initial resources used to implement the RCTs were obtained through collaboration between the researcher, interested politicians, and public and private organizations. In 1991, the US Justice Department initiated a program aimed at reducing the negative implications of poverty on children, entitled Operation Weed and Seed. Through this program $25,000 per city was allocated to different US cities, with the hopes of attracting local organizations that could administer nurse home-visiting programs. Local organizations were responsible for securing the remaining funds needed. Olds approved this method of funding and collaboration, as it "… forced only committed organizations to get involved" (Goodman, 2006, p. 16). This funding process initiated the establishment of nurse home-visiting programs in California, Florida, Missouri, and Oklahoma.

The exact means of allocating resources varies from site to site locally and among states. For example, following the establishment of the Nurse Home Visitor Act in 2000, sites were financially supported by tobacco settlement funds in Colorado. Louisiana also has a state NFP initiative, supported by block grant funding. The county health department system supports the program in Oklahoma. In Pennsylvania, Temporary Aid to Needy Families (TANF) originally funded the NFP in 1999. In 2006, NFP expanded further in that state due to Governor Tom Ridge's Community Partnership for Safe Children program (Goodman, 2006). Other communities use a variety of local, state, and federal funding sources to support the program, including Medicaid, welfare-reform, maternal and child health, and child abuse prevention dollars. One benefit of having several funding bodies for a program is that if one reduces the level of support, another is available to compensate, thereby promoting financial sustainability (Jones & Offord, 1991).

Being long term and intensive, the NFP is more expensive than many other prevention programs. The average per-family cost during the first 3 years of program operation was estimated at $3200 per year, increasing to $4100 in 2011 (Center for the Study and Prevention of Violence, 2004; HVEE, 2011). Fortunately, the NFP encourages economies of scale by housing the program in already existing agencies in the implementing community, including state and county departments of public health, community-based health centers, or hospitals (NFP, 2007d). For a fee, the national office offers training, support, and evaluation services to local sites in order to encourage their success (Olds, 2002). In spite of the program's expense, external and internal cost-benefit analysis have deemed that the program saves expenditures in the health care, criminal justice, and social services realms in the long run (e.g., Karoly, Kilburn, & Cannon, 2005; Olds et al., 1993).

28.3 Implementation

Each stage of sustainable implementation can be characterized by specific tasks. The model is sustained through well-defined principles, guidelines, role and task delineation, an ongoing system of communication between all levels of the system, as well as flexibility in certain areas (P. Hill, personal communication, September 4, 2007; NFP, 2007a). These facilitators to sustainability are discussed below at the planning, training, and maintenance phases of program implementation.

28.3.1 Implementation Planning

The guiding principle of fidelity to the original and tested model is upheld by the application of specific guidelines that are systemically transferred between each level of the organization. Guidelines are altered to suit the various levels of implementation, including initiating, establishing, maintaining, and reinforcing implementation. Sites are approved by the national office to initiate, develop, and maintain the program in their communities. Interactions with the administrative and research levels of the organization influence service providers at all levels of implementation (NFP, 2007a, 2007h; P. Hill, personal communication, September 4, 2007).

Agencies or individuals interested in implementing the NFP program apply to the national office. An agency aspiring to implement the NFP must display a genuine interest in advancing the quality of care to first time mothers and their families and demonstrate that it will adhere to the ideals, policies, and standards associated with the central program. The national office supplies the interested parties with information and guidelines for application. Strict selection criteria have been designed to ensure that only suitable agencies are approved. The criteria ensure that potential providers will follow the program's evidence informed practices and design. The potential implementing agency must demonstrate that the demographics of the community include a sizable proportion of young first-time mothers with low SES. The potential implementing agency must also demonstrate that the NFP will not duplicate existing services in the community; that it has the ability to liaise, coordinate, and accept referrals from existing health and social service agencies in the area; and that it has a plan for sustained funding. The potential agency must have ample physical storage and meeting space as well as be able to recruit and maintain qualified staff that will be able to implement the program in accordance with the predetermined standards (NFP, 2007c, 2007h; P. Hill, personal communication, September 4, 2007).

28.3.2 Establishing a Program: Selection and Training

The central administration directs potential program sites to hire nurses. Each center is required to employ registered nurses to act as supervisors and front-line home visitors. Nurses and nurse supervisors are selected based on strict criteria. The rigid hiring criteria demonstrate the principle that well-defined professional standards and skills contribute to sustainability (Johnson et al., 2004; Nutter & Weiden, 1988). The importance of employees' characteristics is evident by the description of an ideal nurse for NFP, being able to work independently, ability to be patient, to be able to understand and accept client perspectives, and to work with clients with various presenting issues (P. Hill, personal communication, September 4, 2007). The literature implies that the nurses must display maturity, an ability to work independently, and possess a psychosocial approach to clinical interaction. The selection of appropriate clinicians is facilitated by interviews. The NFP site in Rochester ensures that there is a good fit between the potential employee and the site by enabling nurses to experience home visiting during the hiring process (P. Scott, personal communication, October 31, 2007). Although applicants are interviewed and hired by the on-site program developers, interview guides are designed by the national office to help the on-site program developers consider all relevant hiring criteria (NFP, 2007h; P. Scott, personal communication, October 31, 2007).

The national office continues to cooperate with the program sites as they establish the NFP program in their area. Internal coherence is managed by transferring the principles of the NFP program to the front-line team through a training protocol. This protocol facilitates future workers' ability to internalize principles, goals, and methods of interaction with clients. Concepts associated with reflective practice, maternal and child development, attachment theory, as well as maternal self-efficacy are central to the material covered (NFP, 2007f; P. Hill, personal communication, August 14, 2007).

Job training is divided into several phases reflecting the trainees' level of familiarity and experience with the NFP. The national office remains available during the first phase when trainees engage in self-learning processes facilitated through manuals and online material. At the same time that nurses study self-learning manuals, they also undergo an intense orientation at the site where they are guided by experienced nurses. Following the completion of the self-learning module, all trainees attend an intense training session that extends over a few days in the national office in Denver. All future nurse supervisors and front-line nurses attend the seminars as well. Following these sessions, the national office monitors the learning process through the provision of periodic courses to nurse supervisors in Denver, on-site in-services, ongoing communication with nurse supervisors, and written material (NFP, 2007c, 2007i; P. Hill, personal communication, September 4, 2007).

The Home Visit Experience. Each nurse carries a maximum caseload of 25 families. The frequency and order of home visits, the supportive style, and the subject matter covered in each visit are determined by the central administration of the NFP program and are based on principles of maternal and child development. Home visits usually begin between week 13 and 28 of pregnancy. Ideally the nurses' visits include:

- Four weekly visits after enrollment in the program
- Weekly visits for 6 weeks after birth
- Visits every other week through the child's 21st month
- Monthly visits for months 22–24

Although visits do not extend beyond month 24, some NFP graduates may choose to keep in contact with their nurses on an informal basis after the program terminates (NFP, 2007c).

The educational material focuses on six main domains including personal health, environmental health, life course development, maternal role, family and friends, as well as human services (California Evidence-Based Clearinghouse for

Child Welfare, 2008). These topics reflect the evidence about the changing developmental needs of pregnant clients, first-time parents, infants, and toddlers. The nurses' task is to emotionally support and to scaffold clients' learning processes as they internalize novel concepts. Both key informants emphasized that nurses practice reflective rather than directive interactions with clients. The key informants' similar views not only demonstrate the centrality of this point however also illustrate the joint ownership of concepts throughout various levels of the system (NFP, 2007c; P. Hill, personal communication, August 14, 2007; P. Scott, personal communication, October 31, 2007). This reflective interaction validates mothers' feelings and encourages them to come up with solutions to problems on their own. While nurses follow predetermined guidelines carefully, they are also encouraged to use their judgment and read client's cues as a means of suiting learning goals to the client's readiness for learning, in addition to her emotional state. Nurses will address the material the client wants to cover but will also access the program's injury prevention guidelines if they see a concern in the home during that visit (P. Scott, personal communication, October 31, 2007).

The goal of supporting and educating parents is to enhance the interactions between parents and children. The nurses teach parents to understand their child's perspective and thereby identify safety hazards that coincide with their child's developmental level. Consequently, these teachings will help parents base their interactions with their children on child-centered needs, cues, and child-focused interventions (NFP, 2007c; P. Hill, personal communication, August 14, 2007; P. Scott, personal communication, October 31, 2007).

28.3.2.1 Implementing Injury Prevention

The nurse-client relationship and the principles associated with education and support influence the prevention of injury in these families. Salient areas of injury prevention in the target population include the prevention of falls, ingestions, burns, asphyxiation, and car accidents (Safekids Worldwide, n.d.). Similar to other areas of parent education, nurses scaffold learning and respect parents' processes of self-efficacy as they aspire to create safe environments. The concept of self-efficacy is central to the injury prevention aspect of the program. Nurses provide clients with information and resources that enable them to apply the concepts learned and to create safe environments without direct intervention. Modeling and applying appropriate behaviors are aspects of the educational process that allow nurses to provide clients with information without directing them (P. Hill, personal communication, September 4, 2007; P. Scott, personal communication, October 31, 2007). In Table 28.2, key injury prevention teaching techniques are expressed by a nurse supervisor.

Parents are educated about babyproofing through discussions and written material. They are guided to resources providing safety devices such as window guards, stair gates, and car seats. Families unable to purchase devices on their own may be referred to resources providing financial assistance or donations. Box 28.1 below represents the injury prevention teaching guidelines for a nurse home visit during the toddler stage.

Note: P. Scott, personal communication (October 31, 2007)

Table 28.2 Key injury prevention teaching techniques

Teaching technique	Example
Reflexive practice	Questions asked by the nurse such as "What are you going to do if you put the baby on the couch?" or "What do you think made your child calm down?"
Active listening	Clients verbalize their thoughts, feelings, and plans back to the nurse, in order to confirm the content of the nurse's message
Modeling	Dolls or the baby may be used for demonstration purposes
Education	Discussion of the consequences of a young child falling Discussion of child's developmental cues and limitations

Note: P. Scott, personal communication (October 31, 2007)

Box 28.1 Teaching Guidelines of Childhood Injury Prevention During Toddler Stage

Discuss that injuries are the leading cause of childhood death

Review with the client measures she has taken to childproof the home

- Always use safety gates and window guards.
- Never allow toddlers to stand up in a stroller, high chair, or shopping cart.
- Never leave toddlers on a table or counter or any surface where their feet do not touch the floor.
- Arrange furniture so that it is not placed near cabinets or open windows.

Examples of the principle of self-efficacy are evident when nurses teach clients how to provide a safe home environment. According to the key informants, obstacles impeding injury prevention are associated with clients' inability to apply the information provided by nurses. Language barriers are a possible obstacle to successful program implementation. There is a shortage of nurses who possess both the appropriate clinical skills and ability to speak the languages spoken by some clients (P. Hill, personal communication, September 4, 2007; P. Scott, personal communication, October 31, 2007). Even if the clients speak English, they might not understand the injury prevention material; this lack of understanding may be due to misconstrued messages or intervention of family members with conflicting views. If a client has not followed through on a installing a safety device in the home, the nurse would inquire into the client's barriers to implementing the safety device rather than challenging the client. Any parenting interventions that the mother undertook to enhance safety are celebrated. Further problem-solving would occur around the remaining steps necessary to install the safety device. Nurses promote client independence by encouraging clients to identify and travel to an agency that offers free or discounted safety devices (NFP, 2007c; P. Hill, personal communication, September 20, 2007).

In keeping with the relational focus of the program, most safety education is provided to clients on a one-to-one basis. The expectation to this rule occurs when an NFP site is associated with agencies involved in community programs. In these cases, nurses associated with the NFP might also contribute to community safety awareness programs (P. Scott, personal communication, October 31, 2007).

28.3.3 Maintaining Implementation

Nurses' capacity to continue front-line work is enriched by the opportunities that they are provided with to process their experiences. Nurse home visitors discuss their experiences with their supervisors and peers. In the Rochester site, for example, nurses work in close proximity to one another and often relay their experiences and support one another. This site also has regular team case conferences. In addition, nurses regularly attend one-to-one meetings with their supervisors. Supervisors provide additional support by intermittently accompanying nurses on home visits (P. Scott, personal communication, October 31, 2007). This aspect of the program also provides a means of ensuring that the information about families is shared and appropriate feedback is provided (NFP, 2007b).

28.3.4 Summary

The NFP program is sustained at the implementation level due to adherence to the model, open systemic communication, and flexibility to change. Professionals from multiple disciplines communicate and work together to sustain the program. Researchers conduct studies and evaluate data reinforcing the NFP model. The administrative level of the program isolates the principles of the NFP model and creates tangible guidelines for implementation at the front-line level. Home visitors and their supervisors internalize and implement program principles and goals and their defined roles and tasks, sustaining the program at the front-line level. Implementation at this level of the system is also sustained by mutual support of workers that changes to reflect their needs.

Flexibility and individuality are also apparent in the formation of trusting nurse-client relationships. Through reflective practice nurses convey information and instill a sense of efficacy in their clients that allows them to raise their children via seeing the world through the child's eyes. These principles, goals, and actions are applied in the injury prevention aspect of the program. Nurses report their experiences to supervisors who send the nurses' data to the national office for analysis. The analysis is returned, and feedback provided to agencies and their front-line home visitors, who alter their actions accordingly.

28.4 Outcome

The NFP program outcomes have short- and long-term results that are explored through a logic model. The previously mentioned RCTs will be looked at as an undertaking to test the model, and community replications tested the translation of the research intervention into clinical practice.

28.4.1 Logic Model

The tasks and objectives of the home visits are clearly delineated in program manuals, teaching sheets, and another program literature. Desired outcomes that are relevant to injury prevention are visually depicted in Fig. 28.1 as the components of the NFP logic model (adapted from O'Brien, n.d.). A logic model provides a visual aid to link program tasks and activities to the desired objectives (Fig. 28.1).

28.4.2 Randomized Control Trials: Results

There was a range of positive health and social outcomes evident in the three RCTs, each contributing to the program's esteem in the eyes of policymakers and practitioners. However, in the following section, the results of the Elmira and

Memphis RCTs will focus only on injury prevention. Furthermore, the results of the community replication will be presented vis-à-vis injury prevention. As the Denver trial did not focus on frequency and severity of injuries, its results will not be presented here.

28.4.2.1 Elmira, NY Trial

The results of the first RCT in Elmira, NY ($n = 400$), indicated that the provision of support and assistance to mothers with young children reduces the frequency of injury in their children (Olds, Henderson, Chamberlain, & Tatelbaum, 1986). The results also suggested that, among the women at highest risk for caregiving problems (i.e., low SES, adolescent mothers without support systems), the women that participated in the program had fewer instances of verified child abuse and neglect in the first 2 years of their child's life when compared to the controls (4% versus 19%; Olds et al., 1986). Moreover, the results of further research indicated that the children whose mothers participated in the program experienced a 56% reduction of emergency room visits from age 12 to 24 months (Olds, 2005). For 1- to 4-year-old children, there was a reduction in healthcare encounters in which injuries were identified, for up to 2 years after the program ended (Olds et al., 1986). The results were concentrated among women at greatest risk of caregiving problems (Olds et al., 1986). At 34 and 46 months, the nurse-visited children were observed to live in homes with fewer household hazards as measured by the Home Observation for Measurement of the Environment Inventory (HOME) score (Olds, Henderson, & Kitzman, 1994). Continued research has spoken to the enduring effects of the injury prevention component of the program to 50 months of age (Olds et al., 1994).

A 19-year follow-up was conducted by Eckenrode et al. (2010), to examine the effect of prenatal and infancy nurse home visitations on the life course development of the same mothers who participated in the original Elmira, NY trial program. It was found that the NFP program reduced the proportion of girls entering the criminal justice system 19 years later (Eckenrode et al., 2010). Eckenrode et al. also

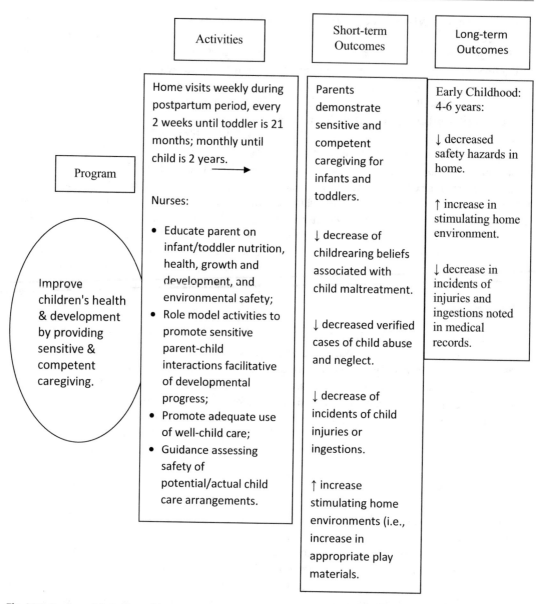

Fig. 28.1 Logic model, the flow of the model from left to right demonstrates how home visit tasks and activities prompt the behavior changes needed to achieve the short- and long-term outcomes of the program. (Adapted from O'Brien, n.d.)

report that girls born to mothers with risk factors (categorized as single and with low-income) had fewer children and were less likely to receive Medicaid than girls with risk factors in the comparison group. These extensive benefits of the NFP program demonstrate the potential it provides to break the cycle-parenting with potential risk factors and negative child outcome.

28.4.2.2 The Memphis Trial

Building on the momentum of the Elmira trial, the Memphis trial was underway in 1987 ($n = 734$). Program effects indicated a 23% reduction in healthcare encounters for child injuries, while the reduction in days hospitalized due to injuries or ingestions was 80% (Kitzman, Olds, et al., 1997). In all, the control group had 15 trips to hospital compared to four trips in the intervention group. The control group suffered two cases of fractured skull and two cases of head trauma. Seven (54%) of the comparison group children were hospitalized with either fractures or head trauma, while none of the nurse-visited children were admitted to hospital for these reasons (Kitzman, Olds, et al., 1997). The difference between the intervention and control groups in terms of injuries was significant. The results also reveal that if the nurse-visited children were hospitalized, they were admitted to hospital when they were older, and their injuries were less severe than the comparison group (Kitzman, Olds, et al., 1997). Similar to the results of the Elmira trial, the program effects on both total healthcare encounters and number of days hospitalized with injuries and ingestions were stronger for the children of women at highest risk for caregiving problems. These results are of the RCT in terms of childhood injuries, and ingestions are summarized in Tables 28.3 and 28.4.

Importantly, the prevention of injuries was achieved in spite of considerable program challenges. For example, a qualitative study of program implementation in Memphis indicates that keeping children away from environmental hazards was difficult. In crowded, busy, and under-resourced homes, nurses found it was difficult for mothers to keep infants away from purses or other storage items that may contain medications. As property owners were often absent or reluctant to improve dangerous housing conditions, safety recommendations were difficult to follow (Kitzman, Yoos, et al., 1997). Nurses had to use their judgment about what hazards needed immediate attention as serious safety concerns and what hazards were minor enough to warrant the nurse assisting the family over time in marshaling the resources needed to address them (Kitzman, Olds, et al., 1997).

These mothers were followed up two decades later to determine the effect of prenatal and infant/toddler nurse home visiting on maternal and child mortality. Olds et al. (2014) found that the women who enrolled in the nurse-visited groups were less likely to have died than women assigned to the control group. It was also reported that by age 20, children whose mothers received

Table 28.3 Diagnoses for hospitalizations in which injuries and ingestions were detected, nurse-visited (treatment group 4)

Diagnosis	Age, months	Sex	Length of stay, days
Burns (first and second degree to face)	12.0	M	2
Coin ingestion	12.1	M	1
Ingestion of iron medication	20.4	F	4

Note: Kitzman, Olds, et al. (1997)

Table 28.4 Diagnoses for hospitalizations in which injuries and ingestions were detected, comparison (treatment group 2)

Diagnosis	Age, months	Sex	Length of stay, days
Head trauma	2.4	M	1
Fractured fibula/congenital syphilis	2.4	M	12
Strangulated hemia with delay in seeking care/burns (first degree to lips)	3.5	M	15
Bilateral subdural hematoma[a]	4.9	F	19
Fractured skull	5.2	F	5
Bilateral subdural hematoma (unresolved)/aseptic meningitis—second hospitalization[a]	5.3	F	4
Fractured skull	7.8	F	3
Coin ingestion	10.9	M	2
Child abuse/neglect suspected	14.6	M	2
Fractured tibia	14.8	M	2
Burns (second degree to face/neck)	15.1	M	5
Burns (second and third degree to bilateral leg)[b]	19.6	M	4
Gastroenteritis/head trauma	20.0	F	3
Burns (splinting/grafting)—second hospitalization[b]	20.1	M	6
Finger injury/osteomyelitis	23.0	M	6

Note: Kitzman, Olds, et al. (1997)
[a]One child was hospitalized twice with a single bilateral subdural hematoma
[b]One child was hospitalized twice for burns resulting from a single incident (Kitzman, Olds, et al., 1997)

home visits during pregnancy and through child age 2 years were less likely to have died from preventable causes compared with their counterparts in the control group (Olds et al., 2014).

These findings suggest that the NFP program interventions may have longer-term effects on health and mortality as the mothers and their children grow older (Olds et al., 2014).

28.4.3 Community Replication

Although there are no randomly assigned control groups with which to compare the community replications of the NFP, the local site data can be benchmarked against objectives gleaned from the clinical trials and national data. The results of this benchmarking have shown that there have been challenges in taking the program to scale. In comparison to the RCTs, women in the community replications present for enrolment later in their pregnancies (Olds, 2002), and caseloads are more varied (O'Brien, 2005). Moreover, average attrition rates are 10–15% higher. The higher attrition rates can be explained by the high rate of mobility among the community participants.

Overall program results for the community replications are promising in terms of maternal and child functioning including child health and development; however, results are somewhat weaker than those of the RCTs (O'Brien, 2005). There have been some promising trends in terms of injury prevention as measured by child hospitalizations (Shores, 2007); however, future research is required to further illuminate the effects of the community replications.

28.4.4 Dissemination

Dissemination activities promote public and strategic awareness of the NFP among the public and stakeholders. There is usually a meeting in a community with local funders at least once a year. A standard presentation template was developed by employees at the national office for NFP sites to use to present program outcomes. National office tailors the basic template to the expected audience with the following steps:

- Helping to organize the meeting to ensure that an optimal mix of policy people and community partners attend. This optimal mix helps foster and preserve key relationships that promote program sustainability.
- Creating the presentation to support the site and ensure the program data are accurate.
- If the expected audience includes policy people or government cost auditors, national office may include a program cost return in the presentation.

28.4.5 Program Sustainability

The NFP has adhered to principles that previous research has shown to be associated with sustainability in community programs (e.g., Johnson et al., 2004). Several strategies used by the NFP that adhere to the principles of sustainability are presented in Table 28.5. As can be seen by Table 28.5, the NFP has focused not only on successful implementation of the RCTs but also on supporting and encouraging local sites to sustain themselves through a series of ordered steps of activities and decisions. The undertaking of such progressive steps is key to a successful sustainability planning model, including a plan for recruiting and engaging staff and clients, finding a niche within the larger community of service providers, as well as regular evaluation of the activities and outcomes of the program (Johnson et al., 2004).

28.4.6 Conceptual Guidelines

Volpe (2004) supports the use of an ecological framework in the context of injury prevention. This framework suggests that change or modifications to prevent injury should be envisaged holistically, that is, both individually/personally and communally/socially. This holistic view accurately reflects the complexity of injury prevention. This complexity is obvious when one considers the myriad of personal and social factors that influence individuals' choices that in turn impact their safety and security and that of their families. Volpe's (2004) life-space model provides a conceptual scheme for the internal and external circumstances that both inform and

Table 28.5 Principles and examples of sustainability, Nurse-Family Partnership

Principle of sustainability	Example
The coalescing of private-public partnerships that facilitate public investment	A variety of funders involved over the years, including the US Public Health Service, foundations, and other nonprofit agencies, corporations, U.S. Justice Department, Medicaid, and other local, state, and federal funders
Response to the needs of the community	Before the mounting of the Memphis and Denver trials, the program model was reviewed by members of the cultural communities that would be involved in the research.
Designing programs with consideration of local capability	For the community replications, there are efforts to hire nurses that reflect the cultural and linguistic composition of the communities served. The community replications are implemented by local sites that must demonstrate that there is a need for the NFP in the community and that they can liaise with existing services in the area
Ongoing internal evaluation of outcomes	Implementing sites pass selection criteria. The sites are encouraged and supported by national office to build the capacity to run the program with fidelity and sustain it themselves
Ongoing external evaluation of outcomes by academics and outside agencies	Long-term follow-up continues for Elmira, Memphis, and Denver RCTs. The results of NFP have been published by Olds and his team in peer-reviewed journals such as Pediatrics and the Journal of the American Medical Association. Local site staff regularly collects process and outcome data that is entered into the web-based clinical information system (CIS). The CIS provides both overall and site-specific monitoring and evaluation
The presence of a program champion	Independent agencies such as the RAND corporation, a nonprofit research organization, and the Brookings Institution, a nonprofit public policy institution have reviewed and recommended the NFP due to its strong evidence base
The presence of a program champion	Several program champions have been involved over the years, David Olds himself. Senators who have advocated for legislation supporting the NFP's expansion as well

Note: Johnson et al. (2004)

constrain individuals' behavior. A consideration of the four divisions of the life space (i.e., sociocultural, interpersonal, physical environment, and internal states) suggest that successful injury prevention corresponds to a combination of legislative, economic, educational, technological, and behavioral practices.

Although many theoretical models imply that service providers instill knowledge and impart change upon a passive individual, the life-space model acknowledges the individuals' roles as active, autonomous agents that impact their environments. A program enhances the possibilities for positive behavior change if it addresses all four life-space divisions that the individual acts within and among. The NFP program components address the four divisions of the life space in a holistic manner.

28.4.7 Implications of the NFP Case Study

The analysis of the NFP has important implications for a program aimed at preventing injury in populations of pregnant women and families with children in high risk situations including but not limited to low socioeconomic environments. An analysis of the model illustrates how these elements ensure that a program continues over time and in various settings. Attention to this design may facilitate sustainability in similar programs.

28.4.7.1 Fidelity

A central feature of this program is the focus on fidelity to the program model. Steps taken to facilitate this element are the creation of a clear mission statement with well-defined goals, objectives, methodology, and feedback cycle. The analysis of this model implies that fidelity to a central model at all levels of the system facilitates sustainability. The review of the NFP organization implies that fidelity to a model is facilitated through careful criteria for membership. Membership requirements for participants, employees, stakeholders, and collaborating agencies are defined clearly and applied rigidly, ensuring an appropriate fit between program goals and members' abilities. Similar steps are taken to ensure that program locations also fit the model.

The NFP implies that, following careful staff and site selection procedures, fidelity to the model is enhanced through the design of explicit procedures which ensure that stakeholders internalize and apply the program model, goals, and methods accurately. NFP demonstrates the importance of defining roles, tasks, and responsibilities. This step clarifies boundaries and facilitates complementary interactions between all members of the system including participants, clinicians, administrators, researchers, financial stakeholders, volunteers, and collaborating agencies. The decision-makers and formats for decision-making are clearly delineated in this program, facilitating feedback and change when necessary. The leadership is strong and highly involved in all levels of the organization while simultaneously enabling independence when applicable. This style of leadership demonstrates that engagement and versatility are necessary components of leadership in a sustainable system.

28.4.7.2 Communication

The design of the NFP demonstrates the importance of open communication for sustainable systems. Open communication enables members of the system to transfer information. The flow of information enables members at all levels of the system to send and receive feedback about the quality of the program. Changes are made based on feedback and in tune with the program model. Information about changes are transferred to subsystems ensuring consistency. According to the review of this case study, open communication also promotes the sustainability of a system by facilitating cohesion and a sense of mutual support between members of the system. Mutual support helps clinicians continue to work in the program. In addition, this structural and functional component instills a joint sense of ownership of the model, enhancing further fidelity to the model. The sense of ownership is also perpetuated at the client level, enhancing participation and promoting the growth of program when families promote it to others in their communities.

The NFP demonstrates how communication is used to influence the macrosystemic and exosystemic interest and collaboration. Communication with external systems increases interest, collaboration, and support of the program by community agencies, fundraisers, and financial donors. Several levels of the organization are involved in ensuring ties with systems external to the organization. The research subsystem, the administration, community sites, and front-line workers collect and share data with different parties. Program needs and successes are shared widely with others in order to ensure that external sources have realistic expectations of the program. This factor contributes to mutual efforts and long-standing relationships between the program and members of the macro- and exosystems. Shared information is always accurate, although the method of communicating is altered to suit the interest of varied target groups including communities, policymakers, and government agencies. Thus, a review of the NFP demonstrates means of communication with sources outside of the organization and implies that these interactions contribute to sustainability of the program.

The NFP's communicative interaction with external sources also demonstrates how fidelity to the model is upheld during interactions with external sources such as donors. Potential donors are considered when their function or goals are congruent with the aims of the program. Fidelity to the model is also upheld by carefully defining the tasks and responsibilities of donors and ensuring that boundaries are respected.

Thus, a review of the implementation of the NFP in various communities over a long period of time has important implications for organizations attempting to create sustainable programs. This program suggests that creating steps enabling fidelity to the model is essential at all levels. The accurate definition of program aims, goals, objectives, and means of implementation is transferred to subsystems through a structure with defined boundaries, carefully designed internal procedures, and a well-developed system of communication.

28.5 Conclusion

The NFP is a long-standing program facilitating effective injury prevention in target populations of young children and their families presenting with risk factors that may impair parenting. The growth of this nationwide project from a research study to replication in varied settings is facilitated by a design that takes several measures into account. The program paradigm manages to successively meet the injury prevention needs of target populations in growing settings over time due to strongly defined goals and attention to structural organization and processes. These elements help the organization remain true to the original model while integrating evidence-informed changes that suit the needs of the target population and objectives of the program while reducing the risk of injury to children in high risk contexts.

Acknowledgments The authors would like to express sincere appreciation to the key informants for this case study—Peggy Hill of the Nurse-Family Partnership National Office in Denver, CO, USA, and Pam Scott of Monroe County Department of Public Health in Rochester, NY, USA—whose consultation made this project possible.

BRIO Model: Nurse-Family Partnership

Group Served: Low-income women, pregnant with their first child.

Goal: Improve pregnancy outcomes, improve child health and development, as well as improve the economic self-sufficiency of the family.

Background	Resources	Implementation	Outcome
High-risk neighborhoods in Baltimore were observed to have poor housing, a lack of safe play spaces, high crime levels, and other threats to children's safety and well-being. David Olds began developing a nurse home visitation model in 1977 to address problems and improve the health of children. Three separate clinical trials were conducted and confirmed positive outcomes regarding child injury rates and other child health and developmental outcomes. Positive effects for parents are also noted. Program disseminated to six US sites in 1996. In 2000 the program expanded and became an initiative of the National Centre for Children, Families, and Communities	Developing and sustaining the model with fidelity require considerable time and effort from both the national office and the local site. The NFP is often embedded in already existing community agencies, which promotes economies of scale. Collaborating agencies are responsible for their own funding sustainability plans. The exact means of allocating resources varies from state to state	Currently there are more than 260,000 families served in 42 states. A state-based approach to program expansion was selected by Olds and his team after research and consultation. The Nurse Home Visitor Act (2000) supports the program in Colorado. Similar legislation has passed in Texas and Tennessee to promote Nurse-Family Partnership program development. A bill for the New Healthy Families Act (2007) promotes the Nurse-Family Partnership nationwide	Results of three clinical trials were positive in terms of decreased injury rates and other health and social outcomes. Elmira program effects for injuries: 56% reduction in emergency room visits. Reduction in child maltreatment 80% Memphis program effects for injuries: reduction in healthcare encounters for injuries was 23%, and reduction in days hospitalized was 80%. In all, control group had 15 trips to hospital compared to four in intervention group. Significant difference between the two groups. Denver trial indicated that the program model was transportable to a variety of community and cultural contexts

Life-Space Model: Nurse-Family Partnership

Sociocultural: civilization/ community	Interpersonal: primary and secondary relationships	Physical environments: where we live	Internal states: biochemical/ genetic and means of coping
Acknowledge the limited resources of the target population. Strategize with client about a plan for long-term economic self-sufficiency Marshal grassroots support for legislation (e.g., through the nonprofit organization Invest in Kids) Approach program expansion with a state-based financial sustainability plan Embed the program in already established community organizations such as public health agencies and health centers Involve the cultural communities served through consultation and inclusive hiring practices	Educate clients to use safety devices according to program guidelines Engage family members of the client in the program activities Explore supportive social networks with the client. Link the client to community resources Ensure staff has the time and ability to develop a personal relationship with client and her family Meet both expected and unexpected needs of the client and her family through a flexible and individualized service plan	Recognize the unsafe housing and living conditions of the population served Attain appropriate safety devices (e.g., window guards, safety gates, car seats, and smoke detectors) through grants and liaison with community agencies	Assess client's knowledge, experience, and beliefs around baby care and child development Empower the client, using self-efficacy theory, to impact her environment and problem-solve around child safety issues Enhance the client's level of responsiveness and ability to read child's developmental cues through attachment theory Help the client reflect on the impact of her own caregiving experiences on her present child rearing

References

Bandura, A. (1977). Self-efficacy: Toward a unifying theory of behavioral change. *Psychological Review, 84*, 191–215.

Bowlby, J. (1969). *Attachment and loss: attachment* (Vol. 1). New York, NY: Basic Books.

Bronfenbrenner, U. (1979). *The ecology of human development: Experiments by nature and design*. Cambridge, MA: Harvard University Press.

California Evidence-Based Clearinghouse for Child Welfare. (2008). *Nurse-family partnership (NFP)*. San Diego, CA: Author. Retrieved from http://www.cebc4cw.org/program/nurse-family-partnership/detailed

Center for the Study and Prevention of Violence. (2004). *Blueprints model programs: Nurse family partnership*. Boulder, CO: Author. Retrieved from http://www.colorado.edu/cspv/blueprints/model/programs/NFP.html

Children's Healthy Policy Centre (2019). Nurse-Family Partnership is being tested in Canada. Retrieved from https://childhealthpolicy.ca/nurse-family-partnership/

Columbia Broadcasting Station Evening News. (2007). *A partnership for a brighter future: The nurse-family partnership provides a life-changing lesson in motherhood* (p. 101). New York, NY: Columbia Broadcasting Station. Retrieved from http://www.cbsnews.com/stories/2007/07/11/eveningnews/main3045638.shtml

Eckenrode, J., Campa, M., Luckey, D. W., Henderson Jr., C. R., Cole, R., Kitzman, H., et al. (2010). Long-term effects of prenatal and infancy nurse home visitation on the life course of youths: 19-year follow-up of a randomized trial. *Archives of Pediatrics and Adolescent Medicine, 164*(1), 9–15.

Goodman, A. (2006). *The story of David Olds and the nurse home visiting program. Robert Wood Johnson Foundation grants results special report*. Princeton, NJ: Robert Wood Johnson Foundation.

Home Visiting Evidence of Effectiveness. (2011). *Implementing nurse family partnerships (NFP)*. Washington, DC: HHS. Retrieved from https://homvee.acf.hhs.gov/Implementation/3/Nurse-Family-Partnership%2D%2DNFP%2D%2DEstimated-Costs-of-Implementation/14/5

Howard, D., Husain, F., & Velji, J. (2005). *Nurse-family partnership: Organizing for national expansion*. San Francisco, CA: The Bridgespan Group.

Invest in Kids. (n.d.). *Nurse-family partnership: Program overview*. Denver CO: Author. Retrieved June 27, 2007, from http://www.iik.org/nurse_family_partnership/

Johnson, K., Hays, C., Center, H., & Daley, C. (2004). Building capacity and sustainable prevention innovations: A sustainability planning model. *Evaluation and Program Planning, 27*, 135–149.

Jones, M. B., & Offord, D. R. (1991). *After the demonstration project*. Hamilton, ON: McMaster University. Unpublished paper.

Karoly, L. A., Kilburn, R. M., & Cannon, J. S. (2005). *Early childhood interventions: Proven results, future promise*. Santa Monica, CA: Rand Corporation.

Kitzman, H., Olds, D., Henderson Jr., C. R., Hanks, C., Cole, R., Tatelbaum, R., et al. (1997). Effect of prenatal and infancy home visitation by nurses on pregnancy outcomes, childhood injuries, and repeated childbearing: A randomized controlled trial. *Journal of the American Medical Association, 278*(8), 644–652.

Kitzman, H., Yoos, H. L., Cole, R., Olds, D., Korfmacher, J., & Hanks, C. (1997). Prenatal and early childhood home-visitation program processes: A case illustration. *Journal of Community Psychology, 25*(1), 27–45.

Nilsen, P. (2005). Evaluation of community-based injury prevention programmes: Methodological issues and challenges. *International Journal of Injury Control and Safety Promotion, 12*(3), 143–156.

Nurse Family Partnership. (2007a). *About us*. Denver, CO: Author. Retrieved October 7, 2007, from http://www.nursefamilypartnership.org/content/index.cfm?fuseaction=showContent&contentID=2&navID=2

Nurse-Family Partnership. (2007b). *FAQ [Fact sheet]*. Denver, CO: Author

Nurse Family Partnership. (2007c). *Home visit experience*. Denver, CO: Author. Retrieved October 7, 2007, from http://www.nursefamilypartnership.org/content/index.cfm?fuseaction=showContent&contentID=47&navID=46

Nurse-Family Partnership. (2007d). *NFP sites*. Denver, CO: Author. Retrieved October 7, 2007 from http://www.nursefamilypartnership.org/content/index.cfm?fuseaction=showContent&contentID=3&navID=3

Nurse Family Partnership. (2007e). *NFP sites: Colorado*. Denver, CO: Author. Retrieved October 7, 2007, from http://www.nursefamilypartnership.org/content/index.cfm?fuseaction=showContent&contentID=110&navID=98

Nurse Family Partnership. (2007f). *Program development*. Denver, CO: Author. Retrieved October 10, 2007, from http://www.nursefamilypartnership.org/content/index.cfm?fuseaction=showContent&contentID=11&navID=11

Nurse Family Partnership (2007g). Ronald Mcdonald house charities provides generous grant *Newslink: NFP National service office, 3*, 6.

Nurse Family Partnership. (2007h). *Program development*. Accessed on Oct. 10, 2007 from the NFP website http://www.nursefamilypartnership.org/content/index.cfm?fuseaction=showContent&contentID=11&navID=11

Nurse Family Partnership. (2007i). *Program development*. Accessed on Oct. 10, 2007 from the NFP website http://www.nursefamilypartnership.org/content/index.cfm?fuseaction=showContent&contentID=10&navID=10

Nurse Family Partnership. (2014). *Research trials and outcomes*. Denver, CO: Author. Retrieved from https://www.nursefamilypartnership.org/wp-content/uploads/2017/07/NFP_Research_Outcomes_2014.pdf

Nurse Family Partnership. (2017). *Overview*. Denver, CO: Author. Retrieved from https://www.nursefamilypartnership.org/wp-content/uploads/2017/07/NFP_Overview.pdf

Nutter, R. W., & Weiden, T. D. (1988). Program evaluation and quality assurance: A reconciliation. *The Social Worker/Le Travailleur Social, Spring*, 18–27.

O'Brien, R. A. (2005). Translating a research intervention into community practice: The nurse family partnership. *The Journal of Primary Prevention, 26*(3), 241–257.

O'Brien, R. A. (n.d.). *Nurse-family partnership: Logic Model*. Denver, CO: Nurse-Family Partnership.

Olds, D. L. (2002). Prenatal and infancy home visiting by nurses: From randomized trials to community replication. *Prevention Science, 3*(3), 153–173.

Olds, D. L. (2005). *Nurse family partnership: Helping first time parents succeed [Power point presentation]*. Denver, CO: University of Colorado Health Sciences Center.

Olds, D. L., Henderson Jr., C. R., & Kitzman, H. (1994). Does prenatal and infancy nurse home visitation have enduring effects on qualities of parental caregiving and child health at 25 to 50 months of life? *Pediatrics, 93*, 89–98.

Olds, D. L., Henderson Jr., C. R., Phelps, C., Kitzman, H., & Hanks, C. (1993). Effect of prenatal and infancy nurse home visitation on government spending. *Medical Care, 31*(2), 155–174.

Olds, D. L., Kitzman, H., Cole, R., & Robinson, J. (1997). Theoretical foundations of a program of home visitation for pregnant women and parents of young children. *Journal of Community Psychology, 25*, 9–25.

Olds, D. L., Robinson, J., O'Brien, R., Luckey, D. W., Pettitt, L. M., Henderson, C. R. Jr, Ng, R. K., Sheff, K. L., Korfmacher, J., Hiatt, S., & Talmi, A. (2002). Home visiting by paraprofessionals and by nurses: a randomized, controlled trial. *Pediatrics, 110*(3), 486–496.

Olds, D. L., Robinson, J., Pettitt, L., Luckey, D. W., Holmberg, J., Ng, R., et al. (2004). Effects of home visits by paraprofessionals and by nurses: Age 4 follow up results of a randomized trial. *Pediatrics, 114*, 1560–1568.

Olds, D. L., Henderson Jr., C. R., Chamberlain, R., & Tatelbaum, R. (1986). Preventing child abuse and neglect: A randomized trial of nurse home visitation. *Pediatrics, 78*(1), 65–78.

Olds, D. L., Kitzman, H., Knudtson, M. D., Anson, E., Smith, J. A., & Cole, R. (2014). Effect of home visiting by nurses on maternal and child mortality: Results of a 2-decade follow-up of a randomized clinical trial. *JAMA Pediatrics, 168*(9), 800–806.

Peterson, L., & Gable, S. (1998). Holistic injury prevention. In J. R. Lutzker (Ed.), *Handbook of child abuse research and treatment* (pp. 291–318). New York, NY: Plenum.

Safe Kids Worldwide. (n.d.). *Facts about children at higher risk for accidental injuries.* Washington, DC: Author.

Shores, B. (2007). *Investment that pays: Nurse-family program trains young mothers.* Retrieved August 23, 2007, from http://www.spokesmanreview.com/ourkids/stories/?ID=186031

Volpe, R. (2004). *The conceptualization of injury prevention as change in complex systems.* Toronto, ON: University of Toronto. Retrieved from https://legacy.oise.utoronto.ca/research/ONF-SBSPrevention/Background/SBS%20Model.pdf

UCLA Parent-Child Health and Wellness Program: Prevention of Injuries by Parents with Intellectual Disabilities

29

Dara Sikljovan

The UCLA Parent-Child Health and Wellness Program was an evaluated home-based intervention created to explore ways to extend health care and home safety education research to community settings with families at high risk for injuries. The purpose of this program was to establish a community-based model for the provision of self and child health safety/well-being preparatory and preventive education to young or expectant minor or adult parents with cognitive impairments.

29.1 Background

The UCLA Parent-Child Health and Wellness Program was characterized by rigorous adherence to principles and concepts regarding the successful conduct of interventions using all procedures and training from UCLA (Tymchuk, 1996, 1999). Curricula, parent-use materials, and assessment tools used in this program were particularly designed to match the learning needs of the emerging population of parents.

29.1.1 Target Population

A method of describing a particular population must be found for ease of communication (A. Tymchuk, personal communication, 2005). Terms such as "hidden majority" or "invisible disability" have been used to describe individuals with mild cognitive limitations or certain learning difficulties who do not appear to have a "visible" disability. This lack of visibility of a disability has contributed to the difficulties and disadvantages that parents with mild cognitive limitations face (Tymchuk, Lakin, & Luckasson, 2001). Although a variety of terms and definitions exist that can be taken to describe parents with mild cognitive limitations, the needs of a large group of those parents continue to be unaddressed. No service sector has assumed responsibility for providing parenting support to the members of these groups.

The UCLA Parent-Child Health and Wellness Program was designed to meet the needs of these parents; some of these parents had learning difficulties associated with disabilities, and some had children with health-related conditions and associated disabilities (Tymchuk, Lang, Sewards, Lieberman, & Koo, 2003; A. Tymchuk, personal communication, 2005). The program was inclusive and purposively tried to obtain people from the agency identified as having functional parenting needs regardless of a disability label. As different service sectors utilized different labels to

D. Sikljovan (✉)
Hamilton-Wentworth District School Board, Psychological Services, Hamilton, ON, Canada
e-mail: dsikljov@hwdsb.on.ca

© Springer Nature Switzerland AG 2020
R. Volpe (ed.), *Casebook of Traumatic Injury Prevention*,
https://doi.org/10.1007/978-3-030-27419-1_29

essentially describe the same people, the program adopted the label used by a particular service sector when working in that sector. The program recruited low-income and underserved adult and teen parents with an intellectual disability or with a history of intellectual disability or who were presumed to have an intellectual disability, with a health disorder, with another disability, with parents who have a mental illness, and with parents who have been reported for or who are at high risk for child maltreatment.

29.1.2 Program Goals

The overarching goal of the program was to support parents in learning health and safety skills through hands-on experience, illustrations, and language that is easy to understand. Given this goal, one of the major challenges for the UCLA Parent-Child Health and Wellness Program to overcome was to establish and maintain collaboration with four types of community agencies: health care, education, family and children's services, as well as disability services. Along these lines, the related goals of the project were to identify agencies that serve parents with learning difficulties or mild cognitive limitations in several regions in California, to examine the efficacy of a health and safety education program for parents with learning difficulties, and to help decrease the number of preventable illnesses and injuries among children by increasing parents' knowledge base in health and safety.

29.1.3 History and Development

Since the early 1970s, Dr. Tymchuk and his team at UCLA have been examining ways in which they could prescriptively assess home safety knowledge and practices of low-income parents with intellectual disability and/or other individual learning needs. Given the economic recession, federal devolution, and reduction of services for all families in poverty, families in which a parent has intellectual disabilities showed significantly lowered quality of life. Both parents and

their children were shown to be at heightened risk for impaired health status and health outcomes due to unintentional home injuries and injuries from violence (Tymchuk, Llewellyn, & Feldman, 1999). Due to the multiple risk factors that these families face, a multidimensional program that tailored approaches to match the needs of a particular family was considered most likely to be successful.

The Project Parenting was the first special parenting program at UCLA that lasted for about 15 years. A couple of larger grants were obtained that covered the research and the stipends for training the pre- and postdoctoral students across disciplines. Gradually, however, while those dollars stayed the same, their value eroded due to inflation. Although funding still covered the research, it was not sufficient to cover the training. Therefore, in order to sustain both the research and training parts of the program, additional dollars were collected through fundraising and personal financing by Dr. Tymchuk. The success of the Project Parenting program resulted in obtaining additional funding and the initiation of the SHARE/UCLA Parenting Project which was followed by the Wellness Program.

The UCLA Parent-Child Health and Wellness Program study was conducted between January 1995 and December 1999. Within the Wellness Program, child health and safety were identified as critical parenting domains. Health was conceptualized as ranging from an understanding of basic health concepts and how a body changes during illness to parental response to the most common childhood emergencies. Safety was conceptualized as both identification and remediation or prevention of child home dangers as well as precaution implementation. It is important to realize that rather than being distinct entities, both health and safety are intertwined with understanding of child development, being able to plan as the child develops, to make decisions, and to cope when things go awry while using supports as needed.

The Health and Wellness Program: A Parenting Curriculum for Families at Risk by Alexander Tymchuk (2006) has since been seen as a foundation and was even widely disseminated as a part of the Australian national strategy Healthy Start (a national capacity building strategy which aims to improve health and well-being outcomes for children whose parents have learning difficulties). *Healthy and Safe: An Australian Parent Education Kit* took their lead from UCLA Parent-Child Health and Wellness Program, in order to provide a home-based education resources which are tailored to the unique learning needs of parents with learning difficulties (California Evidence-Based Clearinghouse for Child Welfare [CEBC], 2017). This was designed to equip parents who have young children with the knowledge and skills necessary for managing home dangers, accidents, and childhood illness (CEBC, 2017).

29.1.4 Behavioral Approach to Injury Prevention

Analogous to Haddon's model (1980), which recognizes the importance of an examination of injury pre-events, of the injury event itself, and then post-injury events, the Wellness Program adopted the behavioral framework within which an injury may be seen as having an antecedent, or series of antecedents, and a consequence, or series of consequences. If antecedents that occur earlier in the chain can be identified for types of injuries, interventions can lead to elimination of antecedents earlier on, thereby preventing the occurrence of those injuries. Furthermore, if a direct antecedent, through person, time, place, or action proximity, to a specific injury can be identified, efforts can be directed toward changing that antecedent and thus preventing the occurrence of a similar injury. Referred to as the process approach (Peterson, Farmer, & Mori, 1987), it also can be utilized for injury prevention planning that is specific to individual families. Such individualization has been shown to be more effective in injury prevention, than simple dissemination of information. In the establishment of a Wellness Program, the importance and how-to of planning as well as problem anticipation and solving methods are presented. Within the program model, antecedents can be related to

characteristics of the environment, to characteristics of the caregiver (or of the caregiver's behavior), or to characteristics of the child or to the interaction of these factors (A. Tymchuk, personal communication, 2005).

Environmental factors that have been associated with greater child injury risk include general quality of the home including the frequency and types of hazards observed in the home, whereas maternal factors associated with greater child injury risk include the degree to which the mother is able to identify hazards in her home, her perception of the risk to her child of each danger, her vigilance in child care, her injury prevention knowledge, and the degree to which she believes injuries can be prevented. It has long been recognized that specificity is required in order to increase the efficacy of preventive efforts. This approach works very well within the Wellness Model for parents with intellectual disabilities.

29.1.5 The Wellness Program Model

There are four content areas within the program model: (1) fundamental knowledge and skill areas for parents, (2) infant and child health care, (3) promotion of home safety and injury prevention, and (4) parent and child enjoying each other. Table 29.1 lists internal consistency for each of the four component areas considered to be critical for assessment and education. Within the Wellness Program, fundamental knowledge and skills for parents form the basis for parenting on other three areas and as such may significantly influence the health and safety of parents and of their young children. Since few parents at risk have never received either formal or informal instruction about injury prevention, the lack of familiarity with and understanding of home dangers will significantly hamper their ability to ensure the safety of their child and of themselves (A. Tymchuk, personal communication, 2005). In particular, if they do not know what dangerous, young parents will be unable to prevent or remediate a danger's occurrence. Further, lowered educational achievement of young at-risk parents often results in their not having sufficient

Table 29.1 Internal consistency of component measures critical for parenting adequacy

Component areas considered to be critical for assessment and education (alpha)	
Fundamental knowledge and skills for parents (0.81)	(a) Support relationships (b) Effective short- and long-term planning (c) Effective decision-making (d) Effective coping (e) Effective observational skills (f) Finances and budget (g) Meal planning (h) House Cleanliness (l) Hygiene
Parent health behavior (0.69)	(a) Body works (b) Diagnostics (c) Life-threatening emergency (d) Calling the doctor (e) Medicine
Safety (0.99)	(a) Partner safety (b) Safety in the home/apartment (phone safety, door safety, on vacation) (c) Community safety (going out, in the community, returning home, reporting a crime) (d) Home safety (home dangers, fire, electrical, danger of choking from small objects, suffocation, firearm and other projectile weapons, poisons, falling heavy objects, sharp objects, clutter, inappropriate edibles, dangerous toys/animals, cooking, general dangers, yard/outdoors, danger safety maps)
Parent and child enjoying each other (0.80)	(a) Child safety (b) Parent and child playing (c) Parent reading and singing to child

Note: A. Tymchuk, personal communication (2005)

reading recognition or comprehension experience in order to utilize available materials (Tymchuk, Groen, & Dolyniuk, 2000).

29.1.6 Focus on Information Processing

To address differences in learning and application of received information, the three-phase framework was adopted: (1) The input phase (presentation) refers to how parents become prepared for new information and skills and how they obtain or are presented with information and skills; (2) the assimilation phase (learning) refers to how parents take new information and assimilate it with their current knowledge or skills bases; and (3) the output phase (immediate and delayed use) refers to how parents make use of new information and skills as well as how they maintain knowledge and skills for later use.

Each of these individual phases are influenced both by parental factors and by environmental factors which influence learning and use of information which can further inform modification. The following parental factors have been shown to influence how well a parent does in each phase: (1) physical functioning (with or without any corrective devices that may be needed), such as vision, hearing, motility, and coordination; (2) previous experience and background; (3) availability of social supports; (4) personal values, interest, and motivation; (5) processing capacity; (6) memory capacity; and (7) reading recognition and reading comprehension ability, speech recognition, and speech comprehension in English or in their primary language.

29.1.7 Focus on Parental Strengths

Within the Wellness Program, a focus on parental strengths is done in order to redirect focus from risk factors only. While there have been previous projects that have shown success in their intent to help at-risk parents attain knowledge in home injury prevention (Mandel, Bigelow, & Lutzker, 1998; Tymchuk et al., 2003), none has specifically addressed parental needs and life circumstances. The importance in their identification is to develop programs that increase the influence of the advantage factors while decreasing the influence of the risk factors. Table 29.2 provides certain enabling factors that provide substantial contribution to the program effectiveness.

29.2 Resources

29.2.1 Human and Financial Resources

29.2.1.1 Stakeholders

The project's originator, neurodevelopmental psychologist Dr. Alexander J. Tymchuk, is an emeritus professor of medical psychology in the psychiatry and biobehavioral science department in the School of Medicine at the University of California, Los Angeles (UCLA). Dr. Tymchuk's

Table 29.2 Factors known to benefit parental/maternal adequacy and facilitate learning

Maternal historical advantage factors	(a) Lived at home (b) Parental approval of marriage/partner/child (c) Older than 18 when first child was born (d) Parenting education (e) Self-health-care education (f) Owen parents are problem free (g) Completed high school (h) Stable partner relationships
Maternal current state	(a) Physically healthy (b) Emotionally healthy (c) Limited stress (d) Adequate self-esteem (e) Reading/speech comprehension >grade 5 (f) No or limited substance intake (g) IQ greater than 60
Maternal current process	(a) Good planning (b) Good decision-making (c) Good coping style (d) Nonpunitive child interaction/some positive interaction (e) Strict child interaction/not idiosyncratic (f) Reinforces (g) Smiles/empathetic (h) Willing to learn/motivated (i) Learns readily/generalizes (j) Recognizes own needs (k) Has done well in other programs (l) Has good adaptive skills
Environmental advantage factors (supports)	(a) Health care (b) Education (c) Friends (d) Psychological (e) Vocational (f) Legal (g) Financial aids (h) Available (i) Comprehensive (j) Frequency (as needed) (k) Duration (as needed) (l) Supports with fair view of capabilities (m) Professionally trained (n) Interventions match learning ability (o) Parental agency contacts through single individual

Table 29.2 (continued)

Family advantage factors	(a) Only one child
	(b) Younger child
	(c) Adequate income
	(d) Adequate/safe/stable housing
	(e) Infrequent moves
Husband/Partner Factors	(a) Current partner as a support
	(b) Emotionally healthy
	(c) Involved in vocation
	(d) Involved in civics
	(e) Relatively stable relationship
Child advantage factors	(a) IQ greater than 70
	(b) Adequate health
	(c) Pleasant temperament
	(d) Few accidents
	(e) Child under the age of 6
	(f) Adequate behavior

Note: A. Tymchuk, personal communication (2005)

interests include competence determination related to parenting, examination of ethical decision-making processes used by professionals, particularly as they relate to vulnerable populations of parents, and development of methods related to ensuring full treatment as well as research assent/consent with vulnerable populations. By necessity, this work has led Dr. Tymchuk to examine as well as address legal and policy issues related to each of these areas. A number of Dr. Tymchuk's assistants contributed to the success of the Wellness Program including his undergraduate, graduate, and postgraduate students: Karen Berney-Ficklin, Rebecca Spitz, Jill Spivac, Elana Evan, Deborah Kanegsberg, Cathy Lang, and Alice West.

29.2.1.2 Collaborators

The program was supported by a grant from the California Wellness Foundation (TCWF) (n.d.), one of the state's largest private foundations. Since its founding in 1992, the foundation has awarded 3858 grants totaling more than $460 million with the mission to improve the health of the people of California by making grants for health promotion, wellness education, and disease prevention. The TCWF defines wellness as a state of optimum health and well-being, achieved through the active pursuit of good health and the removal of barriers to healthy living, both personal and societal, the ability of people and communities to reach their fullest potential in the broadest sense.

Support for the earlier empirical work, within the SHARE/UCLA Parenting Project, was provided by a series of annual grants from SHARE Incorporation interested in funding a groundbreaking research. This support continued within the SHARE/UCLA Center for Family Health, Wellness & Safety. When the Wellness Program was described, local large stores, manufacturers, and distributors provided discounts for safety devices. Fire departments also contributed some recommended fire extinguishers.

29.2.2 Educational Resources

Due to the scarcity of home safety resources available to families in need, Dr. Tymchuk and his team developed and tested methods to improve the knowledge and home safety practices of these parents. In order for the methods of assessment and of intervention to be effective with hard-to-reach families, they determined that those methods had to be more closely matched to the learning abilities and styles of the parents.

29.2.2.1 Tailoring Program to Needs of At-Risk Parents

In response to needs of the parents to primarily understand common words used in critical areas of parenting (i.e., health and home safety), two complementary measures, developed by Dr. Tymchuk and his team, were utilized in the

UCLA program: the UCLA Parenting Reading Recognition List (UPRRL) and the UCLA Parenting Reading Comprehension List (UPRCL). Words were selected from those presented as critical by health-care professionals as well as from those used on labels of products commonly used by parents, including prescription and over-the-counter medications and high-risk household products. Given that the parents' reading comprehension was shown to be predictive of danger identification and reading recognition was predictive of precautions given, assessing a parent's learning ability/knowledge of dangers and precautions seems to be critical step before considering an intervention.

29.2.2.2 Development and Testing Functional Assessment Tools

The ongoing research determined that while some parents could benefit from materials containing only printed words, other parents had difficulty visualizing the situations explained in those documents. Along these lines, several home safety measures were developed and validated by Dr. Tymchuk and colleagues to assess parental knowledge of dangers as well as the safety of the home environment. The development of these illustrations adhered to standards used in the development of written materials in combination with concepts from human learning, information processing, the visual arts (containing medical illustrating), and computer-assisted instruction and multimedia including being viewed by parents at various stages of development (see Table 29.3; A. Tymchuk, personal communication, 2005).

These measures included the Home Inventory of Dangers and Safety Precautions-2 (HIDSP-2) and the Home Inventory of Dangers and Safety Precautions-Illustrated Version (HIDSP-IV); and other measures are the Child Injury Report Form, the Environmental Analysis Form, and the Home Danger Recognition Inventory. Each of these measures provides very useful information for establishing initial goals, monitoring progress, and providing valid feedback to the parent. As an example, the actual results obtained from the HIDSP-IV demonstrate that referred parents are unable to identify the illustrated common home dangers and they are even less able to provide suitable precautions (Tymchuk et al., 2003). Overall, they were able to identify 55.7% of the dangers while only being able to provide 15.9% of the precautions. These results suggested that knowledge and skill cannot be presumed, it should be assessed and that educational efforts to prepare mothers must also ensure that they unlearn harmful knowledge while acquiring accurate information (A. Tymchuk, personal communication, 2005).

29.2.2.3 Development of Curricula

Based upon a behavioral framework, specific health and home safety curricula along with parent-use materials were developed and were efficacy validated through the use of a single-subject multiple baseline procedure with a number of mothers with intellectual disabilities. Curricula used in this project was designed to match the learning needs of this special population. Therefore, to ensure maximum comprehension and understanding, all text was written at an

Table 29.3 Home safety dangers and precautions

Illustration	Dangers	Precautions
Kitchen	Hanging telephone cord	Hook cord on wall hook Always unplug toaster Limit use but store matches in locked drawer
	Metal utensil in plugged-in toaster	Always unplug toaster
	Matches/cigarette on table	Limit use but store matches in locked drawer or cabinet; do not smoke in house
	Open cabinet under sink with poisons	Store up high at back of shelf; store in locked cabinet
Bedroom	Baby with pins at edge of changing table	Place pins away from table
	Cat in baby's room	Never allow cat or other animal in baby's room
	Heavy objects above baby's crib	Do not place anything above baby's crib

Table 29.3 (continued)

Illustration	Dangers	Precautions
Bathroom	Water on in bathtub	Do not leave water on when not in bathroom
	Open toilet lid	Close lid/use lid lock or Velcro tape
	Razor lying on counter	Store razors in high/locked cabinet/drawer
	Hairdryer plugged in near sink	Use hairdryer away from water
Living room	Heavy unfastened unblocked bookshelf	Attach to wall or floor or place table or other heavy object in front
	Tables/fireplace with sharp corners	Use corner covers/tape sponges/towels to block corners
	Plugged in lamp without bulb and shade	Unplug/remove if broken/replace bulb/shade
	Scissors/needles on low shelf	Remove/store in protected area
Stairway	Baby in walker at top	Place gate at bottom/tops of all open stairways
	Toys on stairs	Remove/store in inaccessible container
	Frayed lamp cord	Throw away all devices with frayed cords
Yard/outdoors	Wading pool	Empty/supervise child when in or near pool/open water
	Helmetless child riding bike in street	Let child ride in park; use helmet

Note: Tymchuk et al. (2003)

approximate 5–6 grade level. Adaptations to parent-viewed materials included enlarged, single, and consistent use of font, colored illustrations, use of conceptual groupings, and presentation of single topics. In addition, these curricula were available in both English and Spanish.

Building on Dr. Tymchuk's earlier work, the safety domain of the program was divided into manageable topics. Individual booklets and worksheets followed these topics and included:

- Home Safety: Introduction and Home Safety Tips
- Home Safety: Home Dangers and Precautions Inventory
- Home Safety One: Fire, Electrical, and Cooking
- Home Safety Two: Suffocation, Poisoning, and Things Not Good to Eat
- Home Safety Three: Heavy Falling Objects, Sharp Objects, and Firearms
- Home Safety Four: Toys, Animals, Clutter, and Other Things; and My Home Safety Plan

The safety curriculum was presented in landscape with large black type (30–70 Times New Roman font) on one side of white 8 1/2 × 11 three-holed punched paper and placed in a binder. In addition to being divided into topics, single

ideas were presented accompanied by colored illustrations to facilitate learning. These illustrations were developed after feedback from focus groups to dangers, initial pencil drawings, review by groups, and then by the artist, as were those for the Illustrated Version of the Home Safety Inventory. In addition to the booklets and curriculum, there were separate worksheets as well as black-and-white illustrated, simplified sets of safety and health-care device utilization instructions based upon the original instructions for each device. The safety devices included drawer latches, cabinet locks, electrical outlet covers, cable/cord ties, appliance latches, corner guards, door knob covers, fire extinguishers, and syrup of Ipecac.

There are a number of similarities across all Safety Education sessions including recognition of mother's involvement in education and accomplishments; recognition of the child as well as of others; queries regarding the previous week's events, regarding the circumstances of any accident, regarding the mother's satisfaction with each session; and provision of refreshments. For the purpose of illustration, the home safety sessions 11 and 12 with a focus on falls are provided in Box 29.1 and Box 29.2. Also included is an empirically developed picture of "The Stairway" (Fig. 29.1) and the related worksheet (Table 29.4).

Box 29.1 Home Safety Sessions 11 and 12

1. Recognition of mother's involvement and of her danger remediation, prevention, and maintenance efforts. Review placement of previously provided home safety items. Provide corner guards.
2. Query regarding previous week's events (including things they enjoyed)/circumstances of any accident.
3. Briefly but deliberately review previous session/discuss current topic
4. Review any needs and supports (EP, EDM, EPS, EC).
5. Utilize Safety Curriculum to discuss heavy objects, falls, sharp objects, weapons dangers, and precautions.
6. Complete worksheets and vignettes "The Stairs" and "Prevention Tips".
7. Provide/discuss/facilitate use/maintenance of corner guards/other methods. Provide illustrated instructions/model/generalize/reinforce.
8. Briefly review and talk about next session's topic (place date on parent's and HE's calendar). Give mother Home
9. Safety Booklet Five: Heavy Objects, Falls, Sharp Objects, and Weapons. Query mother regarding her satisfaction with session and what more she would have liked.
10. Provide refreshments.

Note: A. Tymchuk, personal communication (2005)

Note: A. Tymchuk, personal communication (2005)

Worksheet Instructions:

1. Have the parent look at the color/laminated picture called The Stairway and ask them to identify any dangers that they see.
2. Once they have stopped, prompt them once by asking if they see any other dangers.
3. You can ask them why they consider any to be a danger; this is optional.

Box 29.2 Home Safety Sessions 11 and 12 (Falls)

FALLS: A second category is falls. Falls are a major cause of injury to young children. Do you have any places where your children can fall from?

They also may fall and strike their heads or other body parts on the corner of a table or other furniture. Let's find them and make it safe. Look at the windows, where a child can climb and fall, stairs.

Use the observation checklist to ensure that all are addressed. The Living Room picture can be used.

4. Then proceed to ask them about precautions but only for those dangers that they have identified.
5. While the parents may not have a stairway in their home, they may have one in the building or going to the outside. Or the parents must remember when they visit other places that might have stairs so that they must be prepared to handle this.

29.3 Implementation

29.3.1 Pilot Study

During the first half of 1995, each of the assessment devices, curricula, parent education materials, and training manuals that were validated in previous research were re-examined for continued applicability to the UCLA Parent-Child Health and Wellness Program. Gathered information was updated in each component, a series of illustrations to exemplify concepts were develop, and processes were revalidated as needed. Curricula and parent-use materials from earlier work, combined with additionally recommended material, were integrated into "systematic strengths-based injury prevention and health-care development instructional package of assessments, instructional manuals, teaching cur-

Fig. 29.1 Home Safety Illustration: The Stairway (A. Tymchuk, personal communication, 2005)

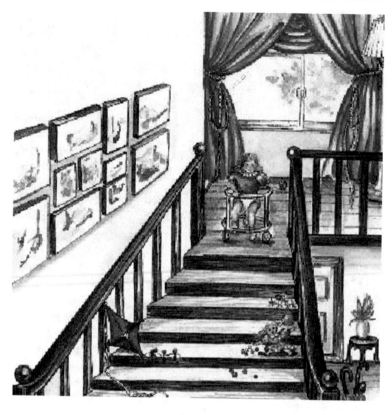

Table 29.4 Home Safety Worksheet for the Stairway Illustration

Dangers	Precautions
(No gate on stairs) Baby at top of stairs/ baby in walker could fall down stairs	Put a gate at the top of (all open) stairwaysWatch child when child is in a walkerCarry child or hold child's hand when walking up and down stairsDo not let child play on stairs Put child downstairs when in walkerYoung child (who is mobile) should not be upstairs unsupervised
Open window accessible to child	Close and lock windows that do not have screens
Skates at bottom of stairs	Store skates where people won't trip overWhen skating:Wear a helmet Wear padding Use safelyWear comfortable clothes Do not skate aloneDo not skate in the streetDo not skate at night
Toys (objects) on stairs Kite, ball, jacks, doll, marbles	Store bigger toys in a toy box or closetStore small objects (marbles, jacks) in a childproof container/put it on a high shelf or in a locked drawerThrow away small objects
Carpet lifted up at bottom of stairs	Repair carpetPlace heavy object over carpet to weigh it downStick/nail it to the floor
Pictures are hung high on wall	Use at least 2 hooks when hanging picture framesDo not hang objects higher than shortest person/do not hang objects high up
Tall lamp	Put tall lamps behind heavy furnitureAttach lamp to floor or wall
Electric cord	Tie up electric cords using cord tiesPut electric cords behind furniture so that child cannot reach them
Open outlet	Use outlet covers in all open outletsPut heavy furniture against wall in front of open outlets
Curtain cords	Tie up curtain cords with cord tiesWrap cords around top of curtain railCut cords shorter
Railings in front of lamp are too wide	Block off with gates or wire mesh
Child is eating an apple that is not cut up	Cut up foods that are hard or big into small piecesFeed child slowly Do not feed child when child is moving around

(continued)

Table 29.4 (continued)

Dangers	Precautions
Frayed electrical cord on lamp	Throw away frayed cords*Do not* use electrical tape on frayed wires
No plate on electrical outlet	Put plate on electrical outlet
Umbrellas are in reach of child	Keep umbrellas out of child's reach
Plant is in reach of child	Keep plants out of child's reach*Do not* grow or buy dangerous (cactus, sharp, poisonous) plants
No screen on window	Put screen on window
Total dangers: _____	Total precautions: _____

Note: A. Tymchuk, personal communication (2005)

ricula, and parent-use materials" (A. Tymchuk, personal communication, 2005).

Matching (or tailoring) of all procedures to maternal learning characteristics and circumstances was done to ensure that intervention results were due to the intervention and not to extraneous (but remediable) factors such as the use of measures or interventions containing complex language presented densely or cluttered either in written or spoken format. Once curriculum and parent-use materials were simplified in English, they were then translated into Spanish. All materials were pilot tested with two samples of 15 parents. One sample was from rural northern California Sacramento County and the other from urban southern Los Angeles County. Only one mother from Los Angeles did not complete participation in this pilot study.

Project staff developed a data management system for evaluation of the project that had the ability to be modified for later use within each agency. They also developed as well as implemented procedures to fulfill legal, regulatory, clinical, and humanitarian requirements across agencies for the recruitment of families and for reporting information while maintaining confidentiality.

In each piloting site, formal collaborative relationships were developed with at least one agency from health care, child protective service, disability/social services, and education from both sites to increase the probability that not only would achievement of the project's goals benefit each agency but also project-developed processes would become an integral part of each agency. Memorandum of understanding (MOU) spells out what each agency agrees to provide at which dates and what each agency will or will not provide and what the research project agrees to provide and what the research project will not provide. In the Wellness Program, MOUs had to be formally approved within specific agencies and signed.

Based from the experience from the pilot study, procedures and materials were modified. Areas of impoverishment and special need were targeted to provide this timely project to those who may need it most. The clinical trial was conducted with 268 families. Referral sources were child protective, disability, education, public and private health care, as well as other social service agencies in Los Angeles and Ventura Counties serving low-income families with whom memoranda of understanding had been negotiated.

29.3.2 Design and Procedures

A three-step recruitment procedure was used, and parents were eligible for this project if (1) they were a first-time parent and/or pregnant with first child (however, parents with more than one child were also considered as participants), (2) youngest child is less than 3 years of age, and (3) parent appears to have difficulty in reading and comprehending written materials, applying new information, retaining information, and/or following through on directions.

Agency workers, or already enrolled parents, informed eligible parents about the project using a parent information sheet prepared for the project where then willing participants were referred to the project team. A member of the project team then contacted these parents to discuss the project, answer any questions, and make an appointment to visit them at home. During this visit, participation was discussed again, an informed consent questionnaire administered, and written informed consent was obtained. The study was approved by the Human Ethics Committee at UCLA. Eligible parents enrolled in this project were randomly assigned to one of two conditions, home instruction or materials in a ratio 3 to 1. Given the nature of this study (intervention to a high-risk population), a no treatment condition was considered ethically inappropriate. The study design is presented in Fig. 29.2. Once parents were assigned to a group, they were assessed of their baseline knowledge in the areas of health and safety. The pre-test measures assisted in determination of the parent current knowledge and skills in accordance with the program framework. Determination of the parent current level of functioning specified the curriculum that would be used in order to address the specific parenting needs, the steps in that curriculum at which the parent would begin, the optimal learning environment, and the person who will provide the education. This was then followed by an intervention period. Parents in group 1 received 15–17 individualized home-instruction weekly sessions, lasting 70 min, covering four components, whereas parents in group 2 received the same parenting booklets and all other items via mail or personal delivery biweekly following the same schedule as group 1. Each topic has a lesson plan with specific goals and objectives, along with ways to meet those goals and objectives individually or in small groups. Materials written in large print and illustrations are used in each, accompanied by booklets to be used by the parents.

Since motivation was an issue that could have been present, the Positive Parenting Attention

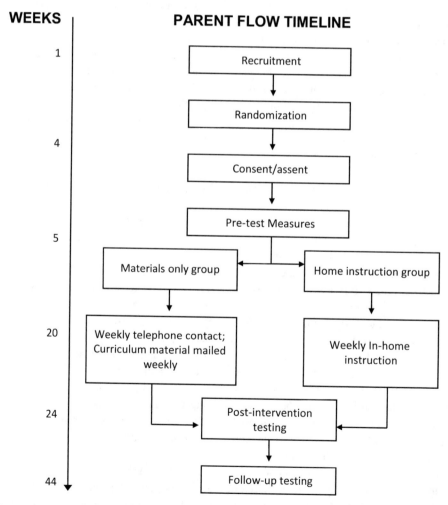

Fig. 29.2 Program framework (A. Tymchuk, personal communication, 2005)

System (+PAS) was devised in which those materials and processes that are most rewarding to the parent were identified. Specific behaviors are targeted for acquisition and maintenance, including attendance, timelines, and actual improvement in knowledge and skills. A schedule of contingencies was developed for providing the materials to the parent, costing in total about $50 per family. Following intervention, parents were then assessed to measure the amount of information that was learned. Five months following the post-testing period, parents were recontacted and assessed again.

29.4   Outcome

Within the UCLA Parent-Child Health and Wellness Program, primary dependent outcomes were maternal health, safety knowledge and skills, number of observed residential hazardous conditions, and number of health items and safety devices available. Statistical analysis showed that maternal health, safety knowledge, and skill scores in both groups improved significantly at post-testing; however, mothers who received interventions in their homes did better on all maternal knowledge outcome variables. Some of the gains attained in both groups remained at follow-up. In addition, both groups did not return to their baseline, and the differences between the two groups were maintained which demonstrated the validity of procedures for general use.

29.4.1 Home Safety Training: Replication Studies

Three home-safety studies were conducted utilizing all of the previously mentioned measures in the resource section. The first home safety training study involved four mothers with mild mental disability who had primary child caregiving responsibilities, substantial, and stable numbers of home dangers of all types that were observed at baseline, with few precautions, if any, implemented. For example, 150 suffocation hazards, 100 poison hazards, and 71 general clutter hazards were observed in the rooms made available for observation in one mother's apartment.

Following baseline observation, weekly group training occurred at a community facility with reassessment and subsequent weekly reinforcement of training in each mother's home following a multiple baseline procedure where one category of dangers and precautions was introduced at a time. Results showed that only after training in each category did reduction in frequency of hazards occur and frequency of precautions increase, however only in the safety category in which training had occurred (A. Tymchuk, personal communication, 2005).

Some of the gains obtained through training were maintained at 1-month follow-up for two mothers; gains were lost for another mother, while one mother did not complete training. Training and maintenance with two mothers were negatively impacted by maternal depression and alcoholism. While reported weekly injury events before and during training were infrequent, none was reported on follow-up. None of the children were removed from any family during the study.

This initial home-safety training study was systematically replicated with a second group of four mothers showing the same results to those on the initial study. Given the complexity of parental supervision in these families, the third study examined whether systematic training of mothers with intellectual disabilities instructing their children about home hazards and precautions would result in any change in observed home dangers and precautions. Following a multiple baseline design, results showed that education was effective in increasing both maternal and child knowledge of home hazards as well as of precautions that could be taken for each hazard.

The implications of these unique series of studies were significant for a number of reasons: (1) a major outcome was the development and validation of a measure that could be reliably used to assess frequency of dangers found in the homes of mothers with mild cognitive impairment that were associated with the most frequently occurring child injuries; (2) a related precautions measure and a structured injury event report also were validated; (3) based upon a behavioral framework, a specific operationalized training program involving curricula and parent-use materials were developed and their efficacy validated through the use of a single-subject multiple baseline procedure with a number of mothers. All these methods formed the basis for the Home Safety Component of the UCLA Parent-Child Health and Wellness Program study.

29.4.2 Process Evaluation

A total of 218 parents within the pilot study (159 in the instruction group and 59 in the materials group) completed the UCLA Parent-Child Health and Wellness Program study. Overall, there were 8500 home visits made. Most of the participants were mothers (95%). The results showed no group differences for maternal age, majority/emancipation status, gender, race/ethnicity, grade completed, cognitive abilities, marital status, or family status. Fifty-one percent of the total sample were minors; 55% indicated that they were depressed; 48% indicated that they were stressed; 30% indicated that they had been physically abused; and 22% indicated that they had been sexually abused at some time in their lives (A. Tymchuk, personal communication, 2005).

Average reported completed school grade was grade 8. Average reading recognition and comprehension grades on study-administered standardized tests were grade 6 and below. Initial reading recognition, comprehension, and self-reported disability status predicted performance at all three measured periods: at in-take, after intervention, and at follow-up. The average score on the IQ test used by the study (the quick IQ test) was 77 (SD 12.3). Cognitive ability and disability status were related to completing the project in that parents with lower IQ scores were more likely to remain in the study. Overall consumer satisfaction was 97% (A. Tymchuk, personal communication, 2005).

29.4.3 Dissemination

The UCLA Parent-Child Health and Wellness Program served as a training model in Colorado as the Colorado Parent-Child Health and Wellness Program (A. Tymchuk, personal communication, 2005). After training and provision of all procedures and materials from UCLA consultation, the project was also successfully experimentally replicated in Australia and evaluated in a randomized controlled trial at the University of Sydney (Llewellyn, McConnel, Honey, Mayes, & Russo, 2003). The original home safety measures, curricula, and parent-use materials, originally developed by Tymchuk and colleagues, were used with some minor modifications to suit the Australian context (Llewellyn et al., 2003; A. Tymchuk, personal communication, 2005). The specific aim of the New South Wales Parent-Child Health and Wellness Program was to assess the effectiveness of a home-based intervention, targeted to identify parents with intellectual disability to promote child health and home safety in the preschool years.

According to Tymchuk (personal communication, 2005), a total of 63 parents with intellectual disability from 57 families were recruited to take part in the study. Forty-five parents (40 mothers and five fathers) from 40 families completed the project. Nearly half (46.6%) of parents self-identified themselves as having some type of cognitive disability. The IQ scores for the sample obtained on the Kaufman Brief Intelligence Test ranged from 40 to 97. Over two-thirds of the sample had IQ scores on this measure <70–79. Almost half (48.9%) left after completing year 10 (Junior High), while only four parents had completed grades 11 and 12 (senior high school).

After taking part in the program, parents learned how to recognize dangers to young children in the family home, to identify appropriate precautions to overcome these dangers, and how to critically implement these precautions in their own home. Moreover, this knowledge and skills were maintained over a 3-month period. The findings from this replication study demonstrate that parents with intellectual disability can learn the necessary knowledge and skills to keep their young children healthy and safe. This finding adds to the extant literature on parent learning which reports successful outcomes but typically uses less rigorous research designs.

Using MANOVA with planned orthogonal contrasts, this randomized control trial resulted in (see Fig. 29.3):

1. A significantly greater number of home dangers identified by parents in home illustrations

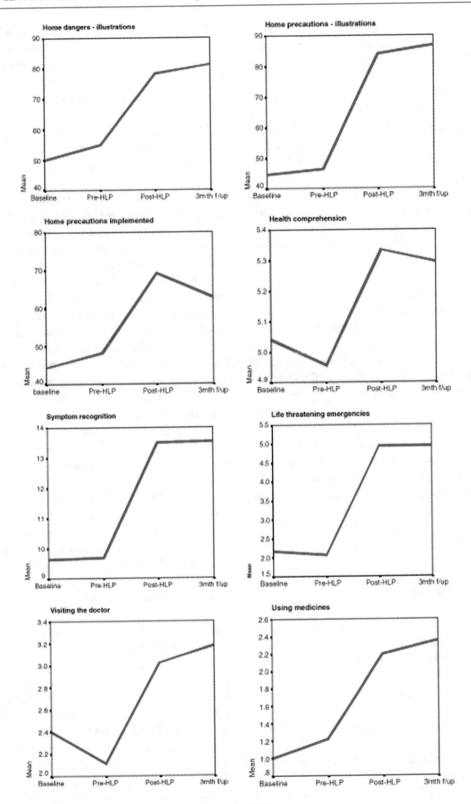

Fig. 29.3 Randomized control trial result (Llewellyn et al., 2003)

compared with other experimental conditions with Visits Only and Current Services Only ($F = 37.27$, $p < 0.001$) and Lesson Booklets Only ($F = 17.92$, $p < 0.001$);

2. A significant increase in the number of precautions identified by parents to deal with the dangers depicted in the home illustrations compared with Visits Only and Current Services Only ($F = 41.29$, $p < 0.001$) and Lesson Booklets Only ($F = 23.95$, $p < 0.001$)

3. A significantly greater number of home precautions implemented by parents compared with Lesson Booklets Only ($F = 27.09$, $p < 0.001$; A. Tymchuk, personal communication, 2005)

These results suggest that the implementation of the program was effective for parents for the most part, regardless of their state of health, literacy skills, or IQ. The positive findings reported here also hold promise in utilizing an intervention to help reduce the disproportionately high removal rate of children from their parents in the early years. Recommendations from the findings using the gold standard of evidence-informed health care in the form of a randomized controlled trial point out the need to (1) identify the knowledge and skills parents require, (2) to select the appropriate instructional materials and strategies, and (3) to implement a specifically designed program in a systematic and structured manner in situ (Llewellyn et al., 2003).

29.5 Conclusion

Three decades of injury prevention work of Dr. Tymchuk and his team have clearly demonstrated that critical aspects of successful interventions for the acquisition, maintenance, and generalization with parents with a cognitive disability include:

1. The behavioral definition of the task(s) to be trained on
2. Functional task analysis of requisite areas
3. Measurement
4. Provision of parent-use materials and curriculum adhering to accepted standards and validated for this population

5. Tailoring of the intervention strategies to mothers, through the use of modeling and role-playing both in vitro and in vivo situations
6. Provisions of supportive feedback and reinforcement, with periodic maintenance training

These requisites for optimal results were independently identified and corroborated in a review of effective parenting programs for parents with intellectual disability, which Feldman (1994) identified several essential elements of exemplary practice. These elements include that wherever possible, teaching and learning needs to take place in situ so that the parent can learn and practice the skills in the situation where these will be used. The instructional techniques must ensure as concrete and practical as possible delivery of material in a systematic sequence. The education process must also incorporate modelling along with the more usual forms of demonstration, verbal instruction, provision of feedback with frequent and regular positive reinforcement to maintain interest, motivation and learning. For many parent's periodic maintenance-training sessions may be required particularly if circumstances change or a different application of already mastered skills is required.

For this review, Feldman (1994) identified 20 intervention studies published in peer-reviewed journals in English which contained full description of methodologies to ascertain adequacy of the study in meeting a number of parameters. Eight of the 16 which utilized a single case multiple baseline procedure and replicated across a number of mothers with intellectual disabilities were conducted at UCLA by Dr. Tymchuk et al. (2003) as were two of the four studies utilizing a grouped design. That is, 50% of the intervention studies worldwide had been done at UCLA (A. Tymchuk, personal communication, 2005). Starting from clinical application, to single case studies following a multiple baseline, to multiple case studies following a multiple baseline, to random clinical trial, to systematic replication and then to randomized controlled trial, Dr. Tymchuk, his team, and colleague fellows demonstrated the utility of evidence-informed program procedures specifically designed to support wellness and injury prevention in populations at high risk.

The UCLA Parent-Child Health and Wellness Program: A Parenting Curriculum for Families at Risk was published in 2006 by the Brookes Publishing Inc, a validated program for professionals who work with vulnerable populations of parents. The book provides the complete program manual with assessment and parent-use materials included on CD for duplication. Offering effective, proven strategies tested with over 800 families, this book assists professionals (psychologists, nurses, social workers, home visitors, parent educators, administrators, and others who work with families at risk) to support parents with a wide range of (dis)abilities or individual learning needs to ensure their children's and their own health, safety, and wellness.

As social, health, and education agencies continue to struggle to meet the increasingly complex needs of multiple risk families, major needs continue regarding how to best prepare parents in ensuring their own home safety and that of their children. In applying exemplary practice criteria, it is realized that multifaceted, comprehensive, evidence-informed programs like the UCLA Parent-Child Health and Wellness Program are most effective in meeting these needs and in reducing injury. Future steps of program evolvement, however, would be to turn the positive finding of program effectiveness under research conditions, reported in this case study, into a similarly positive outcome in inclusive parent education programs offered by service agencies. Only with all levels of the service system working together to support the parents at high risk will the promise of an exemplary practice approach to injury prevention be truly fulfilled.

Acknowledgments The author would like to express sincere appreciation to the key informant for this case study: Alexander Tymchuk of the University of California, Los Angeles School of Medicine in the USA—whose consultation made this project possible.

BRIO Model: The UCLA Parent-Child Health and Wellness Program

Group Served: Low-income and underserved adults and teen parents with intellectual disabilities and other learning difficulties.

Goal: To support parents with intellectual disabilities in learning health and safety skills by focusing on parental strengths as well as exploring ways to extend health care and home safety education.

Background	Resources	Implementation	Outcome
Parenting information in the areas of health and home safety is commonly presented in complex language and format, making it difficult for parents with mild cognitive limitations or individual learning needs to learn and apply	Funded by California Wellness Foundation through a 4-year grant	Multidisciplinary in its approach to injury prevention	Significant increase in parental knowledge and skills on functional measures
	Additional financial resources through in-kind contributions	Two phases of implementation: initial re-examination of all previously developed procedures (pilot) and	The full curriculum has been adopted and instituted across California and pilot tested across sites in Colorado
	Operated under UCLA, department of psychiatry of School of Medicine. Employed multidisciplinary, multiethnic, bilingual staff	clinical random trial phase The program incorporates a perspective that is both	
Strategies take into account the interplay of the host, agent, and the environment at the pre-event (prevention of occurrence), event (severity), and post-event (remediation) level of injury prevention	Over the course of 4 years, program materials were multidisciplinary validated with people who are practicing nurses, social workers, psychologists, physicians, teachers, direct care staff, administrators, and students	flexible and adaptable to address changing needs in diverse populations of parents in families at risk	Replicated as random control trial study at University of Sydney, Australia The complete program with accompanied CD was published in 2006 by the Brookes Publishing Inc.
Education intervention model is based on the principles of empowerment education	Evolved through Dr. Tymchuk's own clinical and community research for over three decades		

Life Space Model: The UCLA Parent-Child Health and Wellness Program

Sociocultural: civilization/community	Interpersonal: primary and secondary relationships	Physical environments: where we live	Internal states: biochemical/genetic and means of coping
Substantial evidence shows that low-income mothers with or without intellectual disabilities do not have basic information about injury prevention. Need for supportive programs that provide accurate information and skills regarding how to act in the event of a child injury. Need for empirically developed program materials addressing parental adequacy at prescriptive level Free, bilingual, community out-reach program, tailored for families with preschool children at high risk for injuries. Nationally and internationally replicated Intervention model is based on the principles of social inclusion and empowerment education Created to explore ways to extend health care and home safety education research to community settings with families headed by parent(s) with intellectual disability	Introduced the memoranda of understanding as formal collaborative relationships between university and at least one agency representing health care, child protective service, disability/social services, and education Successful implementation requires multidisciplinary team coordination including disability, private and public health, welfare, child protection, parenting education, early intervention, mental health, the courts, and other social services The Positive Parenting Attention System (+PAS) has been devised in which those materials and processes that are most rewarding to the parent have been identified	Intervention strategies take into account the transaction of the host, agent, and the environment at the pre-event (prevention of occurrence), event (severity), and post-event (remediation) level of injury prevention Home-safety curriculum is a part of the overall Wellness Program Both in vivo and in vitro identifications of the antecedents (circumstances to injury) and consequences (remediation) of the actual injury event are critical for effective home-safety program implementation since parents may not be aware of either	Intervention addresses changes in parental/maternal information processing A focus on enabling factors is done in order to redirect focus on risk factors only Empirically-based curricula, prescriptive assessment tools, and other educational materials are specifically designed to promote competence in adequate parenting Program efforts were directed to the provision of supports to the parent/mother in order to facilitate self-growth and actualization

References

California Evidence-Based Clearinghouse for Child Welfare. (2017). *Healthy & safe*. San Diego, CA: Author. Retrieved from http://www.cebc4cw.org/program/healthy-safe/detailed

California Wellness Foundation. (n.d.). *About Us*. Los Angels, CA: Author. Retrieved from http://www.cal-wellness.org/

Feldman, M. (1994). Parenting education for parents with intellectual disabilities. A review of outcome studies. *Research in Developmental Disabilities, 15*, 299–332.

Haddon, W. Jr. (1980). Advances in the epidemiology of injuries as a basis for public policy. *Public Health Reports, 95*(5), 411–421.

Llewellyn, G., McConnel, D., Honey, A., Mayes, R., & Russo, D. (2003). Promoting health and home safety for children of parents with intellectual disability: A randomized controlled trial. *Research in Developmental Disabilities, 24*, 405–431.

Mandel, U., Bigelow, K. M., & Lutzker, J. R. (1998). Using video to reduce home safety hazards with parents reported for child abuse and neglect. *Journal of Family Violence, 13*(2), 147–162.

Peterson, L., Farmer, J., & Mori, L. (1987). Process analysis of injury situations: A complement to epidemiological methods. *Journal of Social Issues, 43*(2), 33–44.

Tymchuk, A. (1996). Predicting adequacy and inadequacy of parenting by persons with mental retardation. *Child Abuse & Neglect, 16*, 165–178.

Tymchuk, A. (1999). Moving towards integration of services for parents with intellectual disabilities. *Journal of Intellectual and Developmental Disabilities, 24*, 59–74.

Tymchuk, A. (2006). *The health and wellness program: Supporting families at-risk*. Baltimore, MA: Brookes Publishing.

Tymchuk, A., Groen A., & Dolyniuk C. (2000). Health, safety and well-being reading recognition abilities of young parents with functional disabilities: Construction and preliminary validation of a prescriptive assessment instrument. *Journal of Developmental and Physical Disabilities, 12*(4), 349–366.

Tymchuk, A., Lakin, K. C., & Luckasson, R. (2001). *The forgotten generation*. Baltimore, MA: Brookes Publishing.

Tymchuk, A., Lang, C., Sewards, S., Lieberman, S., & Koo, S. (2003). Development and validation of The Illustrated Version of the Home Inventory for Dangers and Safety Precautions: Continuing to address learning needs of parents in healthcare and safety. *Journal of Family Violence, 18*, 241–252.

Tymchuk, A., Llewellyn, G., & Feldman, M. (1999). Parenting by persons with intellectual disabilities: A timely international perspective. *Journal of Intellectual and Developmental Disability, 24*(1), 3–6.

Indian Health Service Injury Prevention Program/US Department of Health and Human Services

30

Nathaniel Paul

The Indian Health Service Injury Prevention Program (IHSIPP) provides preservice and in-service training to students, community workers, and professionals in the field of injury prevention. It emphasizes creation of innovative training opportunities for federal and tribal employees as part of a system of injury control in American Indian communities throughout the United States.

30.1 Background

Since its inception in 1955, the Indian Health Service (IHS) has acted as both a health advocate and a health provider for Native Americans and has sought to raise their health status to the highest possible level. In pursuit of this goal, the IHS works to provide a multifaceted and comprehensive health services delivery system for American Indians (AI) and Alaska Natives (AN) and emphasizes maximum tribal involvement in developing and managing programs to meet their needs. It is also the responsibility of the IHS to work with the people involved in the health delivery programs so that they can be cognizant of entitlements of Indian individuals, as American citizens, to all federal, state, and local health

programs, in addition to IHS and tribal services. The IHS also acts as the principal federal health advocate for AI and AN people in the building of health coalitions, networks, and partnerships with tribal nations and other government agencies and with nonfederal organizations (e.g., academic medical centers and private foundations (Indian Health Service [IHS], 2000).

30.1.1 Target Population

30.1.1.1 AI/AN Communities

Native American individuals experience injury mortality rates that are 2.4 times greater than other Americans, estimating around $350 million per year for treatment costs (Indian Health Service [IHS], 2017). Reflecting the IHS's general mandate, its Injury Prevention Program (IPP) seeks to reduce the number and severity of injuries in all Native Americans. Potentially, this mandate means a target population of 2.2 million individuals representing more than 567 tribes dispersed over 36 US states (IHS, 2017). As an aggregate, unintentional injury is the leading cause of death among members of this population between ages 1 and 44 and is ranked third overall for all ages (Wallace, 1997; IHS, 2017). While these rates vary only slightly by sex, it is worth noting that for males of all ages, unintentional injury represents the third leading cause of death overall (Indian Health Service [IHS],

N. Paul (✉)
Ontario Justice Education Network,
Toronto, ON, Canada

© Springer Nature Switzerland AG 2020
R. Volpe (ed.), *Casebook of Traumatic Injury Prevention*,
https://doi.org/10.1007/978-3-030-27419-1_30

2015). A great range of injury scenarios are represented within these figures, including many leading causes of neurotrauma. Pedestrian injuries are ranked fourth, and depending upon age range, falls, suffocation, poisoning, drowning, and cyclist injuries are all represented in the ten leading causes of AI/AN deaths (Indian Health Service [IHS], 2002a). All of these tend to figure significantly as major causes of neurotrauma (SMARTRISK, 1998). Finally, while there is some regional variation in these figures, injury and other accidents rank consistently in the top three causes of death in each of the 12 IHS service areas (Indian Health Service [IHS], 2002b).

While it would be a mistake to assume that this diverse population is without resources, it is important to recognize the relationships between socioeconomic status, health outcomes, and intergroup disparity. In addition to disproportionate levels of poverty (approximately twice that of the population in general), many factors have an impact upon the injury status of Native Americans such as tremendous diversity within and between service areas, differences in geographical access to resources, insurance rates, cultural practices, educational resources, and levels, lifestyle, and health beliefs. Additionally, less than half the funding allocated on a per capita basis for healthcare to the US general population is directed toward IHS healthcare (Indian Health Service [IHS], n.d.-b). Former Deputy Director and IPP Manager, Alan Dellapenna, reports that the IHS is funded at approximately 50% of its identified level of need and that within this funding the IPP is funded at approximately 40% of its need (Dellapenna, personal communication, October 10, 2002). Further, the majority of what funding is available to the IHS goes to overhead costs and paying bills for doctors, hospitals, and other medical practitioners for services rendered. Combined with a widespread mistrust of conventional public services following historical violence and marginalization at the hands of state, the diversity and socioeconomic disparity of AI/AN highlights both the challenges and the importance of IHS activities. Injury prevention is doubly valuable as a strategy here; in addition to the immediate rewards associated with reducing injury, prevention stands to reduce the costs and other burdens to be absorbed within a severely underfunded healthcare system.

30.1.1.2 Practitioners

The IHSIPP provides preservice and in-service training to students, community workers, and professionals in the field of injury prevention, with a particular effort to focus upon tribal and IHS employees.

30.1.2 History

Although injury, unintentional and otherwise, has been a significant health issue among US Native people for many decades, there has been more attention drawn to the AI/AN morbidity and mortality statistics, in part a consequence of important gains realized in control of infectious disease. As Robertson (1986) reports, by 1980, injury had become a dominant health threat for Native Americans, whose rate of death from unintentional injury was approximately twice that of the white or black populations. In recognition of the severity of the problem, the IHS commenced developing and implementing specific measures targeting the reduction and prevention of serious injury. The resultant early initiatives mostly focused upon education of the target population about dangerous activities and techniques to reduce the severity of injuries through treatments such as first aid or CPR. Although educational and other prevention strategies premised upon behavioral change are normally most successful when combined with other measures (such as engineering or legislative changes), it is noteworthy that in servicing populations and areas that have had relatively minimal exposure to preventive self-care information, such initial outreaches can have a dramatic and sudden impact. Thus, Robertson's (1986) evaluation of IHS injury prevention activities between 1980 and 1984 documents significant reductions in hospitalizations due to falls (from about 6 to about 4 hospitalizations per 100 population) and motor vehicle accidents (from 4.4 to 2.6), in association with injury control efforts.

As the 1980s progressed, the IHS increased both the breadth and the sophistication of their activities, including more detailed surveillance and data collection in partnership with its service area units and hospitals and the creation of innovative training methods for injury prevention professionals. Launched in 1987, the IHSIPP represents an important next step in preventive education, combining advanced data collection and analysis with training programs designed to produce dedicated individuals with not only a strong background in general injury epidemiology but also with highly specialized skills appropriate to different areas and types of intervention.

30.1.3 Identifying the Problem

This emphasis upon both diversity and educational rigor can be understood as a response to a number of central problems identified in professional training. Most significantly, there has been a critical shortage of injury control professionals with field-specific preparation in the United States. For example, one national study conducted in 1990 estimated that "as many as 75% of state and regional health department managers had never taken a graduate-level course in the epidemiology or prevention of injury" (Smith, Dellapenna, & Berger, 2000, p. 176). Most injury control practitioners were therefore working at a community level with minimal guidance from the specialized public health disciplines and focusing upon "common-sense" approaches and public awareness campaigns, with little emphasis upon program evaluation. Similarly, environmental and enactment/enforcement were largely underutilized as control strategies.

Further, where appropriate education was available, it required lengthy time commitments, minimally several semesters, or, more frequently, multiyear degrees (Shepard, 2000). While clear benefits exist in association with this type of training, it tends to exclude the possibility of educating individuals to make effective simple interventions with immediate impacts at the grassroots level. This exclusion in turn tends to exacerbate the already wide gulf between academic and local initiatives and lead to isolated, rather than collaborative, strategies. Additionally, the cost of these programs presented its own challenges. Long-term courses of study are expensive, potentially prohibitively so for members of the native communities they intend to serve. Similarly, public agencies were understandably reluctant to pay these costs for professional development of their employees if that meant the loss of these individuals from their already strained posts for extended durations of time (Shepard, 2000).

30.1.4 Model

These considerations pointed to the need to develop a model for creating training programs that would attend to the following priorities:

- The reduction of injury and its associated social, emotional, and economic costs among AIs and AN
- The provision of a cadre of practitioners to implement strategies in support of this goal
- The development of curricula designed to guide both local and regional level efforts and to foster collaboration between academic- and community-based approaches
- The reduction or removal of time and expense barriers to accessing this training
- The encouragement of participation by individuals representing the communities to be served
- Provision of resources necessary for realizing, evaluating, and adapting the particular efforts that would emerge in conjunction with this program

The above are clearly reflected in the IHSIPP, which emphasizes the creation of the following:

Innovative training opportunities for federal and tribal employees as part of a system of injury control in AI communities throughout the United States. The IHSIPP offers technical assistance to tribes, evaluates injury control projects, funds local interventions, advocates for tribal injury control at the federal and regional levels, and provides data for action at the community level. The training program provides a cadre of individuals to implement the program at regional and local levels (Smith et al., 2000, p. 176).

The geographic distribution of IHS regional offices makes for accessibility throughout the continental United States and Alaska, creating widespread opportunities for community development in connection with the program's mission:

To raise the health status of AIs and AN to the highest possible level by decreasing the incidence of severe injuries and death to the lowest possible level and increasing the ability of tribes to address their injury problems (IHS, 2017).

In practical terms, this goal means providing courses and other training opportunities that cater to a wide range of cultural, educational, and professional backgrounds, levels of interest, and types of intervention. Specifically, the IPP offers courses that range in duration from a half-day to a full year and utilizes "experiential instruction, preceptors, and community case studies to … promote community empowerment" as a mode of intervention (Smith et al., 2000, p. 175). Its graduates have therefore launched a broad spectrum of initiatives, far too numerous to mention here, that have addressed both primary and secondary intervention, combined elements of enactment, and environmental change with education and innovation, and engaged with injury through both immediately workable projects and longer-term studies and strategies drawing from and creating new knowledge for the field.

30.2 Resources

30.2.1 Stakeholder Participation

Due to the breadth of the population it aims to serve, identifying particular groups as unique stakeholders in the IPP may be somewhat misleading. In addition to the obvious target population of all AI/AN, it is important to note that non-Aboriginal people residing in proximity to IHS service areas shared certain aspects of their injury profile due to similar life circumstances

and stood to benefit from many of the efforts that would be launched under the auspices of the program. In considering the resources available to the IHS for its injury prevention activities, it is helpful to be able to locate the agency in relation to other public offices in US governance. The IHS was created under the auspices of the Federal Department of Health and Human Services and is divided into three distinct offices.

30.2.1.1 The Office of the Director (OD)

The OD is chiefly responsible for administrative matters such as budget, payroll and personnel, as well as some advocacy and congressional liaison.

30.2.1.2 The Office of Self Determination (OSD)

This office was created in response to Bill 93-638, the Indian Self-Determination and Education Assistance Act, which stipulates that federally recognized tribes have the option to either assume the administration and operation of health services and programs in their communities or remain within the IHS direct health system. Under this legislation, each of the 567 recognized tribes may opt out of any program provided by the IHS and take the proportional monetary value of its share of that program to contract an outside provider of an equivalent service. This opting out is known as "compacting," and in the event that a tribe exercises this option, the OSD assists in determining the amount of the tribe's allotment, in contracting an appropriate provider and in monitoring the quality of services rendered.

30.2.1.3 The Office of Public Health (OPH)

This third division is directly responsible for all IHS direct healthcare provision, maintaining an extensive system of hospitals and clinics, as well as a smaller public health component. The OPH is subdivided into two branches—The Office of Clinical Services and the Office of Environmental Health—which houses injury prevention activities. The location of the IHS's program under the auspices of environmental health gives it a considerably broader mandate than would be possible were it restricted to a traditional hospital-based program. This location allows the IHS to approach injury as an environmental and ecological problem, rather than an individual, pathological event; therefore, it may be more analogous to a local health department (Dellapenna, personal communication, October 10, 2002).

Thus, the focus of the IHS's broad mandate is comparable to a public health understanding of the epidemiology of injury, with responsibilities ranging from environmental health hazards, water system design, and food safety to motor vehicle and outdoor safety.

Funding for the IHSIPP is channeled from the Federal Department of Health and Human Services through the IHS's annually allotted appropriation and is meted out through national, regional, and local offices. Costs include administrative, salary, and other overhead costs, but many of these are deferred through resource-sharing practices (e.g., colocation) with existing IHS facilities. In turn, the IPP supports the initiatives of its trainees and grantees with up-to-date educational materials and statistical data, funding, evaluation, and other assistance including public advocacy for their efforts and dissemination of their results.

30.2.2 Legislation

Despite a successful, multi-decade commitment to reducing the occurrence and severity of injury in AI/AN communities, the IHS has never had the benefit of authorizing legal language specifically dedicated to injury prevention. Rather, the agency has made effective use of discretionary areas provided in broader pieces of legislation for injury prevention purposes. Several of these have been especially important resources shaping the IHSIPP and training.

The 1955 establishment of the IHS was crucial. Previously, the Bureau of Indian Affairs was responsible for the range of government functions pertaining to AI/AN, but health was not a clear point in their mandate. The service was therefore created as an offshoot of the bureau, in response to massive need and inadequate servicing in areas such as water/sewer systems and sorely inadequate housing. This matter was an important legal development for injury prevention concerns in two ways: first, it helped to bring environmental health into focus, and second, the health gains realized by paying even minimal attention to the systemic health problems of American Aboriginal People meant that the relative profile of injury and its prevention was raised dramatically. This increased attention soon led to the realization that purely education-based strategies for injury control could not address the problem as effectively as a more comprehensive approach could, and in the late 1970s, responsibility for injury was transferred from health education to the Office of Environment and Heritage (OEH). Table 30.1 displays the influential bills and laws that influence the development of IPP.

30.2.3 Retention

As Dellapenna (personal communication, October 10, 2002) notes, retention rates of program participants are made somewhat murky by the unique employment structure of the IHS's injury prevention efforts. The vast majority of trainees are not full-time injury practitioners but rather are employed in a peripheral capacity for which injury is an important consideration. The IHS places a greater emphasis upon seeding its competencies through a network of skilled professionals within the communities it serves than upon rehiring its own graduates on a full-time, per se basis. In other words, many trainees are "retained" to the extent that they cycle through various community agencies or organizations or can bring their training to bear in a variety of community service-oriented activities. Indeed, many of these graduates, and especially fellowship graduates, work as course instructors for the IHS training program, and many go on to hold essential positions as full-time injury control specialists for the IHS or the tribes it serves. As specialists, these people are responsible for conducting and overseeing a comprehensive, regional injury program. This responsibility virtually guarantees a renewable

Table 30.1 Influential bills and laws

Bill/law	Information
Bill 86-121	The Sanitation Facilities Construction Act (Late 1950s–Early 1960s)
	Authorized and funded the IHS to build water, sewer, and wastewater facilities on reservations as part of federal responsibilities to tribes and provided the initial authorizing and funding language that set up the Office of Environmental Health.
	After these systems were built, there was a need for qualified people to work with communities to run them safely. This scenario led to an initial build-up of professional engineers and sanitarians and a focus on the relationship of local communities to environmental health. Injury prevention initially grew out of this concern as a division of environmental health services.
Bill 93-638	The Indian Self-Determination Act
	Provides the authorizing language for federally recognized tribes to enter into "compact" arrangements with the health service providers of their own choosing.
	This "environment of self-determination" shapes much of what the IHS does and can do, by formalizing obligations to tribes and specifying the legal rights and responsibilities that are built into the relationship.
	By introducing an element of competition and performance-based choice into tribal health service provision, this bill encourages the IHS to be service-oriented and to make efforts to be acutely aware of and responsive to the particular character and needs of local communities.
Public Law 94-437	The Indian Health Care Improvement Act
	Serves to confirm the US federal government's commitment to improving the health status of AI/AN and spells out specific objectives to that end.
	This piece of legislation represents an opportunity for the IHS to help shape the direction of care for its constituents and to work for the inclusion of language specifying injury control as a central concern.

Note: Dellapenna, personal communication (October 10, 2002)

supply of well-trained and devoted individuals working to improve the health of their local communities.

Every year, continuing education sessions are offered to graduates of the Injury Prevention Specialist Fellowship program (IPSFP). These sessions take the form of topic-specific colloquia and help ensure that participants in the IPP's most recognized activity have opportunities to keep abreast of current trends and emerging issues, while providing ongoing professional skills and knowledge development. Examples of topics include prevention of impaired driving and the impact of managed care on injury control activities.

30.2.4 Conceptual Guidelines

The initial and continuing development of all IHSIPP courses are organized around four key principles: community input, epidemiologic data, advances in knowledge, and program evaluation. The strength of these principles is such that they ought to be considered program resources in themselves insofar as they provide guidelines for ongoing expansion, refinement, and implementation of its practices.

30.2.4.1 Community Input

This entity helps to ensure both the local relevance of particular initiatives and that implementation methods are sensitive to unique aspects of local cultural communities. These groups' views are important areas that ought to be reflected in curricular materials that are both solicited by the program's specialists and welcomed when they arrive in the form of requests for attention to specific issues. In this way, injury-related trends that may be first identified at the local level can be accounted for in the design of courses. The fact that community members, both AI/AN and non-AI/AN, are attached to the program in steering and learning capacities further reflects the IHS's commitment to community input.

30.2.4.2 Epidemiologic Data

This data is collected in a variety of forums and used for IHSIPP purposes in a number of ways. In some cases, this process involves compiling injury surveillance statistics in partnership with the medical facilities that collaborate with the IPP in some IHS service areas; in others, it involves making use of surveys conducted by other agencies, such as the Centers of Disease Control (CDC) or National Highway Traffic Safety Administration (NHTSA). In this way, both broad (e.g., national) and specific (pertaining to a particular region) figures can be used in the development of course emphases. Further, this data is essential in mapping those priorities that guide the strategies to be developed by students and other concerned parties, for example, by providing demographic data about high-risk groups, environments, or scenarios. The IHS Office of Program Statistics puts out two particularly useful publications on an annual basis, Trends in Indian Health and Regional Differences in Indian Health. These publications can be considered an enhancement of the previous parameter, community input, insofar as they help to yield clear pictures of the state of injury and injury prevention for specific regions or tribes and the strengths and potential challenges these may face.

30.2.4.3   Advances in Knowledge

This principle includes new developments in scientific, medical, and epidemiological knowledge, technical and engineering innovations, and novel approaches to practice, which become central considerations in course design and delivery. For example, the increased focus in recent years upon social marketing in building successful behavioral interventions and the acceptance of environmental or legislative changes is reflected in the inclusion of this perspective in IHS courses and the teaching of research strategies such as focus groups.

30.2.4.4   Program Evaluation

As an element of exemplary practice in prevention of unintentional injury, it is useful to point out that the IHS supports evaluation of not only the initiatives of its own trainees but also of the educational programs it provides. In practical terms, this scenario translates into both participant and external evaluations of IHSIPP courses and operations and published evaluations of particular interventions. These data are further discussed later in the Outcome section. Importantly, some of these reviews have recommended greater attention to evaluation in the course materials, resulting in the creation of core and other courses in research methods and analysis. In this way, trainees have a valuable initial opportunity to learn appropriate evaluation strategies.

30.2.5   Financial Resources

Courses and other training forums offered under the auspices of the program circulate throughout the United States in order to avoid concentrating their availability in only one area. While this rotation does reduce the burden for certain regions in a given year, it necessarily increases this burden for participants from further away. This scenario is compounded by the fact that public service employees and their employers may find it difficult to compensate for their absence due to training attendance or to secure funding to pay the cost. In response to these difficulties, the program has been designed to accommodate various lengths of commitment. In the case of the fellowship, which at a year represents the greatest commitment, travel time is restricted to 6 weeks during the course of the year (Shepard, 2000). During this limited time, fellows are released from their professional responsibilities, and some of the associated costs are allayed because the IHS secures reduced or group travel rates for participants. For the remainder of the year, geographical and professional displacements are less significant issues, because fellowship work can be completed independently, with IPP support. The IHS Headquarters Office in the Office of Public Health provides financial support for fellowship participant travel, per diem, and tuition for required course work and out-of-area field work, excluding participants from self-governance compact tribes which are responsible for paying all expenses for their fellowship participants (IHS, 2002g).

The Tribal Injury Prevention Cooperative Agreement Program (TIPCAP) began to provide funding through a competitive process. Tribes were awarded multi-year funding to hire a full-time injury prevention coordinator who developed programs based on effective strategies in injury prevention. Since 1997, the IHSIPP has funded more than 110 grantees, which are categorized in two programs. Part I is composed of federally recognized tribes new to the IHS IPP ($100,000 for year 1 and $80,000 annually for years 2–5). With Part II, grantees are federally recognized tribes who develop, implement, and evaluate IPPs $20,000 annually for 5 years (IHS, 2017).

30.3 Implementation

The IHS IPP was initially conceived as a response to an identified need for a critical mass of professionals who could draw upon a solid understanding of both local community issues and epidemiology to work for the reduction of the incidence and severity of injury in Native American populations in a variety of ways. An educational approach was identified as the most promising means of meeting this need. By concentrating upon advancing the capacity of an existing workforce, the program provides concrete data and strategies by which these individuals can use their existing expertise in the design and implementation of effective interventions. Further, a Course Revision Committee comprised of existing program staff reviews and revises course materials to keep abreast of new information, strategies, and other important developments in the field (Indian Health Service [IHS], 2002e). However, professional education for community service employees raises its own challenges.

30.3.1 Curriculum

Great care has been taken in the design of educational materials to ensure that they can offer training that is flexible enough to accommodate different intensities, styles, and durations of commitment to preventing injury among Native Americans, while remaining practical and relevant to the field. These courses stand as proof that rigorous and effective training need not alienate grassroots level staff, just as community-based interventions occupy an essential position in academic approaches to epidemiology. This course flexibility makes them accessible and useful for a broad range of individuals that are traditionally enrolled in similar programs:

> Whereas students in academic programs have similar educational backgrounds, students in IHS training courses may include both individuals with master's degrees and those with only a high school diploma. Similarly, while virtually all university faculty have advanced academic degrees, many of the instructors in IHS courses lack advanced degrees but have skills and experience in community-based interventions (Smith et al., 2000, p. 177).

The strength of this approach is evident in terms of both structure and content. The program includes courses that range in duration from 3-h to a full-year fellowship program. Both the short and the long courses of training are designed around the development of key competencies for injury control practitioners in AI/AN communities:

- Project development, implementation, evaluation
- Promote community involvement
- Effective strategies
- Epidemiology
- Data collection and analysis
- Coalition building
- Program evaluation
- Oral/written communication
- Individualized learning experiences
- Field work

These competencies are introduced and elaborated upon cumulatively over three levels of increasingly sophisticated short courses, which then become the prerequisite education for enrolment in two of the year-long fellowships.

30.3.1.1 Level 1

These courses are "mini-courses" in "Introduction to Injury Prevention," which generally cater to tribal program managers, who frequently have very little time to attend longer courses of study.

These short sessions seek to raise the participant's awareness as to the relevance of injury to Native Americans' quality of life and experience with social services and the role that prevention strategies can play in ameliorating these.

30.3.1.2 Level 2
A representation of a series of longer, modular, and cumulative courses, such as "Injury Prevention Data Analysis and Interpretation" and "Translating Information into Action," is required for IHS Community Injury Control (CIC) practitioners. They both review prior content and introduce new and practically oriented material in order to provide a solid background in injury prevention. This core program is offered throughout the year in different areas for CIC practitioners and other individuals whose professional responsibilities or other interest in injury prevention mean that they have a significant involvement in the field. This group tends to represent a broad cross section of backgrounds, ranging from high-placed members of health agencies to tribal community workers.

30.3.1.3 Level 3
This IHS program offers intensive topic-specific workshops throughout the year as well. These either target improving essential skills (e.g., grant writing) or seek to provide training in AI/AN injury control to audiences that might not otherwise receive it, such as conventional medical service providers (Smith et al., 2000).

30.3.2 Fellowship Programs

Whereas the design of Levels 1–3 was guided by the goal that individuals completing all three should be able to oversee a community-based injury initiative, the final and arguably the most successful aspect of the IPP is the 2-year-long IPSFP (Dellapenna, personal communication, October 10, 2002). The first programs of their kind, these Fellowships provide in-depth and advanced training to tribal and IHS staff who have exemplary qualifications and commitment to injury prevention (Rhoades, 1997; Smith, 1988).

30.3.2.1 Epidemiology Fellowship
This program focuses on evaluation, surveillance, data collection, and community-based interventions. A bachelor's degree, completion of Level 1 and Level 2, 3 years in public health, and 2 years in injury prevention are all needed as a prerequisite. Courses cover topics such as project development, epidemiology, field work, and publications and ends with a symposium. The IHS hosts this injury symposium every year, at which graduates present the results from their studies and/or projects to an audience of IHS staff, tribal leaders, and representatives of relevant agencies such as the CDC or the NHTSA (IHS, 2017).

30.3.2.2 Program Development Fellowship
The focus of this program revolves around evaluation, surveillance, data collection, and community-based interventions. Unlike the epidemiology fellowship, an individual does not require a bachelor's degree. However, individuals do need to complete Level 1 and have at least 1 year of professional experience in injury prevention. Courses cover topics such as IPP planning, program implementation and evaluation, field work, marketing, and advocacy. This fellowship also ends with the collaborative symposium (IHS, 2017).

30.3.3 Safe Native American Passengers (SNAP)

Released in 2003, the IHSIPP also offers a culturally appropriate 1-day course introducing child passenger safety (CPS). This program targets individuals who work with families and children in tribal communities. It provides preparatory training for those who are considering taking the certification course, services as an introductory course for CPS, and provides basic overview of the proper use and installation of car seats, addressing issues that are specifically unique to Native American communities. As of 2016, students who complete SNAP will be eligible for 0.6 continuing education units.

Table 30.2 Program mechanisms

Mechanism	Description
Provide technical assistance	Provides expertise in a range of capacities depending on where support is required. For example, the IHS advised on how the techniques of social marketing could be used to build a strategy to increase use of personal flotation devices (PFDs) and reduce extremely high drowning rates in Alaskan waters. This technique "involves utilizing the marketing tools of the business world—focus groups, opinion surveys, mass media—to promote socially valuable causes" (Smith et al., 2000, p. 181). The developed strategy resulted in the creation of a new product, the "floatcoat," which people were far more willing to wear regularly as it was more comfortable and stylish than traditional PFDs, and in new legislation stipulating that all children under age 14 wear PFDs in boats
Evaluate injury prevention projects	Evaluation is a service IHS provides for local initiatives, often arranging that the evaluation of projects be conducted as a special research study for students in the fellowship program. For example, Cook (2000) conducted an evaluation of a comprehensive intervention to reduce the incidence of home-centered child injury on the St. Regis Mohawk Reservation. Cook (2000) used a local hospital patient database to generate a sample of homes with children under age 10 for study for pre- and post-intervention, and a 16-item safety survey was conducted in 94 homes selected to receive the intervention and to 99 nonintervention comparison homes. Following collection, data was analyzed, and a significant reduction in child hazards in the intervention homes was found. Chi-square analysis was used to confirm the strength and the generalizability of this finding
Fund local interventions	The program's design presumes that sensitivity to injury problems is often most acute at the local, everyday level and that with proper support, interventions launched from this perspective can be highly successful. Funding is channeled from the federal agency to local area/regional and community stations, as mentioned in resources
Advocate for tribal IPPs at federal, regional levels	Projects of this scale are ambitious and require the support of powerful offices. Due to the connection to the department of public health, the IHS and the IPP are well-positioned to voice their specific concerns and build partnerships with influential bodies and their efforts. For example, the IHS is a lead federal agency in the Healthy People 2010 initiative, a national coalition of health agencies dedicated to ameliorating public health levels as measured by key indicators, including injury. Tribal injury prevention and other initiatives are encouraged to use the Healthy People guidelines in drafting and implementing their intervention proposals (IHS, n.d.-c)
Provide data for action at community level	One of the IHS's most successful and frequently cited projects, a campaign that sought to increase seat-belt use by combining educational and legislative/enforcement methods, exemplifies how this data has been used. Observational and surveillance studies conducted by the Navajo Area IHS IPP in the 1980s showed that only 14% of Navajo adults and 7% of Navajo children regularly wore appropriate safety restraints while traveling by car (Bill, Buonviri, Bohan, & Garnanez, 1992; Smith et al., 2000). Between 1988 and 1991, the initiative was implemented in successive phases, resulting in a dramatic increase in seat-belt use and a related decrease in car crash fatalities

30.3.4 IHSIPP Activities

In addition to its efforts in professional education and training, the IHS implements its IPP through a series of related but distinct channels (IHS, 2002d). Table 30.2 displays the different mechanisms of the program.

Further evidence of strong practice appears when the IHS standards for reporting and application of data are considered. The core data that all IHS programs rely upon represent a subset of the statistics that are constantly compiled by local IHS providers and information systems in order to manage effective health service programs. These systems include the following:

- Patient Registration System
- Ambulatory Patient Care (APC) System
- Direct Inpatient Care System
- Contract Health Services Inpatient System
- Contract Health Services Outpatient System
- Dental Reporting System

- Pharmacy System
- Environmental Health Activity Reporting and Facility Data System
- Mental Health and Social Services Reporting System
- Alcoholism Treatment Guidance System (ATGS)/Chemical Dependency
- Management Information System (CDMIS)
- Community Health Representative Information System (CHRIS)
- Community Health Activity Reporting System
- Health Education Resource Management System (HERMS)
- Nutrition and Dietetics' Program Activities Reporting System
- Clinical Laboratory Workload Reporting System
- Urban Indian Health Common Reporting
- Fluoridation Reporting Data System

These data are collected locally and regionally and are normally sent through the appropriate area office for analysis and compilation to the IHS Data Processing Services Team in Albuquerque. In addition to the annual publications mentioned above, Trends in Indian Health and Regional Differences in Indian Health, these become the basis of a wide range of other data sources maintained by the IHS Program Statistics Team. These include documents pertaining to the respective health status of Native American women, youth, and elderly people, lists of health facilities operated by AI/AN and their organizations, inpatient and facility utilization statistics, and yearly regional population figures.

30.3.5 Organizational Structure

The organizational structure for implementation of the IPP activities fits within the division of IHS programs more generally, which in turn reflects the geopolitical distribution of AI/AN individuals throughout the United States. The 151 Service Units of the IHS are divided into 12 geographical service Areas—Alaska, Albuquerque, Bemidji, Billings, California, Great Plains, Nashville, Navajo, Oklahoma City, Phoenix, Portland, and

Tucson—each containing multiple districts and tribes (HIS, 2017). In addition to program training, areas conduct their own slate of injury prevention activities, ranging from public awareness campaigns and legislation advocacy to rigorous peer-reviewed studies and conference hosting. There is some variance in the structure of individual area offices, but at each of these, the IPP is overseen by a program manager, typically trained in the fellowship program. Each area also employs Injury Prevention Specialists, who are responsible for comprehensive programs at the area, district, and tribal level. These strictly IPP staff work closely with IHS Environmental Health staff within the appropriate service/district unit. Finally, the program relies upon other IHS and tribal staff, such as health educators, community health representatives, public health nurses, and community/social service workers. Instructors for IPP courses are also drawn from this pool and, in the case of the fellowship, from associated university faculty and community practitioners.

30.3.6 Coalition Building

Partnerships of interests both within and between areas are encouraged, consistent with the IPP's goal of increasing the ability of tribes to prevent injuries within their communities (IHS, 2002e). Building tribal infrastructure remains a priority of the program, and courses designed to teach principles and practices of partnership (e.g., procurement, governance, and evaluation) are offered frequently. Coalition building with other like-minded agencies is another matter entirely, and the IPP relies very heavily on interagency cooperation. It holds, for example, a long-term agreement with the NHTSA to fund traffic safety initiatives and has an officer stationed permanently at the CDC, the US Fire Administration funds its smoke detector programs, and the National Head Start program is a partner on other safety efforts. This resource sharing is critical as while tribes have a legal relationship with the federal government, there is no mandate dedicating any resources of individual States to tribes, so AI/AN are categorically excluded from claims on any resources that are administered at the state level (Dellapenna, personal communication, October 10, 2002). Thus, partnerships with other agencies represent not only a way of maximizing what little funding is there, but it also means accessing some of the State resources that are shared by other agencies.

30.3.7 Steering

A monthly conference call is made between leading representatives of the 12 areas, program headquarters in Rockland, and partner organizations. During these calls, participants discuss ongoing strategies (both mutual and Independent), report on progress, advise one another on obstacles, arrange for future operations, and so on. These individuals are also responsible for collecting feedback on training and other programs that occur in their area. The input of their "frontline" workers such as public health nurses and educators is particularly important as they have the greatest community exposure and so act as an essential conduit between the providers, recipients, and beneficiaries of ongoing programs. However, it is worth noting that the access numbers and passwords for these conference calls are publicly available through the IPP website, making participation ostensibly open to any interested person, not only those formally associated with the IHS or other agencies.

30.3.8 Tribal Steering Committee

Steering participants may also include members of a unique body, the IHSIPP Tribal Steering Committee (TSC) for injury prevention. tribal representation, and governance are essential concerns in the design and implementation of training courses and other IPP initiatives, particularly because of the varied cultural factors that need to be taken into consideration when working with the many different ethnic tribes and nations for whose health the IHS is responsible. The TSC's objectives include the following:

- On a national level, to raise awareness of, and support for, injury prevention activities in Native American and AN Communities
- To enhance the ability of tribes to address injury prevention problems in their communities
- To provide advice and guidance to the IPP of the IHS
- To gather area-specific information on injury problems and activities
- To advocate for adequate funding of IPPs in Native American Communities (IHS, 2017)

The core duties of these members involve the following:

- Working with tribes: Generating a list of injury prevention contacts for their respective area, maintaining contact with these people to obtain feedback on programs and provide information about program activities and opportunities, and providing minutes of TSC meetings to all contacts.
- Working with IHS area injury specialists: Meeting at least quarterly to review local budgets, discuss feedback from tribal contacts, identify training and funding opportunities for tribal programs and review Area evaluations, participate in generating the area's annual budget to increase injury prevention funding, and advocate based on the recommendations made by tribal leaders.
- Participating on regional and national participation: Take part in TSC conference calls, attend TSC national meetings, and respond to TSC communications. Committee members must be tribal employees or community members, but not IHS employees, and are required to have completed at least one course or gained 2 years working experience, in injury prevention. Additionally, to serve as TSC members, they are required to apply with a letter stating their injury prevention interests and qualifications and letters of reference from an Injury Prevention Specialist and a tribal official (IHS, 2001).
- To serve as an advocate and liaison with national partners.
- To enhance the capacity of tribes to address and fund IPPs (IHS, 2017).

30.3.9 Accountability

As a federal body, the IHS is required under the 1982 Federal Managers' Financial Integrity Act to prepare an annual report and justification of expenditures and to make this document available to its stakeholders, the US Congress, and the general public (IHS, 1999). As an IHS function, the IPP provides its fiscal details toward preparation of this document. Similarly, the IPP conforms to the standards of the 1993 Government Performance and Results Act (GRPA), a rigorous protocol for establishing and evaluating performance measures to ensure quality and cost-effective initiatives in federal initiatives (Indian Health Service, 2002f). The GRPA requires that federal agencies demonstrate effective use of funding in meeting their missions. The law requires agencies to develop a 5-year strategic plan describing agency goals for their annual budget and to submit an annual performance plan, including specific performance measures with budget requests. The IHS has established a GRPA Coordinating Committee consisting of representatives from the service unit, area, and headquarters offices to guide the agency's annual performance plan development and implementation as well as annual performance reporting. The committee is coordinated through the IHS Planning and Evaluation Office (IHS, 2002f).

Additionally, the program is responsible to many of its partner organizations about activities related to their respective mandates and missions. The IHS and the NHTSA, for example, worked collaboratively since the early 1990s "to reduce the extraordinarily high injury and death rates associated with motor vehicle collisions among AI/AN people" (IHS, 2002c). The NHTSA has provided funding and technical support for numerous initiatives, and the IHS provides them with an annual report detailing that year's activities and progress in reducing the burden of motor vehicle injury and in building tribal prevention capacity. This phenomenon varies from year to year, but typically includes details of programs concerned with, for example, CPS, youth driver initiatives, and enforcement of driving-related

legislation. As part of the interagency agreement, the IPP is required to submit its own report and provides guidelines for its Area IP Specialists to give details of trainings, programs, conferences, studies, legislation, and other relevant professional activities (IHS, n.d.-a.

30.4   Outcome

A useful initial point to be made regarding the impact of the IHSIPP is that the value of spending years building an infrastructure to train skilled injury prevention professionals with relevant and practical strategies, create new and innovative injury control programs, and support these with rigorous study and evaluation probably cannot be overestimated. An important part of this infrastructure is the fostering of what might be called a culture of exemplary practice and evaluation, reflected in the design, management, and refinement of new and ongoing projects and studies. In keeping with this culture, it is useful to distinguish between outcomes in terms, on the one hand, of projects delivered and, on the other, the evaluated impact of these.

30.4.1 Fellowship Projects

Many individual initiatives in addition to those mentioned in this profile have been launched under the auspices of, or in collaboration with, the IPP Injury Prevention Fellowship and its graduates. While these are too numerous to list here, a very small sample of efforts includes (by title) the following:

- Alcohol legislation and its effect on severe injuries on the North Slope Borough
- An evaluation of an injury prevention project: The Whiteriver Service Unit Child Passenger Restraint Distribution Program
- Assessment of possible detrimental effects of improved highway access through the Alamo Navajo Reservation
- An evaluation of personal floatation device used within interior Alaska

- Reducing motor vehicle crashes on the Crow Reservation
- Rehabilitation of traumatic brain injury
- The evaluation to establish a comprehensive and linked injury surveillance system on the Blackfeet Reservation
- Increasing child car seat usage with home visits
- Implementation and evaluation of a bicycle helmet program at Ysleta del Sur Pueblo

This selection of fellowship projects showcases a range of initiatives including or combining educational, legislative, and environmental strategies to reduce injury. Far more have been conducted and evaluated, and while not all have been equally successful, many have yielded improvement in injury and fatality rates for their targeted populations. For example:

- In the Navajo seat-belt campaign, adult use of restraints rose to 80% (from an initial figure of 14%) by 1998, resulting in 45% decline in hospitalizations in the area. While the program was less successful for children, the increase from 7% to 30% does represent a more than fourfold improvement (Smith et al., 2000). In response, this effort fostered a collaboration between the IHS and National SAFEKIDS Campaign, the Navajo Office of Highway Safety, the Arizona and New Mexico Traffic Safety Bureaus and Governors' Highway Safety Programs, and the New Mexico Department of Health.
- The 1990 Alaska Floatcoat Program has met with steadily increasing success. In the first 2 years of the program, 16 individuals, each wearing one of the new PFDs during boating accidents, reported that the floatcoat had saved them from death or serious drowning-related injury. Moreover, this program was implemented in other communities throughout the 1990s, and a 1998 survey of a 400 mile stretch of the Yukon River found that 90% of boaters were wearing floatcoats.
- Following a 1988 study that showed a pedestrian death rate more than 10 times the national average, funding was obtained to install street-

lights along a 1-mile section of roadway on the White Mountain Apache reservation in Arizona. A follow-up study found that this simple measure resulted in a 36% drop in pedestrian/vehicle collisions and no fatalities in the lit area. The intervention may have also had an unexpected protective effect, as the number of fatalities on surrounding roads also dropped 38% (Akin, 2000).

- A 1992 project found that helmet use among isolated Alaska snowmobile riders increased from virtually nil to statistical significance following an intervention that used community leaders to role-model safer behavior. A decrease in helmet use within the control group suggests that this positive effect was due to the intervention (Welch, 2000).

30.4.2 Internal Evaluations

Evaluations of both the introductory level and the fellowship training programs have been conducted by fellowship candidates. O'Connor (2000) conducted a study of Level 1 (introductory) practitioner courses given between 1992 and 1993. A questionnaire was used to assess what trainees had found most and least useful about the course and to determine whether they would recommend it to others. A total of 97% respondents said they would recommend the course, and 60.7% said they would strongly recommend it. Moreover, O'Connor's (2000) findings were used to advise on course and program development.

A similar evaluation of the IPSFP between 1987 and 1991 was conducted by Shepard (2000) in 1991–1992. Shepard (2000) surveyed all contemporary and former fellows, administering a 16-question instrument to the entire group, and additional 9 questions to program alumni for purposes of investigating what, if any, role the program had played in subsequent professional activities. The integral components of the IPSFP are its academic courses and field surveillance training, and fellows were asked to rate each of the various sessions in these categories on a scale of 1–5, with one being poor and five being excellent, among other more descriptive questions.

Highlights of Shepard's (2000) findings include a mean rating of 4.6 out of 5 for personal and professional satisfaction with the program, an average completion level of 88.8%, 52% of alumni reporting that positive action had been taken as a result of their own final projects (such as guardrails added, legislation introduced, school program funded, pedestrian walkway installed or law-enforcement education), and 37% stating that they had written papers or other reports on injury prevention, including peer-reviewed publications, following graduation.

30.4.3 External Evaluation

Separate long-term evaluations of IHS Injury Prevention activities were conducted by the Injury Prevention Research Center (IPRC) at the University of North Carolina (UNC). These qualitative evaluations have generated a "Stages of Development" assessment tool, which considers 12 criteria of the training programs, rank their level of development as basic, intermediate, or comprehensive, and make recommendations on the basis of these findings. The criteria are as follows:

- Mission/vision
- Resource allocation/Accounting
- Management support
- Staffing/roles and responsibilities
- Training
- Partnerships/collaboration
- Needs assessment/defined service population
- Surveillance data collection
- Injury program planning and implementation
- Marketing
- Evaluation/reporting
- Technical assistance/building tribal capacity (Dellapenna, n.d.)

These criteria, and the evaluations themselves, all represent generative collaborations between the IHS, IPRC, and UNC School of Public Health Department of Health Behavior and Health Education and are funded by the US Public Health Service and Indian Health Service. They are described as follows:

30.4.3.1 IHS Area IPP Evaluations

The overall goal of this evaluation was to assess each of IHS's Service Area IPPs across 12 evaluation components addressing organizational structure, training opportunities, intervention types, marketing and advocacy strategies, and tribal capacity building. Previous years (1997–2001) of this evaluation project have involved evaluating the Oklahoma City, Navajo, Phoenix, Alaska, Bemidji, California, and Albuquerque areas. From October 2001 to 2002, it involved the implementation of the evaluation strategy in three additional IHS areas (Tucson, Billings, and Nashville). Finally, in 2002–2003, it involved the evaluation of the Portland Area and the Great Plains Area, as well as providing overall recommendations, across all 12 IHS Areas, to IHS IPP Headquarters staff. Area Evaluation Reports resulting from the evaluation project document growth, including both the successes and challenges, involved in developing and implementing Area Office IPPs to reduce morbidity and mortality among Native Americans.

30.4.3.2 IHS Injury Prevention Training Program Evaluation

The project was designed to assess the Indian Health Service Injury Prevention Training Program, which included the following activities: (1) Documenting the history of the training program courses, (2) attending selected IHS IP training courses, (3) collecting, reviewing, and summarizing 1990–2000 training course documents, and (4) conducting and summarizing key informant interviews with course instructors and participants. Results of data collection were used with IHS staff to develop a Training Program Action Plan, which will be used as a strategic planning tool to incorporate revisions, modifications, or enhancements to the IHS Injury Prevention Training Program (short courses and fellowship program). This assessment helped to improve the quality of the training program and ensure the long-term success of the IHSIPP.

30.4.3.3 IHS Tribal Injury Prevention Grants Program Monitoring Project

The goal of this 5-year project (2001–2006) was to provide monitoring and training services to 25 tribes or tribal organizations participating in the Indian Health Service Tribal Injury Prevention Grants Program. Project staff conducted the following main activities: (1) develop and publish a project newsletter three times per year, (2) conduct quarterly grantee conference calls four times per year, (3) provide ongoing training and technical assistance, (4) develop and conduct an annual grantee training course, (5) conduct one site visit to each grantee per year, and (6) provide consultation and technical assistance to IHS staff. Completing these activities will enhance the capacity of funded tribes to plan, conduct, and evaluate community-based IPP activities. Under a separate contract, project staff assisted with the development and implementation of a Grant Program Coordinator's Start-Up workshop in February 2001 in Albuquerque, NM.

30.5 Conclusion

Impressive amounts of useful information about the IPP and all its ongoing projects as well as future plans are publicly available through its website at www.ihs.gov/injuryprevention/. Notably, these postings include minutes of previous steering conference calls and other governance matters. The program also generates videotapes and slide presentations, which are useful for training sessions. Due to the relative scarcity of programs of its kind, the IHS training model has attracted the attention of other educational programs and institutions with interests in Aboriginal education, infrastructure building and/or injury prevention and, therefore, is considered an exemplary program.

Acknowledgments The authors would like to express sincere appreciation to the key informants Alan Dellapenna of the Division of Environmental Health Services in Rockville, MD, USA—whose consultation made this project possible.

BRIO Model: Indian Health Service IPP

Group Served: AI and AN.

Goal: Raise the health status of AI and AN to the highest possible level by decreasing the incidence of severe injuries and death to the lowest possible level and increasing the ability of tribes to address their injury problems.

Background	Resources	Implementation	Outcome
AI/AN die due to accidental injury at a rate of two times that of other Americans Program emphasizes creation of innovative training opportunities for federal and tribal employees as part of a system of injury control in American Indian communities throughout the United States	Funding for the IHSIPP is channeled from the Federal Department of Health and Human Services through the Indian Health Service's annually allotted appropriation and is meted out through national, regional, and local offices	Courses and other training forums offered under the auspices of the program circulate throughout the United States The 151 Service Units of the IHS are divided into 12 geographical service areas Area offices employ IPP manager and other injury prevention staff A monthly conference call is made between leading representatives of the 12 areas.	Numerous individual fellowship programs launched as result of IHS IPP training A total of 88% satisfaction with program, 52% report positive action as result of training projects, 37% program participants report having written further articles on injury prevention Replication of efforts and models

Life Space Model: Indian Health Service IPP

Sociocultural: civilization/community	Interpersonal: primary and secondary relationships	Physical environments: where we live	Internal states: biochemical/genetic and means of coping
Directed toward unique AI/AN community's advocacy for prevention programs at regional and federal levels broad interaction with existing health, emergency, and prevention services development of curriculum and training to foster growth of prevention professionals in AI/AN communities, involvement of AI/AN communities through recruitment, and tribal steering committees	Program projects target parenting	Funded projects include safety device initiatives such as "floatcoats," child vehicle restraint use, and bike helmet use evaluation of highway access changes to safety	Empowerment of AI/AN natives to manage and ownership of own health and safety issues/initiatives

References

Akin, D. (2000). Effect of lighting on nighttime pedestrian collisions in the White Mountain Apache Reservation. In L. R. Berger (Ed.), *Indian Health Service Injury Prevention Specialists fellowship program: A compendium of project papers, 1987-1998* (pp. 41–44). Albuquerque, NM: IHS Environmental Health Support Center.

Bill, N., Buonviri, G., Bohan, P., & Garnanez, L. (1992). Topics in minority health: Safety-belt use and motor-vehicle-related injuries—Navajo Nation, 1988-1991. *Morbidity and Mortality Weekly Report, 41*(38), 705–708.

Cook, L. (2000). Evaluation of a child injury prevention program. In L. R. Berger (Ed.), *Indian Health Service Injury Prevention Specialists fellowship program: A compendium of project papers, 1987–1998* (pp. 185–188). Albuquerque, NM: IHS Environmental Health Support Center.

Dellapenna, A. (n.d.). *Overview: The Indian Health Service Injury Prevention Program*. Rockville, MD: Indian Health Service.

Indian Health Service. (1999). *Accountability report, Fiscal Year 1998*. Rockville, MD: Author.

Indian Health Service. (2000). *Trends in Indian health, 1998-1999*. Rockville, MD: Author.

Indian Health Service. (2001). *Seeking members and alternates for the National Tribal Steering Committee for Injury Prevention*. Rockville, MD: Author. Retrieved from https://www.ihs.gov/

Indian Health Service. (2002a). *10 Leading causes of injury death, American Indians and Alaskan Natives 1993-95*. Rockville, MD: Author. Retrieved from http://www.cdc.gov/ncipc/osp/indian/aiinjtbl.htm

Indian Health Service. (2002b). *Demographic and dental statistics section of regional differences in Indian health 2000-2001*. Rockville, MD: Author.

Indian Health Service. (2002c). *Fiscal year 2001 annual report: Interagency agreement DTNH22-XO5252—Indian Health Service and National Highway Traffic Safety Administration*. Rockville, MD: Author. Retrieved from http://www.ihs.gov/medicalprograms/injuryprevention/FY%202001%20NHTSA%20Report pdf

Indian Health Service. (2002d). *Government Performance and Results Act*. Rockville, MD: Author. Retrieved from http://www.ihs.gov/NonMedicalPrograms/PlanningEvaluation/pe-gpra.asp

Indian Health Service. (2002e). *IHS Injury Prevention Program. OEHE Orientation Course, January 29, 2002*. Rockville, MD: Author. Retrieved from http://www.ihs.gov/nonmedicalprograms/dehs/documents/orientation%5Finj%5Fprev%5Fv2.ppt

Indian Health Service. (2002f). *Indian Health Service FY 2003 performance plan, FY 2002 revised final performance plan and FY 2001 performance report. (Congressional justification submission)*. Rockville, MD: Author. Retrieved from http://www.ihs.gov/AdminMngrResources/Budget/index.htm

Indian Health Service. (2002g). *Injury prevention specialist fellowship program class of 2003 information packet*. Rockville, MD: Author. Retrieved from http://www.ihs.gov/medicalprograms/injuryprevention/2002%20IPF%20packet.pdf

Indian Health Service. (2015). *Indian Health Focus: Injuries 2015 Edition*. Rockville, MD: Author. Retrieved from https://www.ihs.gov/dps/includes/themes/newihstheme/display_objects/documents/Injuries2016Book508.pdf

Indian Health Service. (2017). *Injury Prevention Program*. Rockville, MD: Author. Retrieved from https://www.ihs.gov/injuryprevention/

Indian Health Service. (n.d.-a). *Indian Health Service report to the National Highway Traffic Safety Administration: Guidelines for Area IP Specialists*. Rockville, MD: Author. Retrieved from http://www.

ihs.gov/medicalprograms/injuryprevention/nhtsa%20
reporting%20guidelines.pdf

Indian Health Service. (n.d.-b). *Notice of availability of
funds for Native American research centers for health.
(Program Announcement).* Rockville, MD: Author.
Retrieved from http://www.ihs.gov/publicinfo/publi-
caffairs/pressreleases/pressrelease2000/researchprg-
mannounce2000.asp

Indian Health Service. (n.d.-c). *Tribal management grant
program: Announcement information.* Rockville, MD:
Author. Retrieved from http://www.ihs.gov/nonmedi-
calprograms/tmg/original%5Ffiles/announcement.
htm

O'Connor, M. B. (2000). In L. R. Berger (Ed.), *Evaluation
of the IHS injury prevention practitioner level 1 course*
(pp. 149–152). Albuquerque, NM: IHS Environmental
Health Support Center.

Rhoades, E. R. (1997). Reflections on a decade as the
director of the IHS. *The IHS Primary Care Provider,
22*(1), 1–4.

Robertson, L. S. (1986). Community injury control programs of the Indian Health Service: An early assessment. *Public Health Reports, 101,* 632–637.

Shepard, C. (2000). In L. R. Berger (Ed.), *Evaluation
of the IHS Injury Prevention Specialists Program,
1987-1991* (pp. 85–88). Albuquerque, NM: IHS
Environmental Health Support Center.

SMARTRISK. (1998). *The economic burden of unintentional injury.* Toronto, ON: Author.

Smith, R. J. (1988). IHS fellows program aimed at low-
ering injuries, deaths of American Indians, Alaska
Natives. *Public Health Reports, 103,* 1263–1269.

Smith, R. J., Dellapenna, A. J., & Berger, L. R. (2000).
Training injury control practitioners: The Indian
Health Service model. *The Future of Children--
Unintentional Injuries in Childhood, 10*(1), 175–188.

Wallace, L. J. D. (1997). Injuries and the ten leading
causes of death for Native Americans in the U.S.:
Opportunities for prevention. *The IHS Primary Care
Provider, 22*(9), 140–145.

Welch. (2000). Community leaders as role models to
promote helmet use in the Bristol Bay Area. In L. R.
Berger (Ed.), *Indian Health Service Injury Prevention
Specialists Fellowship Program: A Compendium of
Project Papers, 1987-1998* (pp. 93–96). Albuquerque,
NM: IHS Environmental Health Support Center.

ThinkFirst Foundation Canada: A National Brain and Spinal Cord Injury Program

Jelena Zolis

The ThinkFirst Foundation Canada: A National Brain and Spinal Cord Injury Program helps prevent brain, spinal cord, and other traumatic injuries through education, research, and advocacy. It aims to help kids realize the importance of making safe choices to lower their risk for injuries.

31.1 Background

ThinkFirst initially started as an American initiative to help prevent brain and spinal cord injuries in teenagers. In the United States, the ThinkFirst National Injury Prevention Foundation, formally known as the National Head and Spinal Cord Injury Prevention Program, was first implemented nationally in 1986. The American Association of Neurological Surgeons (AANS) and the Congress of Neurological Surgeons (CNS) directed two neurosurgeons, E. Fletcher Eyster, MD, of Pensacola, Florida, and Clark Watts, MD, of Columbia, Missouri, to develop a national injury prevention program based on their previous prevention efforts within their own communities (ThinkFirst Foundation Canada, n.d.).

The AANS and CNS initiated the development of the national program due to their frustration at not being able to cure or "fix" brain and spinal cord injured patients. These groups share the belief that prevention is the only cure and that neurosurgeons have a duty to try to prevent these traumatic injuries. Eyster and Watts saw the assignment from the two largest professional neurosurgical organizations as an opportunity to recruit other health professionals to undertake public education prevention efforts and to address public policy issues related to injury prevention.

Each locally established program was sponsored by a neurosurgeon committed to public education and injury prevention. The replicable program materials consisted of a youth-oriented program, reinforcement and public education program, and a program to influence public attitudes and legislative policy. ThinkFirst's initial program, ThinkFirst for Teens, was offered to middle and high school audiences to teach young people about personal vulnerability and risk taking. The tremendous response to the program throughout the country led to its institutionalization by the AANS and CNS. Their support was a statement of the national neurosurgical community's ongoing commitment to public health and injury prevention.

This program has had major influences on public policy initiatives and continues to expand to reach those most vulnerable to traumatic injuries. It offers research-validated, multilevel educational programs that have reached millions of young people nationally and internationally.

J. Zolis (✉)
Hamilton-Wentworth District School Board,
Hamilton, ON, Canada

ThinkFirst was eventually brought into Canada by the Canadian Neurosurgical Society in 1992 with the help of Dr. Charles Tator, who served as one of the initial board members for the American Division of ThinkFirst. ThinkFirst Canada has currently joined with Safe Communities Canada, SMARTRISK, and Safe Kids Canada to create Parachute, a national, charitable organization dedicated to preventing injury and saving lives (Parachute Canada, n.d.). Other countries that are involved in ThinkFirst include Algeria, Chile, Colombia, Guinea, Honduras, India, Italy, Jamaica, Jordan, Korea, Mexico, Nigeria, Peru, Qatar, Senegal, Singapore, and Taiwan (Parachute Canada, n.d.).

31.1.1 Goals and Objectives

ThinkFirst Foundation Canada, the National Brain and Spinal Cord Injury Program, targets children from Kindergarten to 12th grade living in Canada. It also focuses on children specifically engaged in sports including hockey, soccer, equestrian, among others. This nonprofit organization was established to prevent brain and spinal cord injuries in youth by providing school-based programming and general public education and awareness and initiating and creating brain friendly preventative public policy. It strives to promote safe behavior through educational materials while encouraging healthy policy. ThinkFirst conducts research in the causes of injury and on the effectiveness of the programs in order to develop new initiatives to reach communities with ThinkFirst prevention messages (ThinkFirst Foundation Canada, n.d.).

31.2 Resources

31.2.1 Primary Prevention Strategies

ThinkFirst Canada is organized as a network of chapters that attempt to reach children and teenagers through school-based programming. Initially starting with its successful release of a curriculum guide entitled ThinkFirst for Kids

(TFFK) for students from first to third grades in 1993, ThinkFirst Canada has continued to design and distribute comprehensive curricula across elementary and secondary levels in over 5000 Canadian schools since its original inception.

Students are exposed to the ThinkFirst message in a variety of ways; however, one of the most effective and influential method is through the use of multimedia and personal stories. ThinkFirst for Teens (TFFT), the subsequent guide after TFFK, is a high school program that was designed toward the interests and activities of teenagers while using multimedia presentations that are delivered in a classroom or as an assembly for all senior students. The program provides teenagers with an opportunity to meet a "real-life" hero who had survived a brain and/or spinal cord injury and who speaks candidly about their experiences. Together with a health professional, the students are invited to exchange meaningful dialogue about "thinking first" before engaging in any type of risky conduct. The videos shown in the TFFT program include personal stories and testimonies from other young adults and children who have also been affected by brain and spinal cord injury. Finally, students are given a chance to broaden and expand their own knowledge about brain and spinal cord injury prevention by engaging in the in-class activities and cross-curricular lessons provided by the ThinkFirst curriculum package. The TFFK was designed in a similar manner, keeping in mind the interests and developmental understandings characteristic of elementary-aged children.

The TFFK program in Canada was designed by a small team of ThinkFirst stakeholders including a group of teachers from the Greater Toronto Area (GTA), a former superintendent, and principal. The views and opinions of teachers, students, parents, and the ThinkFirst organization were all considered and implemented within this interdisciplinary team approach. The goal of creating a partnership between the ThinkFirst organization, teachers from several school boards across the GTA, and brain and spinal cord research and prevention was one of the main areas of focus for the team. Their initial goal was to create a better curriculum not only to serve the students but also to create a safer community.

The team interviewed several teachers and parents to make sure the needs of the students and fellow teachers who would be delivering the program within the classroom were met. Parents' and teachers' main concerns included the need to stress the importance of prevention education alongside the typical curriculum expectations. Parents were included in the pilot study and were given a chance to provide feedback after the children had completed the modules in class which included an at-home component where parents could help consolidate the prevention message. This partnership and concern helped create a responsible, useful, and sustainable curriculum for the children and the teachers using the ThinkFirst program.

31.2.2 Community Outreach

Community programs organized and implemented by local ThinkFirst chapters also have an impact on the scope and depth of prevention education that can help children make informed decisions. The following are some programs that have come about. Outreach projects have included the Give a Kid a Helmet campaign, which was launched in 2004 as a result of findings from research conducted by the ThinkFirst Foundation of Canada. It was estimated that each year, over 50,000 Canadian children riding bicycles, skateboards, scooters, and rollerblading would be involved in a crash that would require medical attention; a total of 100–130 of these children would die—mostly from devastating head injuries. By simply wearing a properly fitted helmet, over 50 deaths and 6000 injuries can be prevented (Parachute Canada, n.d.). Other community projects include the creation of a public service announcement (PSA) created by McLaren McCann regarding the need for children and youth to wear helmets when engaging in activities such as skateboarding, rollerblading, and bicycle riding. Finally, ThinkFirst has teamed up with junior teachers in the GTA as well as students and staff from the University of Toronto's Department of Neuroscience to develop a community program called Brain Day. This fun and interactive educational program targeted students from fourth to sixth grades that also meet parts of the language and science curriculum expectations. The students not only leave Brain Day with a greater understanding of the brain and nervous system but also absorb critical injury prevention messages that will last them a lifetime.

31.2.3 Funding

ThinkFirst operates as a nonprofit organization and therefore is always looking for new ways to initiate and generate funding. The foundation was originally started with money from the American and Canadian Neurosurgeons Society and continues to hold endorsements from both organizations. Currently, they are supported and sponsored by the TD Bank Financial Group, FedEx Express, Ontario Trillium Foundation, Great West Life, and many others that are listed on Parachute Canada's website. Each of the 24 chapters receives limited support from head office in Toronto; however, they are responsible for raising their own financial support through various fundraising initiatives (J. Russell, personal communication March 5, 2007). TD Bank Financial Group has been funding the revision and redevelopment of the in-school curriculum to ensure that ThinkFirst prevention programs meet the needs of students and fulfill provincial curriculum standards, thus making their program effective, sustainable, and accessible. Many of the sponsors, such as the Trillium Foundation, have been funding ThinkFirst for many years as they believe the value of the programs enhances its sustainability and provides important opportunities to change the lives of children and youth. Funding for ThinkFirst-SportSmart programs come from TD Waterhouse, Ontario Ministry of Tourism and Recreation, Canadian Ski Council, The Krembil Foundation, and many others to make certain that the SportSmart programs are available and accessible in both French and English versions. In 2007, ThinkFirst and Aviva Insurance teamed up to prevent brain and spinal cord injury. Aviva Canada Inc. is one of Canada's leading property and casualty insurance groups, making the partnership between ThinkFirst and Aviva a good match to spread the prevention message (J. Russell, personal communication, March 5, 2007). Aviva's role in the funding formula within the ThinkFirst Foundation is to help support local chapters and fund special events by providing financial support and volunteers at various community events across Canada.

31.3 Implementation

The comprehensive TFFK program is available for teachers to order in every school board across Canada. The curriculum is provided free of charge and is designed for grades K-6; it is neatly and conveniently packaged in a binder format. The K-8 curriculum is broken down into binders that include Kindergarten, first to third grade, fourth to sixth grades, and seventh to eighth grades. Each binder contains lesson plans, background material, and exercises needed for each module and are also made available on the Parachute Canada website. The lessons for each binder are also aligned with specific curriculum expectations for each province, therefore, making it extremely easy for teachers to integrate instruction into their existing program. Likewise, all visual and audio components for each lesson are included in the binder. The curriculum was initially created with teachers primarily from the Durham District School Board and then pilot tested in 50 classrooms. The data from these pilot tests suggest that the TFFK program resulted in a significant increase of knowledge regarding safe practices, especially in the area prevention of brain and spinal cord injury (Cusimano et al., 2000).

The curriculum's design allows it to be taught as one entire unit or integrated into class schedules according to teacher's discretion or preference. The nature of the lessons lets them easily be implemented and taught during health and physical education time within the school day. However, they also include small group tasks and brainstorming activities that could be part of various language arts activities when teachers and students discuss personal safety and making smart choices when engaging in physical activity. Furthermore, there is a musical component included with the primary TFFK program that consists of a CD with songs and jingles. These can be enjoyed and used to further teach and consolidate the smart choices taught within previous lessons by using a more interactive approach during music and drama lessons.

The only requirement is that the first lesson on the anatomy of the brain and spinal cord be taught prior to any of the safety lessons, in order to provide a rudimentary understanding of the need for safety practices. Lessons are also enhanced by the addition of experts or community resource personnel—the police or fire services, public health, and various medical personnel: doctors, nurses, paramedics, swimming instructors, and lifeguards. Each school has ties within the community with various departments and organizations, such as local public health and police services, whose staff support programs such as anti-bullying and bus safety. The ThinkFirst program is therefore a well-designed addition to safety and prevention education, which is already being promoted across schools in Canada. The more involved the community, the stronger the message and subsequently, the greater the long-term benefit to all (ThinkFirst Foundation Canada, n.d.).

The TFFK curriculum is designed to challenge and alter children's cognition, development, and behavior by increasing children's knowledge of risk and injury in a variety of contexts. Exposure to these messages over time and throughout each grade will ultimately impact their ability to make better choices and avoid injury (e.g., wearing a helmet). Some of the areas covered in the TFFK modules include the brain and spinal cord anatomy; vehicular, bicycle, and playground safety; violence and conflict resolution; as well as water safety.

TFFT is a program that was created to reach teens within the school system. The program begins with a curriculum that follows the TFFK program and is available for seventh and eighth grades. There are also wide-ranging presentations that can be delivered to children in this age group and children in ninth to 12th grade. These presentations occur in an assembly or large-group format and target risky behavior in a safe manner through role-playing and a video presentation entitled Dangerous Games. The program contains several reinforcement activities that provide an extension of the concepts introduced during the assembly or group presentation. These lessons address specific curriculum expectations and include cross-curricular activities that can be used as part of science, social studies, language arts, and visual arts classes. Students are exposed to modules such as Shaken baby syndrome (SBS) and other information on hazardous materials; the information in these modules will be useful to them as they complete high school and begin to take on part time jobs, volunteering, and babysitting positions. These modules are topics that can already be found within the seventh and eighth grade Health and Science curriculum in Ontario. Using the hands-on lessons provided within the ThinkFirst module allows teachers to plan more in-depth lessons where they can connect these topics to other areas of the curriculum including Drama and Language Arts, where students are given the opportunity to discuss the repercussions of neglecting safety rules in these situations and the value of prevention education. Moreover, students are encouraged to make educated choices about unsafe behaviors through the TFFT program, as it serves as the first step in educating and preventing brain and spinal cord injury. The program components include user-friendly lesson plans and class games to review concepts; a short film entitled Dangerous Games produced and filmed in Canada that addresses risky behavior and its consequences, including testimonials from teens with brain and spinal cord injuries; anatomy of brain and spinal cord and how injuries occur; and ways on preventing brain or spinal cord injuries as a bystander.

31.3.1 Other Curriculum Developments

ThinkFirst Canada has also taken on several different initiatives, such as developing a Smart Hockey video and the Playing Smart Soccer program as part of their SportSmart division to reach children beyond the scope of the classroom. Programs have been targeted to educate and inform children and teens within the recreational and competitive sport arenas in order to provide even more children with the necessary knowledge and information about preventing brain and spinal cord injury on the field, snow, and ice. Two recent community sports-based programs include The Smart Equestrian DVD and A Little Respect, a new DVD to educate youth on the risks in skiing and snowboarding. SportSmart became its own division of ThinkFirst Canada in 1992, with the goal to create prevention programs and conduct research in sports and recreational activities. The SportSmart division was renamed the ThinkFirst-SportSmart Sports and Recreational Injuries Research and Prevention Centre (TF-SS) in 2003. The videos are available free of charge to coaches, teachers, and parents who would like to promote the prevention message. ThinkFirst has teamed up with several amateur organizations that use the videos as part of their safety lessons, including hockey leagues across Ontario and Equestrian clubs. Moreover, ThinkFirst has an advisory board with representatives from sports organizations, industry, public bodies, and research professionals as board members (ThinkFirstSportSmart Manual, 2006).

They have also continued to revise and update the existing school-based curriculum to meet the needs of individual provincial curriculum standards set out by the Ministry of Education. ThinkFirst's commitment to educate children, teens, and families about the risks of spinal cord and brain injury is growing and continues to evolve (J. Russell, personal communication, March 5, 2007).

31.3.2 Effective Practices

There are many components to the ThinkFirst Foundation that make it an effective, sustainable prevention program. Each aspect of the curriculum or community sports programs has been centered on the prevention of the brain and spinal cord injury through education and awareness.

Each one of the programs has been assessed and integrated to meet the needs of the community it serves and contains all necessary resources to deliver the program. Each program had a working advisory committee comprised of key informants and professionals that have expertise in the specific area. Moreover, the foundation has kept existing partnerships with organizations such as the Durham District School Board, Ministry of Education, Public Health, the Canadian Congress of Neurological Sciences, and the Canadian Association of Neuroscience Nurses. All members that are involved with the research, design, implementation, and delivery of the various programs have been trained and receive support from ThinkFirst local chapters and head office. Each local chapter organizes several in-service training sessions for all staff and their involvement with extended learning opportunities available for children, teens, parents, and other community members through local sponsorship such as the "Community Helmet Fitting" campaign. ThinkFirst's involvement with the community along with their in-school programming is an integral part to the sustainability and delivery of their message to prevent brain and spinal cord injury.

Ongoing research by Michael Cusimano and colleagues suggests that ThinkFirst programs are not only effective but are also highly appreciated by teachers and educators within the school system: 85% of teachers in Ontario rated the TFFK and TFFT program as very good to excellent (Cusimano, Li, et al., 2005). Moreover, the implementation and delivery of the programs are also important. TFFT uses testimonies and an interactive presentation style with young adults to get the message across, in addition to having teachers or other adult's model and instruct healthy behaviors.

31.3.3 Sustainable Assessment and Evaluation

Each local chapter is connected and involved with the programs at the provincial and national levels. The ThinkFirst head office in Toronto coordinates monthly conferences, weekly emails, and the annual general meeting to discuss and update each local chapter with current activities, information, and funding figures. Each program has an advisory board that meets to discuss how to improve and keep ThinkFirst programs effective and sustainable. Members of each program are in place to review curricula, discuss necessary updates, and review evaluation and research examinations.

Committee members include chapter directors, board members, and national office staff (J. Russell, personal communication, March 5, 2007). Decision making occurs at the local, provincial, and national levels with an emphasis on collaboration and communication of needs between each level in order to meet the needs of each chapter and reach as many children as possible. ThinkFirstSportSmart also has its own advisory committee that was developed to ensure that the programs being developed are current and meeting the needs of children and families engaged in sports and recreational activities. The members of the various advisory committees ensure that the ThinkFirst message of prevention is heard throughout the community, whether it is within school-based programs or community events.

31.3.4 Sustainability and Injury Prevention

Shediac-Rizkallah and Bone (1998) have identified several important categories or indicators of sustainable community-based programs. They include (1) maintenance of health benefits achieved through an initial program, (2) level of institutionalization of a program within an organization, and (3) measures of capacity building in the recipient community. More importantly, the community must be involved in the process if sustainable change is to occur. It is suggested that community participation enhances ownership and leads to increased competence and program maintenance (Bracht & Kingsbury, 1990; Flynn, 1995).

In the area of project design and implementation, ThinkFirst has demonstrated its effectiveness through the numerous evaluations that have been conducted by Dr. Cusimano and other researchers. The curriculum started off as a copy of the American version; however, with help from community partners, such as the Durham District School Board, health professionals, and corporate funding, ThinkFirst's in-school program has grown and met the needs of each province and effectively educates students about brain and spinal cord injury. Moreover, ThinkFirst has established many financial partnerships and sources of funding including the Trillium Foundation and TD Canada Trust, which have been with ThinkFirst for many years and have shown their continual belief, respect and support for ThinkFirst programs. Likewise, in terms of program duration, the programs not only have grown but also have initiated several transformations, which include the development and expansion of the ThinkFirstSportSmart programs and research center.

Within the organizational setting of ThinkFirst, its nonprofit design has done a fantastic job reaching children, youth, and families by engaging the public. Making programs for students of all ages and adapting to the needs of each community are keys to the sustainability of ThinkFirst. Additionally, ThinkFirst's support from local school boards and organizations such as the Canadian Neurosurgical Society along with partnership with community members such as neuroscience nurses and teachers are critical. Inviting guest speakers from the community is a powerful and valuable way to educate and inform children about the dangers and impact that brain and spinal cord injury can have on their lives. Finally, ThinkFirst empowers children and families, regardless of socioeconomic status and geographical location, to prevent injury through fun programs such as the helmet campaign and running informative public service announcements.

31.3.5 Dissemination

Research, information, and data are disseminated using a variety of methods including the ThinkFirst website, the Parachute Canada website, newsletters, and many articles published in a variety of neuroscience journals (J. Russell, personal communication, March 5, 2007). Many of the ongoing research projects coordinated and run by Dr. Michael Cusimano and other colleges are also available online.

31.4 Outcome

There have been many changes to the ThinkFirst program and curriculum since its inception in Canada. Researchers in Canada and the United States have conducted many scientific evaluations of TFFK, TFFT, and ThinkFirstSportsSmart programs. Neurologist and researcher, Dr. Michael Cusimano, was part of a three-phase study to test the efficacy of the TFFK curriculum in elementary schools. In the initial phase, Dr. Cusimano and colleagues (Cusimano, Dang, et al., 2005; Cusimano, Li, et al., 2005) conducted an early evaluation of the TFFK curriculum for the first to third grades. It was found that after assessing 584 active students within 25 classrooms, the children showed a significant improvement in knowledge in comparison to the control group (Cusimano et al., 2000). The control group consisted of 596 monitored students over 27 classrooms. Questionnaires were administered to teachers and parents in both active and control schools to assess the degree to which the program objectives were implemented.

The improvement of unsafe decision making did not improve overall according to student self-reports at that time. The researchers concluded that individual choice to engage in risky behavior is influenced by many changing variables including peers, social situations, and individual choice. The only clear message in the report was that information could potentially lead to some students thinking before acting and therefore avoiding unnecessary injury due to their increase in knowledge and understanding of consequences. It is not to be assumed that prevention education causes all students to make safer choices; however, it is clear from the data within this study that safety and prevention education for children is only one of the puzzle pieces in determining how to reduce brain and spinal cord injury. Unsafe decision making did not improve overall according to students' self-reports; however, TFFK delivered at an early age does increase awareness and knowledge and will perhaps influence decision making in the future.

A second phase of the initial study mentioned above was conducted in 2000 (Cusimano, Li, et al., 2005). Questionnaires were administered to 870 students in five schools and served as the pretest for phase 2 of the study (Cusimano, Li, et al., 2005). The questionnaire included sections about the brain and spinal cord injury before the delivery of the TFFK curriculum. Results suggested that there was no change in bike helmet use, although 95% of the students reported having access to a bike helmet (Cusimano, Li, et al., 2005). Phase 3 results showed that over the 6-week period, children in the schools with lower socioeconomic status showed a huge improvement in helmet use and a wealth of knowledge gained in the prevention of brain and spinal cord injury (Cusimano, Li, et al., 2005). The study concluded that awareness and knowledge did increase over the 3 years of the primary curriculum and that the greatest gain in knowledge occurred in the first year (Cusimano, Li, et al., 2005).

Dr. Marni Wesner from the University of Alberta conducted another evaluation study. Dr. Wesner's study aimed to identify youth behavior with regard to injury prevention and to evaluate the impact of the ThinkFirst curriculum delivered in Saskatchewan school programs, which are comparable to the TFFT program in Ontario. The membership of ThinkFirst Saskatchewan is a small but dedicated group of health professionals and brain and spinal cord injury speakers. The ThinkFirst educators used the catch phrase "use your head to protect your body" in order to encourage all school children in the Saskatchewan area to engage in safe behaviors and take any necessary protective precautions (Wesner, 2003). A controlled pre- and posttest design including a self-report questionnaire was used and administered to 1257 sixth and seventh grade students (Wesner, 2003). The participants were from 25 different classes and in 15 different schools

across Regina, Saskatchewan (Wesner, 2003). All schools with scheduled visits from the ThinkFirst team were included in the study. The control group was comprised of 20 classes, demographically matched for age, grade, and SES from both the public and separate schools in the Regina area. Participation was voluntary and anonymous.

This study reported a significant increase in the reported use of protective sporting equipment following the ThinkFirst school visit. The study did not demonstrate a change in risk-taking behavior between male and female respondents; however, potentially dangerous situations may have been altered with the increased use of protective gear. Further, the ThinkFirst program has been shown to develop safer behavior and awareness rather than attempting to alter preexisting practices. Wesner suggested that although it may be difficult to change each student's future behavior by providing exposure and information about safety gear such as helmets and safer choices while engaged in physical activity, students will develop an increased awareness and therefore may chose a safer option (Wesner, 2003).

31.4.1 Community Participation and Feedback

While the quality of the curriculum is valuable and important to the development of a sustainable and effective program, feedback from both deliverers and recipients of the program is also critical in the sustainability of the curriculum. ThinkFirst Foundation Canada is continually seeking reactions from the school community and health professionals who work in partnership with ThinkFirst. Each project such as the TFFK, TFFT, or the ThinkFirstSportsSmart programs has individual teams who gather valuable information from teachers, students, research evaluations, and community health professionals in order to review and update the program each year. These task forces take the values, suggestions, and feedback from each local chapter and reassess the curriculum and its complementary presentation components to meet the needs of each community and each province's curricular standards. It also provides community members across the country with an opportunity to discuss and feel connected to the decisions made at the head office (J. Russell personal communication, March 5, 2007).

ThinkFirst has also made a commitment to integrate beliefs and evaluation from teachers. Since classroom teachers mainly deliver the in-school ThinkFirst program, it is imperative that they value and adopt the ThinkFirst prevention message. Dr. Cusimano, Dang, et al. (2005) conducted a study to examine teachers' perspectives of the effectiveness of the ThinkFirst curriculum from first to third grades. Teachers from both intervention and control groups were asked to complete a questionnaire at the end of each school year. The questionnaire was designed to collect information on observations and perspectives of teachers on many aspects of teaching injury prevention, including the amount of time spent teaching safety lessons, changes in students' daily behavior, and the effect of participation on safety perspectives.

A total of 964 teachers, 399 from the control group and 565 from the intervention group, returned completed questionnaires (Cusimano, Li, et al., 2005). Of these, 461 (48%) reported observing changes in student behavior. Change in student behavior was observed after 1 year of program implementation (Cusimano, Li, et al., 2005). The biggest difference was observed between giving no education (20%) and teaching TFFK lessons for 1 year (66%; Cusimano, Li, et al., 2005). There was very minimal change in student behavior from 1 to 3 years of program implementation. Possible reasons for the 46% increase in changed behavior from zero years of program implementation to 1 year may be the increased awareness of safety issues, increased discussion, and integration of knowledge from the classroom and home settings (Cusimano, Li, et al., 2005). Finally, the presence of teacher turnover and a decrease in the response rate in the third year was cited as possible factors in the limited change observed in the third year of the program (Cusimano, Li, et al., 2005).

31.5 Conclusion

Providing valuable prevention education for children and teens is ThinkFirst's primary mission. With meticulous support and continued research, ThinkFirst Canada not only has made an impact in children's lives and their safety but also has influenced the research community behind brain and spinal cord prevention research.

Unintentional injuries are a major public health problem. As of 2006 in Canada alone, injury was the leading cause of death and disability for Canadians under the age of 45 (Canadian Institute for Health Information [CIHI], 2006). The costs associated with these injuries is estimated at $13.2 billion (CIHI, 2006). Ontario, the largest province in Canada, accounts for about one-third of these injuries (Cusimano, Li, et al., 2005). Therefore, a commitment to ensure that ThinkFirst remains sustainable and includes developing new research projects to further the field of injury prevention and continuing to build the ThinkFirst curriculum.

The impact of ThinkFirst programs, community involvement, corporate sponsorship, and the school-based curriculum is leaving a mark on the brain and spinal cord prevention field. The commitment to reach children and families through a variety of contexts has made the ThinkFirst name a sustainable, reliable, and effective stakeholder in the primary prevention field. While there are many programs that offer a school-based approach, few organizations have grown and developed into a multifaceted prevention program such as ThinkFirst. Their integrative approach to health and the prevention of brain and spinal cord injury within sports, in addition to community efforts to implement educational pursuits, has helped to define how a sustainable program should operate. This outline and examination of ThinkFirst can be used as a foundation and provide information to help make every prevention program exemplary and sustainable.

Acknowledgments The authors would like to express sincere appreciation to the key informants for this case study—Jim Russell of Think First in Toronto, ON, Canada; Charles Tator of the University of Toronto in ON, Canada; Michael Cusimano of St Michael's Hospital in Toronto, ON, Canada—whose consultation made this project possible.

BRIO Model: ThinkFirst Foundation Canada: A National Brain and Spinal Cord Injury Program (Curriculum Manual TD ThinkFirst for Kids 2006a, 2006b, 2006c, 2006d)

Group Served: The ThinkFirst Foundation Canada is a nonprofit organization established to prevent brain and spinal cord injuries in children and youth.

Goal: Their mission is to provide school-based programming, general public education and awareness, and initiate and create brain friendly and preventative public policy.

Background	Resources	Implementation	Outcome
In 2003–2004, within Canada, there were 16,811 hospital admissions for traumatic head injury representing 9% of all trauma admissions for that year, equating to 46 admissions every day in Canada for a traumatic head injury (CIHI, 2006). Children and youth (0–19) were the most highly represented in admissions (30%) ThinkFirst began as an American initiative to help prevent brain and spinal cord injuries for teens. In the US ThinkFirst National Injury Prevention Foundation, formally the National Head and Spinal Cord Injury Prevention Program, was created nationally in 1986. ThinkFirst Canada began in 1992	Curriculum resources include binders from JK–8 with activities, DVDs, and music CDs to engage students in prevention of brain and spinal cord injury. Community members are encouraged to be guest speakers, especially children and youth who have brain and spinal cord injury. Curriculum was created with the help of teachers to ensure that curriculum expectations were being met while providing effective lessons on brain and spinal cord injury Financial resources come from various sponsors. Local chapters receive a set amount of money for program delivery but are encouraged to engage in fundraising to increase their budget	The TFFK curriculum is designed to challenge and alter children's cognition, development, and behavior. Some of the areas covered in the TFFK modules include the following: – Brain and spinal cord anatomy – Vehicular, bicycle, and playground safety – Violence and conflict resolution – Water safety The SportSmart division was renamed the ThinkFirst-SportSmart Sports and Recreational Injuries Research and Prevention Centre (TF-SS) in 2003	Neurologist and researcher Dr. Michael Cusimano conducted an evaluation of the TFFK curriculum for first to third grade and found that children showed a significant improvement in knowledge in comparison to the control group The curriculum has been updated and modified according to the past data collected from teachers and research evaluations Prevention programs have extended and continued to grow and with several community initiatives

Life Space Model: ThinkFirst Foundation Canada: A National Brain and Spinal Cord Injury Program (Curriculum Manual TD ThinkFirst for Kids 2006a, 2006b, 2006c, 2006d)

Sociocultural: civilization/community	Interpersonal: primary and secondary relationships	Physical environments: where we live	Internal states: biochemical/genetic and means of coping
ThinkFirst programs use a multidisciplinary approach by targeting children, youth, and families through in-school education programs, community initiatives, and sports-related programs to reach the largest variety of children and youth Partnerships with other corporate and community members such as TD Bank Financial, Canadian Soccer Association, Ontario Ministry of Tourism and Recreation, Woodbine Entertainment, Aviva Canada, Durham District School Board	The program emphasizes prevention and empowers students to use their brain in order to make a smart choice about any activity Engaging students by using programs that integrate students interests and needs and meeting the prevention message through the use of interactive lessons (DVD, CDs, music) and having real children who have a brain or spinal cord injury talking to the students during classroom and assemblies	ThinkFirst programs extend beyond the classroom and have integrated the community through programs that focus on sport and recreational activities to disseminate the prevention message	ThinkFirst has made changes to ensure that all community members have access to their programs Children, youth, and families are empowered to make healthy, smart decisions to ensure that they have fun while keeping their brain and body safe

References

Bracht, N., & Kingsbury, L. (1990). Community organization principles in health promotion: A five-stage model. In N. Bracht (Ed.), *Health promotion at the community level.* Newbury Park, CA: Sage.

Canadian Institute for Health Information. (2006). *Head injuries in Canada: A decade of change 1994-1995, 2003-2004.* Ottawa, ON: Author.

Curriculum Manual TD ThinkFirst for Kids. (2006a). *Discoverers grades 1, 2, 3.* Naperville, IL: ThinkFirst.

Curriculum Manual TD ThinkFirst for Kids. (2006b). *Explorers grades 4, 5, 6.* Naperville, IL: ThinkFirst.

Curriculum Manual TD ThinkFirst for Kids. (2006c). *Kindergarten Wonders.* Naperville, IL: ThinkFirst.

Curriculum Manual TD ThinkFirst for Kids. (2006d). *Navigators grades 7, 8.* Naperville, IL: ThinkFirst.

Cusimano, M., Dang, M., Bekele, T., Atkinson, J., Hsu, H., Puust, L., et al. (2005). Knowledge translation in communities: Community readiness for injury prevention programming. *Injury Prevention Research Office, St. Michael's Hospital, Toronto, Ontario.*

Cusimano, M., Li, K., Atkinson, J., Bekele, T., Hsu, H., Kalnins, I., et al. (2005). Injury prevention education improves student injury-related behaviours: Feedback from Teachers Implementing ThinkFirst For Kids.

Injury Prevention Research Office, St. Michael's Hospital, Toronto, Ontario.

Cusimano, M., Sharman, A., Coulthard, R., Chipman, M., Freedman, B., & Tator, C. (2000). Injury prevention in the community: An evaluation of the ThinkFirst for kids program. *The Canadian Journal of Neurological Sciences, 27*(2), S22.

Flynn, B. S. (1995). Measuring community leaders' perceived ownership of health education programs: Initial tests of reliability and validity. *Health Education Research, 10,* 27–36.

Parachute Canada. (n.d.). *ThinkFirst Canada.* Toronto, ON: Author. Retrieved from http://www.parachute-canada.org/thinkfirstcanada

Shediac-Rizkallah, M. C., & Bone L. R. (1998). Planning for the sustainability of community-based health programs: Conceptual frameworks and future directions for research, practice and policy. *Health Education Research, 13*(1), 87–108.

ThinkFirst Foundation Canada. (n.d.). *Home.* Retrieved from www.thinkfirst.ca

ThinkFirstSportSmart Manual. (2006). *SportSmart.* Naperville, IL: ThinkFirst. Retrieved from www.thinkfirst.ca

Wesner, M. (2003). An evaluation of ThinkFirst Saskatchewan: A head and spinal cord injury prevention program. *Canadian Journal of Public Health, 94*(2), 115–119.

UCLA-Labor Occupational Safety Program: Youth Project

32

Stephanie Van Egmond

The UCLA-Labor Occupational Safety Program: Youth Project developed a curriculum to educate young people about the hazards they may encounter within the workplace in order to reduce the number of incidences of occupational health and safety hazards for youth.

32.1 Background

The Youth Project that was run out of the University of California at Los Angeles (UCLA) Labor Occupational Safety and Health Program (LOSH) provides an example of an outstanding educational prevention program targeted at Latino/a youth in South-Central Los Angeles (SCLA). UCLA-LOSH was founded in 1978, upon receiving a Federal Occupational Safety and Health (OSHA) New Directions in Worker Training planning grant. Since that time UCLA-LOSH has become a nationally recognized center in Southern California that provides Spanish and English worker training, educational material development, technical assistance, and policy information in workplace health and safety. LOSH works toward its mission of researching and providing education and training in order to improve environmental and safety conditions for workers by collaborating with workers, unions, community-based organizations, and health professionals (UCLA-LOSH, 2002).

In accordance with its mission, LOSH heads projects that focus on hazardous waste workers, immigrant workers, and working teens. A grant report tells that from 1987 to 2002, LOSH was a lead agency of the five-member California–Arizona Consortium, funded by the National Institute for Environmental Health Sciences (NIEHS), to educate workers and communities about the potential health effects of hazardous waste exposure. The immigrant worker project, VOICES from the Plant Floor, involves investigation of workers' perceptions of occupational safety and health in occupations where there is a high concentration of immigrant workers. This project involves documenting workers' experiences, insights, and ideas with the intent of informing policy and interventions that will protect workers' safety and health (UCLA-LOSH, 2002).

32.1.1 The Youth Project: History and Development

The Youth Project (alternately called the Young Worker Project) that ran out of LOSH is exemplary in executing a targeted, developmentally/culturally appropriate, holistic, and community-based educational primary prevention program. The project is collaborative in that it involves a

S. Van Egmond (✉)
Toronto District School Board, Toronto, ON, Canada
e-mail: stephanie.vanegmond@tdsb.on.ca

© Springer Nature Switzerland AG 2020
R. Volpe (ed.), *Casebook of Traumatic Injury Prevention*,
https://doi.org/10.1007/978-3-030-27419-1_32

partnership between a university, schools, and the community. The collaborative nature of this project has lent itself to the development and implementation of a primary prevention program that is both systematic and supported by academic research and flexible and responsive to the specific needs of the target population. Another aspect of its effectiveness is that the project was designed to meet the developmental needs of adolescents with methods that are culturally appropriate with Latino/a populations. The result is a multilevel approach to occupational injury prevention that has resulted in behavioral and environmental changes in the SCLA area.

The Youth Project is targeted toward Latino/a youth in the SCLA area in Southern California. While the primary recipients of the program are high school students, a main goal of the project is to also reach the parents and the wider community through these students. By training and empowering the youth to become health and safety advocates and conduits of information in their communities, this project reaches a much wider population than the youth involved. It is important to note that, historically, a focus on occupational safety for Latino/a youth is warranted in the United States because this group of young workers is especially vulnerable to fatal and severe injuries and has higher rates of employment in hazardous industries such as construction and agriculture (Greenhouse, 2002).

The LOSH Youth Project started in 1996 with a grant from the National Institute for Occupational Safety and Health (NIOSH). NIOSH is part of the Centers for Disease Control and Prevention within the Public Health Service of the US Department of Health and Human Services. Initial funding was provided to three community-based health education projects on young worker issues. The projects were located in three separate sites: Brockton, Massachusetts (Massachusetts Department of Public Health and Education Development Center, Inc.), Oakland, California (University of California at Berkeley Labor Occupational Health Program), and Los Angeles California (Labor Occupational Health and Safety Program) (National Institute for

Occupational Safety and Health [NIOSH], 1999). The projects worked for 3 years (1996–1999) in three different communities, to raise the awareness of young worker issues at the community level. The results of these projects were published by NIOSH in 1999 in a how-to resource guide entitled Promoting Safe work for Young Workers: A Community-Based Approach (http://www.cdc.gov/niosh/99-141.html).

The pilot education project at UCLA-LOSH, initially funded through 3 years from NIOSH, evolved from a partnership between Jefferson High School (JHS), a community-based organization called Concerned Citizens of SCLA (CCSCLA), and the UCLA-LOSH Program. The school and community of Jefferson were selected because they met the target population selection criteria and because the teachers expressed a desire to strengthen school-community links. Early grant proposals and reports reveal that the initial selection criteria were to target populations who had demographic diversity, who also had a socioeconomic need, and where there was the existence of willing community-based organizations that could help to ensure the long-term sustainability of the project (LOSH, 1998).

The relationship between LOSH and the pilot school was nurtured by the eagerness of the teachers at JHS. Moreover, JHS in the Los Angeles Unified School District (LAUSD) is described as a school with a student population of approximately 3400, of which almost 90% are Latino/a and many are recent immigrants to the United States (LOSH, 1998). Both the school and the CCSCLA were already active in the community, and LOSH had collaborated with both organizations on other projects. Thus, the collaborative base for the project was previously established so that focus on integrating the NIOSH-funded work-related curriculum into the LAUSD began immediately.

32.1.2 Professional Affiliations

The Youth Project was affiliated with numerous professional and academic bodies that focus on young worker issues. Two such associations are the National Young Worker Safety and Health Network and the California Partnership for Young Workers Health and Safety. The National Young Worker Safety and Health Network was comprised of researchers, educators, public health professionals, medical specialists, pediatricians, governmental representatives, and others who have, as a common goal, the safety of youth in the workplace. It was founded at the 1996 American Public Health Association's Annual Meeting in New York City and meets annually at that conference, quarterly via telephone conference calls, and on an as-needed basis through a list serve where members would share ideas and resources concerning policy, emerging issues, research, curriculum development, etc. (LOSH, 2002).

The Youth Project was also an active member of the California Partnership for Young Workers' Health and Safety which consists of representatives from governmental agencies, educational institutions, state parent organizations, and other state-wide organizations that are involved with California youth employment and education issues. The group has also been active in sponsoring legislation to improve the state youth work permit system. In 1999, this group was successful in having the governor declare the month of May as the Safe Jobs for Youth (SJFY) Month (LOSH, 2002).

32.1.3 Project Goals

Early grant reports reveal that the overall goals at the outset of the Youth Project were as follows:

1. Understand and describe the work experience of inner-city students in a predominately Mexican immigrant, Korean, and African-American community, where they work, whether they get required work permits, the extent of their exposure to safety and health hazards including stressors such as sexual harassment and the requirement to work too many hours.
2. Integrate curriculum and peer education (PE)/youth leadership program into the schools to educate students about hazards, rights and

responsibilities, and resources and how they can get support to speak up about problems.
3. Reach the broader Spanish-speaking community about workplace health and safety through an educated student population (LOSH, 1998).

Subsequent project reports show that general goals remained consistent throughout the duration of the project with one shift in target population. The original goals show that the project would be aimed at Latino/a, Korean, and African-American students/communities. However, as the project evolved, the focus narrowed to Latino/a youth. Factors that influenced this shift include demographics of the SCLA population (predominately Latino/a), the existence of receptive community-based support, and the responsiveness of the Latino/a community. In addition, the Korean community support agencies were already overcommitted to other projects (L. Delp, personal communication, September 10, 2002).

Over time the scope of the project expanded to include an agenda of environmental health issues in addition to workplace health and safety. Broadening the scope of health and safety issues covered by the Youth Project was in part influenced by funding opportunities available through the California Endowment (L. Kominski, personal communication, August 15, 2002). At the same time, issues of environmental hazards in SCLA posed a significant threat to the community, and its inclusion in the project was warranted and contributed to its overall effectiveness as a health and safety promotion program. In a grant report detailing project activity from 1998 to 2002, broadened project objectives were stated as follows:

- To sustain and significantly expand the university, school, and community collaboration between UCLA-LOSH, CCSCLA, and Jefferson and Fremont High Schools, to fully mobilize available/diverse resources, and to address environmental justice issues in SCLA
- To strengthen the knowledge and skills of students and teachers regarding both workplace and community health hazards and their rights

- To strengthen community organizing and analytical skills of students and to provide leadership opportunities to exercise these skills by developing PE outreach programs and community-based internships
- To strengthen the environmental justice organizing capabilities of CCSCLA and other organizations by developing youth leaders who work within those organizations and who link with other youth environmental leaders in the community
- To document this effort in a variety of ways so it can serve as a model for other school/community agency/university collaborations to enhance community efforts in achieving improved environmental health (LOSH, 2002)

32.1.4 Prevention Model and Methods

32.1.4.1 Empowerment Education Model

This education intervention model is based on the principles of empowerment education. The empowerment education model assumes that prevention efforts must go "beyond the prevailing emphasis on individual behavior change. The threats to occupational and environmental health necessitate a broader approach—one that combines both individual and community empowerment to enhance the health of all residents in a community" (Delp, 2002). The empowerment education approach stresses that participants must use health and safety information to improve their own lives as they analyze the socioeconomic factors that contribute to the problem. From the perspective of this model, health and safety issues are not seen as purely technical issues (LOSH, 1999). The key elements of this model are based on the principles of the listening/dialogue/action model set forth by educator and founder of empowerment education, Paulo Freire. Three critical assumptions of this model are as follows:

1. Education starts from the participants' own experiences. These experiences must include the opportunity for the youth to discuss their collective knowledge and experiences about the problem.
2. Empowerment education must include dialogue to build critical consciousness, i.e., the ability to analyze the root causes of social problems.
3. Education programs must build skills, confidence, and opportunities for individual and collective action (Delp, 2002).

The basic principles of empowerment education guided the general development of this prevention project. An early grant report provides elaboration upon the basic assumptions of empowerment education in the context of the Youth Project as follows:

1. Increased knowledge is a necessary but not sufficient first step to reducing hazards. Students must also have the opportunity to apply information about hazard identification and control to current or potential jobs, to develop confidence and effective communication skills, and to practice speaking up constructively about problems.
2. Social support is an important step in dealing with and resolving workplace problems. Students generally work in nonunion jobs so they cannot rely on union representation if they face problems at work. The curricula are designed to reinforce the importance of talking to coworkers for support to minimize the concern that they will be singled out and fired for raising health and safety issues. This intervention is also designed with the long-term goal of developing an ongoing social support network for young workers within the school and community rather than simply implementing a one-time curriculum unit.
3. Students not only benefit from the existence of a social support network but also help create that network. Peer educators can educate other students and the community through formal presentations and can provide resources and support through informal support networks such as their relationships with friends and family members (LOSH, 1999).

32.1.4.2 PE Methods

The method of PE is a fundamental component of this educational prevention design. It was noted in early grant proposals that teen PE was chosen as a method because it had proven to be effective in raising awareness of other health issues in LA such as AIDS prevention (LOSH, 1998). It was also believed that peer education would build youth leadership skills in the population. By focusing on creating youth leaders, it was hoped that a sustainable knowledge base and community infrastructure would be created. Thus, the prevention effort aimed at affecting long-term behavioral and environmental changes within the target community. Furthermore, peer education methods and youth leadership training address the specific developmental needs of adolescents who rely on their peers as sources of support and identity formation.

The principles of PE as an effective prevention tool are outlined as follows:

- Young people who become peer educators will have integrated health and safety into their consciousness and will enter the workplace with advocacy and organizing skills in addition to knowledge about their rights as workers.
- By targeting Latino/a youth, this emerging immigrant culture will have trained and skilled advocates within their communities to serve as resources and leaders.
- Some peer educators will be inspired to become teachers, health professionals, government inspectors, or community organizers and will carry their knowledge of health and safety issues into their careers (LOSH, 1999).

32.2 Resources

LOSH employs a multiethnic, bilingual staff of ten and (in 2002) had an annual operating budget of approximately $500,000. Of these ten staff, four were employed to work exclusively with the Youth Project, and four LOSH staff were former students of the Youth Project (L. Kominski, personal communication, October 17, 2002). LOSH

is part of UCLA, and the office space is provided for by the university (LOSH, 1998). The operating costs of each LOSH project were funded mainly through external grants. Table 32.1 provides approximations of year-by-year costs and funding sources from the outset of the Young Workers Project until 2002.

The Youth Project was established out of a collaborative base comprised of UCLA-LOSH, Concerned Citizens of SCLA, and JHS. Through outreach efforts, media coverage, and networking between community organizations and project participants, the base of collaboration and support grew to include two more LAUSD high schools, numerous community organizations, students/youths and their parents, elected officials, health professionals, teachers, community members, national and state funding organizations, and evaluation professionals. The participating teachers and schools worked together with LOSH to develop, implement, and evaluate the educational intervention. Community organizations provided internship opportunities for students and advisory support regarding project development, implementation, and evaluation. Elected officials became involved in publicizing May as Safe Work for Youth Month. A private research group conducted project evaluation in the form of focus groups with student interns and surveys of teachers and community-based organizations. NIOSH and a private foundation, California Endowment, provided funding for the project through a series of grants.

The collaborative base grew over time. As was already stated, the project grew to include implementation of the curriculum in two additional schools. LOSH provided numerous in-service teacher-training sessions to facilitate this endeavor. As students became peer educators and interns, community forums were held to inform community members of worker rights and environmental justice issues.

Over time the school-based curriculum was developed and refined with input from students and teachers. The scope of the project expanded its original focus on teen worker health and safety to include a broader concept of health and safety that included environmental health. This flexibility in

Table 32.1 Annual costs and funding for Young Workers Project

Year	Funding sources	Salaries/wages	Goods/services	Evaluation	Total
1996/1997	CA DIR/CHSWC[a] NIOSH/CDC[b]	$63,200	$47,800		$111,000
1997/1998	NIOSH/CDC	$79,200	$74,300		$153,500
1998/1999	California Endowment NIOSH/CDC	$112,500	$167,250	$32,700	$312,450
1999/2000	California Endowment NIOSH/CDC	$211,000	$240,600	$6500	$458,100
2000/2001	California Endowment NIOSH/CDC CA DIR/CHSWC	$181,000	$167,600	$34,800	$383,400
2001/2002	California Endowment NIOSH/CDCCA DIR/CHSWC Sales Contracts Donations	$84,000	$38,800		$122,800
Total		$730,900	$736,350	$74,000	$1,541,250

Note: The categories under which costs are categorized are somewhat arbitrary and have been created for presenting this case. They do not reflect the actual complexity of the Young Workers Project budget breakdown of expenditures
[a]California Department of Industrial Relations' Commission on Health and Safety and Workers' Compensation
[b]National Institute for Occupational Safety and Health of the Centers for Disease Control and Prevention

project goals was a reflection of its commitment to meeting the expressed needs of the target population.

32.3 Implementation

Rather than develop an educational intervention based on a specific injury type, body part, or industry, the LOSH Youth Project takes a community health education approach to promoting workplace health and safety. This approach focuses on empowering youth to protect their workplace rights, to advocate for change, and to act as sources of health and safety information to their families, schools/peers, workplaces, and communities. Early grant proposals show that implementation was planned according to the Community Health Promotion Model created by Bracht and Kingsbury (LOSH, 1998).

32.3.1 Pilot Phase

The initial education curriculum was developed through a joint effort with JHS teachers. It was decided to create a curriculum unit targeted at

ninth grade students who were required to take an education and career planning course. The teachers noted that the curriculum they were using was out of date and not interesting to the students. Based on the needs articulated by the teachers, a 10-h curriculum unit, SJFY, was developed. This unit includes information about how to identify hazards in your workplace, child labor laws, sexual harassment, and workers' compensation. The unit was developed according to the empowerment education model and is participatory in that it engages students with case studies, videos, and role-play activities to help them identify risks and practice speaking-up on the job (NIOSH, 1999).

In addition to collaborating with teachers, LOSH conducted a needs assessment of the target student population. A questionnaire, developed by the University of North Carolina and implemented by LOSH, was given to a random sample of 296 students at JHS during their English classes (Delp, Runyan, Brown, Bowling, & Jahan, 2002). The purpose of the questionnaire was to ascertain the level of student knowledge regarding Young Worker rights, including knowledge of the work permit process in California and workplace health and safety regulatory/advocacy organizations. Subsequently, focus groups were conducted with the youth to learn more about the responses given in the surveys. The information gleaned was used to aid in the development of the curriculum. Results were also used to gain insight into the state work permit process. The results of this research were published (see Delp et al., 2002).

Moreover, an advisory board and steering committee were established to inform and guide the development of the project. The project was directed by the steering committee, which consisted of representatives from each partner organization. A 15-member advisory board, which represented the larger community of students, parents, teachers, government agencies, labor unions, youth groups, and other community-based organizations, also provided guidance. The steering committee met regularly to make decisions about project planning and implementation and to direct the evaluation of its progress. Once the original project goals were met and the curricula were completed, Youth Project at LOSH staff assumed the primary decision-making role, although outside input remains solicited (LOSH, 2002). The Community Advisory Board met biannually (from June 1998 to February 2001) to guide and advise the project. Advisory Board members helped develop and implement the community and media outreach plan; kept the project informed of community involvement opportunities; were directly involved in project activities such as teaching, sponsoring internships, and developing written material; and participated in the evaluation and assessment of the project, including strategic planning for the future (LOSH, 2002).

Prior to the implementation of the SJFY curriculum, four workshops were held as an after-school program, sponsored by a Jefferson social studies teacher, to inform youth about the following:

1. Health and safety on the job
2. Sexual harassment at work
3. Wage and hour provisions under the state child labor law
4. Workers' compensation provisions

The Youth Project reported that most of the youth who initially volunteered for the project had a negative job experience and wanted to know about their workplace rights (LOSH, 2002). This preliminary group of students met weekly and learned about workplace health and safety issues. Then, they participated in a two-session, train-the-trainer, PE class. Next, with support from their teachers and LOSH staff, these youth went to various classrooms and community meetings as peer educators to teach what they had learned to wider audiences in the school and outside community.

32.3.2 Curriculum Development

With a second grant from a private foundation, the California Endowment, the project expanded into regular JHS classrooms and into two additional partner schools: Fremont High School and Manual Arts High School (LOSH, 2002). The ten-session SJFY curriculum had been developed to teach ninth grade students about teen worker rights. Half-day in-service teacher workshops on the curriculum were conducted by LOSH using the exercises contained in the unit. During the period from April to June 2000, SJFY was implemented in 14 Life Skills for the twenty-first century courses (a mandatory 20-week course for all ninth grade students) and reached 250 students at JHS. The SJFY curriculum replaced the earlier education and career planning section that the teachers felt was outdated. Those who used the curriculum were Life Skills teachers, work experience educators, and others who had participated in workshops (LOSH, 2002).

With the California Endowment funds, a semester-long (16 weeks) curriculum was also created for 11th and 12th grade students. A broader focus on environmental safety was incorporated into the project through this curriculum. The resulting Healthy Communities, Healthy Jobs (HC, HJ) curriculum included opportunities for youth to participate in community internships. The youth also received training and experience to become peer educators. This curriculum strived to foster youth leadership within the community, build self-esteem, and believe in their ability to make a difference. Leadership skills were built through hands-on activities, in-class projects, and PE training. In addition, an option was available for students to be involved with a community internship in collaborating community organizations or labor unions. During the internships, students were involved in projects that helped them to develop research, organization, and leadership skills. These were paid internships, and, in some cases, students also received academic credit for their participation.

The same Jefferson teacher who had piloted the after-school program was key to this aspect of the project's success as he agreed to pilot the semester-long curriculum as an elective (LOSH, 2002). An evaluation that included administering written questionnaires to the students and teachers and student focus groups was conducted both prior to participation in the class and upon completion of the class. The curriculum was revised based upon the feedback from the students and the teacher. From 1998 to 2001, the HC, HJ curriculum was implemented at JHS, reaching a total of 57 students (LOSH, 2002). In addition, in 2000, it was implemented in one class at Fremont High School and one class at Manual Arts High School (LOSH, 2002).

32.3.3 Curriculum Description

The semester-long HC, HJ curriculum contains five sections (see below). The introduction to the unit contains five sessions. Students are familiarized with such concepts as environmental justice, workplace health and safety, PE, and the power of collective action. The next unit, HC, focuses on environmental health issues, including air, water, and soil pollution and the health benefits of clean environment. The next unit, SJFY (10 sessions), focuses on workplace health and safety for youth. The following unit, PE (15 sessions), teaches students how to become peer educators and how to educate their families and communities about occupational health and safety information. The last unit contains two sessions

offering activities that provide students an opportunity to summarize and reflect on what they have learned and plan their next steps for doing more work in this area (LOSH, 2002).

32.3.3.1 Curriculum Outline
1. Introduction to healthy communities (HC), healthy jobs (HJ)
   - Using case studies as learning tools
   - Five sessions
2. Healthy communities (HC)
   - Researching and addressing community environmental health concerns
   - Five sessions
3. SJFY
   - Child labor history and laws, identifying and solving hazards in the workplace, resolving problems on the job
   - Ten sessions
4. PE
   - How to Work as a Team; How to Develop Lesson Plans; How to Make Presentations; How to Teach Health and Safety using a Popular Education Approach
   - 15 sessions
5. Conclusion—Healthy Communities, Healthy Jobs: REFLECTIONS and NEXT STEPS for Making a Difference!
   - Ways to Get Involved in Community Health Issues; Evaluation
   - Two sessions

In 2001, the Youth Project's emphasis changed from the previous 5 years pilot phase to expansion. Additional units of the HC, HJ curriculum were added, and the targeted schools and the number of involved community organizations increased. As each curriculum unit was completed, it was made available free of charge for download from the UCLA-LOSH website (www.losh.ucla.edu) or for purchase, at cost, from UCLA-LOSH. During this time, Youth Project staff conducted extensive outreach that included in-service workshops for teachers interested in implementing all or part of the curriculum. In some of the workshops, the teachers could receive a continuing education credit (LOSH, 2002).

32.3.4 Evaluation Methods

Evaluation was an ongoing part of the LOSH Youth Project. Initial methods included the needs assessment in 1996, observations, as well as surveys and focus groups with students, teachers, and interns. LOSH staff, teachers, a UCLA technical assistance group, and a private research group implemented evaluations. The following is a list of historically used methods for evaluating the process and outcome of project activities:

1. Pre- and postworkshop quizzes as well as focus groups for both teachers and students to assess knowledge gained about the topics covered in the trainings (immediate outcome evaluation).
2. Posttraining evaluations from participants regarding their assessment of the training workshops in order to make them more effective (process evaluation).
3. Surveys and interviews of teachers/case managers who attended the workshops to determine who will incorporate the units into their classes, what factors influenced their decisions, and how they plan to teach the units. Those planning to teach the units will be encouraged to contact the Youth Project for any technical assistance they need while teaching the curriculum (process evaluation).
4. Interviews of teachers who have taught classes using the Youth Project curriculum, soliciting their experiences in teaching the curriculum units in the classroom, their opinion of the effectiveness of the curriculum, and recommendations for improving LOSH training methods and/or curriculum content (outcome evaluation).
5. Interviews of teachers who have not implemented any of the curriculum units focusing on their reasons so that a plan for overcoming barriers can be developed for future funding plans (Outcome Evaluation) (LOSH, 2002).

32.3.4.1 Methodological Advantages and Limitations

The primarily school-based nature of this project has advantages and limitations. Implementing prevention programs through schools carries the advantage of reaching potentially large numbers of youth either before they start working or early in their careers. Thus, the advantage of school-based prevention initiatives is that they can reach target populations at the pre-event stage. At the same time, students who drop out of school are missed by such school-based efforts. This scenario is of particular concern with respect to the Latin American population in the United States, as they have a higher dropout rate than other populations (Delp, 2002). Furthermore, mass implementation of the HC, HJ curriculum was impeded due to political and funding issues faced by public schools in California (L. Kominski, personal communication, October 17, 2002).

To address these limitations, the Youth Project began to collaborate with community-based youth training programs outside of schools to assure these youths were informed of their health and safety rights. From May to June 2002, the Youth Project staff conducted five half-day workshops under an agreement with the UCLA Office of the Instructional Development's Community-Based Learning Program. The workshops were presented to Workforce Investment Act Youth Program case managers and UCLA community workers. Under the agreement to train up to 150 individuals, the SJFY curriculum was modified, and a three-session mini-unit for community-based programs was printed. Each participant received a curriculum and video. The sessions were held at the community agencies: Bresee Foundation, Watts Labor Community Action Center, Youth Opportunities, San Fernando Gardens, and Los Angeles Urban League.

One missing component of this project is a connection with employers. Employers are major stakeholders in preventing occupational injuries and legally responsible for providing safe and healthy workplaces. As such, they should be involved in creating/participating in prevention programs. However, it is unclear as to whether it is possible to negotiate the often-conflicting interests of employers and employees into one program. It is also doubtful that the project would have been as free as it had been to empower youth to advocate for their rights had employers been involved as partners. Perhaps a compromise would be to include exemplary employers of youth as partners in order to bring all the required stakeholders together and extend the reach of the project.

Programs such as the LOSH Youth Project are multidimensional in that they link research-based, school-based, and community-based initiatives. Furthermore, they aim to affect change at the level of individuals, communities, and systems—creating a comprehensive approach to occupational health and safety and being able to generate multiple and relevant solutions. One such inherent asset of this design is in providing youth with important health and safety information coupled with developing leadership skills. Such flexibility is an intrinsic strength of multiagency, multidimensional prevention programs over single-focus, single-agency programs.

32.4 Outcome

The LOSH Youth Project sought long-term, sustainable change by empowering the youth to become leaders in their communities. It was designed to be a comprehensive educational program that would create a change in consciousness and behavior to be carried forth throughout the participants' life.

I think our successes were based on our recognition of the unique needs of our immigrant community, and we tailored our work to those needs. For example, the role the students played in the project turned out to be very different from what we expected. Initially, we had planned to reach teens by involving parents in the project. However, in our community, where so many of the parents are not proficient in English and know very little about their own legal rights at the workplace, it went otherwise. The teens ended up educating the parents. In fact, the teens became a very valuable liaison between the project and the entire community, and in the process, they developed their own knowledge, leadership, and communication skills (as cited by NIOSH, 1999, p. 5).

The Youth Project proved successful in reaching its initial project goals of understanding the work experience of Latino/a youth, integrating curriculum into some classes in the LAUSD, and reaching the broader Spanish-speaking community. The LOSH Youth Project was also successful in creating a sustainable community-based prevention infrastructure in numerous ways.

As of 2017, UCLA-LOSH continues to prioritize the education of young workers (UCLA-LOSH, n.d.-a). They now lead a program called Young Worker Leadership Academy in place of their original Youth Project (UCLA-LOSH, n.d.-b). The Young Worker Leadership Academy program is associated with Young Workers (see http://youngworkers.org) and the Young Workers Project run by the University of California, at Berkley Labor Occupational Health Program. These projects continue to work with a variety of community, educational, and government organizations (Regents of the University of California, n.d.). For more information, visit the Young Workers website (http://youngworkers.org/).

32.4.1 Systemic Changes

The full curriculum was adopted and instituted in classes in three schools in the SCLA area and was tried in numerous other schools. During the period from April to June 2000, the SJFY curriculum was implemented in 14 Los Angeles School District schools. Implementation of this portion of the curriculum was most successful in terms of reaching a wider student body. The semester long HC, HJ curriculum section was implemented at JHS where 57 students participated. In addition, in the year 2000, two additional schools offered this course where it reached an additional 36 students (LOSH, 2002). Also, 30 HC, HJ students who had taken the class were hired with community-based organizations as interns (L. Kominski, personal communication, October 17, 2002).

The response to the curriculum and internship programs was positive on the part of teachers and career/work counselors. A growing number of teachers have received in-service training, thereby creating a knowledgeable resource base within the LAUSD. Between 1999 and 2001, a total of 294 LAUSD teachers and career counselors received training in the use and implementation of the curriculum. The SJFY portion of the curriculum was adopted on a larger scale as it was integrated into a mandatory Life Skills course required for all LAUSD ninth grade students (LOSH, 2002).

In addition to training teachers, LOSH staff and interns were successful in offering workshops and community forums to other professional and community stakeholders. For example, health and safety workshops were conducted through two Latino/a community-based organizations, thereby reaching workers outside the reach of the school system. Between 2001 and 2002, professional development training on the SJFY curriculum was offered to approximately 200 professionals associated with youth employment through various agencies (LOSH, 2002). LOSH has conducted research on the effectiveness of the State's Work Permit system and provided these results.

32.4.2 Changes in Consciousness

A comparison of pre-/posttests and follow-up focus group discussions shows a significant increase in students' awareness of their rights and of resource organizations concerned with workplace safety (Delp, 2002). Pre- and posttests were given in 13 ninth grade classes (Delp, 2002). These SJFY students showed significant increases in knowledge gains in the posttest compared to pretest knowledge (Delp, 2002). They also reported that they had gained a sense of confidence because of knowing their workplace rights (Delp, 2002).

The students who were exposed to the semester-long HC, HJ show similar knowledge gains and report being motivated to act in their communities (Delp, 2002). Furthermore, focus group results with these students report that they have developed critical consciousness of workplace hazards as they relate to the greater sociopolitical context (Delp, 2002). In the empowerment education model, this step is necessary for social change/action to occur (Delp, 2002).

32.4.3 Behavioral Changes

The project was successful in that there was an increase in youth involvement in the SCLA community. The development of skills through PE training and the hands-on experience provided through internships resulted in students developing advocacy skills, confidence, and motivation to act as leaders in their community. Thus, the project was successful in facilitating behavioral changes in youth in the SCLA community.

In addition to increased community involvement, students reported that they act as sources of information regarding workplace safety and workers' rights in both their communities and families. Interviews with 35 students showed that these students gave information to 500 community members outside of the 300 students that they reached through PE programs in schools (Delp, 2002).

Finally, during follow-up telephone interviews, intern students reported that their behavior at work had changed. Students reported that they now request safety training and equipment, are aware of workplace hazards, speak to their supervisors about them, know their rights, refuse to work late or too many hours, and have reported injuries, and several students report quitting their jobs because of unsafe work conditions (N. Morales, personal communication, August 17, 2002).

32.4.4 Community Impact

The program goal of empowering youth to act as agents of social change was met, and this phenomenon resulted in direct impact on the SCLA community. Three examples of such changes are as follows: (a) Interns helped create a coalition of youth organizations that advocated for legal, educational, and environmental issues impacting youth. (b) Interns organized to get the Labor Commission to prosecute an employer who violated child labor laws. (c) Students organized to pressure the government to clean up contaminated soil at a middle school and testified in the state capital in support of legislation to prevent building schools on contaminated land (Delp, 2002).

Several of the actions taken by students received regional and national media attention. Articles were published in The Los Angeles Times and Time Magazine. The project was adopted outside of SCLA, thereby broadening its regional impact. The SJFY curriculum was adopted in Dade County, Florida, as part of the after-school migrant workers education program, showing that it is relevant and replicable with student populations outside Los Angeles. In April 2001, UCLA-LOSH gave a presentation about the Youth Project to a community-based organization (Community Voices) in Miami, Florida. As a result, they implemented the curriculum in Homestead, Florida, a very poor farming area with high numbers of Spanish-speaking immigrant workers. One year later, Community Voices piloted the curriculum in the Miami-Dade Migrant Education Program's after-school program at two high schools and two middle schools, reaching a total of 110 youth aged 12–19. The director of the County Migrant Education Program was impressed with the pilot and consequently advocated for it to be included as one of ten themes to be mandated in the Migrant Education Program throughout the State of Florida. It was adopted in five schools (LOSH, 2002).

32.5 Conclusion

The problem of young worker injury, illness, and fatality is complex. The LOSH Youth Project acknowledges that Young Workers injuries are influenced by the broader sociopolitical context. Furthermore, the project recognizes the specific social conditions faced by the Latino/a community in the SCLA district. Their response was to develop a project that sought to empower marginalized youth so that they cannot only prevent injuries but also fully understand their social circumstances and recognize their power to change them. Thus, rather than using an injury-/industry-specific approach, UCLA-LOSH developed a systemic prevention program that targeted change at the individual, community, and societal levels.

In combining the expertise of UCLA, schools, and community organizations, the UCLA-LOSH Youth Project facilitated the development of a primary prevention program that was research-based, responsive to the needs of its target group, and could reach the wider population. By basing the project on prior research about PE and the role of youth in Latino/a communities, LOSH developed a culturally and developmentally appropriate model. This academic professionalism also ensured that the project was developed, implemented, and evaluated systematically and ethically. By conducting ongoing evaluation, a curriculum was developed that was responsive to the needs of the target group. The expertise of LOSH staff in occupational health and safety provided the basis for the development of effective and well-informed prevention measures.

By utilizing the existing infrastructure of schools and community organizations, the curriculum was easily disseminated to the target population. Thus, by integrating the prevention measure into already-existing systems, access barriers were avoided. For example, by using the youth as sources of information within their home communities, language and cultural barriers that potentially exist with prevention programs that rely on outside professionals were avoided. In this project, it became evident that the wider Latin American community trusted the youth from their own communities. This trust resulted in people getting relevant assistance because they divulged more specific information about their individual occupational circumstances—for example, not having legal working papers—without the fear of reprisal (N. Morales, personal communication, August 17, 2002). Lastly, training youth to become leaders in their community carries an element of sustainability to the prevention model in that dependency on outside experts can be decreased over time as the community and schools take on increased responsibility for information dissemination.

UCLA-LOSH's Youth Project provides an example of the preventive potential contained within collaborative partnerships. By bringing together stakeholders, LOSH served to contribute to a sustainable infrastructure that served to support the target community. By empowering the youth to become major stakeholders, the project had a built-in mechanism for longevity. Involved youth were equipped with information and skills that empowered them to advocate for workplace rights for themselves and others. This empowerment education, community-partnership prevention model equipped students to assess the hazards at their workplace and to stand up for their rights. The LOSH Youth Project contributed to the creation of a safety conscious, proactive workforce at the beginning of their careers, and, thus, the potential to change work environments and behaviors throughout their lives.

Acknowledgments The author would like to express sincere appreciation to the key informant for this case study—Laurie Kominski of the University of California, Los Angeles in the USA—whose consultation made this project possible.

BRIO Model: UCLA Labor and Occupational Health and Safety Youth Project

Group Served: Youth aged 13–17, especially targets Latino/a youth.

Goal: To reduce incidence of occupational health and safety hazards for youth.

Background	Resources	Implementation	Outcome
Collaborative project that involves a partnership between a university, schools, and the community Main goal of the project is to reach the parents and the wider community through these students Education intervention model is based on the principles of empowerment education PE is a fundamental component of this educational prevention design	LOSH employs a multiethnic, bilingual staff of ten and has an annual operating budget of approximately $500,000	Initial pilot of curriculum material for ninth grade students SJFY curriculum included in life skills classes in three schools Semester-long Healthy Communities, Healthy Jobs curriculum developed	The full curriculum was adopted and instituted in classes in three schools in the SCLA area and was tried in numerous other schools Significant increase in students' awareness of their rights and of resource organizations concerned with workplace safety Students have reported that they act as sources of information regarding workplace safety and workers' rights in both their communities and families

Life Space Model: UCLA Labor and Occupational Health and Safety Youth Project

Sociocultural: civilization/ community	Interpersonal: primary and secondary relationships	Physical environments: where we live	Internal states: biochemical/ genetic and means of coping
Development of high school curriculum on workplace safety Involvement of schools and teachers in project goals and delivery	Change how young employee responds to employer in terms of health and safety issues	Make explicit the right of having a safe work setting	Empowerment of youth to become health and safety advocates

References

Delp, L. (2002). *Fostering youth leadership to address workplace and community environmental health issues: A university/school/community partnership.* Unpublished manuscript.

Delp, L., Runyan, C. W., Brown, M., Bowling, M., & Jahan, A. S. (2002). Role of work permits in teen workers' experiences. *American Journal of Industrial Medicine, 41,* 477–482.

Greenhouse, S. (2002). Government asked to act on teenagers' job safety. *The New York Times,* A8.

National Institute for Occupational Safety and Health. (1999). *Promoting safe work for young workers: A community-based approach (DHHS-NIOSH Publication No. 99-141).* Cincinnati, OH: Author.

Regents of the University of California. (n.d.). *Young workers leadership academy.* Oakland, CA: Author. Retrieved January 3, 2018, from http://www.young-workers.org/ywacademy/ywacademy html

UCLA Labor Occupational Safety and Health (UCLA-LOSH) Program. (1998). *Young worker health and education project: Los Angeles county [NIOSH grant proposal for 9/30/98-9/29/99].* Los Angeles, CA: Author.

UCLA Labor Occupational Safety and Health (UCLA-LOSH) Program. (1999). *Intervention effectiveness: 1999-01 (NIOSH grant proposal for program announcement 99150).* Los Angeles CA: Author.

UCLA Labor Occupational Safety and Health (UCLA-LOSH) Program. (2002). *Final grant report submitted to the California endowment (Grant # 97-540).* Los Angeles, CA: Author.

UCLA Labor Occupational Safety and Health (UCLA-LOSH) Program. (n.d.-a). *Implementing health and safety classes for youth: "How-to" guide.* Los Angeles, CA: Author.

UCLA Labor Occupational Safety and Health (UCLA-LOSH) Program. (n.d.-b). *Young worker leadership academy.* Los Angeles, CA· Author. Retrieved January 3, 2018, from http://losh.ucla.edu/young-worker-leadership-academy/

MORE^OB: Managing Obstetric Risk Efficiently: A Program for Patient Safety and High Reliability in Obstetrics

Helen Looker

The Managing Obstetric Risk Efficiently (MORE^OB) program is a comprehensive performance improvement program that creates a culture of patient safety in obstetrical units. This program integrates professional practice standards and guidelines with current and evolving safety concepts, principles, and tools with the goal of promoting effective communication and teamwork to reduce the traditional hierarchy in obstetrical units (MORE^OB, n.d.).

33.1 Background

Dr. Kenneth Milne designed this national Canadian program and has led its development and growth from early plans to the expansion into the United States. After nearly 30 years of clinical practice in obstetrics and gynecology, Milne had observed a number of significant events and practices in obstetric care which needed to be addressed to lift the burden of adverse events on all concerned and place patient safety as the central priority and a responsibility shared by accountable members of the obstetric teams within hospitals (K. Milne, personal communication, May 22, 2007). Milne had an abiding interest in education and wanted a program that would

be accessible to a large number of people, relatively short in duration, and a process that was not repetitive.

Milne's personal reflections (K. Milne, personal communication, May 22, 2007) on pivotal issues, his strong interest in education, and the Society of Obstetricians and Gynecologists of Canada's (SOGC) motivation to welcome change coincided with a time of gloomy outlook in obstetrical care as a result of increasing costs for liability insurance from spiraling malpractice rates due to "bad baby outcomes." The SOGC recognized there were a significant number of obstetricians withdrawing from obstetrical care. The society was also aware that something needed to be done to alleviate fears of litigation in practice, attract physicians to the specialty, and be proactive in reducing the frequency of adverse events in Canadian obstetrical units (K. Milne, personal communication, May 22nd, 2007). Considerable skepticism among members about the proposed MORE^OB program failed to dampen Dr. Milne's resolve.

Impetus for change also came from a 1999 US report on preventable harm events, *To Err is Human: Building a Safer Health System*, from the Institute of Medicine, which served to highlight the magnitude of medical harm and induce governmental involvement to fund and oversee improvements in patient safety (Institute of Medicine, 1999). The Clinton administration swiftly responded by ensuring that government

H. Looker (✉)
University of Toronto, Toronto, ON, Canada

© Springer Nature Switzerland AG 2020
R. Volpe (ed.), *Casebook of Traumatic Injury Prevention*,
https://doi.org/10.1007/978-3-030-27419-1_33

agencies were involved in new initiatives to seek strategies to reduce medical mistakes. In the state of Pennsylvania, for example, legislation requires the reporting of "incidents" at all licensed hospitals, birthing centres, ambulatory surgical facilities, and some abortion facilities, giving healthcare workers the means to report anonymously to the Patient Safety Authority (PSA). Reporting systems are also in place for the public and physicians are obliged to report malpractice suits to their professional licensing bodies (Patient Safety Authority, 2006). A similar report from the NHS in the United Kingdom led to the Confidential Enquiry into Maternal and Child Health (Confidential Enquiry into Maternal and Child Health [CEMACH], 2005). Black and Brocklehurst (2003) remarked that there is some evidence that obstetric emergencies are frequently mismanaged and that the Confidential Enquiry into Maternal Deaths under CEMACH in Britain "has repeatedly identified substandard care in a significant proportion of maternal deaths in the United Kingdom" (CEMACH, 2005, p. 837). Reports testifying for change were also seen in Australia and Canada, although citing this much later (K. Milne, personal communication, May 22, 2007).

33.1.1 System Problems

In a 2006 editorial, William Grobman cited "cultural inertia," the lack of proven methods to assess patient safety and a lack of evaluation when there is imposed change as factors constraining the transition to a culture dedicated to patient safety by health care organizations (Grobman, 2006, p. 1058). Grobman noted that there was a consensus among multiple authors of studies that "system problems" underpinned safety issues for patients (Grobman, 2006, pp. 1058–59). System problems may be found in "policies/protocols, access to/transfer of information, communication, discharge procedures/protocols, organization management/culture and record-keeping" (Davis et al., 2001, pp. 4–5). System error, on the other hand, may result from "defective equipment/ supplies, equipment/supplies not available,

Table 33.1 Root causes of perinatal death and permanent disability

Cause	Percent
Communication	72%
Teamwork/organizational culture	55%
Staff competency	47%
Orientation and training	40%
Inadequate fetal monitoring	34%
Lack of monitoring equipment/drugs	30%
Credentialing/privileging/supervision physicians and nurse midwives	30%
Staffing issues	25%
Unavailable/delayed physician	19%
Unavailable prenatal information	11%

Note: Percentages reflect the amount of which are considered a problem to perinatal death or permanent disability (Joint Commission on Accreditation, Health Care Certification, 2004)

inadequate reporting/communication, inadequate training or supervision of doctors/other personnel, delay in provision/scheduling of services, inadequate staffing, inadequate functioning of hospital services, or no protocol or failure to implement a protocol/plan" (Davis et al., 2001, pp. 4–5). Analyzing the 40 perinatal deaths and seven cases of permanent disability reported to the Joint Commission on Accreditation, Health Care Certification, between 1996 and 2004, poor communication was identified as the prime cause, followed by lack of teamwork due to the organizational culture, which are both system problems. Other causes are listed in Table 33.1 (Joint Commission on Accreditation, Health Care Certification, 2004). Recommendations for action stemming from the two major causes of perinatal death and injury from ranked strategies to reduce high risk events reported by healthcare organizations are already embodied in the MORE[OB] program (JCAHO, 2004).

33.1.1.1 High Reliability Organizations (HROs)

All of these issues are addressed within the MORE[OB] program and applied based on principles of HROs. HROs engage in operations and activities where the potential for error is great and consequences of errors often lead to catastrophic results (Baker, Day, & Salas, 2006). Environments for such organizations are typically complex in structure and technology, where employees have highly stratified roles and interdependent responsibilities (Baker et al., 2006). Many HROs serve the general public and are, therefore, held accountable for mistakes causing personal harm by external groups and internal authorities (Carroll & Rudolph, 2006). High reliability is achieved through a preoccupation with all failures or emergency situations possible so that multifactorial strategies are applied to maintain safety for as long as possible (Baker et al., 2006; Issel & Narasimha, 2007). HROs operate through highly trained teams, which adapt to time constraints when routine activities become problematic (Baker et al., 2006). The regular exchange of feedback is critical to team functioning and development (Baker et al., 2006). An important aspect of HRO teams is that decision making is not linear or tied to hierarchy, as team members on the frontline may be the first to recognize signs of risk or problematic implications (Carroll & Rudolph, 2006; Issel & Narasimha, 2007).

33.1.2 Patient Safety

The SOGC drew attention to slipped rankings for Canada among the Organization for Economic Cooperation and Development (OECD) countries for maternal mortality, perinatal mortality, and infant mortality, according to data reported in June 2006, which was compared to data reported in 1990. By 2006, maternal mortality rates fell from second place to 11th, perinatal mortality rates fell from 12th place to 14th, and infant mortality rates dropped from sixth to 21st (Society of Obstetricians and Gynecologists of Canada's [SOGC], 2006; SOGC, 2007). This scenario captured politicians' attention and was ranked high on the research agenda years after important publications and studies from other countries influenced risk management in healthcare. The Canadian Patient Safety Institute was created in 2002 by the Canadian Federal government who funded the organization with $50 million over 5 years (Baker et al., 2004). Baker et al. (2004) conducted the first study in Canada to report on

the incidence of adverse events nationally by reviewing charts at different types of hospitals in five provinces, but the study excluded obstetrical and psychiatric adverse events and restricted review to adult patients.

In Ontario, some perinatal deaths are reviewed by the Obstetrical Care Review Committee for The Office of The Coroner of Ontario with the aim of generating discussion on the status quo of obstetrical care in the province (Acheson, 2004). Cases are brought to the attention of the review committee by staff within the Coroner's office, as they may be indicative of a noticeable trend occurring. Cases reported on are not absolutely representative of all cases of perinatal origin reported to the Coroner (M. Dunn, personal communication, April 29th, 2007). The Tenth Annual Report for cases reviewed in 2003 reflects a disturbing trend compared to the eighth and ninth report, where recommended changes in three important categories increased in frequency, especially problems in obstetrical management. This alarming report demonstrated the need for improvement in these areas. Drawn from three annual reports, Table 33.2 shows three obstetrical care issues and a comparative analysis of recommendations by category frequency.

In 2000, adverse events within the NHS in the United Kingdom were scrutinized by a group of experts, chaired by the Chief Medical Officer of Health (Department of Health, 2000). The resulting report entitled *"An Organization with a Memory"* not only revealed the breadth and depth of weaknesses and failures in patient safety but analyzed many underpinning factors that contributed to poor standards of patient safety that were systemic in nature due to the organizational culture within the NHS (Department of Health, 2000). The status quo of healthcare in the NHS

Table 33.2 Changes in recommendation category frequency

Recommendation category	Eighth report	Ninth report	Tenth report
Documentation	29%	34%	40%
Fetal monitoring	41%	28%	40%
OB management	47%	59%	80%

Note: Acheson (2004)

was appalling yet enlightening, and the critique clearly identified areas for improvement and provided the rationale for necessary changes.

33.1.3 Medical Training

The use of forceps is on the decline as evident from the literature; however, they remain an optional tool applied at the discretion of an obstetrician (Bofill et al., 1996; Cheong, Abdullahi, Lashen, & Fairlie, 2004; Edozien, 2007). In a 1996 survey of residency programs in Canada and the United States where the response rate was 73%, respectively, 68% of programs favored the use of forceps in instrumental deliveries, while 32% favored vacuum cups, mostly the soft rather than metallic type (Bofill et al., 1996). At this point in time (1996), European obstetricians had already moved away from forceps as a primary choice in difficult births due to the potential for severe maternal injury, and North America followed suit (Bofill et al., 1996; Johanson & Menon, 1999). Instrumentally assisted birth using one of many types of vacuum cups is also known as "ventouse." It is important to note that perineal trauma is more likely to occur with the use of forceps; there is, however, increased maternal concern with the use of ventouse (Talukdar, Purandare, Coulter-Smith, & Geary, 2013).

According to Cheong et al. (2004), formal, multifaceted education and training of junior medical staff over 4 months failed to improve the rate of successful instrumental deliveries. The multifaceted educational package covered theory without accumulated experience (Cheong et al., 2004). Significantly, the vacuum cup was preferred by staff at a ratio of 2:1 over forceps, but failed ventouse in this study was followed by forceps delivery. Although successful in the cases cited, Towner reported that it is widely acknowledged that sequential use of instruments invites a high risk of injury to the mother and baby (as cited in Cheong et al., 2004). Significant reductions in the amount of time spent in medical training with the intent of improving patient safety have served to reduce skill acquisition

among medical professionals in the United Kingdom and the United States (Sau, Sau, Ahmed, & Brown, 2004). Because it is unlikely that obstetric complications and serious errors can be completely eliminated, team training and drills are particularly valuable for capacity building since the focus is on error correction and management to minimize harm to patients (Department of Health, 2000). Error management partnered with error prevention initiatives "is one of the most fundamental differences between success and failure" (Department of Health, 2000, p. 28).

33.1.4 Mode of Delivery

Operative assistance, short of a caesarian section, is the choice between using forceps or vacuum cups for extraction. Forceps have been found to be a greater risk factor for head and neck injuries than ventouse (Hughes, Harley, Milmoe, Bala, & Martorella, 1999). The training for, and use of forceps has dramatically declined for reasons associated with maternal and neonatal morbidity as well as consequential medicolegal concerns. The Canadian Institute for Health Information (CIHI) reports that the primary choice of instrumental delivery method has reversed from forceps to ventouse between the early 1990s to 2001 at a 2:1 ratio, a trend paralleled in the United Kingdom, United States, Australia, and New Zealand (Canadian Institute for Health Information [CIHI], 2004). In a 1996 study surveying residency training in Canada and the United States, Bofill et al. (1996) found that 36% of survey respondents had ceased instruction of mid-pelvic instrumental delivery, with 74% of these respondents preferring caesarean delivery as a safer alternative (Bofill et al., 1996). A total of 38% of directors canvassed in this group also admitted that potential litigation was a reason for eliminating the teaching of mid-pelvic instrumental delivery (Bofill et al., 1996).

Although vacuum extraction appears to be safer than forceps, Treffers determined that application at upper stations of the birth canal has been strongly opposed, as this process was associated with multiple severe birth traumas and deaths (as cited by Hankins, Clark, & Munn, 2006). O'Mahoney, Byrne, and Donnelly (2005) had similar findings but cranial or cervical spine injuries were the predominant evidence of trauma in a study reviewing neonatal deaths. Shoulder dystocia, cephalohematoma, and low Apgar scores (7 or less) after 5 minutes tend to be common with ventouse, while maternal third or fourth-degree perineal and vaginal lacerations and facial nerve damage to newborns occurred more with the use of forceps. Consensus on the danger of applying rotational forces on the fetal head is well established; forceps, in fact, are considered "a lethal instrument in unskilled hands" (Clarke, 2004 and Yoong, Milestone, & Sahana, 2004, p. 24, in rapid response to Patel & Murphy, 2004; O'Grady, Pope, & Hoffman, 2002). Spinal injury to the fetus as a consequence of rotation occurs in approximately 1/1000 rotations (O'Grady et al., 2002). Outlet and low-pelvic forceps operations are "simple operations" considered reasonably safe to mother and baby; mid-pelvic operations compare favourably with caesarean delivery if clinical indicators qualify both patients and if the physician has skill (O'Grady et al., 2002, p. 9). An eminent obstetrician, Ian Donald, called the use of forceps before complete cervical dilation an "obstetrical crime", but ventouse under similar circumstance "much less of a crime" (Edozien, 2007, p. 642).

33.1.5 Major Types of Birth Trauma

33.1.5.1 Brain Damage

Subgaleal hematomas (SGH) are severe, potentially fatal extracranial injuries that are a result of forceful traction or shearing against the scalp which may happen by improper use of vacuum extraction cups in instrumental deliveries (Parker, 2005; R. Sherwood, personal communication, May 9, 2007). Extreme complication of SGH has been recognized, throughout the years, which requires prompt surgical intervention and extracranial cerebral compression as a consequence of large volume SGHs (Amar, Aryan, Meltzer, & Levy, 2003).

33.1.5.2 Spinal Cord Damage

It has been estimated that injury to the spinal cord may be considered a cause in roughly 10% of neonatal deaths (Sorantin, Brader, & Thimary, 2006). There are three distinguishable clinical presentations of spinal cord injury (SPI): stillbirth or death soon after birth, respiratory failure in the neonatal period, and markedly diminished tone and weakness manifested as spasticity or "cerebral palsy," also seen within the neonatal period (Sorantin et al., 2006, p. 202). Onset of spasticity later in life following SCI, however, can be mistakenly ascribed to cerebral palsy, and report of this misdiagnosis was made in 1979 by Koch and Eng (Brand, 2006; Ruggieri, Smarason, & Pike, 1999).

There is evidence that epidural analgesia contributes to the need for instrumental delivery by prolonging labour (Thorp & Breedlove, 1996). Saunders, Patterson, & Wadsworth, (cited by Thorp & Breedlove, 1996) reported that epidural analgesia is also significantly associated with postpartum infection and postpartum hemorrhage, secondary Apgar scores under 7, maternal hypotension, and fever, to name a few risks (Ploeckinger, Ulm, Chalubinski, & Gruber, 1995). Swedish researchers, however, also concluded that low-dose epidural analgesia was not associated with risk of instrumental delivery for nulliparous women, but the 16% rate of instrumental delivery for the majority of maternity units administering epidural analgesia to 40–49% of women did not include caesarean deliveries and is a much higher rate than reported elsewhere (Eriksson, Olausson, & Olofsson, 2006). Sherwood, (personal communication, January 9, 2008) commented that shifting evidence is common in obstetrical issues but noted that epidural analgesia may be expected to delay the second phase of labour, primarily due to a reduction in maternal expulsive efforts, secondary to the motor block which accompanies effective epidural pain relief. This phenomenon then leads to the need for instrumentally assisted birth. If epidural analgesia is administered, then a longer, more tolerant allowance for the second stage of labour is a technique that reduces the likelihood of an instrumental delivery (Johanson & Menon, 1999).

33.1.6 Emergence of MORE^OB

At the time when the MORE^OB program was emerging, Black and Brocklehurst (2003) performed "a systematic review of training in acute obstetric emergencies" (p. 837). They reported six programs as poorly described with training delivery that were mostly remote from labour wards and inadequately evaluated due to the lack of performance assessments and differences in specific outcomes in maternity units (Black & Brocklehurst, 2003, p. 840). The MORE^OB program fulfills the criteria suggested by Black and Brocklehurst (2003) for components of a training program to improve outcomes of obstetrical emergencies including on-site and team training, a long-term program, multiple training mediums, tailoring of program to deal with local issues, reasonable cost, a focus on communications, national standards, and professional evaluation techniques to improve standards and outcomes of obstetrical care.

33.2 Resources

Milne (personal communication, May 22, 2007) produced his own skeleton drafts of the MORE^OB program in 2000, presenting them to the executive and council of the SOGC in 2001. Working full-time at the SOGC, Milne (personal communication, May 22, 2007) found it difficult to recruit others, but had a dedicated volunteer working group by the fall of 2001. This group produced the program content by spring 2002, which was accessible to SOGC members on the website. The SOGC provided substantial financial support for the start-up of the program; Milne (personal communication, May 22, 2007), however, pitched his concept to several insurance companies in order to secure funding for a pilot project. Though insurance companies were attentive, Milne formed a partnership with the Health Insurance Reciprocal of Canada (HIROC) as the response time was efficient and they "stepped up to the plate" (K. Milne, personal communication, May 22, 2007). HIROC had access to hospitals

since these institutions were clients with complex insurance needs. HIROC gave support in the way of consulting and funding when they partnered with the MORE^OB initiative, with their financial commitment being $3,000,000 to start (E. Morton & M. Boyce, personal communication, May 3, 2007). The most appealing aspect of the program to HIROC was that one of the major goals of MORE^OB was to promote effective communication and teamwork to reduce the traditional hierarchy in obstetrical units. Because obstetrical care was to be provided by a team approach by healthcare professionals, this method promised a synergistic improvement in performance with expected declines in rates of malpractice claims as a consequence (E. Morton & M. Boyce, personal communication, May 3, 2007).

When the hospitals contracted to implement the program, it was agreed that there would be an 80% plus participation rate. HIROC specified particular criteria as important signposts to exemplary practice from their standpoint of risk management: address problems, place greater emphasis on charting, stress education, improve and standardize transfer of care, and achieve fuller understanding of individual abilities by all team members (E. Morton & M. Boyce, personal communication, May 3, 2007). Budget reallocation or new sources of funding have to be founded by hospital administrators interested in implementing MORE^OB. Hospitals, therefore, need to identify strategies to release nurses from direct patient care responsibilities in order to participate in selected MORE^OB activities. In addition to this, hospitals are challenged to provide funding support for the core team (E. Morton & M. Boyce, personal communication, May 3, 2007).

33.3 Implementation

Milne (personal communication, May 22, 2007) attributes HIROC's leadership role in eagerly initiating the MORE^OB program to the corporate culture already established at HIROC. HIROC has an education department that exists for the benefit of its clients to reduce financial losses

(E. Morton & M. Boyce, personal communication, May 3, 2007). A sense of fiduciary responsibility may also have influenced HIROC's interest and investment (K. Milne, personal communication, June 26, 2007). Senior management at HIROC conveyed that the MORE^{OB} program was an excellent opportunity to make use of the wealth of data and analysis carried out by actuaries and risk managers (E. Morton & M. Boyce, personal communication, May 3, 2007).

33.3.1 Locations

HIROC executives met with Dr. Milne to review the proposal before the start of the program, which was then taken to HIROC's board of directors (E. Morton & M. Boyce, personal communication, May 3, 2007). Dr. Milne was introduced to key business colleagues by HIROC executives, and introductory letters describing the program were sent to hospital clients by HIROC

(E. Morton & M. Boyce, personal communication, May 3, 2007). HIROC responded to questions about the program, insisting that hospitals subsidize participation costs and help determine required levels of participation by the medical professions involved in obstetrics (E. Morton & M. Boyce, personal communication, May 3, 2007). Milne (personal communication, May 22, 2007) organized a pilot run for the program in 21 healthcare organizations, representing 33 hospital sites in a variety of settings. As of 2010, the MORE^{OB} program is within 211 hospitals involving over 10,000 participants, showcased in Fig. 33.1 (Milne and Salus Global Corporation, 2010). Figure 33.2 demonstrates the expansion into the United States in 2005, and St. Joseph's Hospital Health Center in Syracuse New York became the first hospital in the United States to actively engage in the Program (Milne and Salus Global Corporation, 2010). Following this, there has been a steady increase in the number of hospitals adopting MORE^{OB} in the United States,

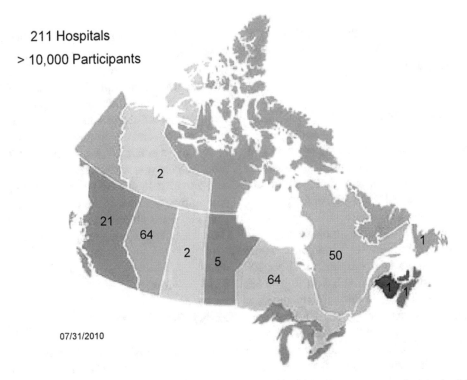

Fig. 33.1 Total number of hospitals that have participated in Canada, separated by provinces and territories (Milne & Salus Global Corporation, 2010)

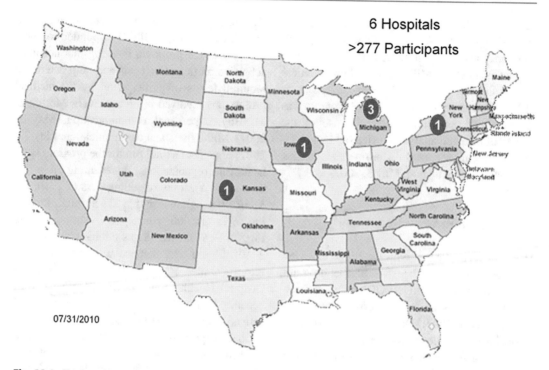

Fig. 33.2 Total number of hospitals that have participated in the United States separated by state (Milne & Salus Global Corporation, 2010)

leading to six hospitals with 277 participants on board as of 2010 (Milne and Salus Global Corporation, 2010).

33.3.2 Participants

The professional discipline continues to be consistent within participating hospitals, consisting of nurses, obstetricians, family physicians, and midwives (Milne and Salus Global Corporation, 2010). There are interdisciplinary "core teams" which are responsible for implementing and administering the MORE^OB program within obstetrical units. A large hospital with over 200 participants, for example, may have a 30-member core team. An interdisciplinary instructor team provides a 2-day training program at a hospital site at the initialization of the program, returning at the beginning of each subsequent module to introduce progressive phases of the program, which allows for continuous learning. The six emergency drills that the program covers are

for shoulder dystocia (delivery of the shoulders), cord prolapse, postpartum hemorrhage, emergency fetal bradycardia, breech delivery, and management of multiple births. The MORE^OB program also provides ongoing client support through regional representatives and head office staff, building and a website was made available to the public in late 2003. Overall, the MORE^OB program goal was for at least 80% of the healthcare providers in obstetrical care units to participate in the activities of the program; this target percentage was surpassed in all sites as of 2010 (Milne and Salus Global Corporation, 2010).

33.4 Outcome

33.4.1 Pilot Phase

The pilot phase of the MORE^OB program comprised of 33 hospitals and over 2000 participants as seen through Table 33.3. Feedback from these institutions and participants confirmed positive

Table 33.3 Healthcare providers who participated in program pilots and rates of participation

Profession	No.	%
Nurses	1830	69%
Obstetricians	345	13%
Family physicians	265	10%
Midwives	216	8%
Total participants	2656	

Note: MORE^OB (n.d.)

improvements in "culture" change regarding patient safety and professional interrelationships, with significant upgrading of clinical knowledge across all disciplines. Other information was used to modify the program for a planned national launch. Executives from HIROC saw the six emergency drills as the most valuable part of the practicum sessions as it created a level playing field for all involved (E. Morton & M. Boyce, personal communication, May 3, 2007). In testimonials reported by Dr. Kenneth Milne, process evaluation rather than judgment of individuals, multidisciplinary involvement, and trust in coworkers built through achieving parity of core knowledge and skill drills were outstanding facets of the MORE^OB program (Milne & Lalonde, 2007). Nursing, from its inception, was deliberately organized on a military model of subordination by Florence Nightingale, and the imperative to abide by doctors' decisions remains integral to practice (Fahy, 2007). To achieve and maintain a culture of safety, however, the MORE^OB program harmonizes the traditional nurse/physician relationship to function on egalitarian terms.

33.4.1.1 Identifying Gaps and Improvements

The program enables hospitals to identify gaps and addresses specific issues such as charting, oxytocin administration, and fetal heart monitoring. Information from audits is shared and used internally by hospital participants. In 1987, the largest settlement for an infant case involving malpractice was around $1 million, while in 2003, a similar case resulted in $9.3–$12 million as a settlement award for a catastrophic injury (E. Morton & M. Boyce, personal communication, May 3, 2007). Inflation rates have doubled in

the estimation of settlement awards, some awards exceeding a compounded 3% inflation rate (E. Morton & M. Boyce, personal communication, May 3, 2007). According to HIROC, numbers for poor obstetrical outcomes are low, and while some claims are clearly due to negligence, many claims for negligence are attributable to other birth-related issues (E. Morton & M. Boyce, personal communication, May 3, 2007). Since the MORE^OB program has been in place, there has been a significant drop in the time taken by hospitals to report adverse events (K. Milne, personal communication, June 26, 2007).

The hospitals identified a number of improvements within their clinical outcomes. The most commonly reported improvements included a reduction in the incidence and severity of postpartum hemorrhage, a reduction in the number of babies requiring transfer to neonatal intensive care unit (NICU) and of women requiring transfer to ICU, and a reduction in the incidence of brachial plexus injury resulting from shoulder dystocia (K. Milne, personal communication, May 6, 2008). Initially, Milne (K. Milne, personal communication, June 26, 2007) found that colleagues were reluctant to accept the numbers of harmful events associated with obstetrical management. Milne cited relevant examples as proof, however, to gain understanding and support for a patient safety culture, attributing low awareness levels to organizational structure and reporting of cases singularly.

33.4.2 Sustainability Tests

The assessment of a program to be considered an "exemplary practice" depends on whether evaluation is a component of the program that meets the test of sustainability represented by the four "E"s rubric (i.e., education, economics, enactment, and engineering), in which at least three of the four "Es" must be reached (Volpe, 2002). Empowerment and evaluation have been added to the test of sustainability since they are closely interwoven with the human resources and funding associated with program success and continuance. The MORE^OB program qualifies in every "E" category, as briefly outlined below.

33.4.2.1 Education

The adult learning principles deployed in the program include repetition to make actions and behaviours second nature; relevant, useful content and activities; hands-on and interactive experiences; and interesting material for the professionals involved. Both the Royal College Maintenance of Certification Program and the College of Family Physicians of Canada recognize the continuing medical educational components of the MORE[OB] program for purposes of accreditation (N. Whitelaw, personal communication, May 1, 2007). The central educational topics in the clinical chapters include a combination of guidelines from professional societies such as the SOGC's own obstetrical management guidelines, material from American Congress of Obstetricians and Gynecologists, and other guidelines related to obstetrical events, namely, Patient Safety Theory, Behavioural System Theory, and research articles deemed as exemplary current evidence on obstetrical management, which is reviewed annually (K. Milne, personal communication, May 22, 2007). The delivery of education for MORE[OB] is a 3-year program delivered in three modules through secure web access available at any computer, whereas structured, interdisciplinary workshops are usually held on site (C. Davies, personal communication, July 10, 2007). Facilitating a team approach to problem-solving and opportunity for discussions, the workshops reinforce the HRO paradigm for patient safety and clinical competency (K. Milne, personal communication, May 22, 2007).

33.4.2.2 Economics

The status quo for HIROC in liabilities is that 14% of malpractice suits filed are from adverse obstetrical events, but at least 47% of reserves must be set aside to potentially settle such lawsuits (E. Morton & M. Boyce, personal communication, May 3, 2007). The amount a court may award for a successful case, especially a catastrophic claim, is also disproportionately larger than it was 25 years ago, substantially more than a 3% compounded inflation rate. In light of these trends, funding the MORE[OB] program is a sound business investment for insurance companies. A variety of cost-sharing arrangements are in place between the hospital and their insurance liability provider.

33.4.2.3 Enactment

As mentioned, the program's contract requirements specify that 80% + of all obstetrical care providers in a hospital must participate. Creation of the core team at the start of the program provides leadership to ensure that controlled progression through the program occurs. Some larger hospital sites have added a part-time coordinator role to assist the core team in program implementation. From the outset, MORE[OB] trainers external to each site come to give intensive training days. MORE[OB] Regional Representatives provide ongoing follow-up, support, and mentoring to the core team to help them achieve the program goals. An external consultant helps to educate the trainers and remains accessible to these staffs to facilitate quality delivery of the program and motivate participants. Well-grounded financial incentives also encourage hospitals and governments to support the program (K. Milne, personal communication June 26, 2007).

33.4.2.4 Engineering

Interactive software was developed from scratch by an Ottawa, Ontario, company for the specialized content necessary for professional accreditation, knowledge testing, reference materials, and other facets of program delivery to multiple users. Other media materials from Partnership for Patient Safety (p4ps®) were also made available. The comprehensive website gives a good overview of the MORE[OB] program and the kind of content participants will encounter. In Toronto, through a research initiative, MORE[OB] was involved with a simulation program studying team function in emergency clinical scenarios (C. Davies, personal communication, July 10, 2007). Information from this research provided direction for the type of technology that was integrated in the MORE[OB] program (C. Davies, personal communication, July 10, 2007). From the United Kingdom, a simulation-based training course geared to obstetric emergency situations called Managing Obstetric Emergencies and Trauma (MOET) showed early success when first applied in Bangladesh and Armenia (Maslovitz, Barkai, Lessing, Ziv, & Many, 2007). Simulation training originates with the aviation industry and the HROs consisting of major international airline companies (Maslovitz et al., 2007).

33.4.2.5 Empowerment

The MORE^OB program refines the training of multidisciplinary professionals so that synergy is achieved through teamwork. The program's intent is to change a culture of hierarchy and autonomous practice to one of collaboration and mutual respect where critique is open and encouraged. Any member of the caregiver team who recognizes less than optimal care delivery is encouraged and supported to voice concerns, opinions, or judgments to assure patient safety. Empowerment for women who give birth at hospitals to be "the locus of control during labor and delivery" in the obstetrical suite is important in culture change designed to improve patient care (Cherouny, Federico, Haraden, Leavitt Gullo, & Resar, 2005, p. 2). The MORE^OB program emphasizes the importance of including women as full and active partners with the healthcare team in decision-making regarding the safe care of themselves and their babies. This goal is achieved through the following components that are embedded within the program:

- An underlying philosophy of patient-centered care, for example, "nothing about me without me," understanding the patient's perspective.
- Specific communication and teamwork strategies to include women and families in the care process: this includes, for example, incorporating women's birthing plans into the plan of care, daily collaborative rounds which include the patient, ensuring informed consent, patient question cards that facilitate comfort in raising concerns with caregivers.
- Patient satisfaction survey that includes questions about the care team's responsiveness to patient needs and preferences.

33.4.2.6 Evaluation

Within the MORE^OB program, evaluation is one of the four principal components that reinforce other elements such as reflective learning, which emphasizes continuous learning over the course of professional careers. At each hospital site, the core team looks at results from reports and audits. Audits may be performed on specific aspects of obstetrical care such as the management of labour and cases ending in C-section following spontaneous labour which may be very time-consuming (C. Davies, personal communication, July 10, 2007). There are four levels of evaluation which include reaction, learning, application, and business as seen through Table 33.4 (Milne and Salus Global Corporation, 2010). The MORE^OB program uses a balanced score care approach,

Table 33.4 Four levels of evaluation

Level	Method	Measures
1 Reaction	Questionnaire Focus groups	Overall satisfaction, perceived value and recommendations Effectiveness of tools and activities
2 Learning	Questionnaire Focus groups Core knowledge pre- and post-test	Gains in core clinical knowledge Caregiver confidence Caregiver competence Patient safety knowledge
3 Application	Questionnaire Focus groups CAS Environmental scan	Culture change Practice change Work processes
4 Business	Questionnaire Focus groups Claims statistics	Hospital accreditation Patient satisfaction, caregiver satisfaction Liability cost reduction Work-related stress Worthwhile investment

Note: Milne and Salus Global Corporation (2010)

an adaptation of the Kirkpatrick–Phillips model of training evaluation (Milne & Salus Global Corporation, 2010). This method gathers trend information in knowledge enhancement, cultural change, and an annual environmental scan (Milne & Salus Global Corporation, 2010).

33.4.3 Analysis

Ownership, leadership, and ongoing support by the SOGC and HIROC are significant factors in the MORE[OB] program's sustainability and credibility beyond the Canadian border (MORE[OB], n.d.). Recruitment of American nationals and opinion leaders to be the support contacts for hospitals in the United States has been a wise decision as the model of healthcare is quite different, and insurance options for hospitals are highly varied in the United States.

The use of feedback, gathered by formal means and spontaneous response, is actually a heuristic effectively used to reveal opportunities for better strategies. The iterative use of feedback is directly borrowed from HROs where the heuristics of reduce/reveal/focus are applied to maximize coordination of practitioners, their support systems and tools, and the work environment (Patterson, 2007). Within a large urban hospital, the MORE[OB] program was initially met with much resistance because "extra work" was the first impression, and doctors felt it was a "fad." This definitely changed, however, due to the quality of the program material and involvement which motivated people to have an appreciation of knowledge consistency and enhanced working relationships (C. Davies, personal communication, July 10, 2007).

Team behaviour as a strategy to reduce error in healthcare settings was integral to strategies promoted by the Institute of Medicine in the United States. Morey et al. (as cited by Rice Simpson, James, & Knox, 2006, p. 547) reported that much evidence exists to show "teams accomplish more safety-critical tasks better than individuals," leading to improved patient safety (Nielsen et al., 2007). Although a randomized control trial of crew resource training in obstetrics failed to show a detectable impact, continuation of interdisciplinary team training made it apparent that almost a year was needed to demonstrate "a significant decline in the Adverse Outcome Index" (Nielsen et al., 2007, p. 54). This information supports the need for a long-term program such as MORE[OB] and also advancing with MORE[OB] to effect lasting change, not only in adverse events but also in behavioural and attitudinal change in obstetrical team members. The program embodies recommendations and strategies from acclaimed healthcare reports and the aviation sector, a leader among HROs. Learning from litigation has also shaped the MORE[OB] program and provided the powerful economic incentive of reduced claims and lawsuits to participating hospitals.

The importance of communication cannot be overstated and common understandings together with communications protocol have been prime recommendations for patient safety cultures (Kohn, Corrigan, & Donaldson, 1999). In a study of communication between labor nurses and obstetricians in four large community hospitals in the United States averaging 2800–6500 births annually, communications amounted to between 2 and 4 min per routine labour, although this was often deliberate to keep obstetricians away for as long as possible (Rice Simpson et al., 2006). Obstetricians favoured a hierarchical order and defied unit policies, a culture which rarely enhances patient safety (Kohn et al., 1999 cited in Rice Simpson et al., 2006). Because neither discipline in this study of four sites held mutual understandings of how best to interpret fetal heart rate readings, patient safety could have been compromised. This example of clinical practice underscores one of the fundamental MORE[OB] educational objectives: to have shared knowledge in interdisciplinary teams and the proven benefits of an adaptive hierarchy, especially in emergency situations (JCAHO, 2004; Roberts & Tadmar, 2002). Open communication promoted by the program is also a defence against the loss of situational awareness—"the attribution of being involved in and aware of what is going on" (Edozien, 2007, p. 648). Failure to follow guidelines, poor recognition of risk factors, and use of excessive traction are examples of lost situational awareness in instrumental deliveries, any of which place patients at risk (Edozien, 2007).

While it is possible to train and educate health professionals to work as teams in a culture of safety, reconfiguring a hospital to an HRO requires ongoing "productive tension" for a number of "dualities," such as having strong controls in place but preserving flexible approaches (Carroll & Rudolph, 2006, p. i5). This process must involve leadership in hospital administration by executives, especially to maintain a surplus of human resources to analyze, audit, and review operational standards rather than thinking that high reliability will be sustained without such resources (Carroll & Rudolph, 2006). HRO principles, particularly concerning culture, have been shown to raise reliability in a large sample of intensive care units in the US state of Michigan (Pronovost et al., 2006).

33.4.4 Sustainability

The US healthcare arena is heterogeneous throughout the states and quite different from Canada. Assuring credibility for the program means that Americans will be hired to provide program support. Milne (personal communication, May 22, 2007) has used professional consultants at times when expertise was needed to move the program forward or assist with evaluation complexity, thereby not overtaxing his own reserves or his team's resources to function effectively.

The MORE^OB program does not necessarily end after the initial 3-year program is completed; evaluations at the end of the program may highlight areas needing concentrated further development. A tailored program "Advancing with MORE^OB" could then be designed for a hospital to follow. The advanced programming would be funded by the healthcare organization or in partnership with a liability provider. The centrality of organizational change is highly appropriate because an informed culture of safety endures over time despite practice adaptations and staff changes (Department of Health, 2000).

Organizationally, the MORE^OB program is no longer reliant on dedicated volunteers and has become highly professionalized as it now employs specialists in evaluation, IT, and curriculum development. In addition, using a medical research analyst has facilitated rigour and timeliness in selection of the best evidence available (K. Milne, personal communication, May 22, 2007). Milne (personal communication, May 22, 2007) is particularly conscious about succession planning and actively recruits new team members, seeking those with executive potential.

Hanson and Salmoni (2007) reported on the following important factors influencing sustainability, most of which apply to the MORE^OB program:

- Dr. Milne is the program "champion" who works tirelessly to develop and promote the program, creating synergy along the way.
- The program is flexible to different sized institutions in a variety of locations.
- Evaluation data will be used strategically.
- MORE^OB has become an entity embedded in the healthcare industry.
- The program "fits" with values and objectives of professional organizations and health ministries.
- Benefit is derived by all participants and stakeholders.
- Alternative funding has been secured to reduce financial burdens to those involved with the program.
- Growth continues with recruitment of hospitals across Canada and out of country.
- The medical community is more organized through drills and a team approach and more skilled through clinical education and practice.
- Different strategies have been used to target individuals, organizations, and institutions.

33.5 Conclusion

Dr. Kenneth Milne is a self-proclaimed evangelist when it comes to patient safety in obstetrics and is driven to bring a culture of safety to an important area of healthcare. As with other sectors, Milne draws on organizations such as the military, nuclear power generation, and aviation where safety is paramount and where the short run approach to address issues will not suffice. Real and permanent change in climate and culture must become embedded in obstetrical practice, and the MORE[OB] program is commended for this primary objective as favourable results to date remain elusive elsewhere. MORE[OB] is an exemplary practice as current practices are critically reviewed, and the transfer of evidence-informed research in obstetrics, organizational behavior, reliability science, and risk management constantly revitalize the program. The literature reverberates with recommended interventions to address deficiencies in obstetrical emergency management; problematic areas are consistently reported to be communication, human factors, and system failures, which teamwork, constant rehearsal, feedback, and self-evaluation overcome.

Acknowledgments The author would like to express sincere appreciation to the key informants for this case study— J. Kenneth Milne of Salus Global Corporation in London, ON, Canada; Eleanor Morton of Healthcare Insurance Reciprocal of Canadain Toronto, ON, Canada; Mike Boyce of Healthcare Insurance Reciprocal of Canadain Toronto, ON, Canada; Rupert Sherwood of The Royal Australian and New Zealand College of Obstetricians and Gynaecologists in Melbourne, VIC, Australia; M. Dunn of Sunnybrook Health Sciences Centre in Toronto, ON, Canada; Mike Vezina of Salus Global Corporation in London, ON, Canada; Sharon Huber of Regina General Hospital in Regina, SK, Canada; Cynthia Davies of Mount Sinai Hospital in Toronto, ON, Canada; Nancy Whitelaw of Salus Global Corporation in London, ON, Canada, and Rebecca Attenborough of the Reproductive Care Program of Nova Scotia in Halifax, NS, Canada—whose consultation made this project possible.

BRIO Model: MORE[OB]: Managing Obstetrical Risks Efficiently

Group Served: Obstetricians/family physicians/nurses/midwives.

Goal: To change culture in obstetrical practice in order to improve safety and quality care.

Background	Resources	Implementation	Outcome
Development initiated by Dr. Milne from observations of 29 years of clinical practice Collaboration with multiple key stakeholders: Surgeons of Canada, College of Family Physicians of Canada, The Association of Women's Health, Obstetric and Neonatal Nurses, the Canadian Association for the Canadian Council on Health Services Accreditation	Funding from hospital liability providers Hospital administration Provincial government funding support Collaboration with American Society of Obstetricians & Gynecologists Actuarial data years providing compelling data of poor risk record Core teams Patient safety model	Piloted in 33 hospital sites in Canada Interactive software developed specifically for training requirements of the program Simulation training Educational credits recognized by ACOG Address problems Diligent charting Education Transfer of care when appropriate. Emergencies rehearsed Multidisciplinary review of routines.	HIROC supported 80% blended participation rate for involved health professionals Committees formed in regions of Canada to modify program and craft the program content Expansion into the United States Empowerment to question actions in delivery of care by all health professionals Currently implemented in 211 hospitals Iterative process to improve the safety model; first 3 years of data to be used for program improvements

Life Space Model: MORE^OB: Managing Obstetrical Risks Efficiently

Sociocultural: civilization/community	Interpersonal: primary and secondary relationships	Physical environments: where we live	Internal states: biochemical/genetic and means of coping
Norms and values are aligned with a patient safety culture Shared knowledge Common language and communication Feedback is an important part of process Education is the foundation for training and orientation to a culture of safety	Minimum 80% of obstetric personnel participate in the program Teamwork builds cooperation Hierarchy is flexible to foster egalitarian decision-making Rehearsal of emergencies through drills means less stress facing unexpected problems and builds team capacity	Design improvements made for efficient work flow and patient safety HRO principles of organizational design extend to related services Simulation used to develop/improve clinical skills	Teamwork provides trust, sense of well-being to team members Fear of litigation reduced Pride in reduced errors Contribution to improved systems/procedures through feedback Self-esteem raised in ethical behaviour-greater urgency in reporting of adverse events

References

Acheson, K. (2004). *Tenth annual report of the obstetrical care review committee for the office of the chief coroner of Ontario.* Toronto, ON: Obstetrical Care Review Committee.

Amar, A. P., Aryan, H. E., Meltzer, H. S., & Levy, M. L. (2003). Neonatal subgaleal hematoma causing brain compression: Report of two cases and review of the literature. *Neurosurgery, 52*(6), 1470–1474.

Baker, D. P., Day, R., & Salas, E. (2006). Teamwork as an essential component of high-reliability organizations. *Health Services Research, 41*(4), 1576–1598.

Baker, G. R., Norton, P. G., Flintoft, V., Blais, R., Brown, A., Cox, J., et al. (2004). The Canadian adverse events study: The incidence of adverse events among hospital patients in Canada. *Canadian Medical Association Journal, 170*(11), 1678–1686.

Black, R. S., & Brocklehurst, P. (2003). A systematic review of training in acute obstetric emergencies. *BJOG an International Journal of Obstetrics and Gynecology, 110*(5), 837–841.

Bofill, J. A., Rust, O. A., Perry Jr., K. G., Roberts, W. E., Martin, R. W., & Morrison, J. C. (1996). Graduate education-Forceps and vacuum delivery: A survey of North American residency programs. *Obstetrics and Gynecology, 88*(4), 622–625.

Brand, M. C. (2006). Focus on the physical part 1: Recognizing neonatal spinal cord injury. *Advances in Neonatal Care, 6*(1), 15–24.

Canadian Institute for Health Information. (2004). *Home.* Retrieved May 25, 2007, from http://secure.cihi.ca/cihiweb/dispPage.jsp?cw_page=media_09jun2004_e

Carroll, J. S., & Rudolph, J. W. (2006). Design of high reliability organizations in health care. *Quality & Safety in Health Care, 15*, 4–9.

Cheong, Y. C., Abdullahi, H., Lashen, H., & Fairlie, F. M. (2004). Can formal education and training improve the outcome of instrumental delivery? *European Journal of Obstetrics & Gynecology and Reproductive Biology, 113*(?), 139–144.

Cherouny, P. H., Federico, F. A., Haraden, C., Leavitt Gullo, S., & Resar, R. (2005). Idealized design of perinatal care. In *IHI innovation series white paper.* Cambridge, MA: Institute for Healthcare Improvement, CIHI. Retrieved May 25, 2007, from http://secure.cihi.ca/cihiweb/dispPage.jsp?cw_page=media_09jun2004_e

Clarke, G. C. (2004). Rapid response to Patel, R. R. & Murphy, D. J. (2004) Forceps delivery in modern obstetric practice. *British Medical Journal, 328*(7451), 1302–1305.

Confidential Enquiry into Maternal and Child Health. (2005). *Stillbirth, neonatal and post-natal mortality 2000-2003, England, Wales and Northern Ireland.* London: RCOG Press.

Davis, P., Lay-Yee, R., Briant, R., Schug, S., Scott, A., Johnson, S., et al. (2001). *Adverse events in New Zealand public hospitals: Principal findings from a national survey. Occasional Paper, No. 3.* Wellington: Ministry of Health.

Department of Health. (2000). *An organization with a memory* (Report of an expert group on learning from adverse events in the NHS, chaired by the Chief Medical Officer. Published with the permission of Department of Health on behalf of Her Majesty's Stationary Office). London: Author.

Edozien, L. C. (2007). Towards safe practice in instrumental vaginal delivery. *Best Practice & Research Clinical Obstetrics & Gynecology, 21*(4), 639–655.

Eriksson, S. L., Olausson, P. O., & Olofsson, C. (2006). Use of epidural analgesia and its relation to caesarean and instrumental deliveries – A population-based study of 94,217 primiparae. *European Journal of*

Obstetrics & Gynecology and Reproductive Biology, 128(1-2), 270–275.

Fahy, K. (2007). An Australian history of the subordination of midwifery. *Women and Birth, 20*(1), 25–29.

Grobman, W. A. (2006). Editorial: Patient safety in obstetrics and gynecology, the call to arms. *Obstetrics and Gynecology, 108*(5), 1058–1059.

Hankins, G. D. V., Clark, S. M., & Munn, M. B. (2006). Cesarean section on request at 39 weeks: Impact on shoulder dystocia, fetal trauma, neonatal encephalopathy, and intra-uterine fetal demise. *Seminars in Perinatology, 30*(5), 276–287.

Hanson, H., & Salmoni, A. (2007). *The sustainability of the stay on your feet demonstration project* (Prepared for the Ontario Neurotrauma Foundation). Toronto, ON: ONF.

Hughes, C. A., Harley, E. H., Milmoe, G., Bala, R., & Martorella, A. (1999). Birth trauma in the head and neck. *Archives of Otolaryngoly Head and Neck Surgery, 125*(2), 193–199.

Institute of Medicine. (1999) In L. T. Kohn, J. M. Corrigan, & M. S. Donaldson (Eds.), *To err is human: building a safer health system*. Washington, DC: The National Academies Press.

Issel, L. M., & Narasimha, K. M. (2007). Creating complex health improvement programs as mindful organizations, From theory to action. *Journal of Health Organization and Management, 21*(2), 166–183.

Johanson, R. B., & Menon, V. (1999). Vacuum extraction versus forceps for assisted vaginal delivery. *Cochrane Database of Systematic Reviews*, (2), CD000224.

Joint Commission on Accreditation of Healthcare Organizations. (2004). Sentinel event alert issue 30-- July 21, 2004. Preventing infant death and injury during delivery. *Advances in Neonatal Care, 4*(4), 180–181.

Kohn, L. T., Corrigan, J. M., & Donaldson, M. S. (1999). *To err is human: Building a safer health system*. Washington, DC: National Academic Press.

Maslovitz, S., Barkai, G., Lessing, J. B., Ziv, A., & Many, A. (2007). Recurrent obstetric Management mistakes identified by simulation. *Obstetrics & Gynecology, 109*(6), 1295–1300.

Milne, J. K., & Lalonde, A. B. (2007). Patient safety in women's health-care: Professional colleges can make a difference. The Society of Obstetricians and Gynaecologists of Canada MORE^OB program. *Best Practices & Research Clinical Obstetrics and Gynecology, 21*(4), 565–579.

Milne, J. K., & Salus Global Corporation. (2010). *Performance improvement in patient safety and risk reduction with participation in the MORE^OB Program. A review of the national data from hospitals participating in the SalusMore^OB obstetrical patient safety program*. Mississauga, ON: Salus Global Corporation. Retrieved from http://www.moreob.com/images/pdfs/en/july2010impactofmoreob.pdf

MORE^OB. (n.d.). *Home*. Retrieved from https://www.moreob.com/

Nielsen, P. E., Goldman, M. B., Mann, S., Shapiro, D. E., Marcus, R. G., Pratt, S. D., et al. (2007). Effects of teamwork training on adverse outcomes and process of care in labor and delivery, a randomized controlled trial. *Obstetrics & Gynecology, 109*(1), 48–55.

O'Grady, J. P., Pope, C. S., & Hoffman, D. E. (2002). Forceps delivery.Best Practices & Research. *Clinical Obstetrics and Gynecology, 16*(1), 1–16.

O'Mahoney, T., Byrne, G., and Donnelly, A. (2005). *The Environment Protection Agency's SEA experience in Ireland – The first twelve months*. Paper presented at the IAIA SEA Conference, Prague.

Parker, L. A. (2005). Part 1: Early recognition and treatment of birth trauma: Injuries to the head and face. *Advances in Neonatal Care, 5*(6), 288–297.

Patel, R. R., & Murphy, D. J. (2004). Forceps delivery in modern obstetric practice. *British Medical Journal, 328*(29), 1302–1305.

Patient Safety Authority. (2006). *Reporting medical errors*. Harrisburg, PA: Author. Retrieved May 25, 2007, from http://www.psa.state.pa.us/psa/cwp/view.asp?a=1147&q=440863&psaNav=|

Patterson, E. S. (2007). Communication strategies from high-reliability organizations, translation is hard work. *Annals of Surgery, 245*(2), 170–172.

Ploeckinger, B., Ulm, M. R., Chalubinski, K., & Gruber, W. (1995). Epidural anesthesia in labour: Influence on surgical delivery rates intrapartum fever and blood loss. *Gynecologic and Obstetric Investigation, 39*(1), 24–27.

Pronovost, P. J., Berenholtz, S. M., Goeschel, C. A., Needham, D. M., Sexton, J. B., Thompson, D. A., et al. (2006). Creating high reliability in health care organizations. *Health Services Research, 41*(4), 1599–1617.

Rice Simpson, K., James, D. C., & Knox, G. E. (2006). Nurse-physician communication during labor and birth: Implications for patient safety. *Journal of Gynecological Neonatal Nurses, 35*(4), 547–556.

Roberts, K. H., & Tadmar, C. T. (2002). Lessons learned from non-medical industries: The tragedy of the USS Greenville. *Quality & Safety in Health Care, 11*(4), 355–357.

Ruggieri, M., Smarason, A., & Pike, M. (1999). Spinal cord insults in the prenatal, perinatal, and neonatal periods. *Developmental Medicine and Child Neurology, 41*(5), 311–317.

Sau, A., Sau, M., Ahmed, H., & Brown, R. (2004). Vacuum extraction: Is there any need to improve the current training in the UK? *Acta Obstetricia et Gynecologia Scandinavica, 83*(5), 66–470.

Society of Obstetricians & Gynecologists in Canada. (2006). *Pre-budget consultation executive summary*. Ottawa, ON: Author.

Society of Obstetricians & Gynecologists in Canada. (2007). *A national birthing strategy for Canada*. Ottawa, ON: Author.

Sorantin, E., Brader, P., & Thimary, F. (2006). Neonatal trauma. *European Journal of Radiology, 60*(2), 199–207.

Talukdar, S., Purandare, N., Coulter-Smith, S., & Geary, M. (2013). Is it time to rejuvenate the forceps? *Journal of Obstetrics and Gynecology of India, 63*(4), 218–222.

Thorp, J. A., & Breedlove, G. (1996). Epidural analgesia in labor: An evaluation of risks and benefits. *Birth, 23*(2), 63–83.

Volpe, R. (2002). *A compendium of effective, evidence-based best practices in prevention of neurotrauma.* Toronto, ON: University of Toronto Press.

Yoong, W., Milestone, N., & Sahana, G. (2004). Rapid response to Patel, Roshini R and Murphy, Deirdrie J. Forceps delivery in modern obstetric practice. *British Medical Journal, 328*(7451), 1302–1305.

Safe Babies New York: The Upstate New York Shaken Baby Syndrome (SBS) Education Program

34

Cheryl Hunchak

The Safe Babies New York: The Upstate New York Shaken Baby Syndrome Education Program is a statewide effort to educate all parents about normal infant crying, stress management, and safe sleep in order to decrease Shaken baby syndrome (SBS), injuries, and sudden unexplained deaths in infancy.

34.1 Background

Pediatric neurosurgeon Dr. Mark Dias was working at the Children's Hospital of Buffalo in Western New York in the 1990s. His extensive experience treating infants with SBS had led him to conduct a retrospective study in serial radiography for SBS patients. When his own son was born in 1997, Dias experienced firsthand the frustrations that parents are faced with in caring for an inconsolable infant (Lewandowski, 1999). He realized the ease with which exasperated parents or babysitters could impulsively direct their frustrations onto a crying child. Dias resolved to share his expertise in inflicted infant head injuries with new parents to provide them with the necessary knowledge and coping skills to prevent a

bout of frustration from resulting in a case of shaken baby syndrome.

Dias' original study provided 6 years of reliable incidence data for SBS cases in Western New York. The Children's Hospital of Buffalo, the sole tertiary referral center for pediatric neurosurgical cases in the region, provided an ideal location for launching his envisioned program. It was to be a comprehensive, hospital-based, universal prevention program that educated parents at the time of the infant's birth about the dangers of violent infant shaking. Outcome measures were defined as the regional incidence rate of SBS, the number of parents reached by the program, and parental pre- and post-program knowledge about SBS. This format was intended to improve upon the multitude of fragmented, unevaluated programs previously in operation. It was also unique in being the first to determine whether improved public knowledge could translate into a reduction in the incidence rate of SBS.

Dias' original study revealed that a total of 33 infants were diagnosed with SBS at the Children's Hospital of Buffalo between 1992 and 1998, with an average incidence rate of 7.2 infants per year (Dias, Backstom, Falk, & Li, 1998). Ranging from 1 to 26 months, the average victim age was 6.7 months (Dias et al., 1998). This data, along with Dias' experience in treating infants with SBS, shaped the following hypotheses that guided the ultimate program design:

34

C. Hunchak (✉)
Department of Family and Community Medicine, Schwartz-Reisman Emergency Medicine Centre, Mount Sinai Hospital, Toronto, ON, Canada

© Springer Nature Switzerland AG 2020
R. Volpe (ed.), *Casebook of Traumatic Injury Prevention*,
https://doi.org/10.1007/978-3-030-27419-1_34

1. SBS differs from other forms of child abuse in that it seems to result from impulsive acts of adult rage due to infant crying that may be modifiable with timely parental education.
2. Education efforts must be targeted at parents and, particularly, at males, since 71% of perpetrators are parents and paramours, and males comprise the majority.
3. Due to increased public awareness about SBS from public education campaigns and highly publicized infant fatalities, many parents are already aware that violently shaking an infant is dangerous. Therefore, the aim of the education campaign should be to remind parents about SBS at the appropriate time—during a mother's postnatal stay in the hospital—after which both parents will soon be immersed in the challenges of infant care.
4. Parents are optimal advocates for infant safety/care and may be most effective at disseminating information about SBS to caregivers that will be in contact with their child.

Dias conceived that an SBS education campaign could act as a "vaccine" to "inoculate" parents with information and protect infants from acquiring shaking injuries during the first years of life, when they are most susceptible. Given that the average age at which infants incur inflicted head injuries ranges from 5 to 9 months, the goal that parents retain the program information for at least the first year of each child's life seemed both effective and attainable (Dias & Barthauer, 2001a).

The Upstate New York Shaken Baby Syndrome (SBS) Education Program has since changed its name to Safe Babies New York. This program still includes the hospital-based, postnatal intervention envisioned by Dias, for parents of all newborn infants to learn about SBS, however added information about Safe Sleep in 2014 which informs parents about safe sleeping environments to prevent sleep-related infant deaths (California Evidence-Based Clearinghouse [CEBC], 2016).

34.1.1 Western New York Demographics

Dias remarks how Western New York was ideal for first implementation and evaluation of an SBS education program for the following reasons:

1. Accurate historical incidence data from 6 years' prior at the Children's Hospital of Buffalo was readily available.
2. The Children's Hospital of Buffalo was virtually the exclusive referral site for all pediatric neurosurgical cases in the region.
3. Western New York is geographically discrete, as it is bounded by Canada and Pennsylvania on three sides and had predictable patient referral patterns.
4. The population base was stable, with little immigration or emigration in the region.
5. A regional Perinatal Outreach Program providing tertiary infant care in conjunction with Western New York hospitals was already in full operation (Dias, Mazur, Li, Smith, & DeGuehery, 2002).

The Perinatal Outreach Program consisted of a network of nurse managers from the maternity wards of all hospitals in Western New York. It provided an effective vehicle for disseminating the intended educational materials to new parents. Nurse managers were assigned to receive and distribute the program materials within their respective hospitals. They were to be educated about inflicted infant head injuries and how to implement Dias' Shaken Baby Syndrome Parent Education Program. In turn, the nurse managers at each hospital would convey the program information to the obstetrical ward nurses.

34.1.2 Program Objectives and Goals

Dias' original program aimed to accomplish the following four main goals: (1) to provide educational materials about SBS to the parents of every new infant in Western New York, (2) to verify parents' comprehension of the dangers of violent infant shaking, (3) to track the distribution of information through the collection of the returned commitment statements, and (4) to evaluate the program's effect on the regional incidence of SBS (Dias & Barthauer, 2001a). While continuing to implement those objectives, the overall goals of the updated Safe Babies New York program are as follows:

1. To educate parents about the normalcy of infant crying, the dangers of violent infant shaking, how to calm a crying infant and reduce caregiver frustration and anger, and how to wisely select other caregivers for the infant.
2. Reduce the frequency of abusive head trauma.
3. Educate parents about safe sleeping environments, the dangers of co-sleeping, and sudden unexplained deaths in infancy (CEBC, 2016).

34.1.3 Program Tracking

Within Dias' first implementation, nurse coordinators at each hospital would be instructed to return all signed commitment statements (which parents would sign affirming their receipt of the SBS material) to the program office on a monthly basis, where the information would be entered into a database. An exhaustive monitoring strategy for identifying new cases of SBS were outlined as follows: (1) all admissions of inflicted infant head injury to the Children's Hospital of Buffalo during the program would be identified and recorded; (2) nurses at each hospital were to notify the program coordinators of any known cases that were not referred to the children's hospital; (3) regular contact with regional child fatality teams, child protective services workers, law enforcement officials, and medical examiners would be established; and (4) regional media sources, including television and newspapers, would be periodically reviewed (Dias et al., 2002). A child abuse specialist working at Strong Memorial Hospital in Rochester, New York, was also to be regularly contacted to identify any

additional new cases, in the unlikely event that Western New York patients were referred outside of the region. Based on these investigations, the incidence of inflicted infant head injury in Western New York would be calculated and compared with the historical incidence rate from the previous 6 years (Dias et al., 2002). Upon identifying a case of SBS, the infant's birth date and birth hospital would be identified and then cross-referenced with the mother's last name. This tracking method would indicate whether the parents had participated in the program and whether or not they had signed a commitment statement.

34.2 Resources

The Shaken Baby Syndrome Parent Education Program began in December 1998 with a 2-year grant from the New York State Office of Children and Family Services. Funding came from the William B. Hoyt Memorial Children and Family Trust Fund and allotted Dias $8000 in 1998 and $11,000 in 1999 to initiate the program. The grant money was predominately used to purchase and distribute program materials to participating hospitals (Dias & Barthauer, 2001a).

By 2000, more funding was required to maintain and effectively coordinate the program. Dias applied for and received a much larger grant from the William B. Hoyt Memorial Children and Family Trust Fund. This new 4-year grant provided $132,000 each year for the first 2 years, followed by a decrease in funding to 50% and 25% of the original amount in the third and fourth year, respectively. The grant was intended to finance the operation of the existing program in Western New York and also to fund a major program expansion into the adjacent Finger Lakes Region. These additional finances enabled Dias to hire two nurse project coordinators, registered nurses Kim Smith and Kathy DeGuehery, to run the expanded program. With the anticipated involvement of 33 hospitals spanning the two regions, the total program budget reached over $450,000. The remaining funding needs were addressed by the Matthew Eappen Foundation, the Children's Hospital of Buffalo, Strong

Children's Hospital in Rochester, the State University of New York at Buffalo, the University of Rochester, and other participating hospitals in the form of various in-kind donations (Dias et al., 2005; Dias & Barthauer, 2001b).

The William B. Hoyt Memorial Children and Family Trust Fund continues to be a financial contributor to the Shaken Baby Syndrome Parent Education Program even as it adapted to the Safe Babies New York Program. In 2005, the Upstate Shaken Baby Syndrome Prevention Education Program was replicated and honored at the 15th National Conference on Child Abuse and Neglect for its strong commitment to the safety and well-being of children as an effective strategy for preventing shaken baby syndrome, having a total budget of $564,228 (Roach, 2005). Within the 2008 Trust Fund report, funds of $387,893 were allocated, while in 2011 there was $193,947 (Cuomo & Carrion, 2011; Paterson & Carrion, 2008). As of 2014, when the program changed to Safe Babies New York, Cuomo and Poole (2014) found that nurses engaged with over 100,000 families; therefore, funds of around $200,000 were allocated to Westchester Medical Center and Kaleida Health, a women and Children's Hospital of Buffalo.

34.2.1 Educational Materials

Program materials are to be distributed by obstetrical and neonatology nurses to all new parents during their postpartum stay in hospital. All mothers and as many fathers as possible would be presented with an information brochure from the Department of Health and the American Academy of Pediatrics that describes both SBS and safe sleep. It provides suggestions for coping with infant crying, describes the dangers of shaking an infant, and urges parents to seek immediate medical attention if they suspect that their child has been shaken. In addition, parents are to watch two videos: one on shaken baby ("Never Ever Shake a Baby") and one on safe sleep ("As Simple As: Alone, Back, Crib"). The former video discusses the dangers of violent infant shaking, describes the mechanism of shearing

brain injury, and portrays the stories of three infant victims of SBS, while the latter communicates how to lay a baby down to sleep in a safe environment. Finally, parents would be asked to voluntarily sign a commitment statement to verify that they received the program information. All materials are made available in English, Spanish, and Chinese and accessible through the Safe Babies New York Website (Dias et al., 2002).

In addition to providing a record of every parent's participation in the program, the commitment statement would ask parents several brief demographic questions regarding age, education level, marital status, insurance coverage, city of residence, and the zip code of the infant's primary residence. Parents would also be asked to answer the following three questions:

1. Was this information useful to you?
2. Was this the first time you've heard that shaking an infant is dangerous?
3. Would you recommend that this information be given to all new parents?

Nurses administering the materials were to sign the commitment statement to witness parents' receipt of the information, even when parents refused to sign the commitment statement themselves. The final source of information provided to parents would come from an educational poster ("Never, Never, Never, Never Shake a Baby," SBS Prevention Plus; Pueblo, CO). The posters were intended for display along the hallways of obstetrical wards, in full view of parents and outside visitors. Nurses would be encouraged to provide the information about SBS separately from other standard hospital discharge information (Dias & Barthauer, 2001a).

The inclusion of the commitment statement in the program design was a key improvement over virtually all other existing SBS prevention programs. The commitment statement was designed to accomplish two main objectives: (1) to actively engage parents in their own education about SBS and (2) to facilitate program data collection and tracking. By signing a commitment statement, parents would feel that they were entering a "social contract" with the hospital, their infant, and their community in protecting their child against SBS.

34.3 Implementation

From 1998 to 2000, Dias served as the sole program coordinator and principal investigator. He took responsibility for tracking new cases of SBS, building the program database, and fulfilling all program roles outside of those within each specific hospital. Participating hospitals were gradually phased into the program over the 2-year period. Most nurse managers were enthusiastic and cooperative in initiating the program in their hospitals. Within the first 2 months, all hospitals in Western New York were providing parents with the program materials. Collecting and returning signed commitment statements was set in place; however, it was a slower process to instill. From a logistical standpoint, smaller hospitals were able to embrace and implement the program more rapidly than larger centers, due to lower daily delivery rates and timely approval by hospital Institutional Review Boards. Dias found that personal contact with nurse managers was essential for establishing each hospital's commitment to the program and ensuring consistent participation from hospital staff.

In 2000, a survey of maternity nurses revealed that the program was virtually unanimously well received (Dias & Barthauer, 2001a). Nurses reported routinely providing program materials to new parents and having them sign the commitment statements. The video was being regularly shown in over half of the hospitals, and over 2/3 of participating hospitals were displaying the posters (Dias & Barthauer, 2001a). Feedback from parents was also very positive; over 90% claimed that they already knew about the dangers of shaking an infant but felt that the program information was helpful (Dias & Barthauer, 2001a). A total of 95% of parents that signed a commitment statement felt that SBS information should be provided to all new parents (Dias & Barthauer, 2001a). The exceedingly small proportion of parents who felt that the program

information was not helpful mostly perceived it to be redundant, while only 1% of parents refused to sign a commitment statement (Dias & Barthauer, 2001a).

34.3.1 Staff Roles and Responsibilities

The two principal investigators serve as overall program coordinators and oversee the data tracking within their respective regions. They also act as a valuable resource for staff regarding program innovations, troubleshooting, and the provision of feedback. Additionally, they supervise and communicate directly with the two project coordinators, who are responsible for the bulk of the administrative tasks associated with routine program operations. The project coordinators orchestrate the purchase, receipt, and delivery of all program materials to the hospitals and conduct obstetrical and perinatology nurse training sessions. Additionally, they communicate regularly with the nurse managers and assist them in tackling local logistical problems. They also monitor the monthly collection of signed commitment statements and maintain the program database. As active participants in the vigilant tracking of new SBS cases, project coordinators regularly contact hospitals, the media, and other child abuse professionals to identify new cases. They also conduct the 7-month follow-up phone calls, assist with the preparation of program data for statistical analysis, and provide program updates for a monthly newsletter distributed to all participating centers regarding ongoing concerns, progress reports, and project status. Finally, the project coordinators are public speakers and community advocates for the prevention of SBS, as requested by local public service groups, researchers, and other regions interested in replicating the program (Dias & Barthauer, 2001a).

On the on hand, every participating hospital has one nurse manager and a network of obstetrical and neonatal nurses that deliver the program to parents. The nurse managers are mainly responsible for the following:

1. Educating the maternity nurses about SBS and about how to implement the program.
2. Receiving and delivering all program materials.
3. Collecting and delivering all signed commitment statements from the maternity nurses to the project coordinators each month.
4. Providing the project coordinators with monthly delivery statistics to be used in future incidence rate calculations. Any logistical difficulties that arise are solved through direct communication with the project coordinators.

On the other hand, maternity ward nurses are trained to educate parents, distribute program materials, and collect signed commitment statements from a maximal number of parents, especially fathers if possible. They return signed commitment statements to the nurse managers for delivery to the project coordinators each month. These nurses are the "frontline" program workers, directly interacting with the target population and delivering the primary prevention information.

34.3.2 Expansion of the Program: The Finger Lakes Region Hospitals

Hospitals in the Finger Lakes Region were phased beginning in January 2001. Because the Finger Lakes Region shares many of the same population and geographical features as Western New York, the expansion effort did not require any major structural changes to the program. Strong Children's Hospital in Rochester is analogous to the Children's Hospital of Buffalo in that it is the sole tertiary referral center for pediatric neurosurgical cases in the region. A similar Perinatal Outreach Program was also in full operation; its staff network and hospital linkages were used to introduce and run the program. Dr. Linda Barthauer, a pediatrician specializing in child abuse from Strong Children's Hospital, was appointed to be the principal investigator (Dias & Barthauer, 2001b). The two new project coordi-

nators assumed many of the administrative roles that Dias had previously fulfilled.

During the expansion phase, the commitment statement was amended to include a request that parents' consent to receive a follow-up call 7 months after their infant's birth. The call was intended to assess parents' recollection of the information received in the hospital and to solicit program feedback. The timing of the follow-up call coincided with the midpoint in the peak incidence of SBS and was designed to test the hypothesis that parental retention of the program material could endure for a minimum of 7 months (Dias et al., 2002).

With the addition of the Finger Lakes Region, 35 hospitals in 20 counties would be participating in the program with over 35,000 families educated per year and over 120,000 families since its inception (Dias & Barthauer, 2001a). The following quantitative program performance goals were set at the outset of the expansion: (1) to establish a regional program including all counties in Western New York and the Finger Lakes Region, (2) to educate at least 70% of new parents about shaken baby syndrome prior to discharge from the hospital, and (3) to reduce and maintain the incidence rate of SBS in each region to 50% of the historical baseline figures, whereas qualitative program goals remained unchanged. All other aspects of the program, including staff infrastructure, program materials, and incidence-tracking strategies, were introduced in the same manner as in Western New York (Dias & Barthauer, 2001b).

34.3.3 Initial Feedback

The start-up period for the Finger Lakes Region hospitals was remarkably smooth. Within several months, nearly all hospitals were fully participating and returning commitment statements to the program office. The project coordinators were invaluable in ensuring consistent, open communication with nurse managers, diligently tracking returned commitment statements, and providing prompt assistance for hospital staff in tackling logistical hurdles. The smooth expansion can likely be attributed to two main factors: (1) the creation of the two nearly full-time project coordinator positions and (2) the demographic similarities shared by the two participating regions. The Finger Lakes Region program was just as well received as that in Western New York, and the program performance goals were consistently met. The 7-month follow-up questions provided valuable insight into parental retention of program information, and the feedback from parents was overwhelmingly positive. A survey of nurse managers in 2001 revealed that nearly every hospital was routinely providing brochures, posters, and commitment statements to parents (Dias et al., 2002). Most impressively, the project coordinators' persistent efforts in improving the percentages of returned commitment statements produced an increase in return rates from 46% in Western New York before 2001 to 77% from the combined Upstate New York program (Dias & Barthauer, 2001b).

34.4 Outcome

The program's impact on the annual incidence rate of SBS in Upstate New York was unprecedented. From 1998 to 2005, the average annual incidence of inflicted infant head injury decreased from 8.2 to 3.8 cases per year or from 41.5 cases per 100,000 live births to 22.2 cases per 100,000 live births (Dias et al., 2005). In just a 3-year period of the start of the program, all of Western New York had experienced a 47% drop in the incidence of SBS (Dias et al., 2005). Of the 21 infants that did incur shaking injuries during the study period, less than half of the parents participated in the program and signed a commitment statement. Preliminary data from the Finger Lakes Region in 2003 revealed that the number of reported cases of SBS had dropped by 41% (Dias et al., 2005; National Association of Children's Hospitals and Related Institutions [NACHRI], 2003). These results likely represent a minimum drop in incidence, due to the increased vigilance with which cases have been tracked during the program (Dias et al., 2002).

Other child abuse statistics suggest that the dramatic and temporal reduction in SBS cases in Western New York can be directly attributed to the Shaken Baby Syndrome Parent Education Program. The incidence rates of other forms of child maltreatment referred to the Children's Hospital of Buffalo remained stable throughout the duration of the program, and no congruent decline was observed in the number of cases of SBS reported in neighboring regions of New York State. Finally, a documented sharp decline in the incidence of SBS is not known to have occurred in any other region in the world at the time, as investigated by the Special Interest Group on Child Abuse (Dias et al., 2002). The results support the overall program hypothesis that a primary prevention program providing timely education about SBS to new parents can be effective in preventing inflicted infant head injury.

The returned commitment statements revealed that 93% of parents were previously aware of the dangers of shaking an infant. However, 95% still felt that SBS educational materials should be provided to all parents (Dias et al., 2005; Dias & Barthauer, 2001b). Over 90% of parents found the information helpful, regardless of their level of prior knowledge about SBS (Dias et al., 2005). These results support an additional program hypothesis—that most parents are already aware of SBS and merely need to be reminded at the right time to ensure their child's safety and protection.

The 7-month follow-up calls revealed that, without prompting, nearly one in three parents in Western New York recalled receiving information about SBS at their infant's birth hospital (Dias et al., 2002, 2005). When asked directly, 98% of parents remembered receiving the program information. The video was the least remembered component of the program, although a survey revealed that less than two thirds of hospitals regularly showed the video to parents (Dias et al., 2005). This information offers valuable guidance for improving the design of the Upstate New York program for replication in other jurisdictions and confirms that parents are retaining the program information for at least 7 months, during the period of highest risk for infant abuse.

34.4.1 Community Reactions

The success of the Upstate New York Shaken Baby Syndrome Education Program quickly earned the attention of both the media and state politicians. After the New York Times published an article about the program's successes in 2001, the project coordinators in Upstate New York were flooded with inquiries about the potential for program expansion to other regions (Foderaro, 2001). New York Assemblyman Sam Hoyt sponsored a bill stating that all new parents in New York State were to receive an informational leaflet detailing, "the effect of shaking infants and young children, appropriate ways to manage the causes of shaking infants and young children, and a discussion on how to reduce the risks of shaking infants and young children" (Lithco, 2004). As this was well received, several other states have introduced similar legislation.

Effective policy making has been said to require an "iron triangle": an effective lobbying organization, congressional "champions," such as Sam Hoyt, and inside help from a supportive bureaucracy (Krugman, 1999). Parent victims and healthcare workers in contact with shaken children have formed the most powerful lobby for the prevention of SBS in the United States, and it is encouraging that policy makers have been receptive to their efforts. With evidence supporting the effectiveness of a primary prevention program against SBS, politicians, healthcare providers, and affected families were eager to introduce Dias' program in their own jurisdictions.

34.4.2 Program Expansions

The program involves three distinct phases, including (1) a planning phase lasting from 6 to 9 months, (2) a start-up phase lasting 18–24 months, and (3) a maintenance phase beginning in the second year of the program. Tasks in the planning phase include establishing a staff network, eliciting program participation from hospitals, and obtaining approval from hospital Institutional Review Boards. During this phase, program materials are ordered, staff are hired/trained, and a program start date is set. Efforts are also made to establish the regional baseline incidence rate of shaken baby syndrome. In the start-up phase, the selected staff implement and coordinate the new program. This period is devoted to solving logistical problems, communicating regularly with hospital staff, and working diligently to achieve the program performance goals. The principal investigator is most active during the planning and start-up phases, campaigning for program support and acting as the ultimate contact person for fielding questions from hospital staff and professionals. After approximately 2 years, the maintenance phase begins. By this time, the program should be firmly established and consistently meeting targeted program performance goals. The role of the project coordinators shifts predominantly to involve data input, follow-up calling, incidence tracking, and public relations. The following are samples of the locations where the Upstate New York Shaken Baby Syndrome Parent Education Program was implemented.

34.4.2.1 Utah

The success of the Upstate New York Shaken Baby Syndrome Parent Education Program prompted a group of professionals from the Primary Children's Medical Centre, the National Centre on Shaken Baby Syndrome (NCSBS), and the University of Utah's Intermountain Injury Control and Research Centre to replicate it in Utah in 2000. The program was unique in being the first to receive joint funding from private healthcare insurers, Utah State agencies, and Medicaid (Herman et al., 2000). The format is nearly identical to that in Upstate New York, with the exception that parents are also offered additional materials from the NCSBS, including an information card about "The Period of Purple Crying" and a video called "Elijah's Promise." Three-month follow-up phone interviews were conducted to determine how much of the program information was retained by parents and what aspects of the program were most useful, and preliminary results suggest that the video was most remembered by parents (A. Wicks, personal communication, 2005).

34.4.2.2 Pennsylvania

In 2001, Dias relocated to Central Pennsylvania and personally spearheaded the Pennsylvania expansion effort. The new site was chosen based on its challenging demographic and healthcare system characteristics. Central Pennsylvania contains several major neurosurgical care centers with ill-defined referral patterns extending into neighboring states and regions. It also lacked a well-organized regional Perinatal Outreach Program. Central Pennsylvania offered an opportunity to test the effectiveness and applicability of the Upstate New York Shaken Baby Syndrome Parent Education Program in a region lacking a centralized healthcare system (Dias et al., 2002).

The program began in 2002 with funding from the Pennsylvania Commission on Crime and Delinquency and the Children's Miracle Network (Dias et al., 2002; NACHRI, 2003). All operational design aspects of the program remained unchanged, with one exception. The Central Pennsylvania Shaken Baby Syndrome Education Program formed a partnership with the Pennsylvania Department of Children, Youth, and Families, which maintains a state-wide database of reported child abuse cases (Dias et al., 2002). This registry has the ability to track cases of inflicted infant head injury according to the county in which the abuse took place. This specificity is advantageous for tracking cases in a decentralized region, where it is possible for infants born in Central Pennsylvania hospitals to receive treatment in outlying regions. The database can also query cases based on several other location characteristics, including birth county, enabling the project coordinators to isolate and identify new cases arising specifically from the Central Pennsylvania region.

Legislation was passed in 2002 mandating the provision of SBS prevention materials to parents of newborns in all hospitals in Pennsylvania (NACHRI, 2003). Dias' program had been exclusively operating in Central Pennsylvania, but after the legislation was introduced, all 130 hospitals in the state were required to participate. Although the full program had only been running for 1.5 years, the project coordinators had achieved an 85% commitment statement return rate, and 125 hospitals were fully participating in all aspects of the program (C. Rotman, personal communication, 2005). The Pennsylvania governor, the Pennsylvania State University College of Medicine, the Pennsylvania Children's Partnership, and several other state and regional child welfare agencies strongly support the program (Dias et al., 2002). With academic, governmental, and community endorsement, it represents a multi-institutional partnership that embraces the concepts of collaboration and cooperation in reducing child maltreatment.

34.4.2.3 Minnesota

In 2002, the Children's Hospitals and Clinics in Minneapolis formed a task force of local experts to bring the Shaken Baby Syndrome Parent Education Program to Minnesota. Program materials were translated into several languages, including Hmong, Russian, Spanish, and Somali, to cater to the ethnic diversity of the target population. Efforts to determine the preexisting incidence rate of SBS in the region were undertaken by the Minnesota Department of Health, funded in part by a grant from the Centers for Disease Control and Prevention (NACHRI, 2003).

34.4.2.4 Ohio

Dias' program was launched in 2002 in Columbus, Ohio, by an enthusiastic group of volunteers from the Ohio chapter of the National Council of Jewish Women. Initial funding came from the Ohio Children's Trust Fund. In addition to the standard program materials, parents receive a gift bag containing educational fridge magnets, baby bibs, and brochures with the "Love Me, Never Shake Me" and "The Period of Purple Crying" slogans from the NCSBS (NACHRI, 2003; L. Carroll, personal communication, August 2005). A media awareness campaign and community outreach component complement the hospital-based program. People in local correctional facilities, public schools, home visitor programs, and teen parenting agencies also receive information about SBS. Incarcerated women have even participated in the design, assembly, and distribution of program materials to Ohio hospitals. This unique initiative aims to empower the women to make a positive contribution to the society and to educate them about SBS, while simultaneously creating a supply of program materials. Some hospitals in Ohio have placed the provision of program materials on the hospital discharge nursing summary sheet. On-going funding for the Ohio program has come from state agencies, the Ohio Attorney General, and private foundations, although program leaders have also focused on empowering parents and members of the local community to take an active role in preventing shaken baby syndrome.

34.4.2.5 New York State

The Upstate New York region has truly paved the way for other states to expand their shaken baby syndrome education to new parents and caregivers. The program in New York has also been updated and expanded from its original foundation. Currently, at every infant's first visit to pediatric care providers, parents are given advice regarding how to cope with infant crying and are reminded of the dangers of infant shaking, in addition to signing a second commitment statement (Dias et al., 2005). It is hoped that the repeated information will help parents responsibly cope with the stresses of infant care and, ultimately, further reduce the incidence rate of shaken baby syndrome.

34.4.2.6 Other Additions

The Shaken Baby Syndrome Parent Education Program has been introduced to other regions as well such as the Grand Rapids, Michigan, and Phoenix, Arizona (NACHRI, 2003). At the start, both states did not have legislation mandating the provision of program materials and had encountered difficulties in establishing the baseline incidence rate of SBS. In Arizona, severe nursing staff shortages and liability concerns had prevented the formation of a hospital-based program, and so program materials were delivered primarily through private physician's offices and parent education classes (NACHRI, 2003). The commitment statements had also been omitted from the program. While information about SBS is likely valuable in any context, the lack of program centralization in the birthing hospitals and

the omission of the commitment statement significantly alter the nature of the program and limit the capacity for evaluation.

This program has also been looked at as a template for implementation internationally. In Ontario, Canada, the University of Toronto and the Ontario Neurotrauma Foundation have collaborated to implement the Shaken Baby Syndrome Parent Education Program in a variety of different hospitals and within community-based settings. The integration of the program in Ontario was divided into three phases: the planning phase; the implementation phase, where participating project sites administer the education to parents and families; and the maintenance phase, where sustainability issues are addressed and program refreshers are administered (Volpe et al., 2009). Each program site has a coordinator, which was often a nurse, to oversee the research in their community, and to reach a variety of different personnel, a website was developed and can be reached at http://legacy.oise.utoronto.ca/research/ONF-SBSPrevention/index.htm. In a study done by Volpe et al. (2009), it was found that participants from six different sites implementing the program in Ontario and completed a commitment form, 96.53% of them found the information to be helpful, and 98.99% indicated that the information should be provided to all new parents. Out of those six sites, 6.5% of respondents reported that the SBS education provided to them was the first time they had heard of inflicted infant head trauma. Upon follow-up (at 6- and 12-month postpartum), participants were asked if they remembered the information provided to them (see Table 34.1) and questions regarding supplementary education and dissemination of SBS information (see Table 34.2; Volpe et al., 2009). Overall, the SBS program in Ontario has replicated the original hospital-based work in Upstate New York and extended those findings to include community-based work. There have even been replications of the SBS program in Australia that have shown remarkable results. The Shaken Baby Prevention Project in Western Sydney was implemented by the Westmead Children's Hospital in 2002 and revealed that those who

Table 34.1 Participant memory of SBS education

	Hospital-based sites	Community-based sites	Total
Do you remember receiving care of child info?	96.02%	94.07%	95.18%
Do you remember receiving SBS info?	98.54%	93.34%	96.31%
Do you remember receiving a healthcare professional talk about SBS?	87.59%	94.16%	90.40%
Do you remember receiving SBS materials?	92.27%	92.18%	92.23%
Do you remember the video?	89.33%	91.78%	90.38%
Do you remember the consent form?	61.48%	67.41%	64.02%
Do you remember an SBS posters?	55.13%	68.27%	60.76%
Did you receive [site specific] info?	50.08%	64.82%	56.39%
Do you remember signing the form?	94.62%	91.74%	93.38%

Note: All responses indicate percentages of respondents replying "yes" (Volpe et al., 2009)

received education not only recalled the information in times of stress but also communicated their knowledge to other caregivers in their home environment (Tasar et al., 2014).

34.5   Conclusion

The Safe Babies New York/Western New York Shaken Baby Syndrome Parent Education Program has emerged as an exemplary practice in the prevention of inflicted infant head injuries. The program is fully operational in several states and is expanding into other areas such as Canada and Australia. It has been well-received by the public, the media, healthcare workers, governments, and public and private institutions and funding agencies. It has the potential to be successfully implemented in regions with varying demographic characteristics, provided that the

Table 34.2 Supplementary education and dissemination of SBS information

	Hospital-based sites	Community-based sites	Total
Did you receive SBS materials after leaving the hospital?	31.34%	49.17%	38.98%
Did you receive SBS information from your doctor?	23.79%	41.75%	31.48%
If the baby's father/father-figure is living in the home, did he receive information on SBS in the hospital?	94.51%	72.11%	84.91%
If the baby's father/father-figure is not living in the home, did you share the SBS information with him?	81.49%	80.40%	81.02%
Do you ever leave your baby in care of another adult?	73.98%	80.50%	76.77%
Have you shared SBS information with your caregivers?	47.39%	65.56%	55.18%

Note: All responses indicate percentages of respondents replying "yes" (Volpe et al., 2009)

necessary financial and professional resources are available.

The original goals developed by Dias in 1998 remain outlined as components of the program. These goals include the following: (1) the program is universally applied, operating in all maternity care hospitals within a given region; (2) information is consistently provided to parents at the same point in time—in the hospital, following the birth of their child; (3) the participation of fathers and father figures is actively sought, even though program materials are presented to both parents; (4) the commitment statements engage parents in their own educational process and instill in them a sense of responsibility and commitment toward preventing shaken baby syndrome; (5) the dissemination of program materials is effectively tracked using the returned commitment statements; (6) the 7-month follow-up calls provide research data on parents' recollection and retention of program information; and (7) clearly defined, quantifiable outcome measures enable staff to assess the effectiveness of the program (Dias et al., 2002).

The available evidence demonstrates that this simple program saves infant lives, and conveniently, it also has the potential to save money. Cost-benefit analyses have strongly indicated that the costs of preventing SBS are far less than the costs of treating shaken infants. Dias estimates that the overall program costs are equivalent to $10 USD per child, which is comparable to the cost of routine childhood immunizations. The program expenditures could be reclaimed if the average cost of caring for injured infants was $21,925 per child per year, which is well within published estimates (Dias et al., 2005).

While Dias' program is the first to demonstrate a quantifiable decrease in the incidence rate of SBS, the challenges in producing this evidence cannot be overemphasized as there has been minimal improvement in the area of child maltreatment surveillance. Although the International Classification of Diseases finally introduced a specific code for shaken infant syndrome in 1996, it is largely underutilized and unknown, resulting in a persistent underestimation of the magnitude of the problem (SBS, 2005). Until centralized surveillance systems are functional, regions aiming to effectively prevent SBS will continue to encounter incredible difficulties in establishing baseline incidence rates of inflicted infant head injuries. Without this data, the long-term impact of these programs will remain unknown.

Inadequate financial support has also been a critical factor, limiting program dissemination to other regions (Dias et al., 2002). Public interest and demand far outstrip available funding opportunities. Even existing programs have been unable to secure long-term funding to ensure program sustainability. States such as Pennsylvania are at risk of being in a future position where program provision is required by law, but funding is inadequate to support program operations. As evidence for the program's effectiveness mounts, it is hoped that the challenges of obtaining financial backing will diminish. Increased participation from private health insurers appears to be a realistic hope for the near future, with the Utah and New York programs currently benefiting from this innovative partnership. Health insurance companies stand to save a significant amount of money by funding the program, and it is hoped that they continue to recognize the financial and social value of their support in the future.

The following are two key factors that have been identified for successful program replication: (1) finding capable project coordinators and (2) maintaining a manageable pace of program implementation. Kim Smith and Kathy DeGuehery's consistent, enthusiastic, competent leadership has been vital to the long-term success of the Upstate New York program. The importance of these qualities in project staff cannot be overemphasized. Regions that have encountered the greatest difficulties in program implementation have either lacked devoted, experienced project coordinators or have attempted to introduce the program at an unsustainable pace.

The success of the original program has been enthusiastically embraced, but the replication process has been partial, undermining the evidence for the program. Many new regions adopting the program have failed to incorporate a research component into the planning, startup, and maintenance program phases. To benefit from the proven effect of this exemplary practice in the prevention of SBS, program leaders should strive to uphold the evaluation component to facilitate accurate assessment of the program's applicability and efficacy in a variety of social contexts. Rather than rest on the laurels of the success in Upstate New York, program coordinators must persist in effectively educating parents about SBS by assessing the value of their innovations in terms of its impact on the incidence rate of this tragic form of abuse. The program is unique in its proven effectiveness and can only evolve into an optimally transportable, efficacious entity with a continuous commitment to evaluation and innovation.

It is encouraging to note a progression toward increasingly evidence-informed endeavors in the field of SBS prevention. Having a variety of published studies that embody different approaches to primary prevention in the field of SBS will certainly stimulate future research and raise the bar on the standard of prevention work currently being conducted. One example of this is the important joint initiative between researchers in Washington State, United States, and British Columbia, Canada. Barr et al. (2009) undertook the first randomized controlled trial in the primary prevention of shaken baby syndrome. This study compared the effectiveness of delivering parent education materials in various healthcare settings including hospital delivery wards, pediatricians' offices, and prenatal classes (US National Institute of Health, 2005). Barr's approach to prevention focused on the normalization of persistent infant crying and on encouraging parents to develop effective coping strategies to deal with the feelings of low self-efficacy, depression, and frustration that can be associated with infant crying. His materials about the "Period of PURPLE crying" describe the timing and characteristics of persistent infant crying behavior. It was found that those who used the PURPLE education materials seemed to lead to higher scores in knowledge about early infant crying and the dangers of shaking and in sharing of information behaviors considered to be important for the prevention of shaking (Barr et al., 2009).

Given the success of the Safe Babies New York: Upstate New York Shaken Baby Syndrome Parent Education Program, it is anticipated that regions across North America will continue to embrace and deliver this highly effective primary prevention program to all new parents. Its goal to reduce child abuse is universally applauded, and the fact that it has produced valid, quantifiable results is immensely promising. If the efficacy of the program can be established in a variety of social venues, it is both desirable and possible for this program to capture the attention of health departments and professionals around the world and be incorporated into routine postpartum hospital visits. Clearly, the evidence suggests that it is possible to prevent this devastating form of child abuse using a simple and comprehensive parent education program.

Acknowledgments The author would like to express sincere appreciation to the key informants for this case study—Mark S. Dias of the Penn State University; Milton S. Hershey Medical Centre in Hershey, PA, USA; Kim Smith of Upstate New York in Buffalo, NY, USA; and Kathy DeGuehery of Upstate New York in Buffalo, NY, USA—whose consultation made this project possible.

BRIO Model: Safe Babies New York: The Upstate New York Shaken Baby Syndrome (SBS) Education Program

Group Served: Parents and caregivers of newborns.

Goal: To educate parents about the normalcy of infant crying, the dangers of violent infant shaking, how to calm a crying infant and reduce caregiver frustration and anger, and how to wisely select other caregivers for the infant in order to reduce the frequency of abusive head trauma.

Background	Resources	Implementation	Outcome
95% of severe neurotrauma cases in infants less than 1 year of age are the result of nonaccidental causes Initial in-patient hospitalization costs for the care of a shaken infant can approach $70,000 USD, $300,000 for the next 5 years, and in excess of $1 million over long term for one shaken infant	Funding from grants and participating hospitals provided more than 450 $US in funds and in-kind donations Educational material developed from Dr. Dias' own research Program materials were to be distributed by obstetrical and neonatology nurses to all new parents during their postpartum stay	Hospitals in different areas phased in the program overtime and made adaptations to fit their environment Project coordinators work with nurse managers to distribute and collect project material and data Maternity ward nurses trained to deliver program material Parents asked to confirm receiving materials and to commit to follow-up phone call about materials	The average annual incidence of inflicted infant neurotrauma has decreased from 7.0 to 2.2 cases per year Other child abuse statistics suggest that the dramatic and temporal drop in SBS cases in Western New York can be directly attributed to the Shaken Baby Syndrome Education Program Replication in Central Pennsylvania

Life Space Model: Safe Babies New York: The Upstate New York Shaken Baby Syndrome (SBS) Education Program

Sociocultural: civilization/community	Interpersonal: primary and secondary relationships	Physical environments: where we live	Internal states: biochemical/genetic and means of coping
Educational materials to all Western New York parents of newborns Involvement of community nurses, public health, and hospitals	Create expectation that the parenting relationship will act as protective system Strengthening parenting relationships and caregiver to child relations	Address the implications of sound as a source of stress Identifying and educating caregivers about unsafe sleeping environments	Parental commitment statement acknowledging education about SBS Follow-up calls to refresh coping mechanisms

References

Barr, R. G., Rivara, F. P., Barr, M., Cummings, P., Taylor, J., & Lengua, L. J. (2009). Effectiveness of educational materials designed to change knowledge and behaviors regarding crying and shaken-baby syndrome in mothers of newborns: A randomized, controlled trial. *Pediatrics, 123*(3), 972–980.

California Evidence-Based Clearinghouse. (2016). *Safe babies New York program.* San Francisco, CA: Author. Retrieved 2017, from http://www.cebc4cw.org/program/the-upstate-new-york-shaken-baby-syndrome-education-program/detailed

Cuomo, A. M., & Carrion, G. (2011). *Looking upstream: New York State Children and Family Trust Fund, 2011 Annual report.* New York, NY: New York State Office of Children and Family Services.

Cuomo, A. M., & Poole, S. J. (2014). *William B. Hoyt Memorial Children and Family Trust Fund 2014, Annual report.* New York, NY: New York State Office of Children and Family Services.

Dias, M. S., Backstom, J., Falk, M., & Li, V. (1998). Serial radiography in the infant shaken impact syndrome. *Pediatric Neurosurgery, 27,* 77–85.

Dias, M. S., & Barthauer, L. (2001a). *The infant shaken impact syndrome: A parent education campaign in Upstate New York (First Year Summary).* Unpublished manuscript, State University of New York at Buffalo and University of Rochester School of Medicine.

Dias, M. S., & Barthauer, L. (2001b). *Western New York/Finger Lakes regional shaken baby education project.* Unpublished grant application to William B. Hoyt Memorial Children and Family Trust Fund.

Dias, M. S., Mazur, P., Li, V., Smith, K., & DeGuehery, K. (2002). *Preventing shaken baby syndrome: A hospital based parent education program.* Manuscript submitted for publication, State University of New York at Buffalo.

Dias, M. S., Smith, K., DeGuehery, K., Mazur, P., Li, V., & Shaffer, M. L. (2005). Preventing abusive head trauma among infants and young children: A hospital-based parent education program. *Pediatrics, 115,* 470–477.

Foderaro, L. W. (2001). A simple hospital video may prevent shaken baby syndrome. *The New York Times,* B1.

Herman, B., Corwin, D., Sandberg, M., Olson, L., Bradshaw, J., & Brechlin, T. (2000). *Preventing shaken baby syndrome in Utah: Replication and evaluation of a promising program to reduce the incidence and associated medical cost of shaken babies.* Unpublished program proposal.

Krugman, R. (1999). The politics. *Child Abuse and Neglect, 23*(10), 963–967.

Lewandowski, J. (1999). Dias works to prevent shaken babies. *University at Buffalo Reporter, 31*(8). Retrieved July 5, 2002, from http://www.buffalo.edu/reporter/vol31/vol31n8/n4.html

Lithco, G. (2004). *Testimony concerning the establishment of a statewide shaken baby syndrome education and prevention program.* Submitted to the New York State Senate Task Force on Children's Health Safety.

National Association of Children's Hospitals and Related Institutions. (2003). *Children's hospitals at the frontlines confronting child abuse and neglect. A simple model, a vital purpose: Preventing shaken baby syndrome.* Alexandria, VA: Author.

Paterson, D. A., & Carrion, G. (2008). *New York State Children and Family Trust Fund: Annual report.* New York, NY: New York State Office of Children and Family Services.

Roach, T. (2005). *New York State Children and Family Trust Fund 1984-2005. Supporting children, adults, caregivers, and the elderly to live free of violence strengthening families through prevention.* New York, NY: New York State Office of Children and Family Services.

Shaken Baby Syndrome. (2005). *Surveillance in Massachusetts.* Retrieved July 13, 2005, from http://www.sbscentralmass.com/MoreInformation.html

Tasar, M. A., Sahin, F., Polat, S., Ilhan, M., Camurdan, A., & Dallar, Y. (2014). Long-term outcomes of the shaken baby syndrome prevention program: Turkey's experience. *Turkish Archives of Pediatrics, 49*(3), 203–209.

U.S. National Institute of Health. (2005). *Prevention of Shaken baby syndrome.* Bethesda, MD: Author. Retrieved July 17, 2005, from http://www.clinicaltrials.gov/ct/show/NCT00105963

Volpe, R., Davidson, C., Sheard, E., Bell, R., & Members of the University of Toronto Research Coordinator Unit. (2009). *Preventing inflicted infant head trauma: A best practice implementation. Life span adaptation projects.* Toronto, ON: University of Toronto. Retrieved from http://legacy.oise.utoronto.ca/research/ONF-SBSPrevention/documents/SBSRPTFIN18JN09PH1.pdf

New Zealand Injury Prevention Strategy

35

Daria Smeh and Nick Bonokoski

The New Zealand Injury Prevention Strategy's vision was for New Zealand to become injury free by achieving a positive safety culture and creating safe environments. This strategy focused on the areas of drowning, the workplace, motor vehicle crashes, suicide/self-harm, falls, and assault. Its implementation provided a "framework for injury prevention policy development and services delivery activities" as facilitated by the feedback provided from government agencies, local government, nongovernment organizations, communities, and individuals involved in program development (Safe Communities Foundation of New Zealand, p. 4).

35.1 Background

The idea to develop a national injury prevention strategy was created based on two major factors. First, the views and comments made in the injury prevention sector between 1999 and 2001 informed the need for a nationwide strategy. In fact, not only did the Associate Ministers of Accident Insurance realize the need, but researchers also underscored the importance for a more coordinated approach and the necessity to build capacity and capability if a major improvement in New Zealand's injury prevention performance

was to be seen. Initial ideas for the nationalized strategy were informed by the experiences to improve road safety in which several central government agencies (i.e., Ministries of Transport, NZ Police, Land Transport NZ, Transit NZ, and ACC) combined their efforts to develop road safety enforcement, education, and engineering initiatives (G. Wilson, personal communication, January 7, 2008).

Second, the development of the New Zealand Injury Prevention Strategy (NZIPS) was informed by the election of a labor-led coalition government in late 1999, who intended to re-nationalize the accident compensation scheme in New Zealand. Subsequent to their election, amendments were made to legislation for the accident compensation scheme with an emphasis that injury prevention would become a key focus for the Accident Compensation Corporation (ACC). The party's platform also complemented the views emerging from the injury prevention sector and contributed to the ideological momentum to develop the NZIPS (G. Wilson, personal communication, January 7, 2008).

35.1.1 Emergence of New Zealand Injury Prevention Strategy

Planning for the NZIPS began in 2001 and continued until implementation in 2004 (G. Wilson, personal communication, January 7, 2008). It primarily

D. Smeh (✉) · N. Bonokoski
LoyalTeam Environmental, Toronto, ON, Canada

© Springer Nature Switzerland AG 2020
R. Volpe (ed.), *Casebook of Traumatic Injury Prevention*,
https://doi.org/10.1007/978-3-030-27419-1_35

involved Hon. Ruth Dyson and Hon. Lianne Dalziel and Associate Minister for the ACC in 2001, the two NZIPS program champions, who observed extensive work in injury prevention by many local community agencies prior to the formation of the NZIPS. In addition to improving involvement of communities and agencies, the Associate Ministers aimed to identify the inadequacies in the existing system (see Table 35.1) in order to understand what would impact the efficacy and sustainability of injury prevention initiatives in place at the time (C. Coggan, personal communication, July 25, 2007). By identifying the four deficiencies of the existing injury prevention initiatives, the program champions were able to ensure that lessons were learned from past experience and a reformed approached was included within the NZIPS.

The NZIPS was also grounded in the philosophy of the Haddon's Matrix which is the interaction between agents and factors during pre-event, event, and post-event, explaining injury and their prevention. It was adopted as a strategy as its implementation plan was targeted to address risk of injury pre-event, event, and post-event and encouraged an understanding of the host, agent/vehicle, physical environment, and social environment of where injury takes place. By addressing injury risk at every stage and understanding the environment in which injury risk takes place,

the NZIPS was able to promote sustainable and effective injury prevention by using a combination of intervention approaches (Haddon, 1972).

However, the collaborators subsequently worked together to reformulate the first draft of the NZIPS as it was seen to rely too heavily on the Haddon Matrix theory. The vision in the original draft was incongruent with the vision and mission of some of the stakeholders involved. Thus, changes to the NZIPS were agreed upon in this respect. Additionally, the government felt that the financial commitment required to implement the first draft was unrealistic and unfeasible (C. Coggan, personal communication, July 10, 2007). Ultimately, the NZIPS was seen to be more likely to be sustained if stakeholders were willing to modify it to the needs of the partners.

35.1.2 Flexibility Model

Flexibility for and adaptability of stakeholders was recognized as highly important from the outset of the development process. In fact, stakeholder collaboration was grounded in a "flexi-model" (or approach) and a range of criteria for its success (see Fig. 35.1). The flexi-model encourages the interaction between skilled, passionate, and dedicated local and regional coordi-

Table 35.1 Deficiencies in New Zealand's injury prevention approach and lessons learned

Deficiency in previous efforts	Lesson learned
Fragmentation of effort Broad range of involvement by multiple injury prevention agencies and organizations could translate into inconsistent messages and unnecessary duplication of effort	Injury prevention activity needed to be integrated through coordination and collaboration between government agencies and other organizations
Gaps in injury prevention activity Some important injury issues had attracted limited attention relative to their impact (e.g., fall prevention and drowning prevention), while some coverage in certain areas was patchy. For example, New Zealand had a Youth Suicide Prevention Strategy, but lacked a cross-sectoral suicide prevention strategy covering all age groups	National strategies have been outlined to define where coverage took place; however, a lot of work had to be done to implement these new strategies
Workforce capability issues Injury prevention workforce was diverse, often isolated, and has limited access to training opportunities	Capability of the injury prevention workforce needed to be strengthened
Quality of, access to, and dissemination of injury information Dissemination is fragmented; overall access to and type of data collected needed to be improved	A need for better, more accessible and improved dissemination of injury data and information on injury prevention activity must be met

Note: Government of New Zealand (n.d.-e)

Fig. 35.1 Flexi-model established to enhance collaboration and coordination (GNZ, n.d.-c)

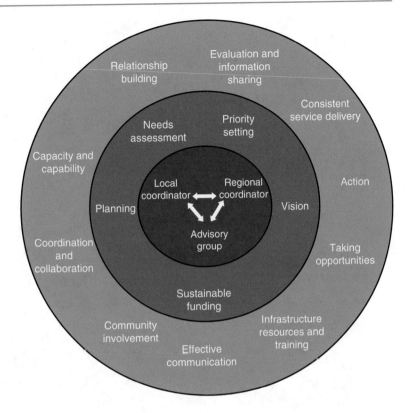

nators and experts, as well as connected and well-informed advisory group with a strong needs-assessment process, sustainable funding, sound infrastructure, expert capability and capacity, information sharing, and evaluation. Recognizing and incorporating stakeholders early ensures community buy-in and ownership (Government of New Zealand [GNZ], n.d.-c).

Feedback was incorporated through consultation with stakeholders across the injury prevention sector including researchers and practitioners, as well as local and central government and communities throughout all of New Zealand. With the efforts to organize the NZIPS during the initial stages of planning by two program champions in well-placed positions in government, the NZIPS was able to become well established and entrenched within a variety of sectors around the country that required interventions. That is, individuals in positions of power at the senior level in government, Hon. Dyson and Hon. Dalziel, were able to legalize the NZIPS. Furthermore, they worked tirelessly, amicably, and openly with stakeholders to realize

legalization and develop the foundation of the program. Hon. Dyson became Minister for ACC in August 2002 and retained a strong interest and support to address the successful implementation and evolution of NZIPS (G. Wilson, personal communication, January 31, 2008).

35.1.3 Vision, Goals, Objectives, and Principles of NZIPS

Since its development, the vision, objectives, and goals of the NZIPS were established (see Fig. 35.2). The NZIPS integrated sustainability into the goals and objectives of their strategy, with initiatives developed and implemented specifically to foster that sustainability (Shediac-Rizkallah & Bone, 1998). Moreover, not only were the objectives, goals, and strategies developed considering sustainability to ensure success in the long-term, but the NZIPS was also developed to account for deficiencies in main parts of the injury prevention approach utilized in the past.

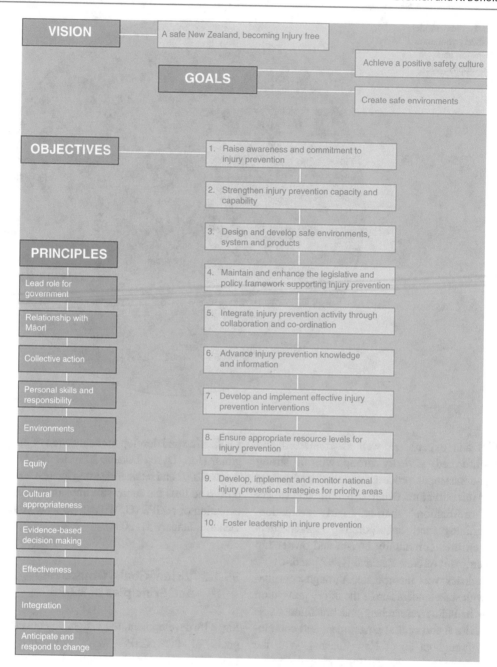

Fig. 35.2 The NZIPS vision, goals, objectives, and principles (Government of New Zealand [GNZ], 2004a)

35.2 Resources

Among stakeholders, responsibilities were delegated in accordance with the injury prevention area relevant to each specific government department, agency, or ministry (e.g., workplace injury under the guide of the Department of Labor, advocacy of legislation guided by governmental and nongovernmental agencies, approval of legislation under the authority of governmental agencies) (G. Wilson, personal communication, January 14, 2008).

Overall, there are 12 key agencies that contributed financially to injury prevention initiatives under NZIPS, some having a lead role involving substantial budgets, while others have smaller contributory roles with smaller budgets (G. Wilson, personal communication, January 7, 2008).

35.2.1 Human Resources

At the time of development, the national government assembled governmental agencies to oversee decision making and assemble stakeholders to be involved in the formation of the NZIPS, including the following:

- The NZIPS Secretariat (which was made up of four staff within the ACC's Strategic Policy and Research Group)
- The Stakeholder Reference Group (22 members formed to ensure input from a variety of governmental and nongovernmental agencies and organizations within the field of injury prevention in New Zealand)
- The Expert Advisory Panel (assembled group of academics and experts in the injury prevention field whose role was to complete an outcome evaluation, which quantified injury rates and fatalities, and to deliberate the potential methods that could be used to measure safety culture and safe environments; GNZ, 2004a)
- The Government Interagency Steering Group (comprised of 13 representatives of government agencies who possessed responsibilities and interests in injury prevention)

The key stakeholders and governance structure and general information flows and communication channels is demonstrated through Fig. 35.3.

Formal leadership within governmental sectors was allocated to the agencies based on the priority areas of NZIPS. Examples are as follows:

- ACC (NZIPS Secretariat) was responsible for administering the NZIPS.
- Assault (family violence and community violence) was under the Ministries of Social Development and Justice.

- Motor vehicle traffic crashes were under the leadership of the Ministry of Transport.
- Falls prevention and drowning prevention were the responsibilities of the ACC Injury Prevention Group.
- Suicide prevention was under the direction of the Ministry of Health.

In addition to existing government agencies, nongovernmental organizations, sector interest groups, community organizations, the research community, industry, and the general public were consulted to develop the NZIPS. These stakeholders include community agencies from all over the country, and the role that they played was informed by the nature of each organization's aims and funding requirements. For example, the Injury Prevention Network Association of New Zealand (IPNANZ) provided support and leadership for individual injury prevention practitioners, while the Safe Communities Foundation NZ provided leadership to community organizations and local government. Researchers such as the Injury Prevention Research Unit at Otago University and the Auckland University School of Population Health had consistently provided leadership through knowledge and dissemination of research findings. Overall, many of the nongovernmental organizations that were central to the planning of the NZIPS still play critical roles in its evolution and implementation.

35.2.1.1 Accident Compensation Corporation's Role

As discussed earlier, the ACC played a particularly central role as it was financially responsible for compensating injured people. Their collaboration with agencies and the national government was considered pivotal over the lifespan of the strategy, its implementation, and evaluation. The ACC administered New Zealand's accident compensation scheme, which supplied personal injury coverage for all New Zealand citizens, residents, and temporary visitors to the country. As this system is available, people do not have the right to sue for personal injury, other than for exemplary damages. The ACC is a crown (or governmental) entity that is responsible for the following:

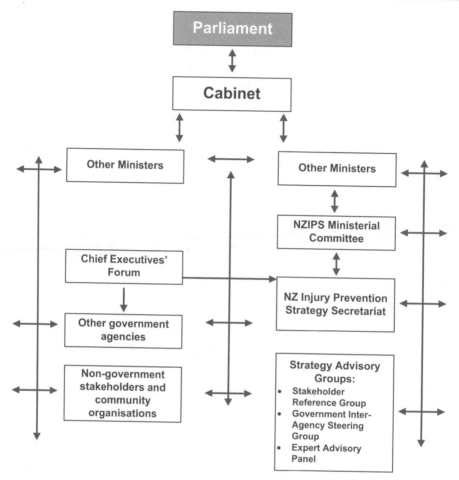

Fig. 35.3 Key Stakeholders and governance structure and general information flows and communication channels (Government of New Zealand, n.d.-g)

- Preventing injury
- Collecting personal injury cover levies
- Determining whether claims for injury are covered by the scheme and providing entitlements to those who are eligible
- Paying compensation
- Buying health and disability support services to treat, care for, and rehabilitate injured people
- Advising the government
- Providing accident coverage, injury prevention services, case management, medical and other care, and rehabilitation services

The NZIPS was led by the ACC through the NZIPS Secretariat, which operated within the Corporation's Strategic Policy & Research Group (Allen, & Clarke Policy and Regulatory Specialists Ltd, Gribble, Mortimer, & Smith, 2006). The ACC specifically partnered with government agencies, such as the Department of Labor, ministries of health, justice, social development, and transport, and community agencies to formulate approaches for the six injury areas (Accident Compensation Corporation, 2007b). The ACC also used their authority to bring stakeholders together and be actively involved as a stakeholder itself. For example, in January 2006, the ACC convened the Implementation Management Group (IMG), made up of the ACC and several regional and water safety agencies; as a result, they devised the Drowning Prevention

Strategy's Implementation Plan 2007–2011 (Accident Compensation Corporation, 2007a).

Dr. Keith McLea, director of injury prevention at the ACC, specifically acted on behalf of the NZIPS project team between 2001 and 2002 to mobilize government support and facilitate community ownership and buy-in into the proposed strategy within the six national priority areas (K. McLea, personal communication, April 26, 2007). In August 2006, McLea was appointed as General Manager Levy and Scheme Management in the ACC. McLea acted as a strong source of support for the secretariat and labeled a champion for the NZIPS (Injury Prevention News [IP News], 2006).

35.2.1.2 Collaboration

To ensure high-level leadership for the NZIPS and to promote government agency coordination in injury prevention, Hon. Dyson established an Injury Prevention Ministerial Committee, which first met in April 2006. Coggan (personal communication, July 10, 2007) attended this meeting and reported that "seven ministers showed up to the first meeting; they were engaged in the committee work and they were collaboration-focused," producing productive and positive outcomes. The work of the ministerial committee strengthened through the establishment of a Chief Executives' Forum made up of Chief Executives from ACC and the other agencies that have lead responsibilities under NZIPS, covering road safety, workplace, falls prevention, drowning prevention, assault, and suicide. The forum was established in February 2006 and provides a focus on improving alignment of activities by government agencies in each of the strategy's priority areas. Proactive actions by the development agencies, as well as the response from the collaborative agencies, demonstrated a continual interest to commit to the objectives of NZIPS. On a broader scale, a continual renewal and openness to increase stakeholder accountability within the NZIPS enhanced the quality, type, constancy, and continuity of a top-down and bottom-up flow of information among all stakeholders. Ultimately, improved dialogue with the upper level government officials led to

more secure funding, while improved interaction at the community level encouraged buy-in, education, awareness, and strong positive perceptions about the NZIPS initiatives.

According to Coggan (personal communication, July 10, 2007), the formation of the strategy and its implementation plan was a "real community focused approach." She admitted to being "surprised" and "pleased" at the large number of people who attended the consultation meetings during the development stage of NZIPS and the over 70 written submissions that were received during the consultative meetings, suggesting changes to the NZIPS. McLea (personal communication, April 26, 2007) described the process of communication to develop the strategy and facilitate implementation as "fluid" because the stakeholders were continuously engaged in a dialogue until all of the collaborators came to an agreement. In addition, Coggan (personal communication, July 10, 2007) describes consultation for the strategy eventually bringing "all facets of injury under one umbrella," which strongly encouraged "government departments to talk to each other"— an important aspect of a collaborative effort toward injury prevention on such a grand scale.

35.2.2 Financial Resources

Financial support was crucial to facilitate the development of the NZIPS and to provide avenues and venues for relationships to form. Some of the funds dedicated by the GNZ to the development and implementation of NZIPS are outlined in Table 35.2.

Each agency working to implement the plans of the NZIPS was allocated a specific budget to fulfill their responsibilities. For example, the NZIPS Secretariat (within ACC) was funded from

Table 35.2 Funding issued to implement the NZIPS between 2003 and 2007

Year	Funding amount ($)
2004/2005	$506,111
2005/2006	$541,593
2006/2007	$571,383

Note: G. Wilson, personal communication (January 7, 2008)

ACC's operating budget. A second example was the budget allocated to the ACC Injury Prevention Group, which in 2007 had an operating budget of $40 million for interventions to reduce the cost of injuries on the accident compensation scheme; included within this budget were initiatives supported by NZIPS. Other agencies that had lead responsibilities for priority areas within NZIPS had their own budgets allocated to them by the GNZ and similarly utilized these finances toward NZIPS-supported initiatives.

Three of the most important factors of sustainability with regard to resources are a stable source of funding, procurement of alternate funding or in-kind services, and creative use of human resources. If programs lack multiple resource sources, then initiatives at the community level suffer from fragmentation and proper training to adequately prevent injuries. A survey conducted among injury prevention workers in 2005 by the Safe Communities Foundation of New Zealand found that, prior to the implementation and grounding of the NZIPS mandate within agencies, over half of the respondents felt that the level of funding they had for their work was minimal. Not surprisingly, the same percentage of injury prevention workers felt that this minimal funding affected the sustainability of their injury prevention efforts. Injury prevention workers were open in support of and collaborate with the NZIPS stakeholders to implement NZIPS initiatives; that is, the same survey described above indicated that 61% of people stating that they use the NZIPS indicated that it has reduced duplication of injury prevention efforts in their organization or community (Coggan & McKay, 2005).

With this in mind, in 2005–2007, the ACC significantly increased its expenditure on injury prevention programs, while the Department of Labor received additional funding to include implementation of the workplace Health and Safety Strategy. Specifically, in 2007, the government allocated $4.5 million over the next 4 years to help implement the new suicide prevention strategy. Funding tended to mainly be granted by appropriation from Parliament to government agencies. In the case of the ACC, funding was approved by the ACC Board of Directors and was funded from ACC's operating budget, which was derived from ACC income (G. Wilson, personal communication, January 7, 2008).

Several of the NZIPS priority areas, such as motor vehicle crashes, each not only possessed a relative degree of financial independence from the ACC body but also received reliable financial assistance from it (Hanson & Salmoni, 2007). That is, although they provide budget details for injury prevention work to ACC, the leading agency of a priority area was able to distribute and allocate funds among the collaborating agencies to implement initiatives. Since planners and administrators of NZIPS developed realistic views of expenditures, they were able to account for the costs required for the NZIPS, its implementation, and its dissemination throughout New Zealand (Jones & Offord, 1991).

35.3 Implementation

Shifting individual's thinking about injuries so they are seen to be preventable rather than an inevitable and unavoidable part of life is key to implementation (Government of New Zealand [GNZ], 2003, p. 13). A way to do so is to raise levels of motivation and skill among individuals/organizations to create safer environments and support protective behaviors (GNZ, 2003, p. 13). The first NZIPS Implementation Plan took effect in July 2004. As already mentioned, within the implementation plan were six national priority areas for injury prevention as follows:

1. Drowning: Drowning Prevention Strategy Framework, Drowning Prevention Strategy: Towards a Water Safe New Zealand
2. Workplace: Workplace Health and Safety Strategy
3. Motor Vehicle Crashes: Road Safety/Safer Journeys
4. Suicide and Self-Harm: New Zealand Suicide Prevention Strategy

5. Falls: Preventing Injury from Falls: The National Strategy
6. Assault: Action Plan to Reduce Community Violence & Sexual Violence

The purpose of this section is to provide a brief overview of each strategy separated into the Tables 35.3, 35.4, 35.5, 35.6, 35.7, and 35.8 containing a brief description of the various agencies and their successes in their priority area.

Table 35.3 Drowning prevention strategy framework, drowning prevention strategy: towards a water safe New Zealand

Focus/vision	Focused on the planning requirements needed to address the challenges for water safety and facilitated the implementation of initiatives that enhanced water safety
	A water safe New Zealand, free from drowning
Goals	Provision of effective leadership by the water safety sector and government
	Delivery of exceptional water safety services
Objectives	To provide strategic direction and effective coordination by and for the water safety sector
	To ensure an appropriate water safety infrastructure
	To ensure an appropriate level and distribution of resourcing for water safety initiatives and agencies
	To improve water safety knowledge through research and development
	To provide quality water safety emergency rescue services
	To provide quality water safety education and awareness
	To create safer environments in, on, under, and around water
	To enhance community and sector engagement in water safety initiatives
Implementation	ACC was the lead agency to support implementation of this strategy, which implemented the following initiatives: bathroom and laundry safety, BoatSafe, Child safety—preventing drowning, Maori Water Safety, Maritime New Zealand, PoolSafe, Recreational water activities, RiverSafe, Swim for Life, Surf Life Saving New Zealand, Waka Safety Guidelines, Water Safety and WaterSafe Auckland Inc.
	An IMG was convened by ACC to provide input to the strategy and to collaborate with various stakeholders to implement the initiatives under the strategy
	Stakeholders included ACC, Injury Prevention Research Unit (University of Otago), Maritime New Zealand, NZIPS Secretariat, New Zealand Recreation Association, New Zealand Search and Rescue Council Secretariat, Royal New Zealand Coastguard, Surf Life Saving New Zealand, Swimming New Zealand, WaterSafe Auckland, and Water Safety New Zealand (Government of New Zealand, n.d.-a)

Table 35.4 The workplace health and safety strategy

Areas of national priority	Airborne substances; workplace vehicles; manual handling; psychosocial work factors; slips, trips, and falls; vulnerable workers; small business; and high-risk industries
Goals	To promote prevention, participation, responsibility, and practicability in the effort to reduce injuries in the workplace and make people more productive
Objectives	To promote government leadership and practices
	Create preventive workplace cultures
	Encourage industry leadership and community engagement
Implementation	The Department of Labor undertook the lead role in implementing this Strategy. To achieve the objectives, the following are seven main intervention approaches within the strategy:
	1. Effective regulation
	2. Appropriate incentives
	3. Capability development
	4. Good governance
	5. Social dialogue
	6. Better design and technology
	7. Sound research and evidence
	An example of one initiative was Site Safe New Zealand, which is described in Box 35.1 (WHSS, n.d.)

Box 35.1 Site Safe New Zealand

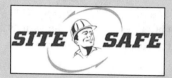

Site Safe New Zealand is dedicated to reducing deaths and injuries in construction and is headed by an independent, not-for-profit, industry-wide organization of the same name. Site Safe has a range of sector-specific induction "passports," which ensure that everyone on a construction site has a basic understanding of the health and safety hazards they are likely to face in their industry, ensuring no one endangers themselves or others. Site Safe regularly offers consultation, sector-specific training, supervisory certification, height safety courses, high-level management courses, and construction management training. To enable smaller businesses to implement health and safety management systems easily, the organization has also developed a safety plan for small business: it follows that the courses are an easy, cost-effective way to manage risk in any industry organization (Hines-Randall, 2005).

Table 35.5 Road safety/safer journey strategy

Updates	This strategy was updated to a 2010–2020 "safer journey" strategy
Vision	A safe road system increasingly free of death and serious injury
Goals	An affordable, integrated, safe, responsive, and sustainable transport system was the goal for 2010 (King, 2007)
	The new goal is to improve the safety of roads and roadsides to significantly reduce the likelihood of crashes occurring while minimizing the consequences of those crashes that do occur
Objectives	Make the road transport system more accommodating of human error
	Manage the forces that injure people in a crash to a level the human body can tolerate without serious injury
	Minimize the level of unsafe road user behavior
Implementation	The implementation of this initiative is overseen by the Minister of Transport and coordinated by the National Road Safety Committee (NRSC).
	The NRSC is a group of chief executives from the ACC, Land Transport New Zealand, Local Government New Zealand, Ministry of Transport, New Zealand Police, and Transit New Zealand (Government of New Zealand, n.d.-f)

Note: Ministry of Transportation (2017)

Table 35.6 New Zealand suicide prevention strategy

Vision	For individuals to achieve the following:
	– Feel valued and nurtured
	– Value their own life
	– Be supported and strengthened if they experience difficulties
	– Not want to take their lives or harm themselves
Goals	Promote mental health/well-being and prevent mental health problems
	Improve the care of people who are experiencing mental disorders associated with suicidal behaviors
	Improve the care of people who make nonfatal suicide attempts
	Reduce access to the means of suicide
	Promote the safe reporting and portrayal of suicidal behavior by the media
	Support individuals that are affected by a suicide or an attempt
	Expand the evidence about rates, causes, and effective interventions
Objectives	Aimed to reduce the following:
	– Rate of suicide and suicidal behavior
	– Harmful effect and impact associated with suicide and suicidal behavior on families, friends, and the wider community
	– Inequalities in suicide and suicidal behavior

(continued)

Table 35.6 (continued)

Implementation	Although the Ministry of Health headed the campaign, the suicide prevention strategy also encompassed a comprehensive array of additional governmental support
	This included the Ministry of Youth Development, New Zealand Police, Ministry of Education, Te Puni Kokiri, ACC, Ministry of Social Development, Child, Youth and Family, Department of Internal Affairs, Ministry of Pacific Island Affairs, Department of Corrections, Ministry of Justice, and Ministry of Women's Affairs
	The strategy also encouraged engagement by local nongovernmental organizations and the media. All stakeholders were required to report to the Ministerial Committee on Suicide Prevention (Government of New Zealand, n.d.-d)

Note: Associate Minister of Health (2006)

Table 35.7 Preventing injury from falls: the national strategy

Vision	Primarily addressed falls prevention in the locations where they most commonly occur at the home, during sports and recreation activities, in social settings, at schools and early childhood education centers, and in facilities for older adults (e.g., nursing homes and hospitals)
Goals	Aimed to promote initiatives that reduced the incidence and severity of injury from falls and the social, psychological, and economic impact of fall-related injuries on individuals, families, and the community
Objectives	Build effective leadership and coordination in the prevention of injury from falls
	Improve the gathering and dissemination of knowledge about the prevention of injury from falls
	Develop and implement program and interventions that focus on the prevention of injury from falls, based on exemplary practice
	Create safer environments to prevent injury from falls
	Ensure appropriate resources for the prevention of injury from falls
Implementation	The ACC Injury Prevention Group undertook the lead role in implementing this strategy.
	The stakeholders ranged from the ACC, to New Zealand ministries that dealt with health and aging, to nongovernmental organizations that working with youth and the elderly

Note: GNZ (2005)

Table 35.8 Taskforce for action on violence within families and action plan to reduce community violence and sexual violence

Vision	Two national valence prevention strategies
	For all families to have healthy, respectful, stable relationships, free from violence
	The Action Plan to Reduce Community and Sexual Violence was developed to address attitudes to violence, alcohol-related violence, violence in public places, and sexual violence
Goals	The goal of the Taskforce for Action on Violence within Families was to work together to provide leadership to stop family violence and promote stable and healthy families
	They advised the Family Violence Ministerial Team on how to make improvements to the way family violence is addressed and to eliminate family violence in New Zealand
Objectives	Leadership—leadership at all levels in order to transform society into one that does not tolerate family violence
	Changing attitudes and behavior—reducing society's tolerance of violence and changing people's damaging behavior within families
	Safety and accountability—swift and unambiguous action by safe family members and the justice sector increases the changes of people being safe and of holding perpetrators to account
	Effective support services—individuals and families affected by family violence need help and support from all of us so they can recover and thrive
Implementation	The Ministries of Social Development and Justice, respectively, led these areas of work
	Actively involved stakeholders include government agencies that dealt with social services and crime and organizations that represented local people and local violence-related issues

Note: Government of New Zealand (2004b), Ministry of Social Development (2006)

35.3.1 Factors Facilitating Implementation in the Priority Areas

According to Wilson (personal communication, January 7, 2008), various mechanisms were used to ensure that feedback was exchanged among partnering agencies and that active participation was maintained. From a national perspective, the NZIPS Secretariat used information dissemination, which was undertaken through the following:

- Distribution of an electronic bi-monthly newsletter
- "IP News"; delivery of regional workshops for community and regional government injury prevention providers
- Update briefings provided to the strategy's advisory groups

The NZIPS Secretariat also communicated through a mandate included within the Memorandum of Understanding (MoU) among the ACC, IPNANZ, Land Transport New Zealand, Ministry of Health, and the NZIPS Secretariat. The MoU encouraged them to meet three to four times each year to review past projects, develop the next phase of objectives, and fund the initiatives (V. Norton, personal communication, February 5, 2008). Furthermore, the NZIPS Secretariat compiled an annual report on progress of NZIPS implementation that was then tabled in the national House of Representatives (Parliament). To complete these reports, the NZIPS Secretariat received information from a number of other government agencies, plus national nongovernment organizations, thus demonstrating, once again, the ongoing collaborative sharing of information.

Participation among diverse groups and visible minorities was also highly prioritized. In fact, three of the principles outlined in the NZIPS specifically outlined the importance of recognizing diversity within all of the initiatives, namely, to ensure relationship with Māori, equity, and cultural appropriateness. According to Wilson (2004), Māori people are overrepresented in many serious injury categories but are underrepresented in making minor claims, as their interaction with the ACC was not well established. Fortunately, the NZIPS strategy outlined the need to improve access to information and the fragmentation of effort.

Complementing this scenario was the ACC's interest in establishing a unit to improve the interface between visible minorities and the ACC and to improve people's understanding of and access to the ACC scheme. The process of consultation that led to the creation of the strategy was designed with the intent that different communities would be able to ensure that the NZIPS was useful to them and that the NZIPS, and those involved with it, respected culture. Ultimately, the ACC's intent to readdress their role and improve the ability of people to interact and vocalize their needs reflected organizational maturity and better equipped the organization to respond to the needs of the diverse communities within New Zealand. Moreover, it highlighted the program's intent to be sustainable in diverse types of communities by ensuring community partner and buy-in through proper program fit.

35.4 Outcome

The commitment to injury prevention at a government level through the NZIPS means that as a population, New Zealanders are benefiting from injury prevention initiatives and programs. People are becoming more aware that injuries can be prevented through individual responsibility and actions alongside community, regional, and national responsibility (V. Norton, personal communication, February 5, 2008). As described earlier, the NZIPS was pioneered by a number of program champions, ranging from individual people to agencies as a whole. While Dyson, Dalziel, and McLea were integral individuals from the upper levels of government, Dr. Carolyn Coggan was described as a highly "integral" person in the development process of the NZIPS for her role as Chair of the Stakeholder Reference Group (K. McLea, personal communication, April 26, 2007). She conducted research to ensure that the NZIPS was well grounded in theory and incorporated research-based evidence into the implementation plan, so as to improve injury prevention policy and practice (C. Coggan, personal communication, July 10, 2007). Her influence was seen through NZIPS policy and practice through research. Overall, the presence of well-respected individuals and organizations enables sustainability of NZIPS, as their abilities to influence policymakers to support injury prevention in the national priority areas at all levels.

On an organization-wide level, the ACC has also played a fundamental role by collecting and aggregating all injury data. The collection of the data from one central location allowed for information to be disseminated more uniformly and, in the case of the ACC, with great efficacy. Furthermore, the collaboration with the ACC built organizational, financial, and human capacity that is then available for the stakeholders involved in creating and implementing initiatives for each of the national areas. In fact, the ACC had not only created a centralized database for statistics on the incidence of injury but also facilitated, through the NZIPS Secretariat, the creation of a database where all injury prevention programs in New Zealand, including government agencies and nongovernment organizations, could be searched.

The administration of a formative evaluation also enhances sustainability, as it further facilitated stakeholder participation and buy-in of NZIPS. That is, process evaluations and reviews conducted over the lifespan of the program enabled the developers and evaluators of NZIPS to establish or reestablish the objectives of the strategy, study how the strategy had been implemented, and understand the components of the program that required adjustment. In 2004–2005, the Safe Communities Foundation New Zealand conducted an evaluation of stakeholders' perceptions of NZIPS, resulting in a report entitled Formative Evaluation: Year One Implementation New Zealand Inquiry Prevention Strategy. The evaluation was conducted with key stakeholders

from governmental and nongovernmental organizations. Stakeholders were selected by their level of involvement in the development of NZIPS: it followed that a stakeholder was included if they had high-level influence on its implementation or were representatives of key organizations and were expected to respond to developers during the lifespan of the implementation. Half of the respondents were questioned via telephone, while the other half of respondents were interviewed face to face. A strategy framework logic exercise was also carried out with the senior member of the evaluation team to develop an overview of the outcomes and impacts of the NZIPS (Safe Communities Foundation New Zealand, 2006).

The evaluation concluded that participants applauded the development of the NZIPS and its implementation plan. Respondents recognized that the NZIPS and its implementation had facilitated communities, institutions, and the general public in New Zealand to approach injury prevention in a more defined and proactive manner. According to the Safe Communities Foundation New Zealand (2006), the NZIPS had "created a framework (in which) to galvanize action" and had "moved everyone in the same direction with clear views and shared goals that they were working towards" (p. 69). The role of the ACC was particularly highlighted as it had improved the fiscal and resource infrastructure from which initiatives could be realized and from where decision-making could be facilitated (e.g., the NZIPS Secretariat, Stakeholder Reference Group, the Government Inter-Agency Group and the Expert Advisory Group).

As mentioned earlier, the NZIPS increased access to data collected by the ACC for participating agencies. In fact, the evaluation itself showed an improvement in the collection and dissemination of data. This became quite evident when it was required to document concrete outcomes for the initiatives within the NZIPS. The use of data not only helped complete internal and external evaluations accurately but also the data itself, and subsequent evaluations of programs could enable agencies to obtain alternate forms of financial or other support.

35.4.1 Chartbook

The chartbooks of the NZIPS present indicators of serious injury outcomes to monitor performance in reducing serious injury for the population as a whole, for children, and for Māori (StatsNZ, n.d.). In 2010, the NZIPS Secretariat released the chartbook of the NZIPS serious injury outcome indicators 1994–2009. This chartbook provided a benchmark that was previously unavailable to practitioners, government agencies, and community-based organizations. It presented frequencies and rates of fatal, serious nonfatal, and combined fatal injury, for all injury and for the six NZIPS injury prevention priority areas (drowning, work-related injury, motor vehicle crashes, suicide and self-harm, falls, and assault) (StatsNZ, n.d.). More specifically, the serious injury outcome indicators include the number of deaths, age-standardization injury mortality rate (per 100,000 person-years at risk), number of serious nonfatal injuries, and age standardization serious nonfatal injury rate (per 100,000 person-years at risk).

The purpose of formulating the chartbook was to provide a baseline from which to determine progress and improvement in preventing serious injury throughout the lifetime of the NZIPS. Ultimately, the chartbook concretely defined and redefined goals and objectives achievable in both the short and long term; this scenario was particularly important for the stakeholders involved in the NZIPS not only to measure the cumulative and continuous impact within each of the national priority areas but also to address in a timely manner any barriers to hinder the evolution of the NZIPS and its implementation within each of the national priority areas.

35.4.2 Evaluation and Collaboration

The evaluation conducted of the NZIPS and the Implementation Plan also demonstrated where capacity would need to be further developed and improved. While many grassroots stakeholders played an active role, government ministers and ministries were observed to have provided theoretical, but very little active support. To enhance the effectiveness of the strategy, a broader reach and more active collaboration is required. To facilitate improved ministerial involvement with the NZIPS, an Injury Prevention Ministerial Committee was formed of all Ministers who are responsible for agencies pursuing the advancement and functioning of the NZIPS and its priority area initiatives. To enhance their involvement, their function was explicitly defined to support and facilitate leadership to promote safety, conduct evaluation and progress reporting of the NZIPS and the initiatives implemented for the priority areas, and provide input and direction on policy which reflects the objectives of the NZIPS (including encouraging collaboration and coordination; Government of New Zealand, n.d.-b).

As of 2008, evaluation was a key focus within the initiatives of various key stakeholder agencies. For example, the Ministry of Health, with a contribution from Injury Prevention Network Aotearoa New Zealand (IPNANZ), funded an external evaluation of one of the workplace safety initiatives: The Injury Prevention Workforce Development Project (V. Norton, personal communication, February 5, 2008). In sum, the NZIPS and the six priority area strategies all contain four elements to ensure process and outcome evaluation methods, including evaluation frameworks, regular updates to implementation plans, regular reviews of current programs, and monitoring the effectiveness of communication by receiving and analyzing feedback from contributors and stakeholders of NZIPS for large (e.g., national priority areas, legislation) and small decisions (e.g., editorial of IP News).

The key mechanism to undertake evaluation and conduct reviews is the implementation plan for each priority area. NZIPS Implementation Plans have a life of 3 years before they expire in order to update and reflect recent changes that are adopted from monitoring, evaluations, and reviews (G. Wilson, personal communication, July 12, 2007).

35.4.3 Recognized National Success and Transportability

Success can be measured by examining the improvement in the services offered by the various agencies involved and by the increased involvement and better-delegated responsibility among the various stakeholder agencies. Boxes 35.2 and 35.3 offers insight into the role of NZIPS in already developed initiatives.

Overall, it is apparent that Site Safe's success is sustainable based on a continuous commitment from the industry it serves. Yet, without government departments and industry working together in partnership, the result can be immensely disappointing. Ultimately, although Site Safe may

---

Box 35.2 Outcomes of Site Safe, successes

Since implementation, Site Safe has listed several notable successes as a result of a variety of positive outcomes, including the following:

- The positive relationship between *Site Safe* and the commercial and civil sectors of the construction industry, with notable acceptance from contractors
- A relationship with the residential sector which is continuously growing stronger
- An improvement in Lost Time Incidents (LTI) per 200,000-person hours: in 2006, a median score of 13 LTI occurred, while in 2004 there was a median score of 15 LTI (CIC Update on Health and Safety in Construction 2007—merged Version 2)
- The decrease in ACC average injury cost and the drop in the severity of the injuries affect the average injury cost
- A 60% better cost rate for Site Safe affiliated firms (part of the commercial sector of the construction industry) relative to non-Site Safe companies, whose claims costs are rising

---

Box 35.3 Outcomes of Site Safe, barriers

Main barriers faced through the lifespan of the initiative include (IPNANZ, 2007) the following:

- Lack of communication with architects, consulting engineers, and quantity surveyors
- Difficulty in communicating with the residential sector, as they have demonstrated greater reluctance to adopt safety messages promoted by Site Safe

---

have achieved the same results had NZIPS not been implemented, the strong support from a national body galvanizes this organization and the strategy they are employing (I. Clanachan, personal communication, January 14, 2007).

The NZIPS also provided a forum to recognize the efforts of the initiatives implemented within the national priority areas entitled the New Zealand Community Safety and Injury Prevention Awards. These awards recognized, rewarded, and promoted exemplary-practice community-based injury prevention and safety promotion in New Zealand and were open to all organizations. Figure 35.4 demonstrates a Waimakariri example for the Community Safety and Injury Awards.

According to Coggan (personal communication, January 14, 2008), if it was not for the NZIPS, various outstanding and successful initiatives would not have been highlighted. For example, the Brain Injury Association Northland further adapted a national initiative to improve their collaboration and coordination at the regional level. This program was subsequently highlighted as part of the designation of Whangarei as a World Health Organization/Safe Community. As such the NZIPS provided important support to highlight the efforts of the implementing organization (C. Coggan, personal communication, January 14, 2008). Additionally, prior to the commencement of NZIPS, New Zealand had two communities designated as "International Safe Communities." But at the end of 2007, New

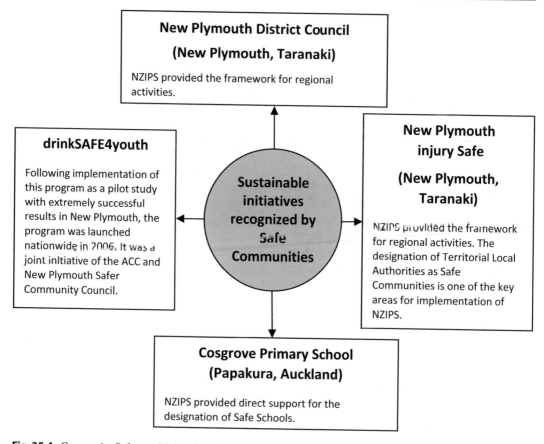

Fig. 35.4 Community Safety and Injury Awards, Waimakariri Example (Source: SCFNZ, 2006)

Zealand had increased that number to six designated International Safe Communities with four more aiming to achieve the criteria for designation in 2008 (C. Coggan, personal communication, January 25, 2008). Box 35.4 is a description of one of the new communities to achieve Safe Community status.

35.4.4 Challenges and Lessons Learned

The following are three main challenges faced since the implementation of NZIPS:

1. Achieving integrated injury prevention across government agencies
2. Raising awareness of safety culture and commitment to injury prevention (NZIPS Objective 1)

3. Strengthening community/regional injury prevention through coordination (NZIPS Objective 5)

35.4.4.1 Challenge One

Achieving integrated injury prevention across government agencies was a major challenge to the overall success of NZIPS as it was reliant on each of the agencies involved remaining committed to both their injury priority area and other areas they support. What needs to be strengthened to improve the NZIPS involvement in the priority areas was the joint accountability for action across agencies.

35.4.4.2 Challenge Two

Raising awareness and commitment to injury prevention to develop a safety culture was addressed by examining injury trends in different

Box 35.4 Wellington City, Safe Community, Accreditation in June 2006

To obtain WHO Safe Community Accreditation, the Wellington City Council (WCC) achieved the following five elements utilizing NZIPS as a guide:

1. Fostered leadership
2. Raised awareness
3. Built capacity
4. Designed the safe community through the use of crime prevention through environmental design (CPTED)
5. Advanced IP knowledge

The Safety Advisory Group established by the WCC meets regularly and helps the WCC to maintain a strong relationship with stakeholders as they have all been meeting since the inception of their initiatives. Stakeholders build capacity and contribute toward the success of Wellington as a Safe Community through the creation of a joint action plan that was developed in cooperation with all stakeholders. The plan outlines the collective and individual responsibilities and roles of each organization to contribute to specific initiatives or projects (e.g., sharing of costs). They are bonded by a common goal of improving community safety and reducing the injury burden.

In their focus toward personal safety, initiatives regarding safety for victims of violence, road trauma, and injury, especially in the central business district, were launched. Evaluation that was completed in 2007 demonstrates a slight reduction in mild to serious injury and an increase in awareness among the target population. Ultimately, to sustain and build long-term success, the WCC values trust and eagerly work toward a common goal. Long-term success is also enforced with evaluation that is built into the programs and initiatives (e.g., the WCC and their partners collect data for evaluation and meet regularly to share information).

From their experiences, the WCC and their partners deal with problems specific to their community. They also have found success in applying programs that are evidence-informed approaches from the past. Additionally, they look to the objectives and actions of the NZIPS to inform a wider range of their community safety initiatives. The NZIPS is a useful tool to accomplish this partly because of its highly informative and flexible approach. The NZIPS has also facilitated a broader level of cooperation and commitment from a variety of stakeholders. The NZIPS Secretariat fosters these relationships because they offer goals, ideas, direction, advice, support, and encouragement.

Note: L. Gabites, personal communication (February 8, 2008)

environments throughout New Zealand. The main challenge in this area was to increase awareness around the social and financial gravity of injuries to the individuals, the ACC scheme, the public health system, and the country as a whole. To address this issue, several actions were taken such as the following: increased focus on building safe communities, better access to information about the cost and consequences of injury, introduction of the national Community Safety Awards in association with a "Safety NZ Week" initiative, development/publication of serious and impairment injury indicators to monitor and evaluate injury trends in NZ over time, and undertaking a population safety culture to develop a baseline from which to measure changes in attitudes to risks over time (G. Wilson, personal communication, March 4, 2008).

35.4.4.3 Challenge Three

Strengthening community/regional injury prevention through coordination was specifically a challenge in the local context. That is, the challenge was to ensure that local support mechanisms are in place and adequately resourced to guarantee support. To encourage leadership at the local level, strong coordination among the central agencies and effective links between central government agencies, community groups, and local government was important. A number of actions were taken to provide local level agencies to develop their leadership roles within injury prevention initiatives, namely, through the work of the Safe Communities Foundation (SCFNZ), regional support and information sharing among injury prevention providers, and agencies such as ACC, Land Transport NZ, District Health Boards, and local Councils who combined their funds to support community injury prevention coordinators (G. Wilson, personal communication, March 4, 2008).

35.4.5 Expansion Beyond New Zealand

In 2005, SMARTRISK devised a national injury prevention strategy for Canada. In consultation with the Insurance Bureau of Canada, SMARTRISK recommended their strategy to the federal government in order to reduce Canada's injury rates. In order for injury rates to be the lowest in the world, the Pan-Canadian strategy had to be implemented. It focuses on six strategic facets including (1) national leadership and coordination, (2) community supports and resources, (3) an effective surveillance system, (4) research, (5) policy analysis and development, and (6) public information and education. In August 2007, the Ministry of Health Promotion in Ontario launched an injury prevention strategy for the province to address this preventable, yet pervasive health challenge. It was entitled the Ontario Injury Prevention Strategy (OIPS).

The ministry invested $2 million between 2007 and 2008 in order to relegate responsibility of policymaking and funding/fundraising to departments of public health throughout the province. This included the following:

- The Ontario Children's Rural Safety Program. The goal was to raise awareness and understanding of farm-related injuries in children and how to prevent them.
- The community-based injury prevention mobilization initiative. It expands the existing model into several communities at greatest risk for injury.
- The Ontario Public Health Association's injury prevention projects.
- The substance abuse prevention mandatory program with the Ontario Neuro-trauma Foundation (Ontario Injury Prevention Resource Centre [OIPRC], 2007)

As the only implemented national strategy, the NZIPS offered insight to the development and implementation of the Canadian national strategy and the Ontario provincial strategy. The experience of developing the NZIPS and subsequently implementing the initiatives in the national priority areas offered national and provincial authorities with effective strategies to improve data collection, ensuring strong consultative communication, and guaranteeing that the initiatives meet the needs of the populations as a whole. Superficial differences between New Zealand as a country and Ontario as a province are obvious (e.g., geography, size, administration); however, Ontario policy and decision makers can stand to learn from the structure and framework, which was outlined for the NZIPS from its inception. That is, the important role that the ACC has played throughout the lifespan of the NZIPS could be translated to a similar institution in Ontario, the Workplace Safety and Insurance Board (WSIB). The WSIB would therefore be required to play an equally strong role in the execution of the strategy—that is, to create sector-specific strategies, reduce injuries, and establish a strong network of stakeholders.

35.5 Conclusion

The objectives of the NZIPS supported the enhancement of social, legislative, and resource capacity, while its principles encouraged community engagement and cultural (safety and ethnic) appropriateness. The few truly remarkable and committed individuals and organizations that spurned the creation of the NZIPS ensured that it could be successfully transported into all settings by soliciting new program champions at governmental and nongovernmental organizations. Their work in the development of the NZIPS and its implementation plan has "provided a framework to support a collaborative, co-operative and inter-sectoral approach to safety promotion and injury prevention in New Zealand" (Coggan & McKay, 2005, p. 10).

Overall, there were three key elements to the NZIPS, including (1) adequate resource, whereby people and funding were available on a long-term basis (i.e., 3-year funding contracts), (2) coordination of local and community actions among key stakeholders, and (3) evaluation that was embedded in day-to-day practice. The NZIPS Secretariat tended to be under resourced for the work they were required to undertake; in response, this resource deficiency had to be rectified, especially since participating agencies would be flexible to change when presented with a sound constructive purpose or rationale for changing (V. Norton, personal communication, February 5, 2008). Although the NZIPS was disestablished in 2013, its injury prevention priorities have become part of the business-as-usual responsibilities of the lead injury prevention agencies. However, the transferability of a strategy like the NZIPS paves the way for other countries to build upon and manipulate to reach the goals of their own environment whilst sustaining the integrity and foundation of NSIPS.

Acknowledgments The authors would like to express sincere appreciation to the key informants for this case study—Carolyn Coggan of the Safe Communities Foundation, New Zealand in Takapuna, Auckland, New Zealand; Keith McLea of the Accident Compensation Corporation in Wellington, New Zealand; and Geoff Wilson of the Accident Compensation Corporation in Wellington, New Zealand—whose consultation made this project possible.

BRIO Model: New Zealand Injury Prevention Strategy

Group Served: New Zealand individuals who are affected by drowning, workplace injuries, motor vehicle traffic crashes, suicide/self-harm, and assault.

Goal: New Zealand becoming injury free.

Background	Resources	Implementation	Outcome
Six national injury prevention priority areas were chosen as follows: motor vehicle crashes, workplace injuries, falls, suicide, assault, and drowning, which accounted for at least 80% of injury deaths and serious injury in NZ Subsequent to the election of the Labor Party, amendments made to legislation emphasized that injury prevention become a key focus for the ACC Developed between 2001 and 2003 and implemented in 2004, the NZIPS was unique for injury prevention worldwide as it was a strategy that was already in effect, which accounts for five main aspects of injury explicitly within its vision, goals, and objectives Flexibility for and adaptability of stakeholders was highly important from the outset of the development process	At the time of development, governmental agencies such as the NZIPS Secretariat (within ACC), Stakeholder Reference Group, Expert Advisory Panel, and Government Interagency Steering Group were formed Dr. Keith McLea, director of Injury Prevention at the ACC, specifically acted on behalf of the NZIPS project team between 2001 and 2002 to mobilize government support and facilitate community ownership and buy-in into the proposed strategy and within the six national priority areas Regardless of changes in the nature of the stakeholders, the efforts of the agencies involved continue to be fluid, collaborative and strongly communicative.	Drowning Prevention Strategy focused on the planning requirements needed to address the challenges for water safety The Workplace Health and Safety Strategy promoted prevention, responsibility, and practicability in the effort to reduce injuries and improve productivity Road Safety to 2010 Strategy aims for an affordable, safe, and sustainable transport system New Zealand Suicide Prevention Strategy aimed to reduce the suicide rate and behavior Preventing injury from falls addressed falls prevention in home, recreation activities, social settings, at schools and childhood/ older adults' facilities Community violence and sexual violence aimed to provide leadership to stop family violence/promote healthy, stable families	Dr. Carolyn Coggan was described as a highly "integral" person in the development process of the NZIPS for her role as Chair of the Stakeholder Reference Group. On an organization-wide level, the ACC has also played a fundamental role by comprehensively collecting and aggregating all injury data on an ongoing basis. The role of the ACC was highlighted as it improved the fiscal and resource infrastructure from which initiatives could be realized and from where decision-making could be facilitated

Life Space Model: New Zealand Injury Prevention Strategy

Sociocultural: civilization/community	Interpersonal: primary and secondary relationships	Physical environments: where we live	Internal states: biochemical/genetic and means of coping
Implementation plans devised for six national priority areas addressed the areas that show where communities are at risk most: Drowning Prevention Strategy Framework: Towards a Water Safe New Zealand Workplace Health and Safety Strategy Road Safety Strategy (Safer Journeys) New Zealand Suicide Prevention Strategy Preventing Injury from Falls: The National Strategy Action Plan to Reduce Community Violence & Sexual Violence Multifaceted approach adapted by specific Ministries with expertise in the priority areas.	On an organizational-wide level, the ACC has also played a fundamental role by comprehensively collecting and aggregating all injury data Participation between skilled, passionate, and dedicated local and regional coordinators, experts, as well as a well-informed and connected advisory group with a strong needs-assessment process, sustainable funding, sound infrastructure, expert capability and capacity, information sharing and evaluation	Drowning, workplace falls, and motor vehicle crashes in addition to the other injury priority areas are a part of urban and rural life in New Zealand and happen to cause the majority of injuries in New Zealand Intervention by multilevel agencies to talk the priority areas as a whole (e.g., for drowning, tackling pool safety, bathtub and washroom safety, and river safety)	Empowerment at national level government as well as provincial ministries and grassroots NGOs and local government agencies Ownership over individual initiatives and participation within national activities—demonstrating a relationship between support at the national level to succeed in initiatives at the local level

References

Accident Compensation Corporation. (2007a). *Drowning prevention strategy, towards a water safe New Zealand 2005–2015, Implementation plan 2007–2011.* Wellington: Author.

Accident Compensation Corporation. (2007b). *Business plan, 2007–2008. Implementation plan.* Wellington: Author.

Allen & Clarke Policy and Regulatory Specialists Ltd, Gribble, A., Mortimer, L., & Smith, R. (2006). *Occupational health and safety in New Zealand. Technical Report prepared for the National Occupational Health and Safety Advisory Committee: NOHSAC Technical Report 7.* Wellington: NOHSAC. Retrieved December 8, 2007, from http://www.nohsac.govt.nz/techreport7/index.php?section=sec4:s1:p070

Associate Minister of Health. (2006). *New Zealand suicide prevention strategy: 2006-2016. The New Zealand Suicide Prevention Strategy.* Wellington: Author. Retrieved from https://www.health.govt.nz/system/files/documents/publications/suicide-prevention-strategy-2006-2016.pdf

Coggan, C., & McKay, J. (2005). *Dissemination of examples of improvements in collaboration and co-ordination of injury prevention across a variety of settings. Safe Communities Foundation New Zealand (SCFNZ), Report Number: 14.* Auckland: Safe Communities Foundation New Zealand (SCFNZ).

Government of New Zealand. (2003). *New Zealand injury prevention strategy, Rautaki Ārai Whara o Aotearoa. Presented by Hon Ruth Dyson, Minister for ACC, Government of New Zealand.* Wellington: Author.

Government of New Zealand. (2004a). *Developing an evaluation framework for NZIPS.* Wellington: Author. Retrieved November 11, 2007, from http://www.nzips.govt.nz/resources/news_04-02_1.php

Government of New Zealand. (2004b). *Safer Communities, Action plan to reduce community violence & sexual violence. Ministry of Justice, June.* Wellington: Author.

Government of New Zealand. (2005). *Preventing injury from falls. The national strategy 2005-2015. Ministry of Justice.* Wellington: Author.

Government of New Zealand. (n.d.-a). *Drowning.* Wellington: Author. Retrieved December 11, 2007, from http://www.nzips.govt.nz/priorities/drowning.php

Government of New Zealand. (n.d.-b). *Implementation.* Wellington: Author. Retrieved December 11, 2007, from www.nzips.govt.nz/implementation/

Government of New Zealand. (n.d.-c). *Integrating injury prevention activity through collaboration and co-ordination.* Wellington: Author. Retrieved December 11, 2007, from www.nzips.govt.nz/resources/news_04-11_4.php

Government of New Zealand. (n.d.-d). *Motor vehicle crashes*. Wellington: Author. Retrieved December 8, 2007, from http://www.nzips.govt.nz/priorities/vehicle.php

Government of New Zealand. (n.d.-e). *Stakeholder relationships*. Wellington: Author. Retrieved December 11, 2007, from www.nzips.govt.nz/implementation/stakeholder.php

Government of New Zealand. (n.d.-f). *Suicide and deliberate self harm*. Wellington: Author. Retrieved December 11, 2007, from www.nzips.govt.nz/priorities/

Government of New Zealand. (n.d.-g). *Why a strategy*. Wellington: Author. Retrieved December 11, 2007, from http://www.nzips.govt.nz/strategy/why.php#why

Haddon, W. (1972). A logical framework for categorizing highway safety phenomena and activity. *Journal of Trauma, 12*(30), 193–207.

Hanson, H., & Salmoni, A. (2007). *The Sustainability of the Stay on Your Feet Demonstration project*. London, ON: University of Western Ontario.

Hines-Randall, H. (2005). *Site safe New Zealand incorporated, (Newsletter), July*. Hamilton: NZIPS. Retrieved January 8, 2008, from www.nzips.govt.nz/resources/news_05-07_2.php

Injury Prevention Network of Aotearoa New Zealand, IPNANZ. (2007). CIC update on health and safety in construction 2007 – Merged Version 2. Internal documentation.

Injury Prevention News. (2006). *Changes at ACC*, Issue 1, August. Retrieved December 5, 2007, from http://www.nzips.m1.co.nz/A.asp?P=149.1.9

Jones, M. B., & Offord, D. R. (1991). *After the demonstration project*. Paper presented at the 1991 annual meeting of the Advancement of Science, Washington, DC.

King, A. (2007), *King launches vision for sustainable transport future*, Beehive, 10 December, [Press Release]. Retrieved December 12, 2007, from http://www.beehive.govt.nz/release/king+launches+vision+sustainable+transport+future

Ministry of Social Development. (2006). *Taskforce for action on violence within families. The First Report*. Wellington: Author. Retrieved from https://www.msd.govt.nz/documents/about-msd-and-our-work/work-programmes/initiatives/action-family-violence/taskforce-report-first-report-action-on-violence.pdf

Ministry of Transportation. (2017). *Action plans - Safer journeys*. Wellington: Author. Retrieved from http://www.saferjourneys.govt.nz/action-plans/

Ontario Injury Prevention Resource Centre. (2007). *Ontario releases injury prevention strategy*, [Press Release], August, 8, 2007. Retrieved February 5, 2007, from http://www.oninjuryresources.ca/ontario_releases_injury_preven.html#more

Safe Communities Foundation New Zealand. (2006). *Injury prevention work wins awards for councils, company and support group, August*. Auckland: Author. Retrieved February 5, 2007, from www.safecommunities.org.nz/safeawds/media2006/2007-05-03.0494725530/download

Shediac-Rizkallah, M. C., & Bone, L. R. (1998). Planning for the sustainability of community-based health programs: Conceptual frameworks and future directions for research, practice and policy. *Health Education Research, 13*(1), 87–108.

StatsNZ. (n.d.). Chartbooks of the New Zealand Injury Prevention Strategy serious injury outcome indicators. Retrieved from http://www.stats.govt.nz/browse_for_stats/health/injuries/chartbooks-of-the-nz-injury-prevention-strategy.aspx

Wilson G. (2004). *ACC and community responsibility, Victoria University of Wellington Law Review, 45*. Retrieved December 5, 2007, from http://www.austlii.edu.au/au/journals/VUWLRev/2004/45.html

Workplace Health and Safety Strategy (WHSS). (n.d.). *Workplace health and safety strategy for New Zealand to 2015. Framework for action*. Retrieved November 5, 2007, from http://www.whss.govt.nz/strategy/section2.html

Index

© Springer Nature Switzerland AG 2020
R. Volpe (ed.), *Casebook of Traumatic Injury Prevention*,
https://doi.org/10.1007/978-3-030-27419-1

Printed
By Ro